Rob & Smith's
Operative Surgery

Surgery of the Upper Gastrointestinal Tract

Fifth edition

Rob & Smith's
Operative Surgery

General Editors

David C. Carter MD, FRCS(Ed), FRCS(Glas)
Regius Professor of Clinical Surgery, Royal Infirmary,
Edinburgh, UK

R. C. G. Russell MS, FRCS
Consultant Surgeon, Middlesex Hospital and Royal National
Throat, Nose and Ear Hospital, London, UK

Consulting Editor

Hugh Dudley CBE, ChM, FRCS(Ed), FRACS, FRCS
Emeritus Professor, St Mary's Hospital, London, UK

Art Editor

Gillian Lee FMAA, HonFIMI, AMI, RMIP
15 Little Plucketts Way, Buckhurst Hill, Essex, UK

Rob & Smith's
Operative Surgery

Surgery of the Upper Gastrointestinal Tract

Fifth edition

Edited by

Glyn G. Jamieson FRACS, FACS
Dorothy Mortlock Professor of Surgery, University of Adelaide, Department of Surgery, Royal Adelaide Hospital, Adelaide, Australia

Haile T. Debas MD
M. Galante Distinguished Professor of Surgery and Dean of the School of Medicine, University of California, San Francisco, California, USA

CHAPMAN & HALL MEDICAL
London · Glasgow · Weinheim · New York · Tokyo · Melbourne · Madras

Published by Chapman & Hall, 2–6 Boundary Row, London SE1 8HN, UK

Chapman & Hall, 2–6 Boundary Row, London SE1 8HN, UK

Blackie Academic & Professional, Wester Cleddens Road, Bishopbriggs, Glasgow G64 2NZ, UK

Chapman & Hall GmbH, Pappelallee 3, 69469 Weinheim, Germany

Chapman & Hall Inc., One Penn Plaza, 41st Floor, New York, NY 10119, USA

Chapman & Hall Japan, Thomson Publishing Japan, Hirakawacho Nemoto Building, 6F, 1-7-11 Hirakawa-cho, Chiyoda-ku, Tokyo 102, Japan

Chapman & Hall Australia, Thomas Nelson Australia, 102 Dodds Street, South Melbourne, Victoria 3205, Australia

Chapman & Hall India, R. Seshadri, 32 Second Main Road, CIT East, Madras 600 035, India

© 1994 Chapman & Hall

Typeset in 10/11 Garamond ITC by Genesis Typesetting, Laser Quay, Rochester, Kent

Printed at The Bath Press, England

ISBN 0 412 53550 5

A catalogue record for this book is available from the British Library

Library of Congress Catalog Card Number: 94-070237

Contributors

I. Braghetto MD
Associate Professor, University of Chile, Department of Surgery, University Hospital, Santos Dumont 999, Santiago, Chile

F. J. Branicki DM, FRCS, FRACS
Department of Surgery, Royal Brisbane Hospital, University of Queensland, Queensland 4072, Australia

R. Britten-Jones
Department of Surgery, Royal Adelaide Hospital, Adelaide, South Australia 5000, Australia

G. F. Buess MD, FRCS(Ed)
Professor of Surgery, Minimal Invasive Chirurgie, Eberhard-Karls University, Schnarrenberg Clinic, D7400 Tübingen, Germany

R. Buhl MD
Department of Surgery, University of Heidelberg, Im Neuenheimer Feld 110, D-69120 Heidelberg, Germany

R. Bumm MD
Senior Resident in Surgery, Department of Surgery, Technical University of Munich, W-8000 Munich 80, Germany

S. H. Carvajal MD
Research Fellow, Department of Surgery, University of California, 513 Parnassus Avenue, S-320 San Francisco, California 94143-0104, USA

J. L. Chassin MD
Chairman, Department of Surgery, The New York Hospital Medical Center of Queens, 56–45 Main Street, Flushing, New York 11355-5095, USA

W. G. Cheadle MD
Assistant Professor of Surgery, Department of Surgery, University of Louisville School of Medicine, Louisville, Kentucky 40292, USA

S. C. S. Chung MD, FRCS(Ed), MRCP
Reader in Surgery, Prince of Wales Hospital, The Chinese University of Hong Kong, Shatin, Hong Kong

A. J. Csendes MD, FACS
Professor of Surgery, University of Chile, Department of Surgery, University Hospital, Santos Dumont 999, Santiago, Chile

H. T. Debas MD
M. Galante Distinguished Professor of Surgery and Dean of the School of Medicine, University of California, 513 Parnassus Avenue, S-320 San Francisco, California 94143-0104, USA

T. R. DeMeester MD
Professor and Chairman, Department of Surgery, University of Southern California School of Medicine, Los Angeles, California 90033-4612, USA

C. Deschamps MD
Senior Associate Consultant, Section of General Thoracic Surgery, Mayo Clinic and Mayo Foundation, Rochester, Minnesota, USA

E. Deslandres MD
Assistant Professor, Department of Medicine, University of Montréal, Division of Gastroenterology, Hôtel-Dieu de Montréal, 3840 Rue St Urban, Montréal, Québec, Canada H2W 1T8

P. G. Devitt FRACS, FRCS
Senior Lecturer, Department of Surgery, Royal Adelaide Hospital, Adelaide, South Australia 5000, Australia

C. Doherty MD, FACS
Assistant Professor, Department of Surgery, University of Iowa College of Medicine, Iowa City, Iowa 52242, USA

F. Dubois
Professor, CMC Pte de Choisy, 6 Place de Port-au-Prince, 75013 Paris, France

A. Duranceau MD
Professor of Surgery, Department of Surgery, University of Montréal, Division of Thoracic Surgery, Hôtel-Dieu de Montréal, 3840 Rue St Urban, Montréal, Québec, Canada H2W 1T8

F. H. Ellis Jr MD, PhD
Clinical Professor of Surgery, Harvard Medical School, and Chief Emeritus, Division of Cardiothoracic Surgery, New England Deaconess Hospital, 110 Francis Street, Boston, Massachusetts 02215, USA

F. Fekete MD
Professor of Surgery and Chief, Department of Digestive Surgery, University Paris VII, Hôpital Beaujon, 100 Blvd du General Leclerc, Clichy, Paris 92118, France

D. Fromm MD
Penharthy Professor and Chairman, Department of Surgery, Wayne State University and Surgeon-in-Chief, Detroit Medical Center, Detroit, Michigan, USA

D. Gavriliu MD
Professor at UNEX-AZ SRL, Universitatea Romana de Stünte si Arte, Bucharest, Romania

J. A. Hagen MD
Esophageal Fellow, Department of Surgery, University of Southern California School of Medicine, Los Angeles, California 90033-4612, USA

C. Herfath MD
Professor and Head, Department of Surgery, University of Heidelberg, Im Neuenheimer Feld 110, D-69120 Heidelberg, Germany

C. A. Hiebert MD, FACS
Chairman Emeritus, Department of Surgery, Maine Medical Center, Portland, Maine, USA

A. H. Hölscher MD
Assistant Professor of Surgery, Department of Surgery, Technical University of Munich, W-8000 Munich 80, Germany

G. J. Huang MD, FRCS
Professor of Thoracic Surgery, Cancer Institute and Hospital, Chinese Academy of Medical Sciences, PO Box 2258, Beijing 100021, People's Republic of China

O. Huber MD
Department of Surgery, University of California, San Francisco, California 94143-0788, USA

G. G. Jamieson FRACS, FACS
Dorothy Mortlock Professor of Surgery, University of Adelaide, Department of Surgery, Royal Adelaide Hospital, Adelaide, South Australia 5000, Australia

S. Johnson MD
Esophageal Fellow, Department of Surgery, University of Southern California School of Medicine, Los Angeles, California 90033-4612, USA

G. W. Johnston MCh, FRCS
Honorary Professor, Queen's University Belfast, and Consultant Surgeon, Royal Victoria Hospital, Belfast BT12 6BA, UK

J.-P. Kim MD, FACS
Professor of Surgery, College of Medicine, Seoul National University Hospital, 28 Yungon-Dong Chongno-Gu, Seoul 110-744, Korea

O. Korn MD
Instructor of Surgery, University of Chile, Department of Surgery, University Hospital, Santos Dumont 999, Santiago, Chile

J. E. J. Krige FRCS, FCS(SA)
Associate Professor, Department of Surgery, University of Cape Town, Observatory 7925, South Africa

Z. H. Krukowski PhD, FRCS(Ed)
Consultant Surgeon, Aberdeen Royal Infirmary, Foresterhill, Aberdeen, AB9 2ZB, UK

B. Launois MD, FACS
Professor, Digestive and Transplantation Surgery, Hôpital Pontchaillou, Rue Henri Le Guilloux, 3500 Rennes, France

T. Lerut MD, PhD, FACS
Department of General Thoracic Surgery, Catholic University Leuven, U.Z. Gasthuisberg, 3000 Leuven, Belgium

A. K. C. Li MA, MD, FRCS, FRCS(Ed), FRACS, FACS
Professor and Chairman, Department of Surgery, Prince of Wales Hospital, The Chinese University of Hong Kong, Shatin, Hong Kong

L. Lundell MD, PhD
Associate Professor of Surgery, Department of Surgery, Sahlgren's Hospital, University of Gothenburg, S-41345 Gothenburg, Sweden

G. J. Maddern PhD, MS, FRACS
Jepson Professor of Surgery, Department of Surgery, University of Adelaide and Queen Elizabeth Hospital, Woodville, South Australia 5011, Australia

J. W. Maher MD
Section of Gastrointestinal Surgery, Department of Surgery, University of Iowa Hospitals and Clinics and College of Medicine, Iowa City, Iowa 52242, USA

M. A. Malias MD
Resident Surgeon, Department of Surgery, University of Louisville School of Medicine, Louisville, Kentucky 40292, USA

A. Mannell FRACS, FRCS, MS
Specialist Surgeon, The Rosebank Clinic, and Consultant Surgeon, Baragwanath Hospital, University of the Witwatersrand, Johannesburg, South Africa

M. T. Marrinan FRCS(Ed)
Fellow in Thoracic Surgery, Mayo Graduate School of Medicine, Rochester, Minnesota, USA

C. J. Martin FRACS
Professor of Surgery, University of Sydney and Head of Surgical Division, Nepean Hospital, PO Box 63, Penrith, NSW 2751, Australia

E. E. Mason MD, PhD, FACS
Professor Emeritus of Surgery, Department of Surgery, University of Iowa College of Medicine, Iowa City, Iowa 52242, USA

N. A. Matheson ChM, FRCS, FRCS(Ed)
Consultant Surgeon, Aberdeen Royal Infirmary, Foresterhill, Aberdeen AB9 2ZB, UK

H. Matthews FRCS
Consultant Thoracic Surgeon, Regional Department of Thoracic Surgery, East Birmingham Hospital, Birmingham and Professor of Surgery, Department of Biological Sciences, University of Warwick, UK

J. E. Meilahn MD
Assistant Professor of Surgery, Department of Surgery, Temple University School of Medicine, Philadelphia, Pennsylvania 19140, USA

R. O. Mitchell MD
Resident Surgeon, Department of Surgery, University of Louisville School of Medicine, Louisville, Kentucky 40292, USA

M. W. Mulholland MD
Associate Professor of Surgery, University of Michigan, 2920 Taubman Health Center, 1500 E, Medical Center Drive, Ann Arbor, Michigan 48109-0331, USA

S. J. Mulvihill MD
Associate Professor of Surgery, Department of Surgery, University of California, 533 Parnassus Avenue, U-122 San Francisco, California 94143-0788, USA

L. K. Nathanson FRACS
Senior Lecturer, Department of Surgery, Clinical Sciences Building, University of Queensland, Royal Brisbane Hospital, Herston 4029, Queensland, Australia

P. E. O'Brien MD, FRACS
Professor of Surgery, Monash University, Alfred Hospital, Prahtan, Melbourne, Victoria 3181, Australia

L. C. Olbe MD, PhD
Associate Professor of Surgery, Department of Surgery, University of Gothenburg, Sahlgren's Hospital, 41345 Gothenburg, Swweden

M. J. Orloff MD
Professor of Surgery, School of Medicine, University of California, San Diego, California 92103, USA

M. S. Orloff MD
Assistant Professor of Surgery, University of Rochester School of Medicine and Dentistry, Strong Memorial Hospital, 601 Elmwood Avenue, Rochester, New York 14642, USA

M. Orringer MD
Professor and Head, Section of Thoracic Surgery, University of Michigan, 2120 Taubman Health Center, Ann Arbor, Michigan, 48109-0010, USA

Y. Panis MD
Department of Digestive Surgery, University Paris VII, Hôpital Beaujon, 100 Blvd du General Leclerc, Clichy, Paris 92118, France

W. S. Payne MD
Emeritus Consultant, Section of General Thoracic Surgery, Mayo Clinic, Rochester, Minnesota 55905, USA

C. A. Pellegrini MD, FACS
Ben A. Reid Sr Professor and Chairman, Department of Surgery, University of Washington, Seattle, Washington 98195, USA

H. C. Polk MD
Senior Professor and Chairman, Department of Surgery, University of Louisville School of Medicine, Louisville, Kentucky 40292, USA

S. C. Rakíc MD, PhD, FACS
Department of Surgery, Leyenburg Hospital, Postbus 40551, The Hague 2504 LN, The Netherlands

W. P. Ritchie Jr MD, PhD
Professor and Chairman, Department of Surgery, Temple University School of Medicine, Philadelphia, Pennsylvania 19140, USA

A. Sali PhD, FRACS, FACS
Clinical Associate Professor of Surgery, University of Melbourne, Parkville, Victoria, Australia 3081

J. R. Siewert MD, FACS
Professor of Surgery, Chairman of the Department of Surgery, Technical University of Munich, W-8000 Munich 80, Germany

A. E. Siperstein MD
Department of Surgery, Mount Zion Medical Center of UCSF, San Francisco, California 94143-1610, USA

J. Terblanche ChM, FRCS, FCS(SA)
Professor and Head, Department of Surgery, and Co-Director, MRC Liver Research Centre, University of Cape Town, Observatory 7925, South Africa

V. F. Trastek MD, FACS
Consultant, Section of General Thoracic Surgery, Mayo Clinic, Rochester, Minnesota 55905, USA

A. Watson MD, FRCS, FRCS(Ed), FRACS
Consultant Surgeon, The Wellington Hospital, London NW8 9LE, UK

Contributing Medical Artists

Antoine Barnaud
11 Rue Jacques Dulud,
92200 Neuilly sur Seine, France

Andrew Bezear
6 Queen Street, Godalming,
Surrey GU7 1BD, UK

Diane Bruyninckx MMAA, AIMI
20 Van Halmaelelei,
B-2930 Brasschaat, Belgium

Angela Christie MMAA
14 West End Avenue, Pinner,
Middlesex HA5 1BJ, UK

Peter Cox RDD, MMAA, AIMI
Canon Frome Court,
Canon Frome, Ledbury,
Herefordshire HR8 2TD, UK

Susan Darrington
P.O. Box 581, Subiaco,
Western Australia 6008 .

Raymond Evans BA(Hons), MMAA
Unit of Art in Medicine,
Department of Cell and Structural Biology,
University of Manchester, Manchester M13 9PT, UK

Diane Kinton BA(Hons)
Gillian Lee Illustrations,
15 Little Plucketts Way, Buckhurst Hill,
Essex IG9 5QU, UK

Gillian Lee FMAA, HonFIMI, AMI, RMIP
Gillian Lee Illustrations,
15 Little Plucketts Way, Buckhurst Hill,
Essex IG9 5QU, UK

Marks Creative Consultants
31 Waddon Road, Croydon,
Surrey CR0 4LH, UK

Gillian Oliver MMAA, AIMI
15 Bramble Road, Hatfield,
Hertfordshire AL10 9RZ, UK

Paul Richardson BA(Hons)
54 Wellington Road,
Orpington, Kent BR5 4AQ, UK

Denise Smith BA(Hons), MMAA
Unit of Art in Medicine,
Department of Cell and Structural Biology,
University of Manchester, Manchester M13 9PT, UK

Contents

Preface

In his preface to the previous edition of this volume, Hugh Dudley commented that 'although gastrointestinal surgery is an old established discipline, it continues to move forward'. Gastrointestinal surgery does indeed continue to move forward, and even the contributors to the last volume (which was published in 1983) would have been surprised at the rapid changes which were about to take place in gastrointestinal surgery. One of the changes, which amounts to a paradigm shift, is thoracoscopic and laparoscopic surgery. Another of the changes which was well established in 1983, but which has gathered momentum in the intervening years, is the separation of general surgery into subspecialties. This edition, for the first time, acknowledges these changes, and this volume is concerned with the upper gastrointestinal tract alone and includes laparoscopic and thoracoscopic techniques.

As with previous editions we have asked experts to describe how they undertake procedures in their field of expertise. The emphasis is always on the practical, with the aim being that a competent surgeon, without great familiarity in an area, in appropriate circumstances would be able to carry out the procedure being described.

Hugh Dudley finished his preface with: 'Here then is how to do it in the gastrointestinal tract by those who know how to do it (with the possible exception, of course, of the editor's own contributions!)' We can think of no better way to finish, but will circumvent Hugh's modesty by paraphrasing his remark to: 'This volume is how to do it in the upper gastrointestinal tract by those who should know how to do it!'

Glyn G. Jamieson
Haile T. Debas
February 1994

Flexible endoscopy of the upper digestive tract

André Duranceau MD
Professor of Surgery, Department of Surgery, University of Montréal, Division of Thoracic Surgery, Hôtel-Dieu de Montréal, Montréal, Québec, Canada

Eric Deslandres MD
Assistant Professor, Department of Medicine, University of Montréal, Division of Gastroenterology, Hôtel-Dieu de Montréal, Montréal, Québec, Canada

Principles and justification

Upper digestive flexible endoscopy has evolved considerably over the last 25 years. It presently plays a dominant role in the evaluation of the upper gastrointestinal tract. Specifically, it provides both direct and complete visualization of the area and direct access for tissue sampling and/or therapeutic intervention. The technique should be mastered by any clinician with a special interest in diseases of the oesophagus, stomach, or duodenum.

Preoperative

Patient preparation

Preparation for upper gastrointestinal endoscopy begins with the initial consultation. Following radiological assessment of the oesophagus and stomach, the indications and advantages of the technique are discussed with the patient. The procedure is explained in simple terms. During the clinic evaluation, allergies, current medication and previous medical history are reviewed. The need for antibiotic prophylaxis is assessed.

The patient should fast overnight before the procedure. Outpatients should be accompanied, particularly if intravenous sedation is to be used.

In the endoscopy suite, the procedure is explained again to minimize the patient's anxiety. Having a calm and relaxed patient avoids to some extent the need for sedation. A tense patient should not be submitted to upper digestive endoscopy under simple topical anaesthesia. Proper sedation dictates the use of pulse oximetry and electrocardiography. Aggressive or uncooperative patients should not be submitted to endoscopy under local anaesthesia.

A lignocaine gargle or spray is used for topical anaesthesia of the pharynx and hypopharynx. The patient is instructed to undertake a Valsalva's manoeuvre in order to protect the larynx from the spray.

It is difficult to be dogmatic about which patients will require intravenous sedation. The advantages of topical anaesthesia are a rapid recuperation after the procedure and a rapid return to normal activities. When this is explained to the patient, it encourages some to undergo the procedure with topical anaesthesia. This is so particularly if the atmosphere and the behaviour of the staff are calm and confident. When needed, adequate sedation may be obtained with benzodiazepines (diazepam, midazolam). Pethidine hydrochloride may be added for relaxation and analgesia. This medication should be administered slowly in small doses until the desired level of sedation is obtained.

Technique

Introduction of the endoscope

Blind insertion

1 The patient sits facing the surgeon or lies in the left lateral decubitus position. The endoscope lies on the right shoulder of the endoscopist. Following appropriate topical anaesthesia, the index and third finger of the left hand are placed on the back of the patient's tongue. Forward traction by the two fingers permits the introduction of the slightly flexed end of the endoscope over the back of the tongue into the buccopharynx.

The endoscopist removes the fingers from the patient's mouth and holds the head of the patient slightly bent forward. The endoscope is gently advanced until resistance is felt. Voluntary swallowing at this point allows the instrument to pass into the cervical oesophagus. The mouthpiece, previously positioned around the shaft of the endoscope, is installed between the patient's teeth and the examination is started.

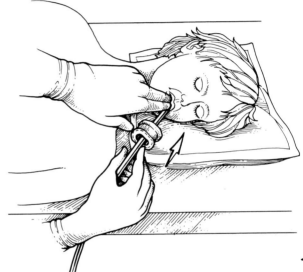

1

Visual insertion

2a–e The patient lies in the left lateral position after buccopharyngeal and hypopharyngeal topical anaesthesia has been applied. A mouthpiece is installed between the teeth or gums and the flexible tip of the endoscope is advanced, taking care to stay in the midline and at the interface between the tongue and hypopharyngeal mucosa. Tongue, uvula, epiglottis and cricoarytenoid cartilages are seen. Passing beside the midline, the cricoarytenoid cartilages are passed and the tip of the endoscope stops on the cricopharyngeus which closes the entry to the oesophagus. Gentle local pressure while asking the patient to swallow allows the tip of the endoscope to pass into the cervical oesophagus.

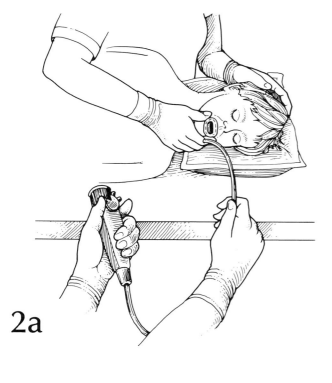

2a

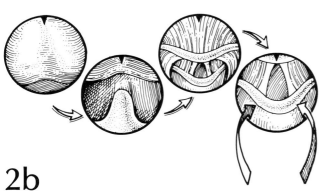

2b

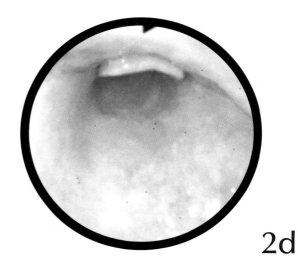

2d

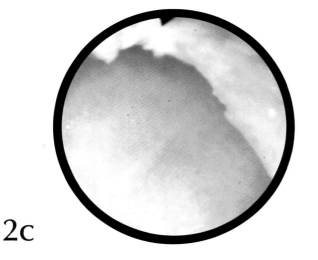

2c

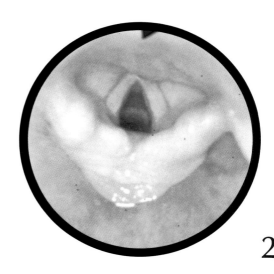

2e

Examination of the oesophagus

The instrument is advanced under direct vision, with the tip of the endoscope always central in the lumen, using optimal insufflation to keep the lumen of the oesophagus well distended. Systematic routine examination of the oesophagus is completed first in order to document as meticulously as possible any mucosal abnormality. This 'first-hand' inspection is important, because no trauma has been caused by manipulation or passage of the instrument. Two rules must always be observed: (1) the endoscope must be advanced with clear vision of the central lumen; (2) if direct vision is obscured or there are any doubts, the endoscope should be withdrawn.

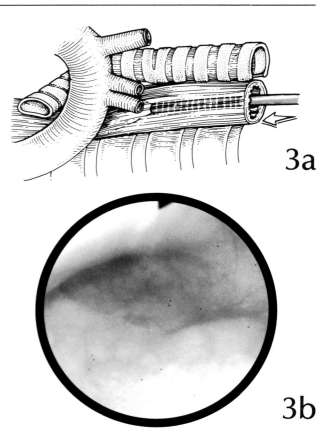

3a, b Distal to the cricopharyngeal sphincter, the first landmark in the oesophagus is the extraluminal compression by the left main bronchus and the aortic arch. Pulsations of the left heart over the distal half are identified. A large oesophagus may be 'moulded' on the descending thoracic aorta.

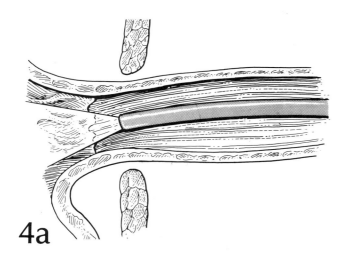

4a−c The gastro-oesophageal mucosal junction is usually identified at 38–40 cm from the incisors. This junction is usually serrated and readily identified by the colour difference between the oesophageal and gastric mucosa.

The position of the oesophageal hiatus in the diaphragm is identified by asking the patient to inhale deeply; the diaphragmatic hiatus during inspiration creates an imprint on the oesophageal or gastric wall. The positions of both the hiatus and the mucosal junction are recorded in order to document the possibility of a hernia or of a columnar-lined oesophagus.

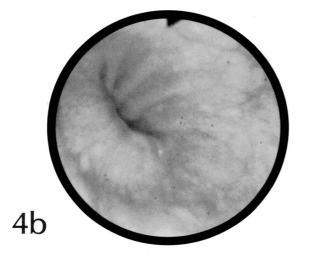

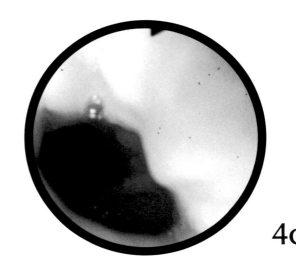

Passage into the stomach

Passage of the endoscope into the stomach requires appropriate observations to be made at the gastro-oesophageal junction. This junction may be closed or widely patulous. Passage into the gastric lumen is usually a simple manoeuvre that occurs without resistance. Occasionally however, mucosal, submucosal, or extrinsic lesions can distort the normal junction and cause difficulty in progression into the stomach. Absence of any mucosal lesion, but a progressive 'giving' of the lower oesophageal sphincter area under pressure, raises the possibility of a motor disorder.

Examination of the stomach

5a, b On entering the stomach, it becomes distended with air and this often causes discomfort to the patient. By tipping the end of the endoscope slightly down and towards the left, a view of the greater curvature and of the posterior gastric wall is obtained. Aspiration of all retained liquid is carried out to decrease the risk of aspiration and also to allow proper examination of the stomach.

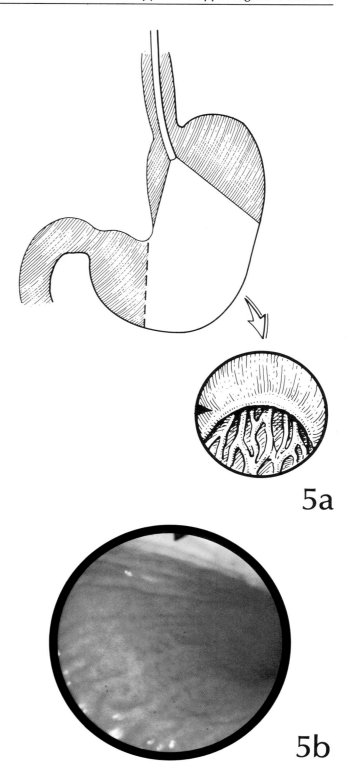

5a

5b

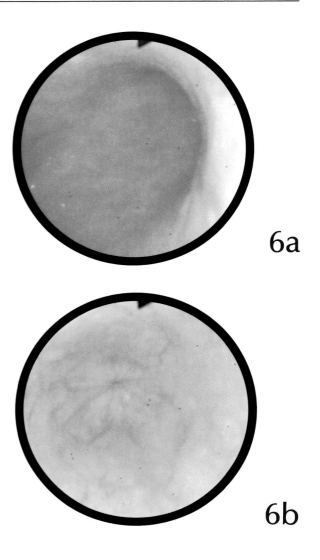

6a

6b

6a–c

A rotation movement of the tip of the instrument allows examination of the anterior and posterior walls of the body of the stomach. The lesser curvature down to the angulus and the greater curvature are viewed by the same motion. The most proximal part of both curvatures are better examined when using the J manoeuvre (see below).

The endoscope is advanced along the greater curvature and the endoscopist rotates the instrument toward the right while angulating its tip. Progression toward the antrum and pylorus is accomplished with the same rotating movement of the tip, allowing complete circumferential assessment of the antrum.

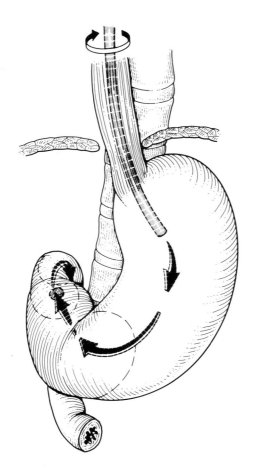

6c

The prepyloric area and the pyloric ring are always approached directly, with passage through the pylorus being done under direct vision. The tip of the endoscope must always visualize the pyloric lumen while pressure is put on the advancing instrument. When the pylorus 'yields', complete assessment of the first part of the duodenum is undertaken as far as the superior duodenal angle. When pathology is thought to be confined to the oesophagus or stomach, the examination is not carried further and the endoscope is pulled back into the distal stomach.

7a–h While the tip of the endoscope lies along the distal lesser curvature and while the stomach is distended, rotation of the instrument is accomplished toward the greater curvature. Complete 180° upwards angulation of the endoscope tip completes the J manoeuvre. The endoscope is pulled back gently while the stomach is distended. Swinging of the retroflexed tip allows proper visualization of the subcardial area and of the fundus of the stomach. Simultaneous rotation of the endoscope gives an excellent view of the lesser curvature from the cardia to the angulus.

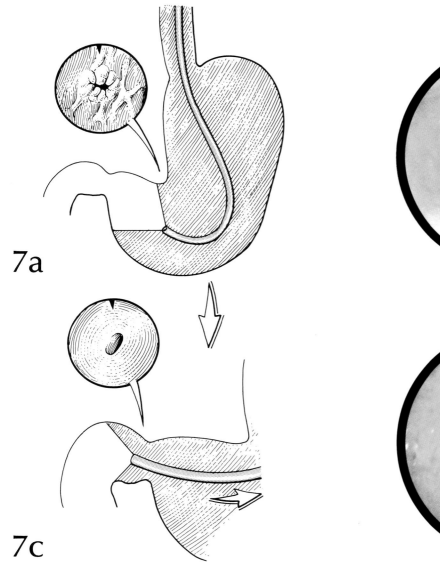

7a

7c

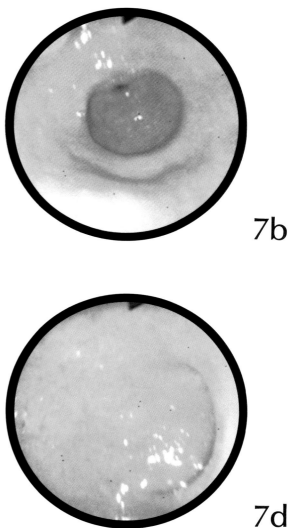

7b

7d

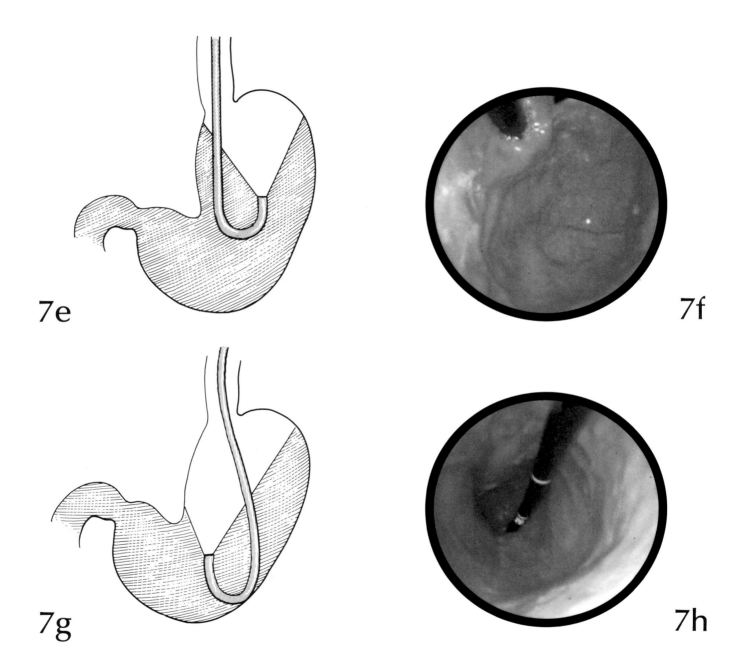

7e

7f

7g

7h

Taking tissue specimens

8a–c Biopsies are taken from any lesion seen in the oesophagus or stomach using cup forceps. The presence of a dependable cytopathology division encourages the use of brush cytology for diagnosis of all mucosal abnormalities. The diagnostic yield of cytology is higher than that of biopsies in the authors' hands, particularly for obstructive oesophageal lesions.

Recovery

Patients are encouraged to avoid drinking or eating for approximately 30 min after termination of the procedure.

The results of the endoscopy should be discussed with the patient immediately if no sedation has been given. If the patient has received sedation, explanations are delayed until the patient has recovered. This information should be given in the presence of the person accompanying the patient, as the effects of sedation on a patient's memory may persist for some time.

Patients are advised not to drive or engage in regular working activities for a few hours if they have been given sedation.

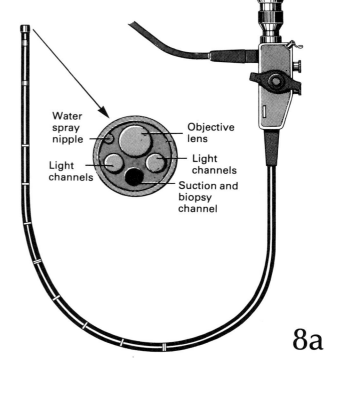

Water spray nipple

Objective lens

Light channels

Light channels

Suction and biopsy channel

8a

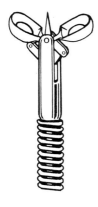

8b

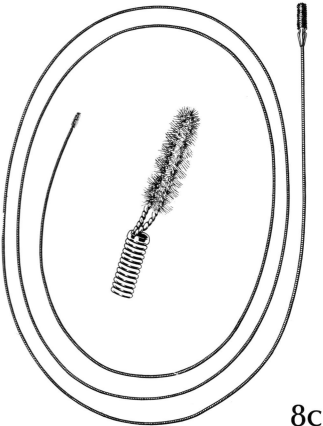

8c

Injection sclerotherapy of oesophageal varices

J. E. J. Krige FRCS, FCS(SA)
Associate Professor, Department of Surgery, University of Cape Town, South Africa

John Terblanche ChM, FRCS, FCS(SA)
Professor and Head, Department of Surgery and Co-Director, MRC Liver Research Centre, University of Cape Town, South Africa

Techniques

The three techniques of injection sclerotherapy are intravariceal, paravariceal and the combination of both intravariceal and paravariceal methods.

Intravariceal technique

Injection of sclerosant directly into the varix to induce variceal thrombosis is the most widely used technique. The injections are localized to the lower 5 cm of the oesophagus. The use of 5% ethanolamine oleate is favoured by the authors.

Paravariceal technique

Sclerosant is injected into the submucosa adjacent to a varix, as described by Wodak[1] and Paquet[2]. The most widely used sclerosant is polidocanol (0.5% or 1% concentration). The sclerosant is administered as 30–40 separate injections (0.5–1 ml each) in a helical fashion, commencing at the gastro-oesophageal junction and extending approximately one-third of the way up the oesophagus. The aim is to produce oedema to compress the varix during acute bleeding and subsequently to provoke tissue reaction, fibrosis and thickening of the mucosa over the varices to prevent bleeding. This technique will not be described further.

Combined technique

The combination of intravariceal and paravariceal injections is used in Cape Town for the emergency management of actively bleeding varices, and in the elective management of large varices to prevent needle-puncture bleeding[3]. The authors use 5% ethanolamine oleate although other agents have been used successfully by other groups. A small volume (1 ml) of sclerosant is injected paravariceally to partially compress the varix, followed by an intravariceal injection of a larger volume (up to 5 ml) to thrombose the varix. As with the intravariceal injection technique, the injections are restricted to the lower 5 cm of the oesophagus.

Equipment

Endoscope

1 Either single- or twin-channel endoscopes are suitable for injection sclerotherapy. The single-channel endoscope should have a large channel so that suction is not reduced after the injector has been inserted. The twin-channel endoscope is useful for acute bleeding because one channel allows unimpeded suction during injection. Either end- or oblique-viewing endoscopes are effective for injection sclerotherapy. For general purposes an end-viewing instrument is more versatile, enabling both diagnostic and therapeutic functions to be performed. The advantages of an oblique-viewing endoscope are better visualization of the greater and lesser curves of the stomach and the built-in forceps elevator which is helpful in aiming the injector, particularly for small varices during elective sclerotherapy.

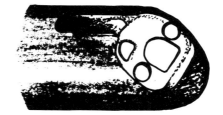

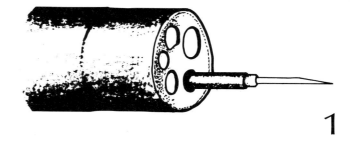

1

Injectors

Several types of sclerotherapy injectors with retractable needles are commercially available (*Illustration 1*). The flexible metal injectors are robust and reusable, but the narrower internal calibre and greater resistance during injection restricts the volume of sclerosant administered per unit time compared with the disposable injectors. Injectors are equipped with either 23 or 25 gauge needles. The larger needle is preferred as it facilitates injection of viscous sclerosant solutions and is not associated with any greater risk of bleeding after withdrawal of the needle.

Sclerosants

Several different sclerosant agents have been successfully used. The Cape Town group uses 5% ethanolamine oleate for both the intravariceal and the combined injection technique[3]. The most widely used alternative solutions are sodium tetradecyl sulphate (1%) and sodium morrhuate (2%) while polidocanol (0.5% or 1%) is used almost exclusively by the proponents of paravariceal sclerotherapy[4].

Operations

ELECTIVE SCLEROTHERAPY

Preparation and positioning of patient

The procedure is explained to the patient and signed consent obtained. Two assistants, including a qualified nurse trained in endoscopy techniques, should be present throughout the procedure. One assistant provides suction of the patient's mouth to avoid aspiration, ensures that the bite guard is not dislodged and comforts the patient. The other assistant advances and retracts the injector needle and administers the sclerosant under the direction of the endoscopist. The posterior tongue and pharynx are sprayed with a local anaesthetic (10% xylocaine). A small butterfly needle is inserted into a superficial hand vein and remains in place for the duration of the procedure. The appropriate analgesia and sedation are administered intravenously according to the medical status of the patient. The desired sedation is achieved by injecting small incremental doses, being cautious to avoid oversedation in the aged and in those with liver compromise. The authors' preference is 2.5 mg midazolam and 25 mg pethidine.

Before passing the endoscope the fully connected instrument should be checked for satisfactory function of the light source and lens, focus and tip deflection controls, air, suction and water channels. The assistants should be familiarized with the technique and equipment. Commands such as 'advance needle' and 'retract needle' should be rehearsed before injection. The endoscopist indicates the volume to be injected and the assistant acknowledges that the desired volume has been injected. It is important that the assistant should comment when more resistance than expected is encountered during injection, because the varix may be thrombosed or the needle incorrectly positioned.

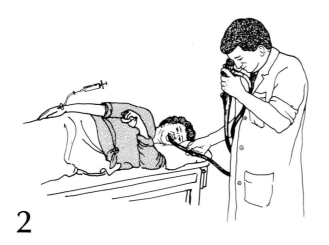

2

2   The patient is placed in the left lateral decubitus position at the top of the bed with the head on a pillow and the neck slightly flexed. The distal endoscope tube is lubricated with a water-soluble medical-grade lubricant, dentures are removed and a comfortable mouthpiece (bite guard) is used in patients with teeth to protect the endoscope.

Endoscopy

3 Passage of the fibreoptic endoscope is initiated by guiding the gently flexed tip over the tongue and then extending the tip in the upper pharynx. The opening of the cricopharynx is identified and negotiated with gentle pressure coinciding with a swallow. The instrument is passed under direct vision, keeping the oesophageal lumen in full view by controlling the tip. Intermittent insufflation of air is used to maintain sufficient distension of the lumen for visibility. Constant or excessive air insufflation should be avoided. Mucus and fluid are removed through the suction channel and the lens cleared with a jet of water when necessary. After passing the cricopharynx, the entire oesophagus is examined for oesophageal varices. The extent, number and size are noted for documentation. Unless varices are bleeding, panendoscopy is first performed to exclude other lesions before commencing injection of varices.

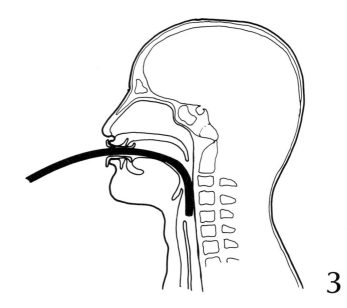

3

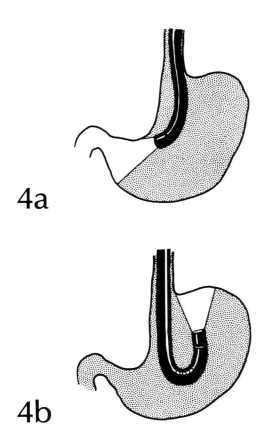

4a

4b

4a, b When the stomach is reached, the tip is passed distally under vision, insufflating only enough air to display the channel ahead. The pylorus is centred in the field of view and air is insufflated to distend the distal stomach and relax the pylorus; as this occurs the tip is gently advanced into the duodenal bulb. The proximal duodenum is carefully evaluated. Thereafter, the endoscope is withdrawn into the stomach and the cardia, gastric fundus and upper portion of the lesser curve are viewed by reversing the tip in the moderately distended body of the stomach. If gastric varices or evidence of portal hypertensive gastropathy are present they are noted and documented.

5   On completion of panendoscopy the endoscope is
    partially withdrawn and positioned above the
gastro-oesophageal junction, and the varices in the
lower 5 cm of the oesophagus are injected.

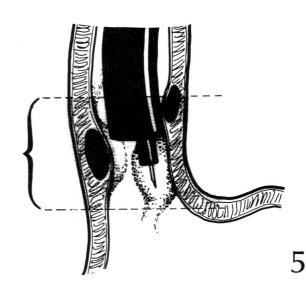

5

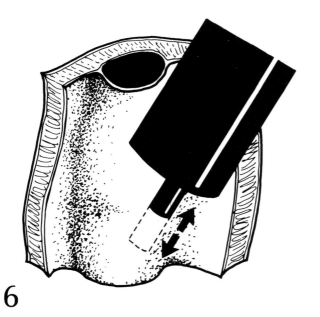

6

Injection technique

6   The endoscope tip is manoeuvred into position and
    the target varix identified. The endoscopist passes
the injector through the channel into the field of view
and the tip is positioned 2 cm beyond the end of the
endoscope. Care should be taken to avoid inadvertent
puncture of the plastic injector sheath and damage to
the endoscope channel by the needle when advancing
the injector. The injector should not be passed through
the channel with the endoscope tip in a position of
acute flexion. The needle should remain in the retracted
position until the tip of the injector has passed through
the endoscope and is visible to the endoscopist. All
movements and manipulation of the injector are
performed *only* by the endoscopist. A practice aiming
pass with the needle retracted is useful to determine the
direction of the advancing needle.

7 The assistant is instructed to advance the needle and a small volume of solution is discarded into the oesophageal lumen in order to fill the injector. The endoscopist inserts the needle directly into the centre and most prominent part of the varix by advancing the injector a further 5 mm: the length of the visible needle and the angle of insertion determine the depth of puncture. If the needle is well placed and appears intravariceal, the assistant is instructed to inject 1 ml of sclerosant. If this is achieved without resistance the assistant injects further sclerosant. With further injection of sclerosant the varix will be seen to distend above and below the injection site and become a paler colour. This is the indication to stop the injection. A total volume of no more than 5 ml is usually required for a large varix: smaller varices will require proportionately less sclerosant. On completing injection of the first varix, the remaining varices are injected. After a previous series of injections, varices will be smaller and less sclerosant is injected. During subsequent endoscopy, varices may be thrombosed and will appear firm and cord-like. If increased resistance to insertion of the needle and injection of sclerosant with leakage around the needle is noted, confirming obliteration of the variceal channel, no further injection should be undertaken.

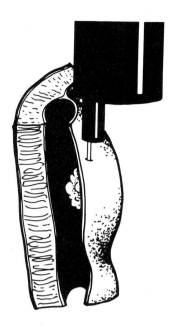

7

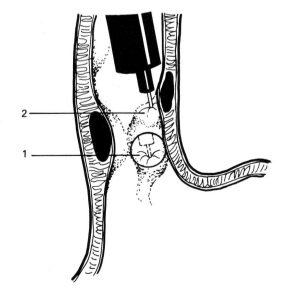

8

8 A second series of injections is performed at a higher level for large varices (site 2). The fibrescope is withdrawn 2–3 cm and the varices injected (usually 2–3 ml of sclerosant is sufficient). As the varices become smaller, after several previous injections, they are injected only at the lower site (site 1).

9 Accurate placement of the needle is critical in obtaining effective delivery of sclerosant and avoiding complications which may follow incorrect injection. A tangential flat angle of insertion as shown in *Illustration 7* is preferable, to avoid a deep injection: a less acute angle with a perpendicular approach may transfix the varix and penetrate the oesophageal wall, resulting in an intramuscular injection. In this situation increased resistance to injection will be noted by the assistant and no blanching or distension of the varix will occur. The injector and needle should be withdrawn and a further injection performed after accurate placement of the needle.

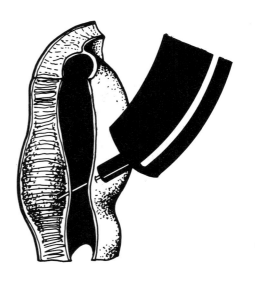

9

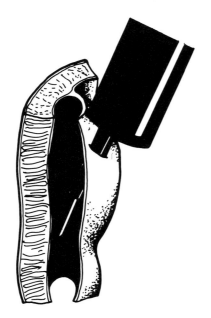

10

10 The needle should not be left protruding while selecting a further varix for injection because inadvertent laceration of a varix with accompanying bleeding may occur, especially with coughing or peristalsis. Needle insertion and variceal puncture requires a delicate wrist action by the endoscopist while manipulating the injector. This provides a limited controlled forward momentum of about 5 mm.

Injection by attempting to spear the varix or forceful jabbing of the varix with the needle may result in deep insertion and cannulation of the varix with entry of both needle and the hub of the catheter sheath and resultant bleeding from the varix on extraction.

EMERGENCY SCLEROTHERAPY

Initial measures

Urgent intravenous fluid resuscitation is started. The authors' group utilizes pharmacological therapy in patients with suspected variceal bleeding, although the efficacy remains controversial[4]. Vasopressin, its synthetic analogue terlipressin, and somatostatin have been used to lower portal pressure[4]. The most commonly used agent was vasopressin, which should be administered as a continuous intravenous infusion. The combination of glyceryl trinitrate and vasopressin reduces the side effects caused by the use of vasopressin alone and potentiates the portal haemodynamic effects. The glyceryl trinitrate can be administered intravenously, sublingually, or transdermally. A combination of continuous intravenous vasopressin (0.4 units/min) and sublingual glyceryl trinitrate (one tablet every half hour for up to 6 hours), was used[4], but currently the authors, like others, have converted to the use of a continuous infusion of somatostatin or octreotide.

Endoscopy

Urgent endoscopy is essential. The patient is positioned as shown for elective sclerotherapy as in *Illustration 2*. One-third of patients with suspected variceal bleeding do not, in fact, have varices. Patients shown to have varices on endoscopy fall into one of three groups although the differentiation may be difficult during active bleeding: (1) those with actively bleeding varices; (2) those whose varices have stopped bleeding; (3) those who have varices but are bleeding from another lesion. At endoscopy, variceal bleeding that has stopped is diagnosed if adherent blood clots are noted on a varix or when varices are present in a patient with upper gastrointestinal bleeding in whom panendoscopy demonstrates no other cause for the bleeding.

Emergency endoscopy should be performed in the endoscopy unit where all the necessary equipment is available. Many units have a fully equipped emergency endoscopy trolley and if necessary this can be taken into the operating room or to the intensive care unit. It is imperative that full resuscitative facilities are available together with skilled staff experienced in dealing with emergencies. Two endoscopy assistants should be present throughout. Adequate monitoring is necessary during the procedure. Emergency endoscopy should not commence until satisfactory venous access and central venous pressure measurement are established and volume replacement and resuscitation procedures with blood transfusions are initiated to correct hypovolaemia. If bleeding is extensive, endotracheal intubation is essential before endoscopy to protect the airway and avoid aspiration.

Intravariceal injection

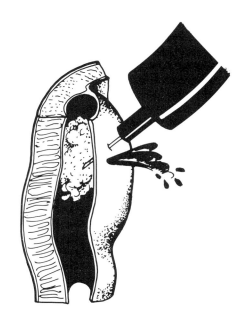

11

11 Active variceal bleeding with a jet of blood or rapid oozing is immediately dealt with by controlling the bleed with intravariceal sclerotherapy. Urgent control of bleeding with accurate placement of the needle and sclerosant should be performed without delay while there is adequate visibility. No attempt should be made to inject distal to the active bleeding site or to insert the needle into the bleeding point, because this may enlarge the hole and aggravate bleeding with extravasation and loss of sclerosant. A technique similar to elective intravariceal sclerotherapy is used with needle insertion proximal to the bleeding site. A total volume of 5 ml of sclerosant is usually sufficient. Distension and blanching of the varix indicate that the needle is in the correct position and that the appropriate volume of sclerosant has been injected. After the bleeding has been controlled, the other variceal channels are sclerosed. A second series of injections is usually performed at a higher level, as depicted in *Illustration 8*. Panendoscopy is undertaken on completion of sclerotherapy to exclude other lesions.

Combined paravariceal and intravariceal injection

12a–c The authors' group prefers this alternative technique to control active variceal bleeding. The needle is inserted in a paravariceal position and sclerosant injected proximal to the bleeding point to compress the bleeding site by raising a weal (*Illustration 12a*). Sufficient sclerosant is injected to control the bleeding (*Illustration 12b*). If this does not completely control the acute bleeding, the paravariceal injection is repeated alongside the bleeding point. The procedure is completed by injecting that particular varix with intravariceal sclerosant as well (*Illustration 12c*). The volume injected in the paravariceal position should not be more than 1 ml at each site to avoid subsequent ulceration of mucosa. The remaining variceal channels are then sclerosed. Panendoscopy is performed on completion of sclerotherapy to exclude other lesions.

If variceal bleeding is profuse, vigorous lavage through the endoscope channel and elevation of the head of the table to 30° may improve visibility and allow identification of the bleeding site. No blind attempts at injection should be used. The procedure is usually performed with the patient on their side as depicted in *Illustration 2*. With profuse bleeding the patient requires endotracheal intubation. The procedure may be facilitated by placing the patient on their back on the bed (or operating table) and adjusting the headpiece to an angle of 45°. If immediate sclerotherapy cannot be performed because of lack of expertise or inadequate visibility, bleeding should first be controlled by balloon tube tamponade before the patient is subjected to further sclerotherapy[4].

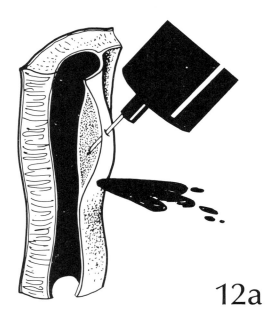

12a

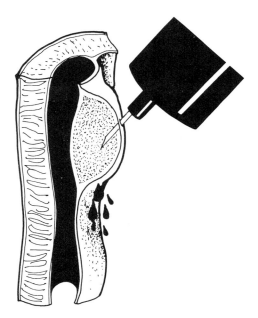

12b

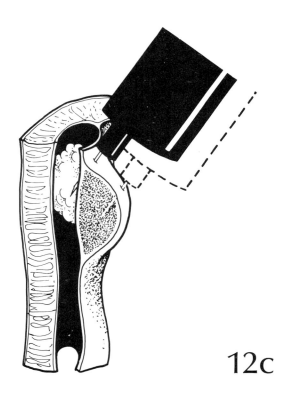

12c

Balloon tube tamponade

13 The four-lumen balloon tube (Minnesota tube) is effective in temporarily controlling variceal bleeding which allows time for resuscitation and management planning[3, 4]. Before inserting the balloon tube in stuporous or comatose patients, the airway should be protected by an endotracheal tube to prevent aspiration. A new tube should always be used and the inflated gastric and oesophageal balloons tested underwater to confirm a complete air seal. The deflated lubricated tube is passed through a bite guard via the mouth after adequate topical pharyngeal anaesthesia. Passage via the nose should not be used because of potential pressure necrosis of the nasal cartilage. The left index finger in the mouth facilitates initial passage of the tube by guiding the tip of the tube over the posterior tongue, through the cricopharynx and prevents coiling of the tube in the pharynx. If difficulty is encountered negotiating the cricopharynx, especially when an endotracheal tube is in place, a McGills forcep and laryngoscope are used to pass the tube under direct vision. The tube is inserted almost fully and the epigastrium auscultated to confirm that the gastric balloon is in the stomach by instilling air with a 50-ml syringe into the aspirating lumen. The gastric balloon is inflated with 50-ml increments of air to 200 ml. If the patient shows signs of discomfort, inflation *must* stop as the gastric balloon may be in the lower oesophagus and the position should be rechecked. When fully inflated, the tube is pulled back until the balloon engages the gastro-oesophageal junction and abuts on the cardia. A partially split tennis ball, secured over the tube, maintains firm traction against the bite-guard and ensures constant compression on the cardia by the gastric balloon.

The oesophageal balloon is inflated only if bleeding continues after traction on the gastric balloon. The oesophageal balloon pressure should not exceed 40 mmHg or be maintained for more than 14 h. Thereafter, preferably within 6–12 h, sclerotherapy should be undertaken to achieve more lasting control because of the high rate of recurrence of bleeding (60%) after removal of the tube. If bleeding persists or recurs after the tube has been placed, the tube should be checked and, if found to be correctly situated, a further diagnostic endoscopy should be performed. A bleeding source that has been missed during the initial endoscopy may be the cause of continued bleeding. Because of associated dangers, a balloon tube should be used only when required to control endoscopically confirmed variceal bleeding[5, 6].

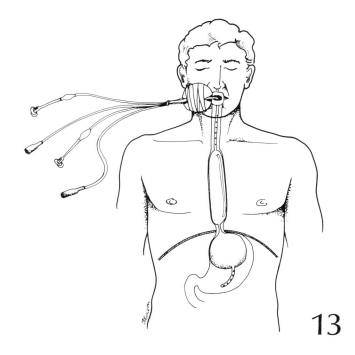

13

Postoperative care

Elective sclerotherapy

After elective outpatient sclerotherapy patients are observed in the endoscopy suite recovery room for an hour before discharge. Bleeding following elective sclerotherapy is rare. Retrosternal discomfort is treated with antacids. After admission for acute variceal bleeding, the first two injection sclerotherapy sessions are performed in hospital. Further injection treatments are performed on an outpatient basis.

Injection sclerotherapy is repeated at weekly intervals until the varices have been eradicated. The first subsequent assessment is performed at 3 months and then repeated at 6-monthly or annual intervals for life[7]. Any recurrent variceal channels noted during repeat endoscopy require a further course of injection sclerotherapy. If ulceration extending over more than one-quarter of the circumference of the oesophagus is present at the site of previous sclerotherapy, further injections are deferred for 2 weeks to allow the ulceration to heal. Minor ulceration or slough is usually ignored.

Emergency sclerotherapy

The patient is returned to an intensive care unit for 24 h after injection. Unless the patient is stuporous or comatose, oral fluids are allowed for the first 24 h and thereafter a regular diet is recommended. Prophylactic antibiotics are not administered routinely in uncomplicated cases. Hepatic encephalopathy and ascites are treated with standard therapy. Mild retrosternal discomfort and low-grade pyrexia may occur for 24 h after injection. If either is excessive or if the patient has dysphagia, a Gastrografin contrast swallow is obtained to exclude an injection site leak[6].

No further bleeding will occur in 70% of patients. If bleeding does recur, vasopressin or somatostatin is commenced and the patient re-endoscoped. Recurrent bleeding from oesophageal varices is treated by repeat injection similar to the initial procedures. If bleeding is massive and satisfactory control is not achieved by sclerotherapy, a balloon tube is placed for acute control and followed by sclerotherapy within 6–12 h. Bleeding from oesophageal ulceration or slough is treated conservatively with oral sucralfate. In the unusual event of persistent bleeding from injection ulceration, intravenous somatostatin is administered.

In patients who have continued acute variceal bleeding after two emergency sclerotherapy injection sessions during a single hospital admission, we recommend that bleeding be temporarily controlled with balloon-tube tamponade followed by a surgical procedure[4,6,8]. Unfortunately, it is not possible to predict during initial evaluation and variceal injection which patients will not ultimately respond to sclerotherapy.

Outcome

Elective sclerotherapy

In the Cape Town 10-year prospective study evaluating the long-term management of patients after oesophageal variceal bleeding[7], oesophageal varices were eradicated in 123 of 140 patients. A median number of five injections were required to eradicate the oesophageal varices which remained eradicated for a mean of 19 months. Varices recurred in 37 patients after a mean of 15 months and were easily re-eradicated by further injection sclerotherapy. Recurrent variceal bleeding was unusual after the varices had been eradicated and occurred in only 13 of the 123 patients.

Acute variceal injection

The success rate of a single injection treatment is 70%[4,6]. The 30% of patients who have further bleeding after initial injection of sclerosant should have a second injection performed: in this group the success rate is more than 90%[4,6].

References

1. Wodak E. Akute gastrointestinale Blutung; Resultate der endoskopischen Sklerosierung von Osophagusvarizen. *Schweiz Med Wochenschr* 1979; 109: 591–4.

2. Paquet K-J, Oberhammer E. Sclerotherapy of bleeding oesophageal varices by means of endoscopy. *Endoscopy* 1978; 10: 7–12.

3. Terblanche J, Krige JE, Bornman PC. Endoscopic sclerotherapy. *Surg Clin North Am* 1990; 70: 341–59.

4. Terblanche J, Burroughs AK, Hobbs KE. Controversies in the management of bleeding oesophageal varices. *N Engl J Med* 1989; 320: 1393–8, 1469–75.

5. Burnett DA, Rikkers LF. Nonoperative emergency treatment of variceal haemorrhage. *Surg Clin North Am* 1990; 70: 291–306.

6. Kahn D, Bornman PC, Terblanche J. A 10-year prospective evaluation of balloon tube tamponade and emergency injection sclerotherapy for actively bleeding esophageal varices. *HPB Surg* 1989; 1: 207–19.

7. Terblanche J, Kahn D, Bornman PC. Long-term injection sclerotherapy treatment for oesophageal varices: A 10 year prospective evaluation. *Ann Surg* 1989; 210: 725–31.

8. Bornman PC, Terblanche J, Kahn D, Jonker MA, Kirsch RE. Limitations of multiple injection sclerotherapy sessions for acute variceal bleeding. *S Afr Med J* 1986; 70: 34–6.

Illustrations by Denise Smith

Rigid oesophagoscopy

Michael T. Marrinan FRCS(Ed)
Fellow in Thoracic Surgery, Mayo Graduate School of Medicine, Rochester, Minnesota, USA

Claude Deschamps MD
Senior Associate Consultant, Section of General Thoracic Surgery, Mayo Clinic and Mayo Foundation, and Assistant Professor of Surgery, Mayo Medical School, Rochester, Minnesota, USA

Principles and justification

Rigid oesophagoscopy is a useful and safe procedure in the evaluation of oesophageal disorders. In recent years flexible fibreoptic oesophagoscopy has enjoyed widespread use, mainly because general anaesthesia is not required, the stomach and duodenum can be examined, and the risk of perforation is lower. Nevertheless, the specific situations outlined below show that a need for rigid oesophagoscopy remains, and the technique should remain part of the armamentarium of all oesophageal surgeons.

In some circumstances, the relatively cheap cost of a rigid oesophagoscope, combined with its greater durability, may make the rigid instrument preferable to the fibreoptic instrument. The greater ease of sterilization of the rigid instrument may also be a factor, particularly where human immunodeficiency virus infection is endemic.

Indications

Removal of ingested foreign bodies is greatly facilitated by the large-bore rigid open tube with appropriately proportioned grasping forceps. When severe oesophageal bleeding is encountered, suctioning is far more efficient. To decrease the risk of aspiration, impacted megaoesophagus should be treated using the rigid endoscope. This allows for liberal irrigation and more efficient evacuation of debris. This technique also facilitates the evaluation of high lesions at or just beyond the cricopharyngeus, an area poorly examined with the flexible endoscope. Whenever the need dictates, larger biopsy specimens can be obtained through the rigid endoscope.

When an endo-oesophageal prosthesis is being considered to palliate intrinsic and extrinsic compression of the oesophagus or malignant oesophagorespiratory fistula, rigid endoscopy is of particular help intraoperatively in dilatation, guidewire positioning and verification of the position of the prosthesis after insertion[1].

While injection sclerotherapy of oesophageal varices is preferably performed under sedation using a flexible oesophagoscope, it is possible and safe to perform chronic sclerotherapy using a rigid oesophagoscope[2].

Contraindications

There are few contraindications to the procedure, but it should not be performed if there is instability of the cervical spine and may be impossible if severe kyphoscoliosis or restricted jaw opening is present. Great care should be exercised if large cervical osteophytes are seen on radiographs of the cervical spine, if there is a large thoracic aortic aneurysm, or if there is a pharyngo-oesophageal or epiphrenic diverticulum. A chest radiograph and barium swallow should be reviewed, and radiographs of the cervical spine may be required if symptoms are present.

Preoperative

Patient preparation

The patient should have taken nothing by mouth overnight or for a minimum of 8 h. This is specifically to decrease the risk of aspiration during the procedure[3]. Dentures should be removed. The oesophagus should be empty, which may require a clear liquid diet for 24 h before the procedure and aspiration of the oesophagus immediately before performing the endoscopy.

Equipment

1   Chevalier–Jackson, Negus, or Moersch-type oeso-phagoscopes may be used. At the Mayo Clinic the preference is for the Moersch oesophagoscope modified to carry a fibreoptic light source. This modification uses a fibreoptic light rod to provide illumination directly at the level of the object being examined.

A full range of sizes, up to 20 mm for a man and 16 mm for a woman, should be on hand. An endoscope with magnification is advisable in children to compensate for the loss of visual acuity associated with the use of a small-bore open oesophagoscope.

Large-bore and small-bore suckers, longer than the overall length of the oesophagoscope, should be available, as well as a variety of long biopsy forceps and a full range of oesophageal dilators and guidewires as described in the chapter on pp. 26–38.

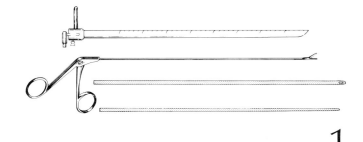

1

Anaesthesia

Premedication consisting of pethidine hydrochloride, 1 mg/kg, and atropine sulphate, 0.4 mg, may be given intramuscularly before the procedure.

General anaesthesia via a cuffed endotracheal tube is employed. Muscle relaxation is helpful for the safe performance of rigid oesophagoscopy, as this reduces the risk of perforation. It is also possible to perform rigid oesophagoscopy under neuroleptanalgesia, although the benefits of complete muscle relaxation are lost.

Throughout the procedure the patient's eyes are kept covered for protection.

During passage of the rigid oesophagoscope through the cricopharyngeal sphincter, the anaesthetist may assist by deflating the cuff on the endotracheal tube and/or pulling forward on the larynx. When insertion of an endo-oesophageal prosthesis is being considered, a smaller endotracheal tube should be used to ease passage of the prosthesis and its introducer.

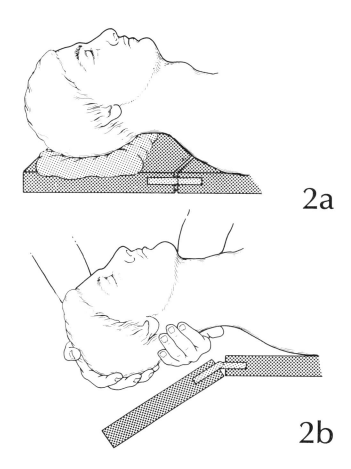

2a

2b

Operation[4]

Position of patient

2a, b The patient is positioned supine on an operating table, the head of which can be raised or lowered easily, with the head stabilized on a foam ring. Alternatively, the head and neck may be entirely supported by an assistant. The surgeon stands during insertion of the oesophagoscope, then sits during the examination.

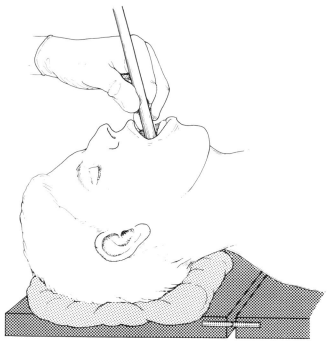

3

Tooth protection

3 The lubricated oesophagoscope is introduced at the base of the tongue with the head in the 'sniffing' position. Throughout the procedure, the upper teeth and gums are protected by a guard and a gauze swab is positioned over the upper lip. The tongue is gently pushed to the left, and the instrument is held at all times between the operator's thumb and fingers, protecting the lips and teeth.

Passage of the oesophagoscope

4a–c The epiglottis is visualized and pushed out of view by the beak of the endoscope. The endoscope is then advanced to the posterior pharynx, and the neck is extended by about 15°. The cricopharyngeal sphincter is identified as a horizontal groove halfway between the posterior larynx and the posterior pharyngeal wall. The oesophagus is entered at this point.

No force should be used as this is an area of high risk for perforation. If resistance is met, the balloon on the endotracheal tube should be deflated, and the anaesthetist can assist by gently drawing forward on the larynx. If there is still difficulty, a small bougie can be threaded through the endoscope into the oesophagus to lead the endoscope through.

As the oesophagus is gently entered the head must be lowered to allow a decrease in the angulation of the instrument, bringing it into alignment with the long axis of the oesophagus.

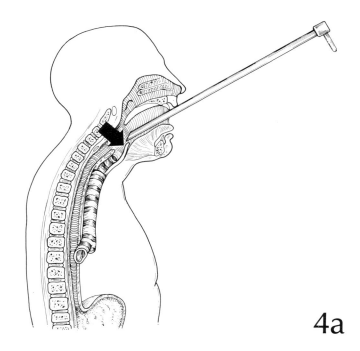

4a

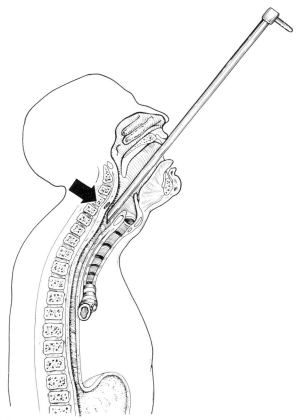

4b

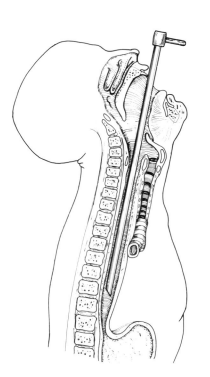

4c

Examination

5a, b The oesophagus is examined under direct vision. The areas of natural constriction of the oesophagus should be borne in mind, as well as the deviation anteriorly and to the left in the lower third of the oesophagus. The position of the gastro-oesophageal junction is of particular importance and should be noted with reference to its distance from the incisor teeth.

The oesophagus should also be examined as the endoscope is being withdrawn, particularly in the area just below the cricopharyngeus, which is poorly seen by other methods. The same care should be taken on withdrawing the oesophagoscope as during its introduction, as the oesophagus can also be injured during this phase of the examination. Those manoeuvres performed on introduction should be replicated in reverse during withdrawal of the instrument.

The opportunity to palpate the abdomen while the patient is anaesthetized and relaxed should be taken.

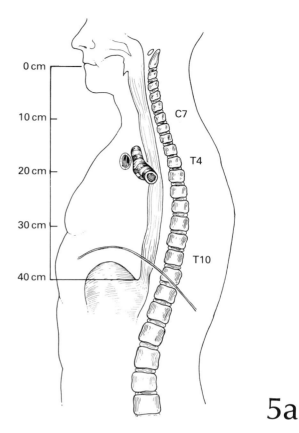

5a

5b

Postoperative care

Apart from aspiration, perforation is the most common major complication following oesophagoscopy[3] and symptoms and signs of this should be sought in all patients in the early postoperative period. The cardinal features of oesophageal perforation are: (1) severe localized pain, (2) subcutaneous emphysema, (3) pneumothorax, (4) pleural effusion, and (5) fever. Even in the absence of any of these features, oral intake should be withheld until the patient is fully recovered from the general anaesthetic. When an endo-oesophageal prosthesis has been inserted, a chest radiograph should be obtained to rule out a pneumothorax and verify the position of the prosthesis. If there is suspicion of perforation, an immediate water-soluble contrast (meglumine diatrizoate) study should be performed.

References

1. Gaer JA, Blauth C, Townsend ER, Fountain SW. Method of endoscopic esophageal intubation using a rigid esophagoscope. *Ann Thorac Surg* 1990; 49: 152–3.

2. Wilson RH, Campbell WJ, Spencer A, Johnston GW. Rigid endoscopy under general anaesthesia is safe for chronic injection sclerotherapy. *Br J Surg* 1989; 76: 719–21.

3. Orringer MB. Complications of esophageal surgery and trauma. In: Greenfield LJ, ed. *The Complications in Surgery and Trauma*. 2nd edn. Philadelphia: JB Lippincott, 1990: 302–25.

4. Fontana RS, Higgins JA. Endoscopic techniques. In: Payne WS, Olsen AM, eds. *The Esophagus*. Philadelphia: Lea and Febiger, 1974: 30–8.

Dilatation of oesophageal strictures

Avni Sali PhD, FRACS, FACS
Clinical Associate Professor of Surgery, University of Melbourne, and Surgeon, Department of Surgery, Heidelberg Repatriation Hospital, Heidelberg, Melbourne, Victoria, Australia

Principles and justification

Significant developments over recent years now enable dilatation of oesophageal strictures with almost no morbidity and mortality in most patients. Numerous dilators are available for selective treatment of various strictures. Wire-guided or endoscopically-guided dilatation with either bougies or balloons has increased success rates, as well as increasing the safety of dilating difficult strictures. Surgical treatment of strictures is now seldom necessary.

Indications

Peptic oesophageal strictures are the most common indication for dilatation, and they are mainly located in the lower third of the oesophagus. Malignant strictures are usually only dilated before the insertion of oesophageal tubes. Strictures due to surgery, caustic ingestion, or radiation, as well as upper oesophageal webs and lower oesophageal rings, can be successfully treated with dilatation.

Types of dilator

Three different types of dilator are in current use:

1. Mercury-filled dilators.
2. Wire-guided dilators.
3. Balloon dilators.

The French gauge (Fr) is most commonly used to indicate the size of the dilator. This gauge is based on circumference size in millimetres, e.g. a 32-Fr bougie has a circumference of 32 mm. The approximate diameter in millimetres of a bougie is obtained by dividing the French gauge by 3.

Mercury-filled rubber bougies inserted without oesophagoscopy

1 Two types of dilator are used, either the Maloney type with a tapered tip, which is widely used in North America, or the Hurst type which has a rounded tip. The tapered tip Maloney dilator is preferred as it is easier to swallow and its tapered tip is easier to pass through a stricture. These dilators are available in 12–60 Fr with each being 2 Fr larger than the preceding one. Mercury provides flexibility and stiffness but its weight is not intended to aid dilatation. Bougies of less than 36 Fr can be difficult to pass because they may be too flexible.

Mercury-filled rubber bougies can be used to dilate mild to moderate strictures. These bougies should not be used for asymmetrical strictures or when a diverticulum is present. The Maloney dilators have been shown to be very safe if patient selection criteria are strictly adhered to. These dilators are best used in

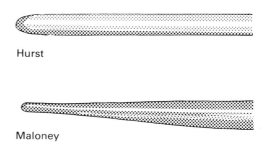

Hurst

Maloney

1

patients who required multiple dilatations. New patients always require oesophagoscopy to assess stricture size and type, and therefore it is more convenient to carry out dilatation at the same time using a wire-guided technique or endoscopically-directed balloon. The Maloney bougie can also be used for self-bougienage.

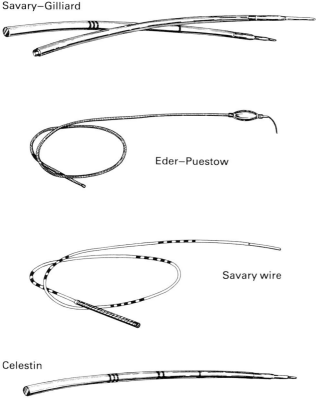

Savary–Gilliard

Eder–Puestow

Savary wire

Celestin

2

Wire-guided dilators

2 The various types of wire-guided dilator are shown.

Savary–Gilliard dilators

3   These are the most recently developed bougies and also the most commonly used, having almost replaced the Eder–Puestow and Celestin dilators. They are smooth, very flexible, incompressible dilators which are made from polyvinyl chloride and are plastic-coated. They vary in length from 70 to 100 cm with diameters ranging from 15 to 56 Fr (5–18 mm).

Distal to the tip and the tapered end is a radio-opaque band in the area of maximal diameter, which can be difficult to see fluoroscopically (*Illustration 2*). In a more recent variant the total length of the bougie is radio-opaque. A central 1.8-mm lumen allows its passage over the guidewire. A metal sleeve at the proximal tip prevents this dilator from passing over the flexible tip of the wire guide. The Celestin dilators do not have this protective metal sleeve.

A guidewire is now available with distance markers (etchings), with the first marker being at 40 cm and subsequent markers 20 cm apart. The total length of the Savary wire (*Illustration 2*) is 200 cm and the etches are 6 mm long and 3 mm apart. The spring tip of the

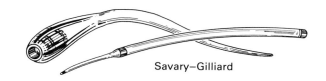

Savary–Gilliard

Celestin

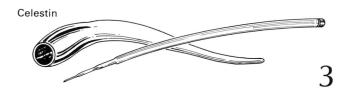

3

wire is reinforced where the spring meets the wire to prevent angulation at this site. This junction could result in complications as occurred with the use of the older Eder–Puestow wire before it was strengthened.

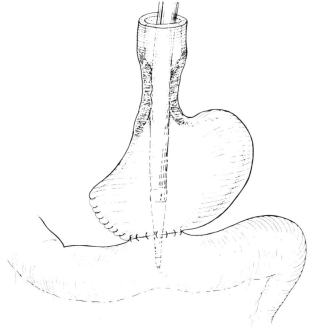

4   The Savary–Gilliard dilators have the disadvantage that multiple dilators have to be passed, but as they are very flexible they can be passed with little difficulty and discomfort to the patient. These dilators also lack feel of the stricture as the dilator passes through. Following partial gastrectomy, it can be difficult to pass the dilator to its widest diameter unless there is enough guidewire distal to the stricture.

4

Eder–Puestow dilators

5 These were the first of the wire-guided dilators and are generally available from 21 to 45 Fr. Larger olives are available. Olives can be secured onto a flexible staff with a flexible spring tip which has a lumen for the guidewire (*see Illustration 2*).

Eder–Puestow dilators can be used to dilate tight irregular strictures. They may be preferable to other bougies for tight strictures, such as those following gastro-oesophageal or oesophagojejunal anastomoses. Their main advantage is that the operator can feel the olive pass through the stricture much more easily than with other dilators. Because they are not tapered, however, they can split the stricture. Eder–Puestow dilators have also been shown to cause more pharyngeal trauma than other dilators.

With these dilators, the guidewire is more often bent during insertion as they do not flow over the wire as well as the very flexible Savary–Gilliard dilators. The guidewire originally available with these dilators was unsafe, but they can be used with the more recently developed Savary wire.

Celestin dilators

These semisolid dilators, of which there are two types, were developed some time after the Eder–Puestow

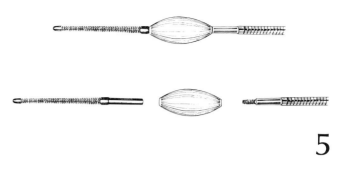

5

dilators and are made of plastic (*see Illustrations 2* and *3*).

The smaller dilator has stepped areas from 4 to 12 mm and the larger from 12 to 18 mm. The main advantage of these step dilators is that only two dilators need to be passed, with the potential of less discomfort for the patient and also fewer guidewires being damaged compared with the Eder–Puestow dilators. The Celestin dilator is much less flexible than the Savary–Gilliard dilator.

A major disadvantage of these step dilators is their very limited flexibility, particularly with the larger diameter dilator, which can meet resistance from the teeth making it difficult to asssess stricture resistance and also necessitating some neck extension. They also lack feel of the stricture as the dilator passes through the stenosis compared with the metal Eder–Puestow olives.

Balloon dilators

6a, b Two types of balloons are used. They may be passed over a guidewire or introduced directly into an endoscope so that they can be viewed through the endoscope. Wire-guided balloons are very occasionally used for oesophageal strictures, although they are ideal for pyloric, biliary, pancreatic and even intestinal strictures. The endoscopically introduced balloon, which is becoming more popular, contains an internal wire which is radio-opaque to stiffen it and allow passage. The shaft of the Rigiflex dilator is made of polyethylene, which offers good torque control.

The diameters of the balloons can vary from 3 to 30 mm, and they are made from a polymer which, if stretched beyond the stated diameter, will burst rather than expand, which is an important safety feature. The size of the endoscopically-guided balloons (18–54 Fr) is limited by the biopsy channel compared with the larger wire-guided balloons (18–60 Fr). The balloons are lengthy (3–8 cm) and have a shaft of 60–200 cm. The longest shafts require a guidewire longer than the standard 200-cm Savary wire.

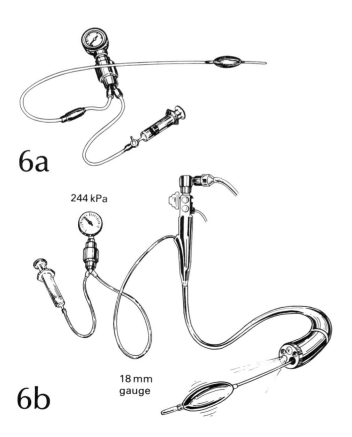

6a

244 kPa

6b   18 mm gauge

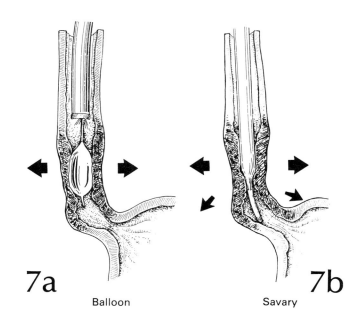

7a, b   Balloon dilators have a theoretical advantage over bougies as the applied force is directed radially against the stricture as opposed to the downward shearing force of bougies. Balloons are ideal for dilating tight, tortuous, long, symmetrical strictures. These dilators are generally preferable for proximal oesophageal strictures.

Disadvantages include difficulty in maintaining the inflated balloon within the stricture and also the high cost of replacing damaged balloons.

Preoperative

Prophylactic antibiotics

The following patients should be considered to be an infection risk: those with prosthetic valves; those with a history of bacterial endocarditis, congenital, or rheumatic heart disease; and those with immune deficiency resulting from chemotherapy or radiotherapy, adrenal steroids, or immunosuppressive drugs. The following prophylactic antibiotic regimens are used:

1. High risk: amoxycillin, 2 g intramuscularly or intravenously, and gentamicin, 1.5 mg/kg, intramuscularly or intravenously, 30 min before the procedures and 8 h after the procedure.
2. Low risk: oral amoxycillin, 3 g orally 1 h before the procedure and 1.5 g 6 h later.

Techniques

DILATATION WITH MERCURY-FILLED BOUGIES

This procedure is ideally carried out with an assistant. All patients must be assessed by endoscopy and biopsy to confirm the presence of benign disease and to ensure that the stricture is mild to moderate in diameter (1.2–1.4 cm).

8 Dilatations can be performed with the fasting patient either seated or in the left lateral position. The pharynx is anaesthetized with topical anaesthetic spray. Very occasionally sedation will be required. A 30-Fr dilator is used initially; however, if the patient has been dilated to 40 Fr on the last occasion, a 40-Fr dilator can be used. With these dilators, the size of the dilated lumen is less than the bougie used because of the flexibility of the dilator as well as the elasticity of the stricture. If the dilator does not pass, a smaller dilator can be used. The distance of the stricture from the mouth is marked on the bougie.

The dilator is held in the right hand, and its lubricated tip is guided to the oropharynx in the direction of the cricopharyngeus muscle with the left hand. The patient is asked to swallow as with passing an endoscope. The distal end of the bougie should be held above the patient's head by the assistant so that the mercury increases tube rigidity. The dilator is advanced until the maximum diameter passes through the stricture. When the stricture is encountered, insertion pressure is increased gently and a give is felt as it passes through. Careful dilatation is carried out with further larger bougies, ceasing if there is pain or excessive bleeding.

If the patient has documented oesophagitis, bleeding is usually seen even with the first dilator, but if there is no evidence of oesophagitis bleeding is a guide to cease dilatation. The amount of resistance to dilatation is also an important guide to the degree of dilatation possible. Generally, no more than three or four dilators are passed in any one session. If there is any difficulty in passing the bougie, the stricture should be dilated using another technique. In the majority of patients dysphagia disappears once dilated to 36 Fr and over. It is best to dilate to the maximum diameter as this is likely to reduce the need for subsequent dilatations.

9 It is possible for the bougie to curl up in the oesophagus proximal to the stricture, and this is more likely to happen with the small bougies.

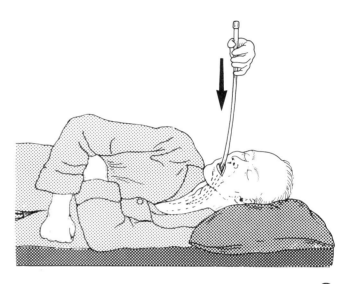

8

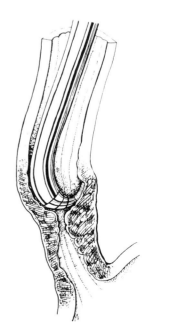

9

SELF-BOUGIENAGE

Self-dilatation can be taught if the patient is intelligent and dextrous and if the stricture is suitable. Dilatation is initially performed with Maloney dilators in hospital until maximum dilatation has been achieved. At the same time the patient is instructed in self-bougienage. Each patient learns to pass a dilator in the sitting position. Most patients can be taught this procedure after two or three practice dilatations on different days in hospital. The distance of the stricture from the mouth is always marked on the bougie as well as a distance 10 cm distal to this, which acts as a guide to the patient of the stricture position and the most distal insertion of the bougie.

10 To insert the Maloney dilator, some patients may prefer to use topical anaesthetic spray on the pharynx. The dilator is introduced by the fasting patient with the tip of the left index finger, and the rest of the dilator is held by the right hand. Once the dilator is in the cricopharyngeal region the patient swallows as the dilator is advanced.

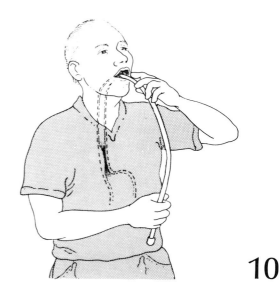

10

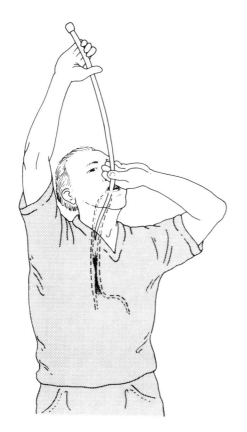

11 When the proximal part of the dilator has been swallowed the distal end is elevated as the patient's head is extended. The elevation of the mercury-containing bougie increases its stiffness.

11

12 The dilator is slowly passed through the stricture using both hands, ensuring that the distal marker on the bougie has reached the mouth.

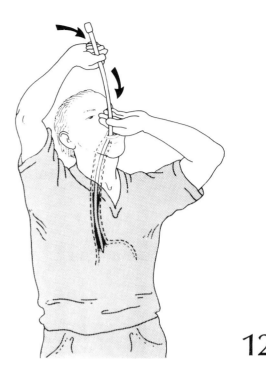

12

DILATATION WITH WIRE-GUIDED DILATORS

These procedures are ideally carried out with two assistants, one assisting the endoscopist with the procedure and the other providing the necessary dilators and caring for the patient. Protective glasses should be worn by all including the patient as the rigid end of the guidewire can cause eye damage. The patient is prepared in the usual manner as for gastroscopy or oesophagoscopy. It is not necessary to admit patients to hospital for the procedure, but this is appropriate when patients are frail or when repeated dilatations are anticipated. Fluoroscopy is generally not necessary, but it is recommended for those with limited experience or in patients where there is a tight or long stricture.

Dilatation is performed with the patient in the left lateral position, which lessens the risk of inhalation of regurgitated oesophageal or gastric contents. The flexibility of the guidewire and the various dilators allows dilatation without extending the patient's neck, although this may be necessary with the large Celestin dilator. Even patients with a severe kyphosis can undergo this procedure. If, for some reason, dilatation is carried out during general anaesthesia, a cuffed endotracheal tube is used and the procedure can be carried out with the patient supine.

If a tight stricture is suspected, a small diameter fibreoptic endoscope is used, whereas a larger diameter instrument can be used if this is not the case. With the finer instrument it may be possible to pass through the stenosis, enabling assessment of the stricture, stomach and duodenum as well as easier and safer insertion of the guidewire. If the stricture does not allow passage of the endoscope, the guidewire may have to be passed with the assistance of fluoroscopy. The larger endoscopes have better suction, which allows better clearance of oesophageal contents and larger biopsies to be taken. For repeat dilatations, it is best to use the shorter flexible oesophagoscope rather than the longer panendoscope, as it is much easier to pass a guidewire as well as balloons. If the endoscope can be passed into the stomach the fundal pool is evacuated before dilatation. Once the stricture is located it is examined diagnostically, taking any necessary specimens for cytology and histology. Biopsy techniques cause bleeding which make visibility poor, and in particular with a tight stenosis, the passage of the guidewire may become difficult or impossible. Biopsies in such circumstances should be undertaken after the dilatation or at a routine second dilatation. The stricture diameter should be assessed and also its distance from the incisors.

13a–c The Savary guidewire with gradations is lubricated before being passed through the biopsy channel of the instrument. The flexible tip of the wire can become impacted in the stenosis, in a diverticulum, or in a hiatus hernia.

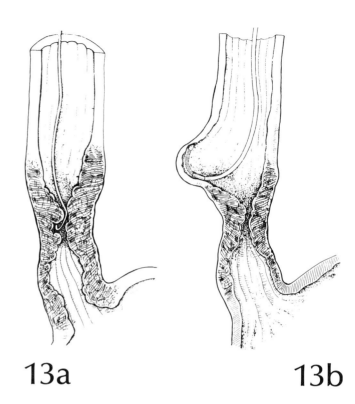

13a

13b

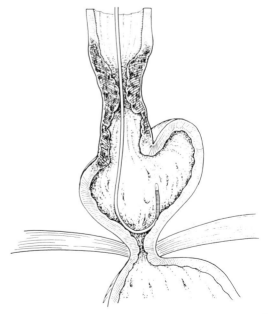

13c

14 The guidewire is placed into the proximal gastric antrum, near the greater curvature but not in contact with it. If it is not possible to pass the endoscope through the stricture, the wire can be passed through the stricture while viewing its progress through the endoscope. If there is resistance in the stricture, which occurs occasionally, fluoroscopy should be used. Once the wire has passed through the stricture, it is further inserted gently until there is resistance against the gastric wall. It is then withdrawn approximately 5 cm to avoid contact of the flexible tip of the wire with the gastric wall. The position of the wire is noted, and it must be maintained in this position.

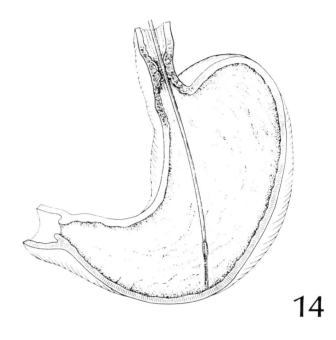

14

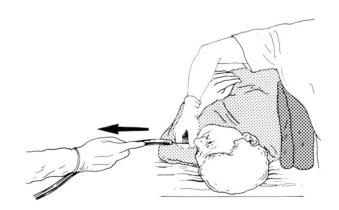

15

15 Once the guidewire has passed, the endoscope is removed by advancing the guidewire and withdrawing the endoscope at the same time. When the wire is visible in the mouth at the tip of the endoscope during its withdrawal, it is held in a fixed position as the endoscope is completely withdrawn by an assistant.

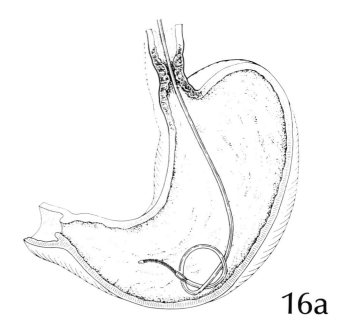

16a

16a, b Withdrawal or insertion of the wire can be dangerous during dilatation. Too much wire in the stomach has the potential of forming a knot. An acute bend can also occur between the flexible tip and the wire if there is contact with the stomach wall.

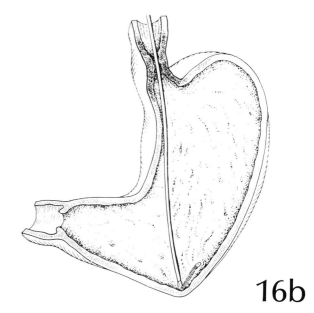

16b

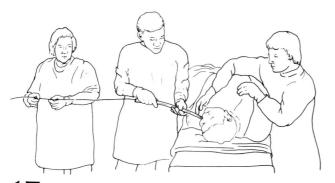

17

17 An assistant holds the proximal end of the wire standing at a fixed point. It is possible to mark the shaft of the dilator corresponding to the distance of the stricture from the mouth. Using this mark, the site of the stricture can be predicted during insertion of the bougie.

Savary–Gilliard dilators

An approximate size of dilator is selected based on the estimated diameter of the stricture. A dilator one or two sizes smaller than the assessed diameter of the stricture is used. The proximal third of the dilator is well lubricated and the wire is threaded into its lumen. If fluoroscopy is being used the position of the dilator is checked when resistance is felt at the stricture site. It is important that the guidewire is fixed by the assistant during all stages of the procedure, as the bougie has a tendency to push the wire forward into the stomach. Once there is excess wire proximal to the dilator, it ceases to serve as a guide and perforation can result. With firm pressure applied, the dilator is gently inserted until the resistance is overcome and the dilator passes through the stricture. The dilator that meets resistance determines the size of the stricture, although with the Savary–Gilliard dilators it is not as easy to feel the stricture as with the mercury-filled bougies and the Eder–Puestow dilators.

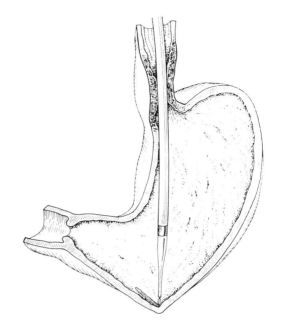

18

18 If the stricture is not felt, the bougie is gently inserted just beyond the mark on the bougie, indicating that the stricture has been passed. If the bougie is unable to pass any further beyond the stricture it has reached the spring tip of the wire. If the bougie is pushed beyond this limit, the end of the wire could penetrate the stomach wall.

Fluoroscopy is particularly important to the inexperienced user at this stage. The number of bougies that are passed at each procedure will vary depending on the severity and the character of the stricture. It is nearly always possible to pass the largest bougie, but occasionally it may not be possible or safe to pass the larger size during the first procedure. With tight strictures that do not allow passage of the endoscope, it is almost always not possible to pass the large dilators on the first occasion. The guidewire is removed at the end of the procedure with the last dilator, which fixes the distal tip of the wire and prevents the wire from injuring the patient's pharynx, mouth, or face. The whole procedure usually takes about 20–30 min to perform.

Diagnostic endoscopy is carried out after the final dilatation if it was not possible to do so initially. At this stage the endoscope has to be inserted very carefully with minimal insufflation in order to reduce the risk of oesophageal perforation. Alternatively, diagnostic endoscopy can be carried out on another occasion, as it is likely that endoscopy immediately after dilatation is more dangerous in those with very tight strictures, where passage of a fine endoscope was not possible initially.

Eder–Puestow dilators

The criterion for selecting the size of the metal olive is similar to that for selection of a Savary–Gilliard bougie. A mouth guard can be used to protect teeth from the metal dilators, but its use is not essential. The olive is attached to the dilating staff (*see Illustration 5*). The lubricated flexible tip and olive are threaded onto the guidewire. If fluoroscopy is used, it is easy to check the position of the dilator. With these dilators it is easier to feel the olive passing through the stricture. It is best to keep the elbows fixed to the trunk with feet apart whilst inserting the dilator (*see Illustration 17*). This position avoids a sudden thrust of the dilator down the oesophagus or stomach when a sudden loss of resistance occurs as the olive passes through a tight stricture. The number of bougies passed at any one session is determined as with the Savary–Gilliard dilators. Less wire is required distal to the dilator than with the Savary–Gilliard and Celestin dilators, so Eder–Puestow dilators can be used following partial gastrectomy.

Celestin dilators

One of the two dilators is chosen based on criteria similar to those for other wire-guided dilators. It is difficult to feel the stricture with this dilator because of its step-like increase in diameter. The patient's neck must be extended, particularly with the larger dilator due to its relative inflexibility. These dilators are seldom used by the author.

BALLOON DILATATION

Wire-guided balloons are inserted in a similar way to the wire-guided bougies, but fluoroscopy is used. The technique used for endoscopically-guided balloons will be discussed.

Endoscopically-guided balloon dilators

Patients are prepared as for wire-guided techniques and are placed in a similar position. Endoscopy is also performed as for wire-guided dilatation. The endoscope is sited just above the stricture (*see Illustration 7a*). The appropriate balloon is selected on a similar basis to selection of other dilators. The balloon, pressure monitor, syringe and stopcock are assembled as shown in *Illustration 6*. The balloon is tested before use; saline is recommended for balloon distension, but for optimal fluoroscopic control dilute contrast medium can be used.

The balloon is fully deflated with a 50-ml syringe before passage. Removal of the rubber valve covering the endoscope biopsy channel can facilitate easier insertion of the larger balloons. Silicone spray is applied to a cytology brush which is passed through the biopsy channel along its entire length to assist balloon passage. Silicone spray is also applied to the balloon. The balloon is then inserted in the biopsy channel like other instruments, with short quick movements.

Under endoscopic vision the balloon is placed through the stricture. It is then inflated with a hand-held syringe while observing the pressure in the balloon with the monitor. Maximum indicated balloon pressure is reached or exceeded briefly while the balloon is inflated. Briefly exceeding the rated pressure during inflation will not burst the balloon. The pressure is maintained for approximately 1 min; if inflation to the indicated balloon pressure becomes difficult and the patient is uncomfortable, the stopcock is closed and pressure is maintained below the maximum recom-

mended for total inflation. Dilatation can be achieved before reaching the recommended maximum pressure. If fluoroscopic monitoring is used, an hourglass deformity of the balloon is seen until the balloon is fully inflated. If the balloon does not pass through the stricture, a small portion of the balloon can be passed into the stricture; it is then inflated to dilate the stricture proximally. By deflating the balloon and then advancing farther into the stricture, it is possible to dilate all of the stricture.

Before withdrawing the balloon, it must be fully deflated and all fluid removed using a 50-ml syringe. It is possible to visualize this deflation with the endoscope. No part of the balloon should be in the biopsy channel while it is being deflated. As the balloon is being withdrawn, suction is maintained to assist withdrawal and protect against balloon damage. If contrast medium is used to inflate the balloon, this must be washed out with water soon after withdrawal.

It is possible to use larger balloons until the patient experiences pain. To dilate beyond 54 Fr, Maloney dilators can be passed up to 60 Fr.

Postoperative care

If sedation is not used, the patient can be discharged following the procedure. The patient should be told to seek medical advice if chest or back pain or fever is experienced or if there is evidence of bleeding. Drinks of water are avoided until the topical anaesthetic has worn off and there is no evidence to suggest perforation. If intravenous sedation has been used, the patient should be observed for 2–4 h before discharge, depending on the difficulty of the procedure and the age of the patient. If oxygen is required during the procedure because of sedation, it may also be necessary following the procedure until sedation wears off.

Preoperative and postoperative management of patients undergoing major upper gastrointestinal surgery

Glyn G. Jamieson FRACS, FACS
Dorothy Mortlock Professor of Surgery, University of Adelaide, Department of Surgery, Royal Adelaide Hospital, Adelaide, Australia

Haile T. Debas MD
M. Galante Distinguished Professor of Surgery and Dean of the School of Medicine, University of California, San Francisco, California, USA

Modern surgery of the gastrointestinal tract is a very safe procedure in patients who are healthy, apart from the specific problem for which they are having their operation. Furthermore, whether a patient is generally fit can usually be ascertained simply from the history. Thus, regardless of age, if patients live an independent existence, do their own shopping and gardening and can walk up several flights of stairs without difficulty, the likelihood of a battery of preoperative tests turning up some abnormality critical to the outcome of an operation is remote.

However, because any major surgery can lead to problems where it may be helpful to know what the preoperative situation was, it is usual to carry out simple investigations in all such patients before surgery. These include determining the patient's blood group and haemoglobin level, obtaining a chest radiograph and, in older patients, an electrocardiogram, and general examination of renal function by measuring the blood creatinine level.

There are other tests which are appropriate to specific operations and these are considered below.

Oesophageal surgery

Preoperative

Diagnosis and operative planning

Today most patients have already had an endoscopy and biopsy by the time they present to the surgeon. If the diagnosis has been made from barium contrast studies, then endoscopy and biopsy should be carried out before surgery. If contrast studies have not been undertaken, they should be carried out as they are helpful in operative planning, giving an anatomical record for observation.

Before surgery all patients should undergo computed tomography to look for both lung and liver metastases, either of which might greatly alter a planned operative approach. Computed tomography may also give information about tumour size and its degree of invasiveness, although the latter is not a sufficiently reliable assessment upon which to base decisions about the operability of a tumour.

If a cervical operation is planned some surgeons advocate an assessment of vocal cord funtion before operation.

It is worth emphasizing at the outset that age is not a significant factor in oesophageal surgery: the major determinants of outcome are the patient's cardiovascular and respiratory fitness.

Cardiovascular fitness

An electrocardiogram is useful for showing any disturbances of cardiac rhythm and sometimes also to reflect past ischaemic events. An exercise electrocardiogram or stress test may uncover incipient ischaemia but the authors prefer to use the cardiac ejection fraction determined by a gated blood flow scan as a means of determining cardiac health. If the ejection fraction is less than 40% this is regarded as a significant risk factor for surgery, and in general terms is a contraindication to a major procedure.

Respiratory fitness

All patients should have an assessment of their lung function and blood gases. Values which should raise concern about a patient's ability to withstand major surgery are: (1) forced expiratory volume of gas less then 1 litre, (2) a vital capacity less that 70% of normal; and/or (3) an arterial oxygen tension of less than 70 mmHg. In patients with marginal lung function it is sometimes best to perform a tracheostomy at the same time as upper gastrointestinal surgery for optimal access to the patient's airways.

Nutrition

Patients with oesophageal cancer are often in a poor nutritional state. The measurement of serum albumin is a relatively crude test of the nutritional state but, taken with the patient's dietary history and evidence of weight loss, it is probably as accurate a measure as is available. Prolonged intravenous feeding is not indicated because any gains in terms of nutrition are usually lost by the complications from the intravenous line. Nevertheless it does seem sensible to commence nutritional support in such patients in the week before surgery and this can be done by a fine nasoenteric tube, an elemental diet or a feeding jejunostomy. The last technique may be used more often in the future with the development of laparoscopic jejunostomy.

Preoperative and perioperative therapy

Neomycin, 200 ml as a 1% solution, is given to the patient orally several hours before surgery in order to reduce oral and oesophageal flora. A broad-spectrum cephalosporin is also given intravenously immediately before surgery. This drug can be continued for 24 h but is then discontinued and subsequent antibiotics are given for specific indications only.

If a non-thoracotomy oesphagectomy is planned it is useful to digitalize the patient the day before surgery as there is a high incidence of cardiac arrhythmias when the surgeon's hands are dissecting behind the heart. Digitalis helps prevent such arrhythmias.

Antithrombotic measures such as intermittent calf compression should always be used, and some surgeons also use minidose subcutaneous heparin.

After the induction of anaesthesia various tubes are passed and monitors and lines established such as nasogastric tube, urinary catheter, intravenous lines, central venous lines and pulse oximetry for measuring oxygen saturation, intra-arterial line for monitoring blood pressure, epidural catheter for pain relief.

Postoperative care

There are few, if any, scientific studies examining the best way of caring for patients after major oesophageal surgery. Surgeons tend to develop their own beliefs, based on their own and others' experience, and sometimes hold to these beliefs as though they are established fact rather than surgical lore. The authors present here an approach which they believe is cautious and has proved effective.

The aim is always to extubate patients as soon as possible after surgery, and preferably while still in the operating theatre. The use of epidural anaesthesia has been very beneficial for pain relief, allowing early extubation. A chest radiograph is taken in the recovery area immediately after the operation, both to check the position of chest drains and particularly to make sure that there has been full lung expansion and that there is no pneumothorax.

Most patients spend their first few days in an intensive care or intensive nursing ward, during which time the patient's haemodynamic and respiratory status is carefully monitored and intensive chest physiotherapy is begun.

The epidural catheter is left in for as long as possible, and the urinary catheter for a further 24 h after the epidural catheter is removed (often on the third or fourth day after surgery).

It is unlikely that a nasogastric tube plays any useful role in these patients but, being creatures of habit and tradition, the authors still tend to leave it in for a few days after operation. It is usually removed some time after the third day.

Chest drains

Two chest drains are left, one anteriorly to remove air and one posteriorly to the region of the anastomosis (if in the chest) to drain blood and pleural fluid. The anterior drain may be clipped after 24 h and removed after a further 24 h. The posterior drain is left until after oral feeding is established, some time in the second week after surgery. Patients should be nursed in the semiupright position to help prevent gastro-oesophageal regurgitation.

Feeding

A feeding jejunostomy catheter is inserted in all patients and means that there is no urgency at all to recommence oral feeding.

Jejunostomy feeds are usually begun (initially with normal saline) on the third day after the operation and full-scale feeding is introduced slowly over the following week.

Patients are allowed to suck ice chips from the first night of their operation but are not given anything else by mouth until after a water-soluble contrast swallow examination has demonstrated anastomotic integrity. This investigation is carried out between the eighth and tenth days after surgery.

Patients then advance slowly through a liquid, to a sloppy to a soft diet. It is worth emphasizing that a normal contrast study 8 days after the operation does not mean that a leak may not become evident at a later time. Such an occurrence is, however, unusual.

Specific postoperative complications

Lung complications such as pneumonia and more severe problems such as adult respiratory distress syndrome may occur after major oesophageal operations and should be treated by antibiotics and respiratory support, as is appropriate (often prolonged ventilation with adult respiratory distress syndrome).

Bleeding from a small mediastinal vessel sometimes occurs in the immediate postoperative period. Frustratingly, even when bleeding is substantial much of the blood does not come out in a chest drain. If haemodynamic stability is easily maintained with fluids, and perhaps one or two units of blood, bleeding usually ceases. If there is haemodynamic instability, reoperation is indicated. With the 'in-between cases' it is often best to return the patient to the operating room, evacuate accumulated clotted blood and deal with any bleeding points (sometimes none are found).

Anastomotic leakage

Anastomotic leakage should never occur in the first few days after surgery as there is really no excuse for the surgeon not ensuring that the anastomosis is 'water tight' at the end of the procedure, as described in the chapters on pp. 84–87 and 108–119.

Leakage occurs when a portion of the anastomosis not only fails to heal but is actually ischaemic and the ensuing necrotic portion of the wall loses its integrity. This process takes several days to develop but is usually evident by the end of the first week. When leakage occurs it may be associated with one of two courses.

Subclinical leak
Sometimes a patient makes steady progress and when the contrast study is performed, about 8 days after surgery, a leak is revealed. If this is a minor leak, i.e. is not associated with a collection of fluid, then no action is taken other than to continue jejunal feeding and maintain ice chips only by mouth. Some surgeons allow fluids by mouth under these circumstances but it seems prudent to limit oesophageal and gastric motility as much as possible to promote healing of the defect. A contrast study is peformed again 5–7 days later, by which time most of these minor leaks will have healed.

If the leak is major, i.e. is associated with contrast medium passing into a fluid collection, then the only difference is that the help of radiological colleagues is sought in order to place a percutaneous drain into the collection. This not only drains the collection but establishes an external fistula, which is an important principle of treatment in leakage from any anastomosis.

Continuing leakage can be monitored partly by the nature of the fluid which is draining (saliva is usually easily recognized) and, if in doubt, a dye or brightly coloured cordial can be drunk to see if egress occurs. When the fistula is thought to have closed it should be checked by another contrast swallow before commencing oral intake.

Clinically evident leakage
'Clinically evident' is something of a catch-all phrase. It should be a maxim for the oesophageal surgeon that whenever a patient is not doing well, whatever the expression of the clinical decline (i.e. respiratory, cardiac, renal failure or combinations of system failure) a leak from the anastomosis should be considered as the primary cause until it is proved otherwise by a contrast swallow.

If a leak is found under these circumstances then percutaneous drainage should be established if possible. If this leads to stabilization and then improvement of the patient, as is usually the case, continued conservative management is pursued. Oral feeding is commenced only after a contrast study has demonstrated that the anastomosis has healed.

On the other hand, if sepsis is uncontrolled in spite of percutaneous drainage and the patient continues to deteriorate, a further operation is undertaken. It is important not to wait too long for this step, no longer then 48 h after insertion of percutaneous drainage for clear signs of improvement. If it does not occur, the patient is returned to the operating theatre. At this time it may occasionally be enough to drain any collection and establish adequate drainage of the anastomosis. On the other hand, it is often the surgeon's last shot at rectifying a disaster and it is therefore usually best to treat the situation as one would a patient presenting late with Boerhaave's syndrome, as described in the chapter on pp. 244–255, with drainage and oesophageal exclusion.

Thoracic duct injury

Injury to the thoracic duct usually becomes manifest when nutritional feeding commences on about the fourth or fifth day after operation. There is a fairly rapid increase in drain losses or in fluid accumulation in the chest. Once suspected, it can be verified by ceasing the jejunal feeds and the fluid loss usually diminishes greatly. Most surgeons undertake a trial of conservative management, which essentially means replacing the enteral with parenteral nutrition for 7–14 days. Occasionally a fistula will close spontaneously, which is why a trial is worthwhile, but usually operative closure of the fistula is required. At operation the use of a dry field and a sharp pair of eyes (which usually means the surgical resident!) is often all that is required to find the chylous leak point. It should be sutured closed without trying to dissect the thoracic duct free. The tissue in the region of the aortic hiatus, excluding the aorta, can also be ligated in continuity as an added means of ligating the thoracic duct.

If difficulty is encountered in finding the chylous leak, Intralipid is instilled into the jejunostomy and the chyle then turns milky, aiding identification of the point of leakage.

A chylous fistula in the neck is seen very infrequently, or perhaps more accurately nearly always resolves spontaneously, and so possibly it occurs more often than is recognized.

Recurrent laryngeal nerve injury

Whenever the cervical oesophagus is mobilized there is the potential for damage to the recurrent laryngeal nerves. This is best avoided by keeping dissection close to the oesophageal wall and using gentle retraction only of the trachea and thyroid gland. In spite of this, between 10% and 20% of patients develop some degree of temporary hoarseness after surgery. Permanent hoarseness occurs in only a very small percentage of patients.

Avulsion of the left recurrent nerve during blunt oesophagectomy is best avoided by allowing the cervical operator to define the plane of separation for the oesophagus down past the aortic arch.

If unilateral vocal cord paralysis proves to be a clinical problem in the postoperative period, injection of the cord with an absorbable material such as Gelfoam can be undertaken.

Gastric surgery

Preoperative

The preoperative management of patients undergoing elective gastric surgery is generally simple. This is particularly true in those operations in which the gastrointestinal tract is not entered, such as Nissen fundoplication and proximal gastric vagotomy. More complex preoperative management is required in the more major operations, particularly when preoperative derangement in nutrition, volume, electrolyte or acid–base status has occurred.

Elective duodenal ulcer surgery

The diagnosis is established from the history, endoscopy and/or upper gastrointestinal contrast studies. When the ulcer is in the stomach malignancy must be excluded with multiple biopsies and brush cytology. Gastric acid secretory studies are unnecessary in most patients because the results have little influence on the selection of operative technique. Two settings in which gastric acid secretory studies are useful include the patient with a recurrent ulcer after a previous ulcer operation and the patient in whom the diagnosis of gastrinoma is strongly suspected but unproven by the secretin test. In the former situation a modified sham feeding test or the measurement of basal acid secretion may provide strong evidence for incomplete vagotomy. In the latter, the demonstration that basal acid output is equal to or exceeds 60% of the maximal acid response to pentagastrin or histamine provides strong confirmatory evidence for the diagnosis of gastrinoma or Zollinger–Ellison syndrome.

Preoperative assessment of the patient being prepared for ulcer surgery is similar to that of any patient undergoing abdominal surgery. Little is required beyond the routine urine and blood tests and assessment of cardiac and renal function, unless an underlying illness necessitates a fuller evaluation. Patients on long-term H_2-receptor antagonist therapy or on omeprazole develop hypochlorhydria or achlorhydria and may have bacterial colonization of the stomach. Such patients have been shown to develop an increased incidence of wound infection after surgery. It is the authors' practice, therefore, to discontinue H_2-receptor antagonist therapy 48 h and omeprazole 5–7 days before surgery. Sequential compression boots are used during the operation in all obese patients and in those over 50 years of age. Low-dose heparin therapy is reserved for patients with a previous history of deep vein thrombosis or pulmonary embolism. A single dose of first or second generation cephalosporin is administered intravenously on transfer to the operating theatre. Some people consider this practice unnecessary in patients with duodenal ulcer, who are generally hypersecretors of acid. Others give prophylactic antibiotics for 24 h. A nasogastric tube is usually placed after the patient has been anaesthetized.

Urgent and emergency ulcer surgery

Complications of peptic ulcer may require urgent or emergency operations. Urgent operation may be required in the patient with gastric outlet obstruction. Preoperative management is directed at preventing aspiration, improving any underlying malnutrition, and correcting any abnormality of extracellular volume, electrolyte or acid–base balance. Nasogastric aspiration is instituted. Some advocate prolonged nasogastric suction in the hope that gastric tone will return before the operation. The value of this practice has not been proven. Treatment with H_2-receptor antagonists or omeprazole will reduce acid secretion and hence limit further fluid loss. Correction of extracellular volume deficit and of hypokalaemic, hypochlorhydric, metabolic alkalosis is generally accomplished by the administration of saline containing potassium chloride. It is exceedingly rare that administration of dilute hydrochloric acid or a solution of ammonium chloride will be required. Ammonium chloride should not be used in the presence of any liver disease. Unless very severe nutritional deficit exists, it is preferable not to institute total parenteral nutrition. Rather, a feeding jejunostomy may be placed at operation so that enteral feeding may be started early after surgery. The stomach is lavaged with saline the night before surgery. After the final wash, 1% neomycin, 200 ml, is inserted into the stomach and the nasogastric tube is clamped. Perioperative parenteral antibiotic therapy is important in patients with gastric outlet obstruction. Postoperative wound infection is significantly reduced with this regimen of antibiotic therapy.

In patients with a perforated ulcer, the essence of preoperative management is to make a prompt diagnosis, institute nasogastric suction and perform early abdominal exploration. It is best to use triple antibiotic intravenous therapy (ampicillin, aminoglycoside and metronidazole) because it is not always entirely clear which viscus has perforated.

The preoperative management of a patient with a bleeding ulcer is that of volume resuscitation with crystalloids and blood. Perioperative antibiotics have been shown to reduce wound infection significantly in patients with a bleeding ulcer.

Gastric malignancy

Once the diagnosis is established by biopsy, the surgeon needs to know the exact proximal extent of the tumour and whether it has metastasized to the liver and regional lymph nodes. The first goal is achieved by the surgeon personally performing or being present at the endoscopy. The second goal is best accomplished with computed tomography of the abdomen to look for hepatic or lymph node metastases. If the patient is nutritionally depleted, enteral nutritional supplement either orally or via nasogastric or nasoduodenal tube is preferable to total parenteral nutrition. Rarely is the latter form of nutritional support used because of the length of time required and the complications attending the procedure. More than 50% of patients with carcinoma of the stomach have hypochlorhydria or achlorhydria. As a result, the stomach tends to be colonized with bacteria and postoperative wound infection is high. In addition, at operation the surgeon may discover unsuspected invasion of the transverse mesocolon, necessitating colon resection. For all these reasons the patient with gastric cancer should undergo

full mechanical and bacteriological preoperative preparation. Mechanical bowel preparation is best achieved with an isosmotic electrolyte solution or magnesium sulphate and enemas. Bacteriological preparation of the bowel is accomplished with a combination of oral neomycin and erythromycin base. Prophylaxis against thromboembolic disease is particularly important in patients with gastric malignancy because they may have a hypercoagulable state.

Postoperative care

Routine postoperative management in gastric surgery is also simple. The major issues revolve around prevention of respiratory complications, management of the nasogastric tube and the timing of oral intake. The general approach to respiratory care in the patient who has undergone surgery has been discussed earlier. The management of the nasogastric tube appears to follow no scientific guidelines and is largely the surgeon's choice. In general, it may be removed 24 h after antireflux operations and by the third day after proximal gastric vagotomy. After vagotomy and drainage or after gastric resection, the tendency is to keep the nasogastric tube in longer. It is generally removed after gastrointestinal function has returned, the 24-h volume of suction is less than 1000 ml, the patient can tolerate two successive 4-h periods of clamping of the nasogastric tube without nausea or fullness, and the residual volume is less than 200–300 ml. Clear fluids are started as soon as gastrointestinal function returns, as evidenced by the passage of flatus or faeces. The diet can then be advanced rapidly to full fluid, soft and normal diet.

After Nissen fundoplication, patients will feel full after a small amount of food and it is therefore preferable to give them six small meals a day for the first few weeks. Patients who have had gastric resection or vagotomy with drainage are susceptible to the dumping syndrome. They should therefore be instructed, at least for the early postoperative period, to take six small meals a day, to take their meals dry, to lie down for 20–30 min after the meal and drink their fluids after that. They should also avoid a high carbohydrate diet. All these patients should be told they may experience diarrhoea but that it is generally short-lived.

Delayed gastric emptying requiring prolonged nasogastric suction may occur after surgery for at least three reasons: a mechanical problem at the suture line such as a haematoma, small leak, too narrow an anastomosis; the development of postoperative pancreatitis; or gastric neurogenic or myogenic abnormality. The stomach should empty well within 4–6 days of a gastric operation. If there is failure of gastric emptying beyond this, the serum amylase should be measured to rule out pancreatitis. If the problem persists to 10 days, a water-soluble contrast study should be undertaken. The study will define the presence of any mechanical problem. If the problem persists for 14 days or longer, a careful endoscopic examination should be performed. Suture-line haematoma and oedema will resolve with time. A technical problem may require surgical revision at some time. If the anastomosis is widely patent and there has been no preoperative atony, computed tomography of the abdomen should be performed to rule out pancreatitis.

A special problem is posed by some patients who have had gastric atony secondary to long-standing gastric outlet obstruction. Such patients, especially if they have also undergone truncal vagotomy, may develop delayed gastric emptying which may sometimes persist for weeks. Such patients rarely respond to prokinetic agents such as metoclopramide. The surgeon must anticipate and prepare for this complication by performing a gastrostomy, if possible, and a feeding jejunostomy. If this is done, the patient can be discharged home in reasonable time and resolution of the problem can be awaited patiently.

Illustrations by Diane Bruyninckx

Technique of cervical approach to the oesophagus

T. Lerut MD, PhD, FACS
Department of General Thoracic Surgery, Catholic University Leuven, U.Z. Gasthuisberg, Leuven, Belgium

The cervical oesophagus can be approached from the right or left sides and there is little to choose between the two sides. The left side is the more common approach, however, as the oesophagus lies a little to the left of the midline in the neck.

Operation

Position of patient

1 The patient is placed supine. General anaesthesia using endotracheal intubation is usually performed. The shoulders are elevated to produce slight hyper-extension of the neck, the head is turned to the right and exposure is accomplished from the left. A right-sided approach is indicated occasionally.

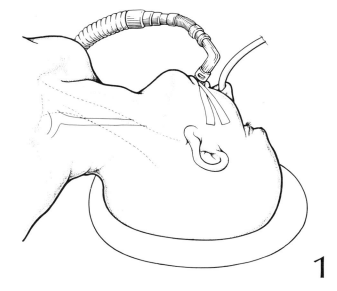

1

Incision

2 The skin is incised along the anterior margin of the sternocleidomastoid muscle approximately on the line connecting the manubrial notch and the angle of the mandible.

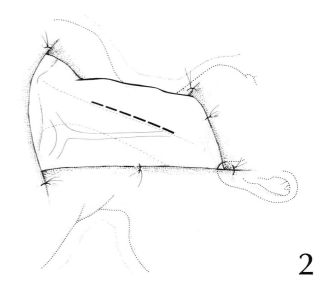

2

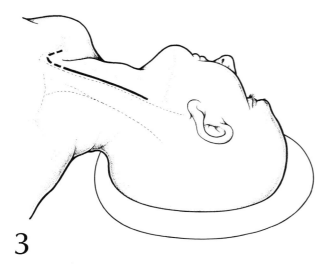

3 For deep lesions an additional J extension of the skin incision above the manubrium sternum is helpful.

3

4 For cosmetic reasons, some authors prefer a more horizontal skin incision, as this may be placed in an even line with one of the skin wrinkles.

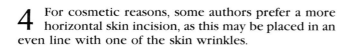
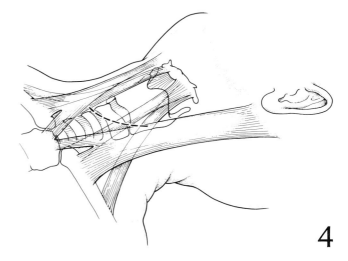

4

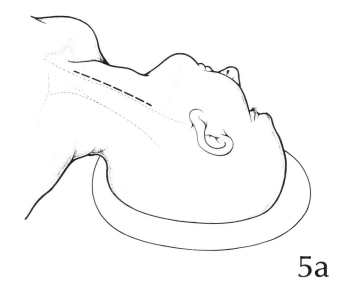

5a

5a, b The incision is deepened through the platysma muscle and superficial cervical fascia until the fibres of the left sternocleidomastoid muscle are visualized.

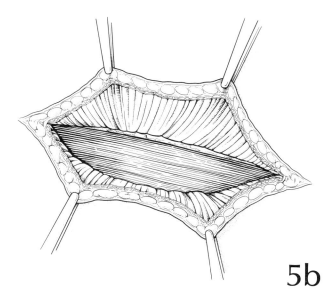

5b

6 The fascia along the anterior border of the sternocleidomastoid muscle is next incised so that the muscle can be mobilized and retracted laterally, allowing exposure and visualization of the carotid sheath containing the jugular vein and the carotid artery. The superior belly of the omohyoid muscle is seen crossing the field from superomedial to lateral. More caudally, the sternothyroid and sternohyoid muscles can be seen.

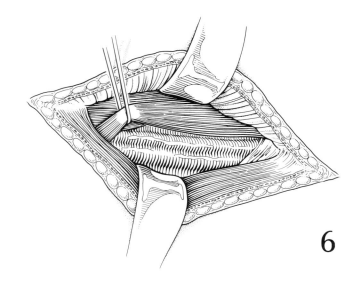

6

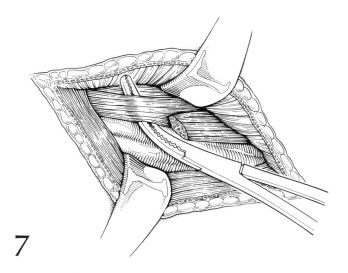

7

7 To reach a more caudally located lesion the operative field can be enlarged by dividing the omohyoid, sternothyroid and sternohyoid muscles with electrocautery.

8 The pretracheal fascial layer of the cervical fascia is incised, exposing the thyroid gland and the contents of the carotid sheath: the internal jugular vein, the common carotid artery and the vagus nerve. The middle thyroid vein is ligated and divided.

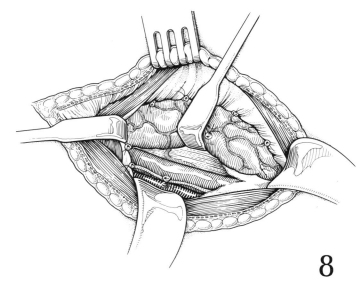

8

9 These structures are retracted laterally, taking care not to squeeze the carotid artery especially in elderly patients. In the cranial part of the operative field it is usually necessary to divide and ligate a tributary vein from the facial region.

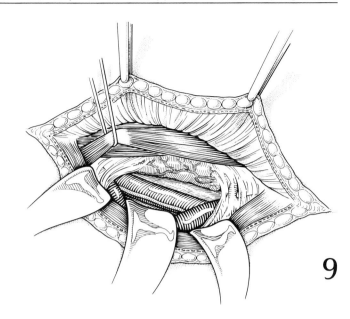

9

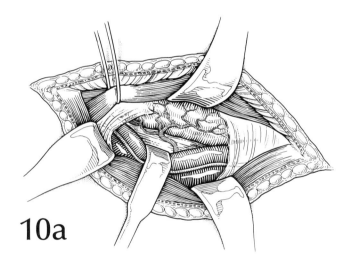

10a

10a, b With the omohyoid and sternothyroid muscles retracted caudally (or sectioned), and the sternocleidomastoid muscle and carotid vessels retracted laterally, the posterolateral aspect of the thyroid gland becomes exposed more clearly. The inferior thyroid artery, a branch of the thyrocervical trunk of the subclavian artery, crosses horizontally beneath the carotid artery. This artery is a useful landmark for identification of the recurrent laryngeal nerve which lies behind the vessel.

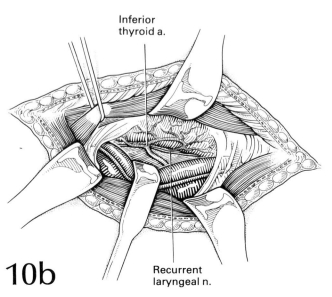

Inferior
thyroid a.

10b

Recurrent
laryngeal n.

11 After double ligation and division of the inferior thyroid artery, the prevertebral cervical fascia is reached. The thyroid is retracted medially to expose the cervical oesophagus, the cricopharyngeal region and the hypopharynx. Great care is taken to locate the recurrent laryngeal nerve to prevent damage caused during retraction.

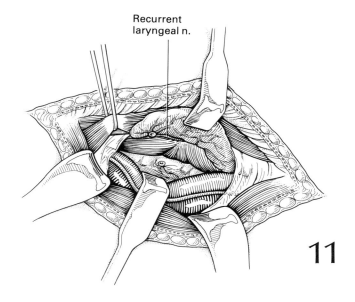

Recurrent laryngeal n.

11

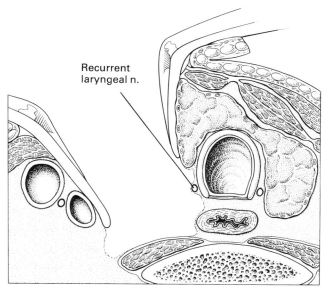

Recurrent laryngeal n.

12a

12a, b The cervical oesophagus is dissected from the pars membranacea of the trachea and encircled by a traction loop, thus exposing the liberated segment. Again, any damage to the recurrent laryngeal nerve is carefully avoided. The cricopharyngeus sometimes causes an indentation at the distal part of the pharynx.

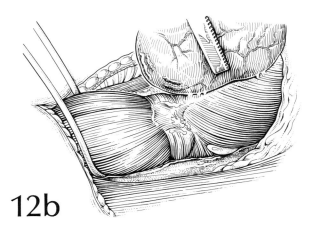

12b

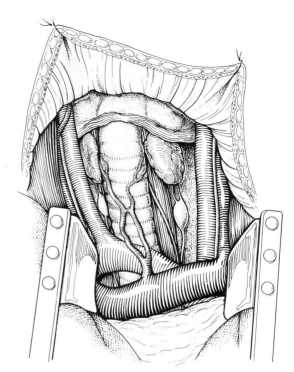

13 If exposure is inadequate the incision can be lengthened by performing a partial proximal sternotomy, exposing the trachea and oesophagus more distally.

13

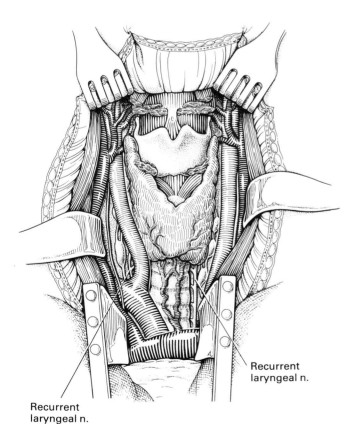

Recurrent laryngeal n.

Recurrent laryngeal n.

14

14 Such an extension is required in the case of carcinoma of the oesophagus if an aggressive lymph node dissection of the neck is undertaken. After completion of the thoracic part of the operation, the patient is turned to the supine position. The neck is hyperextended and a U-shaped incision performed. After incision of the platysma muscle, the anterior border of the sternocleidomastoid muscle is incised at both sides, allowing mobilization and lateral retraction of this muscle. The further steps in the dissection are identical to those already described above.

Omohyoid, sternothyroid and sternohyoid muscles are identified and sectioned on both sides. This allows adequate exposure for cervical paratracheal lymph node dissection. Partial proximal median sternotomy, however, greatly improves further exposure of the brachiocephalic trunk at the right side, and subclavian and carotid arteries at the left side. This approach facilitates the delicate lymph node dissection around both recurrent nerves, giving further access into the proximal part of the chest and its paratracheal lymph node chains at the same time.

Abdominal–right thoracic approach to oesophagectomy

S. C. S. Chung MD, FRCS(Ed), MRCP
Reader in Surgery, Department of Surgery, Prince of Wales Hospital, The Chinese University of Hong Kong, Shatin, Hong Kong

A. K. C. Li MA, MD, FRCS, FRCS(Ed), FRACS, FACS
Professor and Chairman, Department of Surgery, Prince of Wales Hospital, The Chinese University of Hong Kong, Shatin, Hong Kong

Principles and justification

The abdominal–right chest approach is the procedure of choice in the authors' unit for patients with growths of the middle and lower third of the oesophagus. A right thoracotomy gives the best exposure for the extirpation of the oesophagus, and the mobilized isoperistaltic stomach is used to restore digestive tract continuity. After adequate mobilization, the fundus of the stomach can reach as high as the palate. Because of its rich blood supply the stomach is the most reliable organ for oesophageal substitution. It carries the lowest rate of necrosis and anastomotic leakage. Compared with colonic interposition, stomach pull-up is a much simpler operation as only one anastomosis is necessary.

The operation is undertaken with two surgical teams working simultaneously, with the patient in the semilateral position; the thoracic team removes the oesophagus while the abdominal team mobilizes the stomach. In this way there is no need to reposition the patient half way through the operation. With the chest and abdomen open at the same time it is possible to ascertain that stomach mobilization has been adequate to allow a tension-free anastomosis before closing the abdomen. With two teams operating synchronously there is a saving of at least 1 hour in operating time. The surgical team is less fatigued and the incidence of postoperative chest complications may be decreased.

Preoperative

Anaesthesia

The patient is intubated with a left-sided double lumen Robertshaw endotracheal tube. After the right chest has been entered one limb of the Robertshaw tube is clamped to collapse the right lung, improving exposure of the oesophagus. Supplementary epidural anaesthesia allows a lighter general anaesthesia and reduces blood loss by lowering the blood pressure. The epidural catheter can also be used for pain control after the operation. Central venous pressure monitoring is essential for accurate fluid replacement during and after the operation. Invasive blood pressure monitoring by arterial line is advisable because manipulation in the mediastinum may obstruct venous return and lead to wide fluctuations in blood pressure.

Operations

The details of oesophageal resection and reconstruction are described in the chapter on pp. 178–188. The surgical approach to right thoracotomy–laparotomy is described here. In the two-team synchronous approach, surgical exposure may be somewhat compromised. Manoeuvres which facilitate the operation are also mentioned.

1 The patient is positioned in the semilateral position with the right side up. This position is maintained by the use of sandbags behind the patient's shoulders and buttocks. Additional anchorage is provided by an Elastoplast bandage which is taped from under the operating table, over the patient's right shoulder and arm and onto the right arm support of the operating table. The thoracic team stands on the patient's right while the abdominal team stands on the patient's left side.

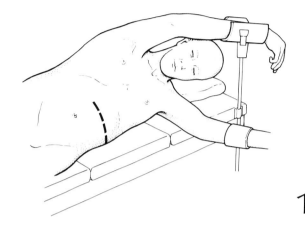

1

ABDOMINAL OPERATION

The abdomen is opened through a left subcostal incision extending across the midline (*Illustration 1*). Compared with a midline incision, a left subcostal incision allows better access to the short gastric vessels. A laparotomy is performed, paying particular attention to the presence of liver secondaries and enlarged lymph nodes around the hiatus. The thoracic team opens the chest if no contraindications to proceed are found by the abdominal surgeon.

The stomach is now mobilized, with preservation of the gastroepiploic and right gastric arcades. The technical details of stomach mobilization are described in the chapter on pp. 178–188. As the patient is in the semilateral position, the viscera fall to the left. Incision of the peritoneal attachments of the second part of the duodenum and extensive Kocherization of the duodenum are facilitated. Surgical access to the short gastric vessels may be somewhat limited with the patient in the semilateral position as the stomach tends to fall towards the left side. Great care should be taken not to put excessive traction on the short gastric vessels during their division as this may lead to avulsion or tearing of the spleen.

The abdomen is closed after the stomach has been pulled up into the chest and the thoracic operator is satisfied that an anastomosis can be performed without tension. Drains are not routinely used.

THORACIC OPERATION

2   When the abdominal operator has confirmed that there are no contraindications for continuation of the operation, the thoracic operator opens the right chest. A long incision skirting the medial border of the scapula is made from the erector spinae muscles to a point just below the right nipple. The serratus anterior and latissimus muscles are divided using diathermy. The division of these muscles is facilitated by developing a plane beneath the muscle and then lifting the muscle between the fingers of the surgeon's hand.

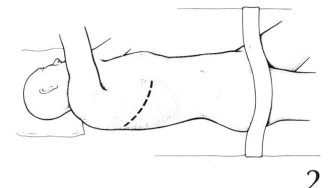

2

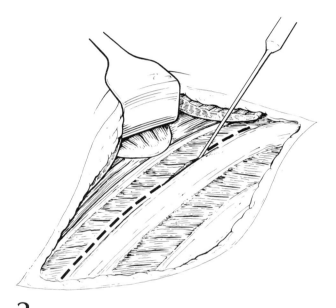

3

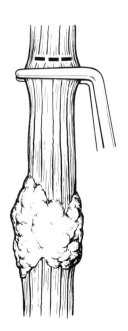

4

3   The scapula is lifted to expose the rib cage. The highest rib that can be palpated is the second, and the fifth rib is identified by counting down. The intercostal muscles and pleura are divided by diathermy, keeping close to the upper border of the fifth rib, and the thoracic cavity is entered. The right lung is collapsed and retracted upwards and medially at this stage, using Allison's lung retractors to expose the posterior mediastinum.

The technique of surgical extirpation of the oesophagus is described in the chapter on pp. 178–188. The entire intrathoracic oesophagus should be excised, and a stapled oesophagogastric anastomosis performed above the level of the clavicle. Some technical tips that make this anastomosis easier and safer are described here.

After the oesophagus and the tumour have been fully mobilized, the stomach is delivered into the chest by traction on the oesophagus. Once the fundus of the stomach is in the thorax, delivery of the stomach should be completed by pulling gently on the greater curvature. A convenient point on the posterior wall of the stomach is chosen for anastomosis. This point should reach the proposed level for anastomosis without any tension.

4   The nasogastric tube (if one has been inserted before operation) is pulled back until its tip lies above the proposed level of oesophageal transection. Downward traction is applied to the oesophagus and a right-angled oesophageal clamp is applied across the oesophagus at the level of the clavicle. If the oesophagus is transected too high, subsequent insertion of the anastomotic gun into the oesophageal stump may be very difficult because of lack of space in the thoracic inlet.

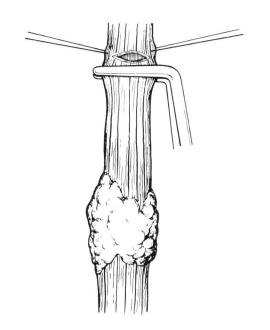

5

5 The anterior half of the oesophagus above the clamp is cut using scissors, exposing the oesophageal lumen. The posterior half of the oesophagus is retained to maintain traction on the oesophagus. Three stay sutures, one at each corner and one anteriorly, are inserted through the whole thickness of the oesophagus. The posterior half of the oesophagus is now divided. A further stay suture is inserted on the posterior wall of the oesophagus.

The key to a successful anastomosis is the accurate placement of the purse-string suture on the oesophageal stump. A 0 polypropylene (Prolene) suture on a round body needle is used and a stapled anastomosis is constructed using the largest diameter anvil that will fit into the oesophageal stump (*see* chapter on pp. 84–87).

The nasogastric tube is positioned in the transposed stomach for decompression in the postoperative period. It may be very difficult to pass a nasogastric tube with the patient in the semilateral position. If a nasogastric tube has been left in the upper oesophagus it is a simple matter to advance it into the stomach. If a fine-bore feeding tube has been used before the operation it is possible to exchange it for an ordinary nasogastric tube by stitching a sterile nasogastric tube to the distal end of the feeding tube and pulling the feeding tube out through the nose.

The opening in the cardia of the stomach is closed with two layers of continuous 2/0 Prolene sutures. The stomach is then placed in the bed of the oesophagus in the posterior mediastinum. Anchoring stitches to fix the stomach into position and manoeuvres to make the anastomosis extrapleural are not necessary.

A final check on haemostasis, with particular attention to the vessels supplying the stomach, is made before closing the chest. Two large-bore chest drains are used, the anterior drain beng placed in the basal position and the posterior drain being placed in the apex of the chest. Intercostal stitches of interrupted 0 Vicryl are employed, followed by layered closure of the muscles using running Vicryl sutures. The skin is closed with interrupted nylon.

Postoperative care

The double-lumen endotracheal tube is exchanged for a single-lumen tube at the end of the operation. The patient is electively ventilated overnight in the intensive care unit. The chest drains are connected to underwater seals. The nasogastric tube is allowed to drain by gravity and is also aspirated hourly. Daily chest radiographs are mandatory until all drains are removed.

Oral feeding is commenced on the fifth day after operation. Contrast studies to exclude anastomotic leaks are not routinely performed before commencing feeding, but this investigation is reserved for cases where there is doubt about the integrity of the anastomosis or if there is clinical suspicion of a leak.

Further reading

Akiyama H, Miyazons H, Tsurumaru M, Hashimoto C, Kawamura T. Use of the stomach as an esophageal substitute. *Ann Surg* 1978; 188: 606–10.

Chung SCS, Griffin SM, Wood SDS, Crofts TJ, Li AKC. Two team synchronous esophagectomy. *Surg Gynecol Obstet* 1990; 170: 68–9.

Wood SDS, McGuire LJ, Chung SCS, Crofts TJ, Li AKC. Intrathoracic stapled anastomosis after oesophagectomy for cancer. *Aust NZ J Surg* 1989; 59: 647–51.

Illustrations by Andrew Bezear

Left posterolateral thoracotomy

H. Matthews FRCS
Consultant Thoracic Surgeon, Regional Department of Thoracic Surgery, East Birmingham Hospital, Birmingham and Professor of Surgery, Department of Biological Sciences, University of Warwick, UK

The exposure described here serves as a general purpose approach to the thoracic oesophagus from the aortic arch to the oesophageal hiatus from the left side. The intercostal incision, however, is made high enough to provide access to the retroaortic and upper thoracic oesophagus if this should be required for mobilization or other reasons. The commonest indications for this approach include the transthoracic correction of gastro-oesophageal reflux, longitudinal oesophageal myotomy for motility disorders, repair of oesophageal perforations or ruptures, excision of oesophageal cysts and duplications and the exploration or resection of oesophageal tumours by oesophagogastrectomy.

Preoperative

General assessment of the patient must include haematological and biochemical tests and assessment of renal and hepatic function. Cardiac status is assessed by chest radiography, electrocardiography and additional tests if indicated. Respiratory assessment requires routine spirometry, with full tests of respiratory function and blood gases if significant abnormalities are found. Smoking must be stopped at least 1 week before operation and all patients instructed by an experienced respiratory physiotherapist in the breathing and coughing techniques that will be required after operation, and in the use of incentive spirometry.

Anaesthesia

After appropriate premedication and induction the patient is intubated with a double-lumen endotracheal tube to permit controlled collapse of the ipsilateral lung during operation. A right-sided Robertshaw tube is generally satisfactory for this purpose, but if it cannot be positioned correctly a right-sided Gordon–Green tube may be preferable. Whichever type of tube is used, its positioning and function must be confirmed after the patient is placed in the lateral position and before the surgical procedure commences. A central venous line is desirable for blood volume control, with radial artery cannulation and pressure monitoring for more complex cases. Prophylactic intravenous or intramuscular antibiotics are given as a single dose soon after induction in order to provide high blood levels during operation.

Operation

Position of patient and incision

1 The patient is positioned lying on the right side with the arm elevated and lying across the front of the face. A superficial incision is then made starting at the anterior end of the sixth intercostal space and extended posteriorly, along the line of the seventh rib, passing 2–3 cm below the point of the scapula, to end at the angle of the rib posteriorly. The subcutaneous fat, superficial fascia and latissimus dorsi muscle are then divided in the line of the skin incision using diathermy.

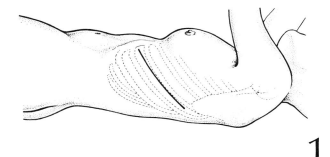

1

2 When this has been done the latissimus dorsi muscle is retracted to expose the anterior serratus. This is not divided in the line of the skin incision. In order to avoid damage to the nerve to the anterior serratus muscle, the muscle is freed along its posterior border and divided 1 cm from its origins on the ribs as shown by the broken line.

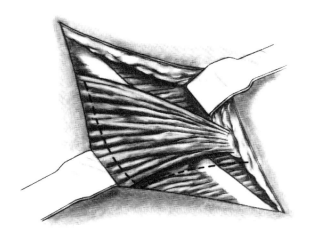

2

Intercostal incision

3 Division of the anterior serratus muscle and posterior connective tissue exposes the full length of the intercostal space and the sixth space is then identified by passing a hand up to the apex of the chest, under the scapula, and counting the intercostal spaces from the first space downwards. When the sixth space has been identified a diathermy incision is made in the intercostal muscles along the upper border of the seventh rib, for the whole length of the intercostal space, so as to leave the periosteum undisturbed. The back end of the seventh rib is then divided with a rib cutter to permit opening of the intercostal space, and a 1 cm length of rib is excised to prevent painful postoperative crepitus. Unless accidentally damaged, the neurovascular bundle to the seventh rib is left undisturbed. The pleura is opened throughout the length of the intercostal space, which is then held open by a self-retaining ratcheted retractor with blades appropriate to the build of the patient.

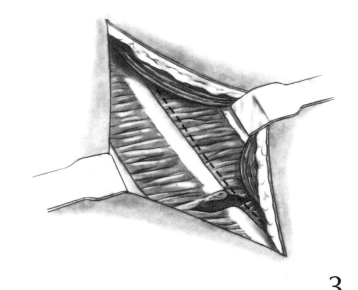

3

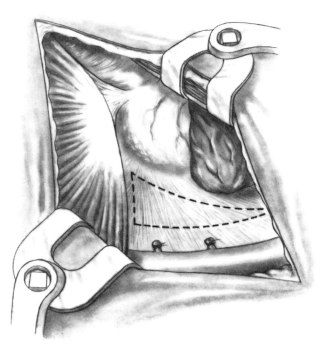

4

Mobilization of the oesophagus

4 Pleural adhesions, if present, are divided and the left lung is then collapsed using the double-lumen endotracheal tube. This exposes the mediastinum from the aortic arch to the hiatus. The pulmonary ligament is divided up to the inferior pulmonary vein and the mediastinal pleura is incised anteriorly in the pleuropericardial angle and posteriorly at the edge of the descending thoracic aorta as shown. These incisions are subsequently extended to meet across the oesophageal hiatus inferiorly and just below the aortic arch superiorly.

5 The oesophagus is mobilized from the mediastinum by blunt dissection of the connective tissue and serial division of the segmental oesophageal branches of the descending thoracic aorta. The oesophagus is encircled with a tape which should include the whole of the oesophageal wall and the vagus nerves, before performance of the definitive part of the operation.

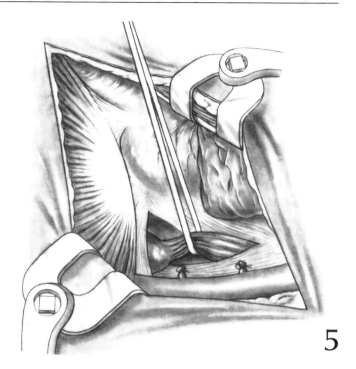

5

Extensions to the abdomen

6 For some purposes it may be necessary to obtain access to the upper abdomen and this can be done in one of four ways as follows:

1. Through the oesophageal hiatus, by division of the pleural and peritoneal covering.
2. By a tangential incision in the central tendon of the diaphragm posteriorly to the phrenic nerve.
3. By a peripheral detachment of the diaphragm about 1 cm from the chest wall in the anterolateral arc.
4. By full thoracolaparotomy, as described in the chapter on pp. 61–69.

Closure of the incision

When the definitive procedure has been completed, haemostasis is achieved and the left lung is reinflated. A small stab incision for the chest drain is made below the skin incision and a deep vertical mattress suture inserted for subsequent closure. A size 32 semi-rigid chest drain with multiple side holes is inserted through the stab incision, positioned well up into the chest, sutured to the skin and connected to an underwater seal.

The chest is then closed in layers using two or three separate strong synthetic absorbable sutures to surround and approximate the sixth and seventh ribs and continuous synthetic absorbable sutures for the muscle and subcutaneous layers. The skin is finally closed with continuous subcuticular synthetic absorbable sutures.

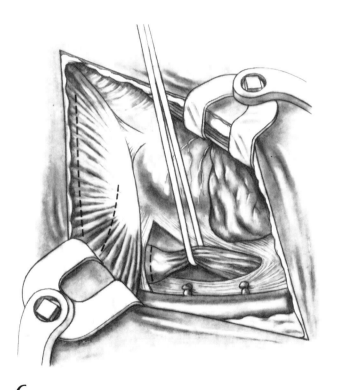

6

Postoperative care

Following operation the patient should be awake, cooperative and breathing spontaneously. Routine cases are admitted to a high-dependency thoracic surgical unit for standard monitoring; only complex cases require intensive care. Postoperative analgesia is by a combination of intravenous low-dose morphine infusion, oral analgesics and analgesic suppositories as indicated by the patient's requirements. Postoperative blood loss is replaced, but intravenous fluid administration is restricted to maintenance requirements of 2 litres of 5% dextrose solution/24 h for an adult, until the patient can resume oral intake. Nasogastric aspiration is not required and oral fluids are commenced from the first postoperative day for patients who have not had oesophageal resection and on the second day for those who have. The chest drain is removed when it has ceased to function, normally between the first and third postoperative day.

Complications

Complications that relate to the exposure are wound infections and wound dehiscence. Wound infection is treated in the standard fashion by drainage, with or without antibiotics as appropriate. Dehiscence should occur very rarely, but if it does it will require formal exploration and resuture, usually with pleural drainage, in order to re-establish integrity of the chest wall.

Late complications may include lung hernia, if the ribs have not been approximated properly, and post-thoracotomy pain. This is an infrequent but serious problem that is poorly understood and difficult to treat. Generally there is no detectable local cause for its occurrence, and further surgical procedures on the wound (e.g. intercostal neurectomy) only serve to make matters worse.

Illustrations by T. Boraine and A. Mannell

Left thoracoabdominal approach for exposure of the oesophagus

Aylwyn Mannell FRACS, FRCS, MS
Specialist Surgeon, Rosebank and Linksfield Park Clinics and Consultant Surgeon, Baragwanath Hospital and University of Witwatersrand, Johannesburg, South Africa

Principles and justification

The left thoracoabdominal approach gives excellent exposure of the cardio-oesophageal junction, the distal thoracic oesophagus and the stomach.

Indications

The indications for this approach include adenocarcinoma of the cardia, squamous carcinoma of the distal oesophagus, connective tissue tumours adjacent to or involving the cardio-oesophageal junction, and gastric cancer involving the proximal half of the stomach.

The left thoracoabdominal approach is also used for the Leigh–Collis gastroplasty, the gastric fundal patch operation described by Thal and for oesophagogastrectomy in the management of early, uncontaminated perforation of the distal oesophagus.

Preoperative

Many patients with obstructing lesions near the cardio-oesophageal junction are in a state of semi-starvation, and preoperative nutritional rehabilitation is extremely important to ensure that wounds and anastomoses will heal. Oral or enteral feeding of a high-calorie, high-protein liquid diet is essential. If necessary, a malignant stricture may be partly dilated to allow passage of a nasogastric tube which, ideally, should be of small calibre and made from Silastic to decrease pharyngeal discomfort which would limit the patient's ability to cough effectively. The patient may also be fed intravenously but gastrostomy or jejunostomy should be avoided. These procedures are associated with a small but real risk of morbidity and mortality and can complicate subsequent major surgery.

Death following oesophagogastrectomy is usually due to pneumonia. Preparation of the patient for surgery is therefore aimed at preventing postoperative pulmonary complications, which are common after thoracotomy. Every effort must be made to improve pulmonary function: the patient must stop smoking and obvious wheezing on auscultation of the lungs is an indication for bronchodilator therapy. Chest physiotherapy is essential to train the patient to cough vigorously and to clear secretions. Incentive spirometry is of great value in preventing and treating atelectasis: training the patient to achieve maximal lung inflation with the incentive spirometer should begin as soon as the decision to operate has been made. Purulent sputum will require appropriate antibiotic treatment based on culture results.

Obvious deficits in hydration, haemoglobin levels and electrolyte balance must be corrected. In patients from countries in which tuberculosis is prevalent active pulmonary tuberculosis must be excluded, and careful assessment of cardiovascular status is required for elderly patients.

Antibiotic prophylaxis

To reduce debris in the oesophagus and stomach, oral or enteral intake should be stopped at least 12 h before surgery. Broad-spectrum parenteral antibiotic prophylaxis is given with the premedication and continued for 24 h after surgery.

Anaesthesia

Deflation of the left lung will improve surgical access for the left thoracoabdominal approach. With the patient supine, a double-lumen endobronchial tube is inserted after induction of anaesthesia and before the patient is positioned for the operation. Careful monitoring of the arterial blood gases is necessary: when the patient is placed in the right lateral position for a left thoracoabdominal procedure the dependent right lung is compressed by the weight of the mediastinum and arterial hypoxaemia, secondary to one-lung anaesthesia, can develop. Arterial hypoxaemia is exacerbated by pre-existing disease in the dependent lung, by significant blood loss and by a long operation. The surgeon must weigh the benefits of improved exposure against the risks of prolonged hypoxaemia and keep the time during which the left lung is deflated to a minimum.

Insertion of nasogastric tube

If not already in place, a nasogastric tube should be inserted after commencement of anaesthesia and before the operation begins. This facilitates rapid intraoperative identification of the intra-abdominal oesophagus and postoperative decompression of the stomach when required. Transanastomotic passage of the nasogastric tube allows enteral feeding to continue in the recovery phase.

Operation

Position of patient

1 The position of the patient on the table determines to a large extent the success of the left thoraco-abdominal approach. A suitable table that can be easily rotated and fitted with chest attachments capable of fixing the patient firmly in position is essential.

The patient's left side is elevated with sandbags under the hip and shoulder to achieve an angle of 60° with the table. The left arm is drawn upwards and forwards, supported by a thoracic arm rest. To fix the patient in this position adhesive strapping is applied across the buttocks to the table and to the left arm in the thoracic arm rest. The operating table is turned to the left side for the abdominal phase and to the right side for the thoracic dissection.

The patient is prepared for abdominal and left thoracic incisions. Application of a clear adhesive drape helps to keep the sterile towels in position during movement of the table.

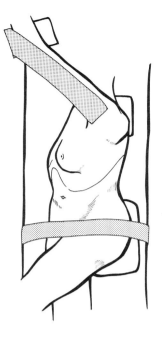

1

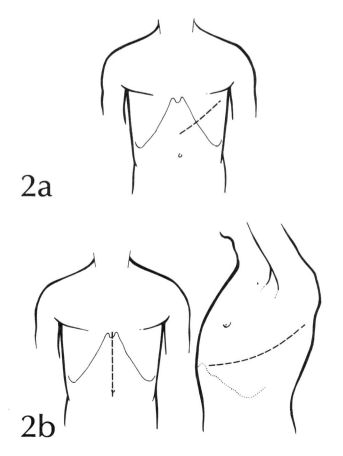

2a

2b

Incision

2a, b Several approaches may be selected. An oblique thoracoabdominal incision begins midway between the xiphisternum and umbilicus, extends across the costal margin over the desired intercostal space or rib and is continued to the inferior angle of the scapula up to the lateral edge of the erector spinae muscle (*Illustration 2a*). This incision is appropriate for the younger patient with good respiratory function.

The midline abdominal incision extends from the xiphisternum to below the umbilicus. The left thoracic incision follows the line of the seventh or eighth rib from the costal margin to the lateral edge of the erector spinae muscle (*Illustration 2b*). These incisions, which preserve the costal margin, are recommended for the frail elderly patient and those with poor respiratory function.

Postoperative instability of the costal margin and extensive incisions into the diaphragm can result in serious impairment of pulmonary mechanics, increasing the risk of postoperative pneumonia.

Exploration of abdomen

Using the oblique incision, the anterior lamina of the rectus sheath over the left rectus muscle is divided. The muscle is transected with electrocautery, the left superior epigastric vessels are ligated and divided and the peritoneum is opened in line with the incision up to the costal margin.

If a separate abdominal midline incision is used the linea alba and parietal peritoneum are divided.

In patients for whom the operation is undertaken for malignancy, a laparotomy is now performed before opening the chest. The liver, general peritoneal cavity and pelvic peritoneum are examined to identify metastatic spread. The coeliac nodes are palpated for evidence of involvement or extracapsular spread. The tumour is examined to assess local infiltration and spread into the diaphragm or stomach. Gross metastatic spread to suprapancreatic, splenic hilar, porta hepatis and para-aortic lymph nodes is excluded.

Thoracic incision

3   If no contraindication to operation is identified the oblique thoracoabdominal incision is continued over the costal margin along the course of the appropriate rib, which is usually the seventh or eighth rib. Serratus anterior and latissimus dorsi muscles are divided with electrocautery along the course of the rib. Bleeding points in the muscles are carefully controlled to limit blood loss.

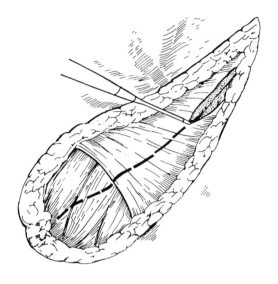

3

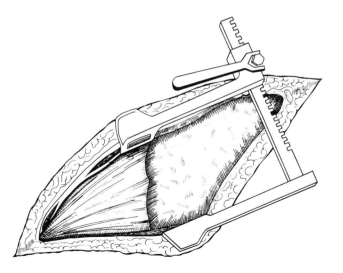

4

Division of intercostal muscles

4   The intercostal muscles are divided along the line of insertion into the superior margin of the rib below, avoiding injury to the intercostal vessels and nerve. This division is continued to the lateral border of the erector spinae muscle. The left lung is allowed to deflate and the pleural cavity opened.

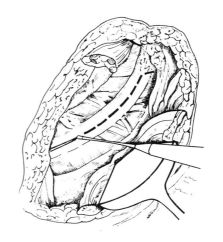

5a

Rib resection

5a–c   If compliance of the chest wall is limited, a rib may be removed and the pleural cavity entered through the bed of that rib. When the rib is exposed, the periosteum is incised with electrocautery and separated from the rib using a periosteal elevator and Doyen's rasparatory. The rib is divided with a costotome and removed from behind the rib angle to its costal end, together with the costal cartilage and a small segment of the costal margin to prevent subsequent overriding on closure of the wound. At this stage, branches of the musculophrenic vessels will require ligation.

5b

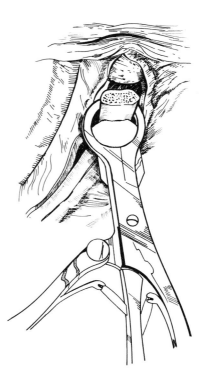

5c

Division of diaphragm

6   The diaphragm is cut from the point of division of the costal margin in line with the phrenic muscle fibres towards the oesophageal hiatus. Haemostasis in the cut edges of the diaphragm is secured by suture ligation, with particular care to ligate the branches of the inferior phrenic vessels near the hiatus. Each leaf of the divided diaphragm is attached to the cut edge of the chest wall muscles with sutures, which improves exposure. A Finochietto retractor is inserted between the ribs and opened widely.

Circumferential incision of the diaphragm may be performed to preserve the phrenic nerve and its branches. After division of the costal margin a Finochietto retractor is inserted to expose the diaphragm, which is then divided circumferentially 3 cm from its insertion into the thoracic margin. The incision should run parallel to the rib cage for about 15 cm.

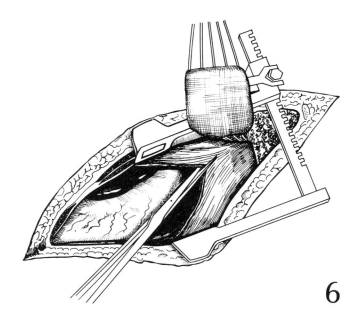

6

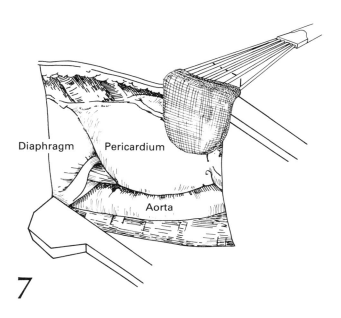

Diaphragm   Pericardium

Aorta

7

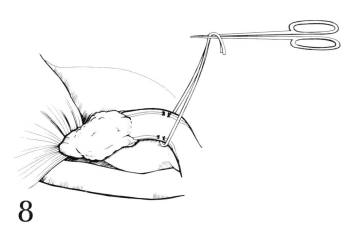

8

Thoracic exploration

7   Any adhesions to the base of the lung should be freed and the inferior part of the pulmonary ligament is divided to facilitate retraction of the lung. The left side of the posterior mediastinum is exposed and, if the operation is being performed for malignancy, it is essential to determine the palpable extent of tumour. The oesophagus must be divided 10 cm above the tumour to ensure complete microscopic clearance. If the upper resection margin is less than 10 cm, the specimen should be submitted to frozen section to confirm that the proximal line of resection is clear of tumour.

Thoracic dissection

8   With the left lung retracted anteromedially, incision of the pulmonary ligament is continued up to the inferior pulmonary vein. The mediastinal pleura overlying the oesophagus is incised and dissected away from the posterior mediastinal contents. The anterior aspect of the aorta is separated from the oesophagus, inferior mediastinal glands, fat and vagus nerves. Small oesophageal arteries arising from the aorta are ligated and divided. Any mediastinal pleura overlying a tumour should be resected with the lesion. Mobilization of the oesophagus is continued to the arch of the aorta; care must be taken to avoid opening the pericardium or injuring the thoracic duct, which may be identified during the dissection. A Jacques catheter is now passed around the mobilized oesophagus for retraction during the next phase of dissection and the vagal trunks are divided above the tumour.

Abdominal dissection

9a–c In cases where the diaphragm has been incised in a radial direction, this is continued into the oesophageal hiatus. However, if a malignant lesion is close to the oesophageal hiatus a cuff of diaphragmatic muscle is removed. The peritoneum on the right aspect of the intra-abdominal oesophagus is incised and the incision continued distally, dividing the lesser omentum close to the liver as far as the gastric antrum. The right gastric vessels should be preserved if gastric reconstruction is planned. The left peritoneal reflection from the intra-abdominal oesophagus is incised, the vagal trunks exposed and divided. For benign lesions and for resection of squamous cancer of the distal oesophagus, where metastases and splenic hilar nodes are found in less than 5% of cases, the gastric fundus is mobilized by ligation and division of the short gastric and left gastroepiploic vessels, close to the splenic hilum. The spleen is carefully preserved to reduce the risk of infective and thromboembolic complications in the postoperative period. With ligation and division of the coronary vein and left gastric artery at its origin from the coeliac axis, mobilization of the distal thoracic and intra-abdominal oesophagus is now complete.

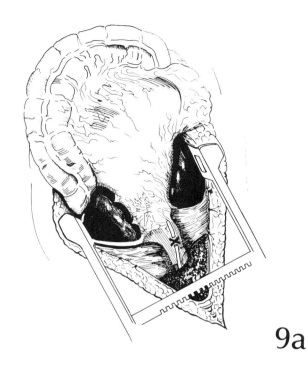

9a

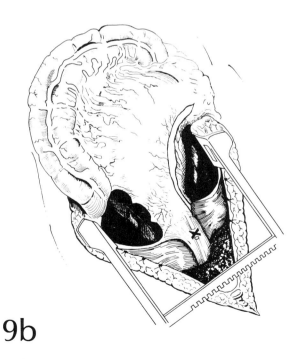

9b

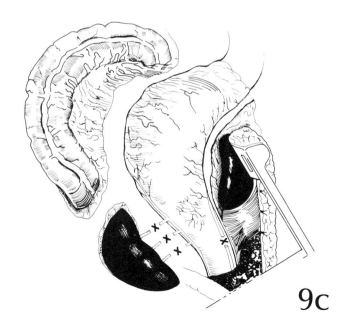

9c

Laparotomy and left thoracotomy

10 If separate abdominal and thoracic incisions have been used, the abdominal dissection should be completed before the abdomen is closed, and the thoracic dissection performed in part through the widened hiatus.

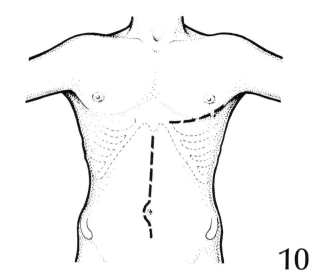

10

Division of left triangular ligaments

11 Following a separate abdominal midline incision the left triangular ligament of the liver is divided and the left lobe retracted to improve access to the cardio-oesophageal area.

Gastric mobilization

The gastrocolic ligament is divided up to the spleen, ligating and dividing the left gastroepiploic vessels and vasa brevia close to the hilum of the spleen. Care must be taken to secure accessory vasa brevia running on the posterior abdominal wall to the gastric fundus. The peritoneal reflection between stomach and diaphragm is divided to complete mobilization of the gastric fundus. This is described in more detail in the chapter on pp. 436–449.

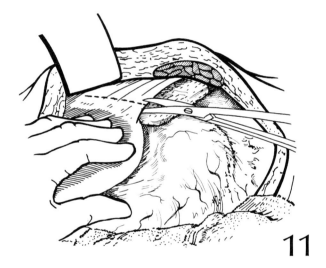

11

Mobilization of cardio-oesophageal junction

The lesser omentum is divided close to the liver, preserving the right gastroepiploic vessels. A branch of the left gastric artery to the left lobe of the liver may need to be ligated and divided. The peritoneum over the intra-abdominal oesophagus is incised and the vagal nerves identified, cauterized and divided. If the operation is performed for a malignancy in the cardio-oesophageal region, the coeliac nodes are gently stripped towards the stomach. The coronary vein and left gastric artery at its origin from the coeliac axis are ligated and divided. A cuff of diaphragmatic muscle may be removed. The left lobe of the liver is retracted and the hiatal musculature is divided, beginning at the left posterior aspect and continuing to the right side. The remainder of the abdominal dissection is determined by the pathology of the lesion and by selection of stomach, jejunum or colon for reconstruction. This procedure is also described in the chapter on pp. 142–153.

Wound closure

Where the thoracoabdominal incision has been used, the diaphragm is now closed with interrupted mattress sutures of 0 Ethibond placed 2 cm from the cut edge. The finished suture line is reinforced with a continuous second layer to reduce the risk of diaphragmatic dehiscence. If the costal margin has been divided, the costal cartilage is repaired with wire sutures. The pleural cavity is irrigated with a warm saline antibiotic solution. Pericostal sutures of 2/0 Ethibond are inserted and an underwater basal drain is led out of the chest in the mid-axillary line. The left lung is allowed to reinflate and the pericostal sutures are tied. The muscles of the chest wall are repaired. The abdominal extension of the thoracoabdominal incision is closed and the skin is sutured.

Postoperative care

The most important aspects of the postoperative care include monitoring of intravenous fluid therapy and the prevention of pulmonary infection. The patient's fluid needs must be carefully titrated against the urine output and central venous pressure readings to avoid fluid overload.

The patient is nursed sitting upright and kept free of pain with regular doses of narcotic analgesics or patient-controlled analgesia. If the operation was prolonged, the patient frail and elderly or the postoperative arterial blood gases unsatisfactory, a nasotracheal tube should be left in place for 24–48 h for intermittent mandatory ventilation and regular tracheobronchial toilet.

Chest physiotherapy is essential to help the patient cough effectively and the preoperative incentive spirometry should be continued in the postoperative period. Prophylactic antibiotics should be continued until the left lung is fully re-expanded, there is no residual haemothorax and the intercostal drain can be removed.

Nasogastric aspirations will keep the stomach empty in patients in whom gastric reconstruction was performed. By the third postoperative day, when the patient has recovered from postoperative ileus, the nasogastric tube may be used for enteral feeding. After a Gastrografin swallow is performed on the sixth postoperative day to exclude anastomotic leakage, the nasogastric tube may be removed and the patient commenced on a graduated oral diet.

Illustrations by Paul Richardson

Abdominal incisions for approaching the abdominal oesophagus and stomach

P. G. Devitt FRACS, FRCS
Senior Lecturer in Surgery, Department of Surgery, Royal Adelaide Hospital, Adelaide, Australia

Principles and justification

The type of abdominal incision chosen and the way in which it is fashioned and closed is often a matter of personal preference, although some important principles can be stated. The most important is that the choice of incision should provide the best exposure of the area to be operated upon so that safe surgery can be performed with the minimum of difficulty. This principle is particularly important in upper abdominal surgery, where access under the costal margin and diaphragm can be difficult. Of secondary importance, the wound should be easy to fashion and close. While attention must be paid to the cosmetic effects of any incision, this is of lesser importance in upper abdominal surgery where the underlying condition is often life-threatening and priority must be given to ease and sometimes speed of access.

Choice of incision

Three types of abdominal incision are commonly used for operations on the stomach and lower oesophagus.

1 A midline incision provides good access for most procedures. The incision is easy to make and access to the abdominal cavity is gained quickly. Neither muscle fibres nor nerves are divided. The wound is easy to extend and easy to close.

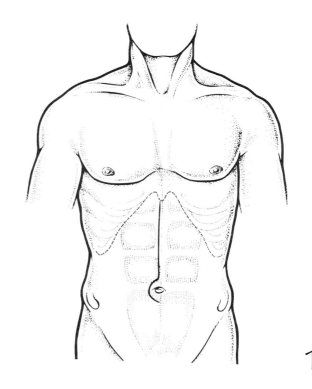

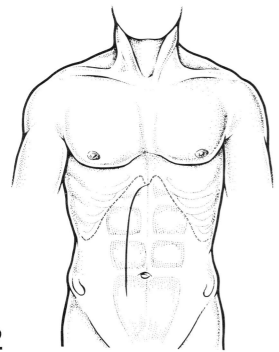

2 The paramedian incision is more time-consuming to make than the midline incision and if it is truly vertical may not give adequate exposure to the subdiaphragmatic region. Exposure can be improved by curving the upper extension of the incision towards the midline. This once popular incision is little used today.

3 A subcostal incision in a patient with a wide costal margin gives good access both to the proximal stomach and duodenum. In addition, the incision can easily be extended across the left costal margin and into the chest.

Method of incision

A scalpel is the instrument of choice for most surgeons, but diathermy can be used for the deeper layers. The skin is held on the stretch and a firm incision is made, the initial stroke going into the subcutaneous fat. All layers down to the peritoneum are usually incised with the knife. The peritoneum is grasped between two forceps and opened with either a knife or pair of scissors. Further extension of this incision in the peritoneum is performed with scissors; blood vessels are coagulated as they are encountered.

Haemostasis

Subcutaneous fat is prone to infection and every effort should be made to control bleeding, minimize trauma and reduce contamination. Many small bleeding points will stop bleeding of their own accord or with gentle pressure from a gauze pack for a few minutes; unnecessary cautery can be avoided in this way. Larger vessels may need to be ligated or cauterized. Excessive use of electrocoagulation increases tissue necrosis and the risk of infection. Despite this, some surgeons maintain that the chance of wound infection is no greater when cutting diathermy is used as the method of incision.

Wound protection/infection

Opening the gastrointestinal tract increases the risk of wound infection. Apart from preoperative preparation with prophylactic antibiotics and the use of bactericidal soaps, the risks of infection may be reduced by covering the edges of the wound with plastic sheeting or gauze packs. Probably of greater importance is meticulous haemostasis and minimization of tissue trauma. The latter is difficult to avoid if fixed retractors are used.

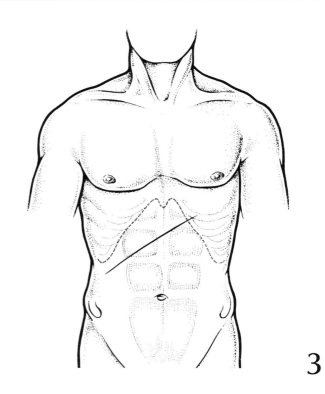

3

Preoperative

Even if it is anticipated that surgery will be performed wholly through the abdominal incision, it is prudent to prepare the patient for possible extension of the operation into the chest or the lower abdomen. This means that the patient should be placed on the operating table in a position which will allow the chest to be opened. In proximal gastric or lower oesophageal surgery this will usually be the left side of the chest and access may be easier if a sandbag or rolled-up towel is placed under the left side of the patient. The skin should be prepared up to the nipples and down to the pubic symphysis. Skin preparation should include the flanks so that drains and feeding tubes may be inserted if required.

Approaches to the upper abdomen

Midline incision

The length of the incision will depend on the shape of the patient and the procedure to be undertaken. It can be taken up to the xiphisternum and down to the pubic symphysis. The xiphisternum can be incised or excised with bone-cutting forceps. When dissecting in this region, terminal branches of the internal mammary artery which will bleed freely and require coagulation are encountered. Even for upper abdominal surgery, it is often necessary to extend the distal end of the incision beyond the umbilicus. If this is to be done, it is more aesthetically pleasing to make the incision around instead of through the umbilicus. The wound is also easier to close if some rectus sheath is left attached to the umbilicus.

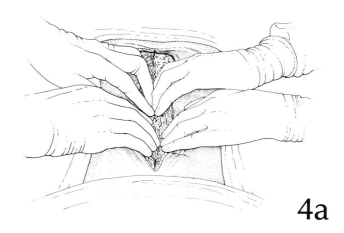

4a

4a, b
The subcutaneous fat is usually incised, but in the obese patient it is easy to stray from the midline and to miss the linea alba. One way of avoiding this problem is to pull the subcutaneous fat away from the midline. There is a relatively bloodless plane of cleavage which can be developed by lateral traction. With the surgeon and his assistant retracting the skin at 180° to the line of the incision, the fat can be split down to the linea alba. The linea alba is then incised using either knife or cautery. The underlying peritoneum is opened to the left of the falciform ligament. To complete the exposure the falciform ligament is ligated and divided. Provided it is sewn up correctly, this incision is no more liable to dehiscence than a paramedian incision.

Paramedian incision

This is more laborious to fashion than the midline incision and involves incision into the right (or left) rectus sheath 2–3 cm from the median decussation. The tendinous intersections of the rectus muscle adhere to the sheath and several of these need to be divided before the belly of the muscle can be retracted laterally. The posterior rectus sheath is incised and the underlying peritoneum opened. The paramedian incision has been superseded by the midline incision, but the former approach should be used where there has been a previous paramedian incision. In such cases the wound is best opened by incising the rectus muscle and splitting it longitudinally. A more laterally placed incision has been described. The approach is the same

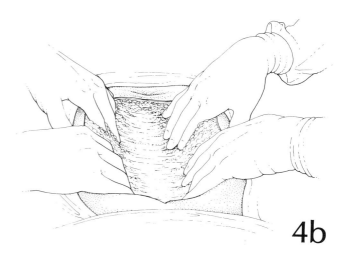

4b

as for the conventional paramedian incision, with lateral displacement of the rectus muscle, but with the incision through the anterior and posterior rectus sheaths placed over the lateral third of the belly of the muscle. This incision is claimed to have a negligible incidence of incisional hernia when compared with midline wounds[1].

Subcostal incision

This is the most time-consuming of the three types of incision. Rectus sheath and muscle must be cut, as well as the oblique and transverse muscles of the anterior abdominal wall. Bleeding is more substantial and difficult to control, as the vessels retract into the cut edges of the muscle. If this exposure is taken from the right flank and across the left rectus muscle, it gives good exposure to both the duodenum and the proximal stomach, and is useful in obese patients with wide costal margins. If necessary, the incision can be taken straight across the left rectus muscle, the costal margin and into the left chest.

The skin incision is made 2–3 cm below the costal margin; if made any less than this, there is insufficient muscle left attached to the costal margin to take sutures when closing the wound. When the rectus muscle is cut, branches of the superior epigastric artery are encountered and coagulated. At the lateral aspect of the wound the segmental dorsal nerves are encountered; the eighth is usually divided, but the ninth should be identified and preserved.

The cut rectus muscle heals to form a fibrous intersection, and as it is segmentally innervated (providing the ninth dorsal nerve has been left intact), it is unlikely that there will be any significant denervation or subsequent weakness.

Exposure

5 Even with an incision in the correct position and a wound of appropriate length, good access is frequently difficult to obtain in upper gastrointestinal surgery. Many different types of fixed retractor are available to improve exposure. Perhaps the simplest and most useful is the sternal retractor. The bridge is fixed as near to the head of the operating table as possible without impeding access for the anaesthetist. It is helpful if the operating table has a separate head section that can be lowered. The bridge should be low; with too steep an angle the blade of the retractor may slip from under the sternum. When the incision has been made, wound protectors (plastic sheeting or gauze packs) are positioned before the retractors; a self-retaining retractor is placed in the wound. If the surgeon operates standing on the right of the patient, the retractor should be placed so that the shaft sticks into the assistant's abdomen instead of his own! The blade of the sternal retractor is placed over a pack on the xiphisternum.

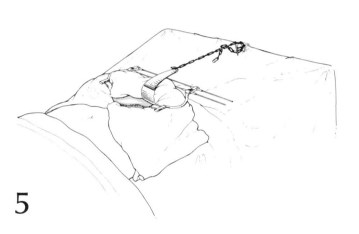

5

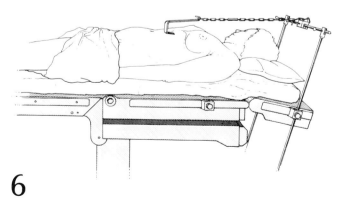

6

6 The retractor may be custom-made; alternatively, the middle blade of a self-retaining retractor may be sufficient. With the blade in position, a length of chain is used to haul the retractor towards the bridge. When the chain has been made fast, further retraction can be obtained by pivoting the bridge backwards by lowering the head section of the table.

7, 8 Other retractors are useful to hold up the liver. These can be fixed to the operating table. Once the retractors are in position, the table can be tilted feet-down (reverse Trendelenburg) so that the contents of the abdominal cavity fall downwards, increasing the access in the upper abdomen.

Wound closure

Wounds heal by formation of dense fibrous scar tissue across cut surfaces and not by re-establishment of the layers of the abdominal wall. The aim of wound closure is to produce apposition of the wound edges and splinting to allow the fibrous tissue to develop and mature. It is unnecessary to close the wound in layers and mass closure is sufficient. Material of sufficient tensile strength and durability must be chosen to keep the wound intact in the postoperative period and to allow fibrous healing to occur. Sutures should be placed at no more than 1-cm intervals and at least 1 cm of tissue away from the wound edge[2]. The sutures should loosely approximate the edges of the wound. If they are too tight, the local tissue oedema and increased intra-abdominal pressure that occurs after operation will cause the material to cut through the tissues. If the wound is closed in a continuous manner, bearing the

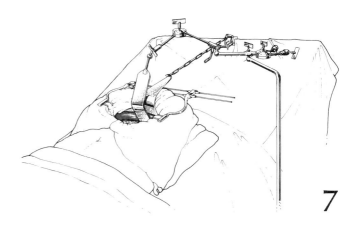

7

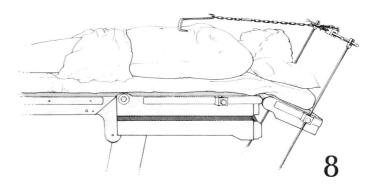

8

above principles in mind, the amount of suture material needed exceeds the length of the wound fourfold.

Early wound failure is usually the result of incorrectly placed sutures or inadequately tied knots. Late wound failure may result from poor choice of suture materials.

Knots

The first suture is placed at the upper end of the wound. Continuous suturing is the most common practice. The knot should be buried in the deep layers; if it is left in the subcutaneous fat it can become a source of sinus formation or irritation to the patient.

9 Alternatively, a loop of nylon swaged onto a needle can be used; this will obviate the need for a knot at the start of suturing.

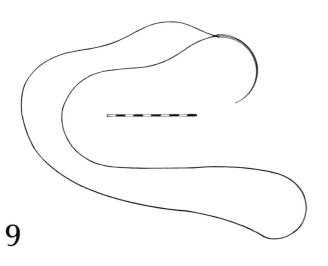

9

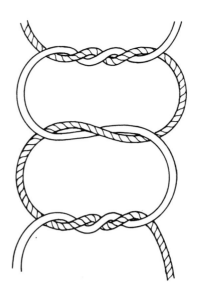

10 Most surgeons use the modified square or reef knot, in which two throws are put on the initial tie. This is followed by a single throw and a third throw which can be double. Coated and monofilament materials tend to slip and at least three throws should be placed.

10

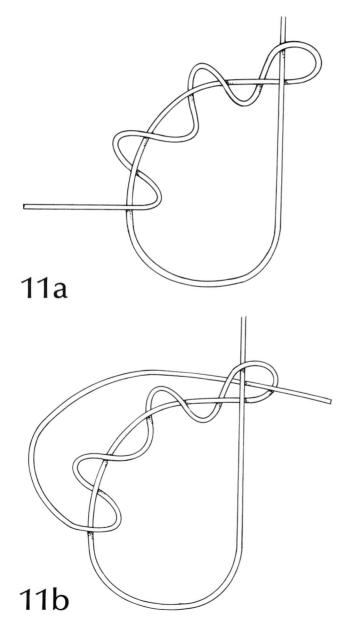

11a

11b

11a, b Used less often, the fisherman's knot is simple to execute and is reliable. It is particularly useful for monofilament materials. The assistant holds the long end of the suture taut and vertical, the surgeon wraps the short end once round the long end and then twists the short end on itself for six or seven turns. The tip of the suture is then passed through the wrap and pulled tight[3].

As each suture is placed, the tip of the needle must be in view to reduce the chance of underlying structures being damaged or caught up in the suture. This can either be done by placing a finger under the wound edge and guiding the needle out of the wound, or by placing forceps on the wound edge and lifting. The latter is safer practice, as most needlestick injuries occur during wound closure.

When the wound is half closed, another suture is started from the bottom end with the aim of making the final closure in the middle of the wound. In this way, what is often a difficult apposition around the umbilicus is made easier, and the final sutures are placed with greater safety by leaving the sutures loose until the last ones are in place. The final knot should be tied so that it can be buried in the deep layers.

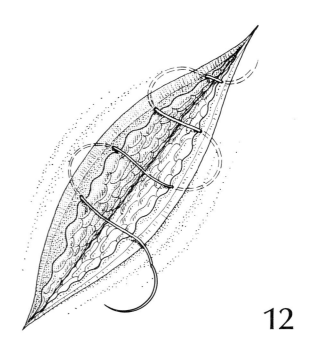

12 The subcutaneous fat does not need to be sutured and a subcuticular stitch provides a cosmetic finish to the closure. Polypropylene on a straight or curved cutting needle is suitable. This material runs easily and excites little tissue reaction. Arguments have been made for the use of skin staples. These are expensive compared with sutures, but may reduce the chance of needlestick injury. It is certainly quicker to close wounds with staples, but the time saved in closing the wound is unlikely to defray much from the overall cost of the operation.

Suture materials

Suitable materials to close the deep layers of the anterior abdominal wall include nylon and polypropylene monofilament sutures and the newer synthetics polydioxanone and polyglyconate. These materials invoke little tissue reaction and maintain their tensile strength. Polydioxanone and polyglyconate have the advantage of dissolution after several months. These sutures should be used for the linea alba and the anterior rectus sheath. Catgut and the synthetics polyglycolic acid and polyglactin do not maintain sufficient tensile strength, with loss of strength by 4 weeks. These materials are unsatisfactory for the linea alba or the anterior rectus sheath, but can be used for the posterior rectus sheath and peritoneum. However, it is unnecessary to close the peritoneum as a separate layer. It does not contribute to the strength of the wound and may even increase adhesion formation.

Single-layer or mass closures

Midline incisions are closed in a single layer. All layers except for the skin and subcutaneous fat are incorporated. If wound failure is a potential problem, such as in severe malnutrition, a 'near and far' technique can be used to close the wound (*see Illustration 15*).

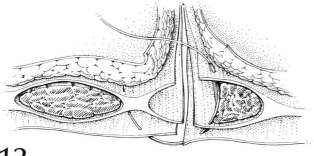

13 The paramedian incision can also be closed in a single layer. The suture is placed through the anterior and posterior rectus sheaths with the belly of the muscle displaced laterally. With the more laterally placed paramedian incision this type of mass closure is not practical and the wound should be closed in separate layers.

Two-layer closures

The paramedian wound is often closed in two layers, the posterior rectus sheath incorporating the peritoneum and being sewn with catgut or a rapidly absorbed synthetic. A monofilament or slowly absorbed synthetic (polydioxanone or polyglyconate) is used for the anterior rectus sheath. Similarly, the subcostal incision can be closed in two layers. A long incision may need two lengths of suture material, but a shorter subcostal wound can be closed with a continuous length of monofilament.

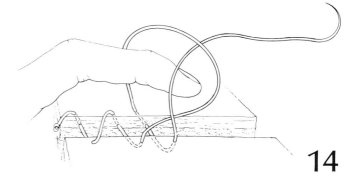

14

14 The knot is placed at the medial end of the wound and the short end held in an artery clip. The deep layer is closed in a continuous fashion and a grocer's knot is tied at the lateral end. With this type of knot the loose end of the suture is grasped through the last loop of suture material placed in the tissues and brought through as another loop. The second loop is pulled up and, in doing so, the first loop tightens down as the first throw of the knot. The process is repeated until several throws have been made and then all the free end of the suture material is passed through the loop and the knot pulled tight. The suture does not need to be cut, and the free end can be brought back, closing the anterior muscle layers and rectus sheath and tied with the original short end.

Tension sutures are mentioned only to be condemned. They are not needed for primary wound closure. Similarly, a dehisced wound can usually be brought together satisfactorily without recourse to these sutures. Tension sutures are painful, unsightly and cut into the tissues. Infection around the sutures and sinus formation is common. The patient is left with an ugly scar. If a wound does split open, it can usually be closed quite satisfactorily by undermining the subcutaneous fat and exposing 4–5 cm of abdominal wall muscle.

15 A 'near and far' technique can then be applied and combined with interrupted sutures to close the wound. Several lengths of monofilament suture material are needed and it is wise to use either nylon or polypropylene. Suturing is started as for a standard wound closure. The first suture is continuous and a 4-cm deep bite of tissue on one side (B) of the wound is married with a 1-cm deep bite on the opposite side (A) of the wound. At the same level the suture is now placed 1 cm from the edge of side B and taken over to be inserted 4 cm deep on side A. The two ends of the suture material are now tied over side B. The suture is now placed 1 cm *down* on side B and the process repeated. It is unlikely that more than two of these sutures will be made with each length of material and an interrupted suture is inserted for every third suture. This technique is laborious but produces a sound repair.

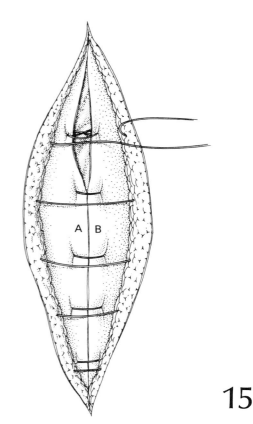

15

The skin may be closed over the repair. Drains and stomas should be brought out through separate incisions otherwise they may weaken the main laparotomy wound.

References

1. Kendall SWH, Brennan TG, Guillou PJ. Suture length to wound length ratio and the integrity of midline and lateral paramedian incisions. *Br J Surg* 1991; 78: 705–7.

2. Jenkins TPN. The burst abdomen: a mechanical approach. *Br J Surg* 1976; 63: 873–6.

3. Wattchow DA, Watts JMcK. The half blood knot for tying nylon in surgery. *Br J Surg* 1984; 71: 333.

Sutured oesophageal anastomosis

Anthony Watson MD, FRCS, FRCS(Ed), FRACS
Consultant Surgeon, The Wellington Hospital, London, UK

Principles and justification

The choice of sutured or stapled oesophageal anasto-moses is dictated largely by personal preference. Such comparative studies as are available show no significant differences in the rates of anastomotic dehiscence[1,2]. Sutured anastomoses are marginally more time consum-ing to perform but are associated with a lower incidence of anastomotic stricture[3], particularly when the smaller staple heads are used. The author's preference has been for hand-sutured anastomoses using the technique described, which has produced reliable results over almost two decades.

The principles involved in the construction of oesophageal anastomoses are similar whether the anastomosis is to stomach, jejunum or colon, and whether the anastomosis is sited in the mediastinum or the neck. Gastro-oesophageal anastomosis is described,

as it is the most widely practised technique and the author's preference following oesophageal resection. Oesophageal anastomoses have a greater propensity for leakage than most gastrointestinal anastomoses, because of the relatively poor vascularity of the oesophagus, the absence of a serous layer, and the high intraluminal pressures generated on swallowing. Consequently, great care must be exercised in ensuring that vascularity is preserved and that the anastomosis is performed with adequate access and without tension. The anastomosis is performed using a single layer of 3/0 silk, as a non-absorbable or delayed absorption material is believed desirable, and the consistency of silk makes it less likely to cut through the fragile oesophagus than some of the newer, synthetic delayed absorption materials.

Operation

1 After construction of a greater curve gastric tube, a horizontal incision is made on the posterior aspect of the gastric tube about 3 cm from its apex, the length of the incision corresponding to the diameter of the transected oesophagus.

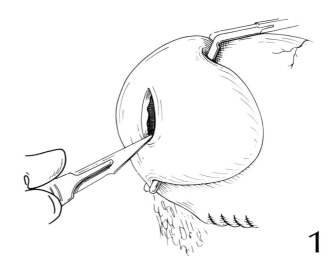

1

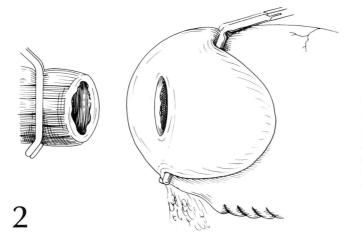

2

2 For mediastinal anastomoses, the proximal oesophagus has usually been divided just below the apex of the mediastinum and the gastric tube is held close to the inferior margin of the thoracotomy wound. The gastric tube and the proximal oesophagus are held in light, non-crushing clamps (such as Satinsky clamps), which are loosely applied about 1 cm proximal and distal to the proposed anastomotic margins. It is vitally important that the mucosa is clearly visible, particularly in the oesophagus where the mucosa and submucosa are the strongest layers and a tendency to retraction of the layers exists, particularly if transection is performed under tension.

3 The proximal oesophagus and the gastric tube are kept separate until the posterior layer of sutures has been placed. Stay sutures are first placed between each corner of the divided oesophagus and the respective corners of the posterior gastrotomy. These are introduced from the serosal aspect of the stomach through to the gastric mucosa, and from the oesophageal lumen through the mucosa and out through the muscular layers, ensuring that an adequate bite of oesophageal mucosa and submucosa is obtained. These sutures are held in the haemostats for later tying by the 'parachute' technique.

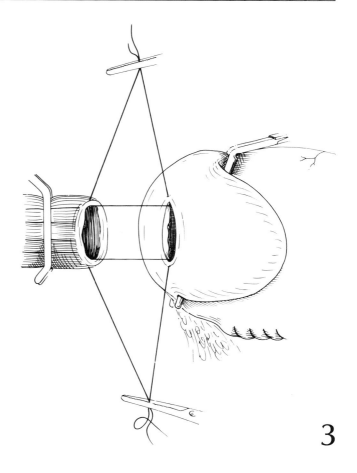

3

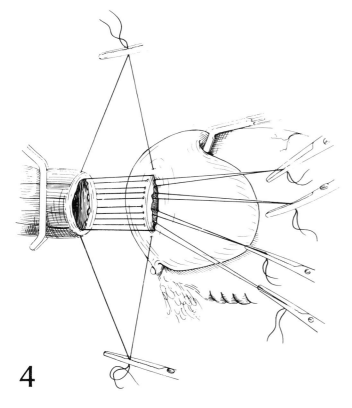

4

4 The posterior layer of sutures is then placed as a series of horizontal mattress sutures 3 mm in width and 3 mm apart. They are constructed as inverting sutures, traversing all layers from gastric mucosa through to gastric serosa, oesophageal muscle and through oesophageal mucosa. Each suture is then returned from oesophageal muscosa to muscle and from gastric serosa to mucosa. Each suture is held in a haemostat for later tying.

5 When an appropriate number of horizontal mattress sutures has been placed in the posterior layer (usually four or five), the luminal surfaces are approximated by bringing the gastric clamp close to the oesophageal clamp. Starting with the corner stay sutures, each suture is then tied sufficiently tightly to approximate the stomach and the oesophagus gently and to avoid undue tension which may cut through or devascularize the oesophagus.

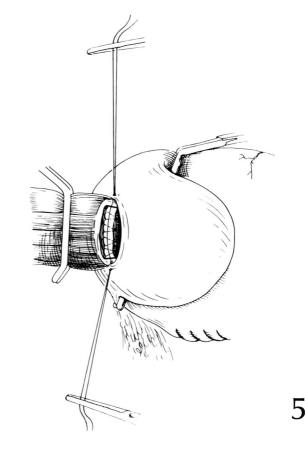

5

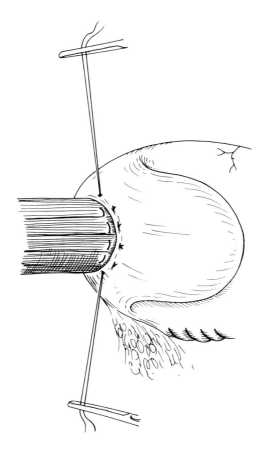

6

6 Once the posterior layer of sutures has been placed, the clamps are removed and the nasogastric tube is fed through the anastomosis and sited in the gastric tube. A similar number of horizontal mattress sutures is placed in the anterior layer of the stomach and oesophagus, in identical fashion to the posterior layer, except that each suture may be tied and cut immediately after placement.

7   The part of the gastric tube proximal to the anastomosis is then placed over the suture line and fixed by two sutures superiorly to the apical mediastinal pleura and by one suture on each side to the posterior mediastinal pleura. This manoeuvre is performed to seal the anastomosis and to divert tension from the anastomotic line to the apex of the gastric tube during postural changes.

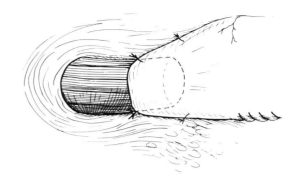

7

Postoperative care

Oral feeding is withheld and the nasogastric tube and basal chest drain are retained until the Gastrografin swallow on the fifth day after operation has confirmed anastomotic integrity. Nutritional status may be maintained by total parenteral nutrition through a peripheral line until the patient's oral intake is adequate, usually within 48 h of commencement of oral fluids.

It is the author's preference to maintain thoracic epidural analgesia during the postoperative period, which enables pain-free cooperation with chest physiotherapy without the need for systemic opiates[4].

Outcome

The technique described has been performed with a clinical anastomotic dehiscence rate of 2.3%, half of which were fatal. This compares favourably with the rates of 3.8% after sutured anastomosis reported by Paterson and Wong and 2.9% using stapled anastomosis[3]. The rate of other complications is low, with an 8% incidence of anastomotic stricture requiring endoscopic dilatation, compared with 13–25% following stapled anastomosis[1,2]. Overall hospital 30-day mortality is 8.6%, which has fallen to 6.6% in the last 6 years coinciding with the routine use of thoracic epidural analgesia[4,5].

References

1. Hopkins RA, Alexander JC, Postlethwait RW. Stapled esophago-gastric anastomosis. *Am J Surg* 1984; 147: 283–7.

2. Wong J. Esophageal resection for cancer: the rationale of current practice. *Am J Surg* 1987; 153: 18–24.

3. Paterson IM, Wong J. Anastomotic leakage: an avoidable complication of Lewis–Tanner oesophagectomy. *Br J Surg* 1989; 76: 127–9.

4. Watson A. Surgery for carcinoma of the oesophagus. *Postgrad Med J* 1988; 64: 860–4.

5. Watson A. Oesophageal neoplasms. *Curr Opin Gastroenterol* 1990; 6: 590–6.

Illustrations by Paul Richardson

Stapling techniques for anastomoses of the oesophagus

Glyn G. Jamieson FRACS, FACS
Dorothy Mortlock Professor of Surgery, University of Adelaide, Department of Surgery, Royal Adelaide Hospital, Adelaide, Australia

Principles and justification

Controlled trials have not established that stapled anastomoses are either better or worse than manually sutured anastomoses. Such trials, however, have usually been performed in units expert in the techniques of oesophageal surgery. It seems quite likely that in the hands of less expert surgeons the stapled anastomosis is safer, because the anastomosis is standardized and it probably has a better blood supply than a manually constructed anastomosis.

Attention to detail is still of paramount importance, however, and the overriding principles of lack of tension and provision of the best possible blood supply apply for stapled anastomoses just as for manually constructed anastomoses.

Technique

The oesophagus receives its blood supply through intramural vascular anastomoses, so that long segments of it can be mobilized without jeopardizing its blood supply. Therefore, 3–5 cm of the oesophagus proximal to where it is to be divided should be mobilized.

1 If an automatic purse-string device is used, it is applied before dividing the oesophagus. If a nasogastric tube lies in the oesophagus it is withdrawn to a point several centimetres above the site of division. The purse-string device is placed in position and closed. A heavy tie is then placed around the oesophagus distal to the purse-string device in order to prevent spillage of oesophageal contents.

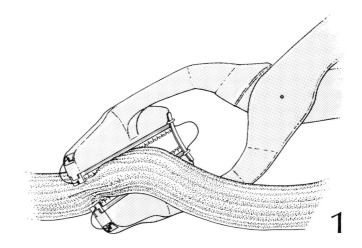

2 The oesophagus is now divided flush with the purse-string device, which is opened and removed. The ends of the purse-string suture are retrieved and held in a pair of artery forceps. Oesophageal contents in the proximal oesophagus are sucked out. There are two points at which the purse-string may not be held optimally close to the oesophagus. These points are at either side where the anterior and posterior rows of staples meet. The author secures the furthest point by placing a single over-and-over suture to incorporate the purse-string. The nearest point is where the purse-string will be tied, and as it lies directly under vision this is not usually a problem. If necessary, an over-and-over suture can be placed here, after the first throw of the knot on the purse-string has been made.

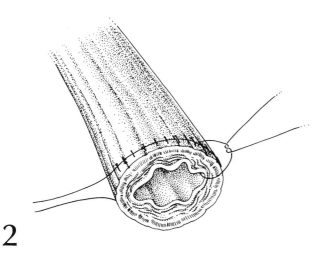

3 The oesophagus contracts and retracts after being divided, and six stay sutures can be used in order to give excellent control of the mouth of the oesophagus. These stay sutures are placed taking a 5–7-mm bite of the full thickness of the oesophageal wall, and they usually pass through the oesophageal wall incorporating the purse-string suture.

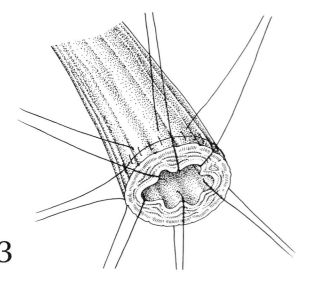

4 Some surgeons prefer to insert the purse-string suture manually. To do this, a 0 polypropylene or monofilament nylon suture on a round-bodied needle is used. The suture begins on the anterior wall of the oesophagus, passing from outside to inside, and then is continued around the oesophagus with an over-and-over running suture taking bites of about 4–5 mm in depth and 4–5 mm apart. When one-third of the circumference of the oesophagus has been traversed, the loop of the over-and-over suture can be held by a pair of Allis' or Babcock's forceps, as this will later be used as a stay suture. Similarly, when two-thirds of the circumference has been dealt with, another pair of Allis' or Babcock's forceps can be used to hold a second loop. The final suture is brought to the outside of the oesophagus, and both ends of the purse-string suture and the two loop stay sutures keep the mouth of the oesophagus open.

The oesophagus is now dilated with either metal dilators or a large Foley catheter with a 25-ml balloon, which the author has found to be very effective. The catheter is lubricated and then inserted well into the oesophagus; the balloon is slowly but firmly inflated and the catheter is pulled down the oesophagus. The bag of the balloon tends to bring a lot of mucus with it, and so a sucker should be held at the mouth of the oesophagus as the catheter is withdrawn.

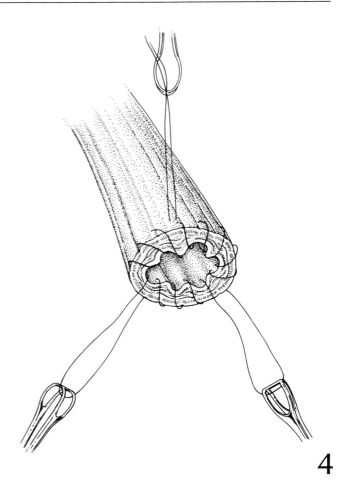

4

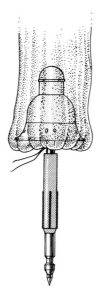

5

5 An appropriately sized staple head is chosen (usually 25 mm or 28 mm). Holding the six stay sutures (or the Allis' or Babcock's forceps) facilitates the placement of the anvil within the oesophagus. Once in position, the purse-string is tied snugly against the shaft of the anvil. If the surgeon is unhappy with the purse-string suture at this stage, a further purse-string can be placed with the anvil in position.

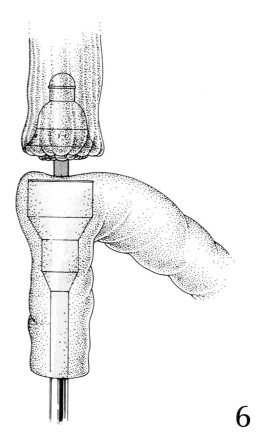

6 The main stapler is introduced into the organ being joined to the oesophagus and the shaft is brought through the wall of the organ.

The anvil is clicked into position on the main shaft of the stapler. The two parts of the stapler are closed, making sure that no extraneous tissue is caught between the oesophagus and the organ to which it is being joined. Closure is completed. A final check is made to see that the tissue is free all the way around the staple head and the instrument is fired.

The parts of the head are separated by turning the appropriate part of the stapler, and the whole device is removed by using a gently rocking motion while at the same time maintaining a pulling traction on the instrument and supporting the anastomosis with the opposite hand. Once the instrument has been removed, the rings of staples are inspected to make sure that they are complete. If there is any doubt about the anastomosis, saline can be instilled into the oesophagus above the anastomosis to check that the join is watertight.

It is debatable whether anything further should be done. If a gastro-oesophageal anastomosis has been constructed in the chest, the author constructs the anastomosis on the posterior wall of the stomach so that the remaining posterior wall can be brought up above the anastomosis to form a partial fundoplication, recreating an angle of His on the opposite side from its 'natural' anatomical angle. In general terms, however, it is better not to place further reinforcing sutures through the anastomosis, as this is more likely to jeopardize the blood supply than to have a beneficial effect on healing.

6

Illustrations by Denise Smith

Hand-sewn techniques for gastric anastomoses

Z. H. Krukowski PhD, FRCS(Ed)
Consultant Surgeon, Aberdeen Royal Infirmary, and Honorary Senior Lecturer, University of Aberdeen, Aberdeen, UK

N. A. Matheson ChM, FRCS, FRCS(Ed)
Consultant Surgeon, Aberdeen Royal Infirmary, and Honorary Senior Lecturer, University of Aberdeen, Aberdeen, UK

Single-layer interrupted anastomosis is preferred to two-layer techniques because it achieves more anatomical realignment of the layers of the bowel, less luminal reduction and less interference with blood supply. It also has the important advantage of simplicity. Single-layer anastomosis is applicable with minor variations throughout the gastrointestinal tract. The standard method described is based on a single layer of interrupted appositional serosubmucosal sutures which consistently achieves satisfactory results[1,2]. Hand-sutured single layer anastomoses are preferred to stapled anastomoses because of their versatility, low complication rate and economy.

SINGLE-LAYER SEROSUBMUCOSAL APPOSITIONAL ANASTOMOTIC TECHNIQUE

1 The basic technique is that each suture incorporates the submucosa but avoids the mucosa. Minor modifications may be made at some sites, e.g. a continuous technique for gastrojejunostomy.

For many years braided polyamide (nylon) 3/0 (2-metric) sutures mounted on proprietary 'Control Release' atraumatic needles have been used. This non-absorbable material is preferred because of its combination of handling, knotting and tissue inertia properties which are presently unmatched by any synthetic absorbable material.

Knots are tied with three throws. The first throw is deliberately crossed, adjusted for tension on the second throw, and the knot locked with the third throw. The tension in the knots should be sufficient to appose the tissues snugly and without strangulation.

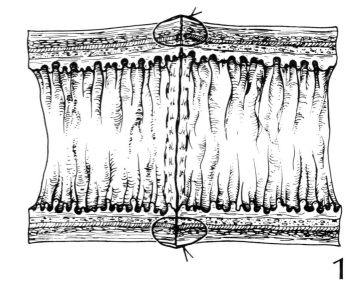

1

PREPARATION OF ROUX-EN-Y LOOP OF JEJUNUM

2 A Roux-en-Y loop is one of the most useful devices in reconstructive gastrointestinal surgery and the ability to fashion it correctly is fundamental. The first step in preparation of a Roux loop is vascular division so that by the time it is to be used for anastomosis any ischaemia at the proposed site of division should be apparent. The distance of jejunal division from the duodenojejunal junction is not critical and depends on the anatomy of the main jejunal vessels supplying the arcades. The first pedicle of sufficient length to permit easy ligation determines the site of division. Transillumination of the mesentery improves accurate identification of the main vessels of the appropriate arcade. The vessels are ligated in continuity after isolation by division of the overlying peritoneum on both sides of the mesentery. According to the vascular anatomy and required length it may or may not be necessary to divide more than one main vascular pedicle.

3 Care must be taken to avoid incorporation of the junctions of blood vessels in bulky ligatures.

4 The jejunum is cleared over a 2-cm length; one or two terminal branches of the jejunal vessels are divided close to the bowel wall to achieve this. After vascular isolation of the proposed loop the rest of the operation may proceed and division of the jejunum is postponed until it is required for anastomosis. The jejunum is cross-clamped at right angles with a Schumacher's clamp and divided distal to the clamp. The distal end is held in a pair of Babcock's forceps and mopped clean with a topical antiseptic.

The distal end is passed, usually in a retrocolic direction, through a convenient window in the transverse mesocolon for the proximal anastomosis to the stomach or oesophagus. This anastomosis is made first (*see* below) and the jejunojejunostomy is the final step in restoration of continuity.

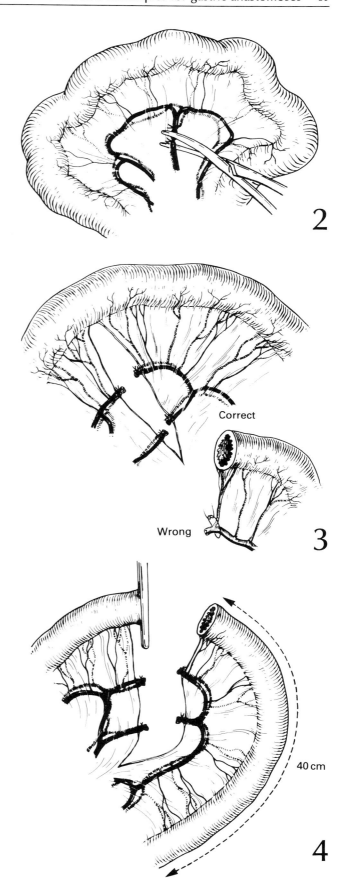

2

Correct

Wrong

3

40 cm

4

End-to-side jejunojejunostomy in a Roux loop

5 Angle sutures are passed horizontally through the proximal jejunum about 5 mm proximal to the Schumacher's clamp, and through the antimesenteric border of the distal jejunum about 40 cm distal to the end of the Roux loop. Care should be taken to place the distal sutures at the appropriate distance apart with the bowel under moderate tension. It is easy to make the enterotomy in the distal bowel too long.

The antimesenteric border of the distal jejunum between the angle sutures is incised with cutting diathermy and the lumen mopped with topical antiseptic.

The Schumacher's clamp is removed and the proximal bowel aspirated and mopped with topical antiseptic. Haemostasis is secured with fine diathermy coagulation. The angle stitches are tied.

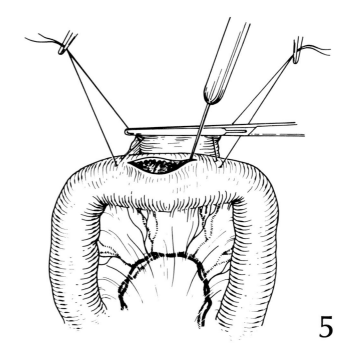

5

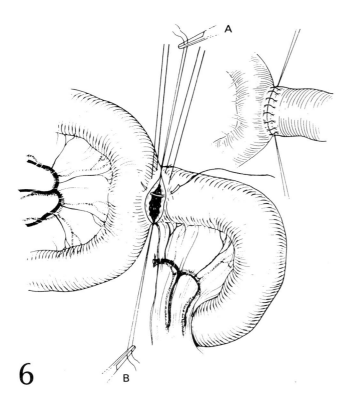

6

6 The anterior sutures are inserted serially into the submucosal plane of the proximal jejunum, piercing the serosa about 5 mm from, and emerging at, the cut edge, entering this part of the distal jejunum just superficial to the mucosa and emerging again about 5 mm from the edge. The sutures are placed about 5 mm apart. A mid point marking suture may be used to aid accurate placement of the whole series. The stitches are held one after the other between the finger and thumb of an assistant.

The anterior sutures are tied serially and cut.

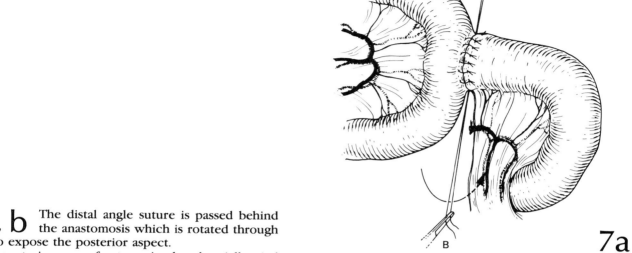

7a

7a, b The distal angle suture is passed behind the anastomosis which is rotated through 180° to expose the posterior aspect.

The posterior row of sutures is placed serially, tied and cut.

Rotation of the anastomosis through 180°, which permits all the knots to be placed on the serosal aspect, depends on mobility. If the site of the jejunal section is close to the duodenojejunal junction, sufficient mobility may be lacking. If this is the case, sutures may be inserted from the anterior aspect.

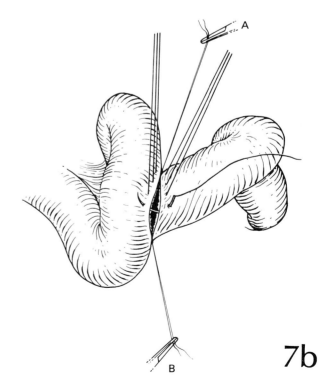

7b

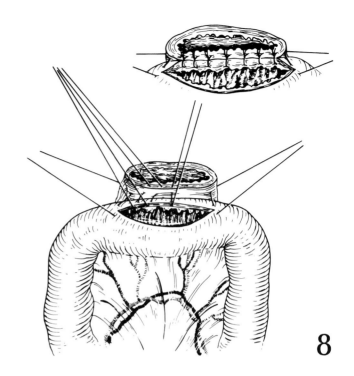

8 The angle stitches in this case are left untied until the first (posterior) layer has been placed. Sutures are inserted serially into the submucosa at the cut edge of the proximal jejunum and emerge at the cut edge of the distal jejunum. As before, about 5 mm of bowel is included on both sides and the sutures are placed about 5 mm apart. A mid point marking stitch may again be used.

The sutures are tied in series with knots on the luminal aspect and cut. The anterior layer is completed as in *Illustration 7a* and *b*.

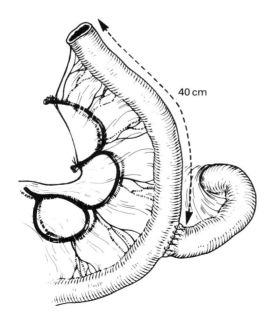

40 cm

RECONSTRUCTION AFTER TOTAL GASTRECTOMY

9 Roux-en-Y oesophagojejunostomy by the abdominal route is the preferred reconstruction after total gastrectomy for malignant neoplasms of the body or antrum of the stomach. Oesophagogastrectomy for malignant tumours at the cardia is not described here.

10 The oesophagus is mobilized for 6 cm proximal to the cardia and two full thickness horizontal stay sutures are inserted 4 cm proximal to the cardia. A right-angled non-crushing clamp (Haughton's) is placed proximal to the stay sutures. The clamp is necessary to relieve undue traction on the subsequent anastomotic sutures. The oesophagus is transected with scissors 1.5 cm distal to the cross-clamp and the lumen mopped with a topical antiseptic.

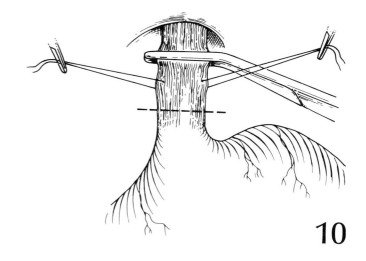

10

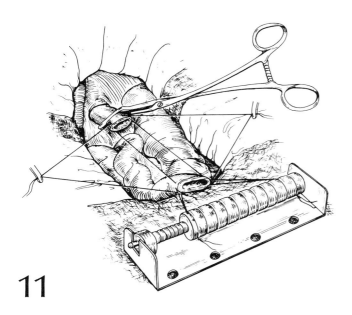

11

11 The previously prepared Roux loop is passed in a retrocolic direction and adequacy of the blood supply is confirmed. To prevent the jejunum slipping into the depths of the abdomen during placement of the posterior row of sutures, two short stay sutures are inserted transversely through the jejunum and are either clipped with artery forceps or held in a suture-holding clamp. A horizontal serosubmucosal angle suture is inserted into the antimesenteric border of the jejunum about 5 mm from the divided end. A corresponding bite of the right side of the oesophageal wall is taken and the suture held in a pair of artery forceps. A similar angle suture is placed on the mesenteric aspect of the jejunum and the other side of the oesophagus.

12 A series of serosubmucosal sutures is placed 5 mm apart on the oesophagus and up to 7 mm apart on the jejunum if there is significant discrepancy in diameter between the two. It is seldom necessary to use a mid point suture because of the relatively narrow diameter of the oesophagus. Care is taken not to pick up the anterior wall of the oesophagus. The sutures are inserted just beneath the mucosa on the cut edge of the jejunum and emerge in the same plane at the cut edge of the oesophagus. If the oesophageal mucosa retracts excessively it may be incorporated in a full-thickness suture. After insertion each suture is held untied in series in the suture-holding clamp.

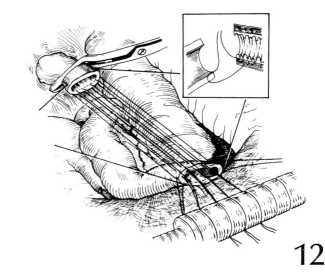

12

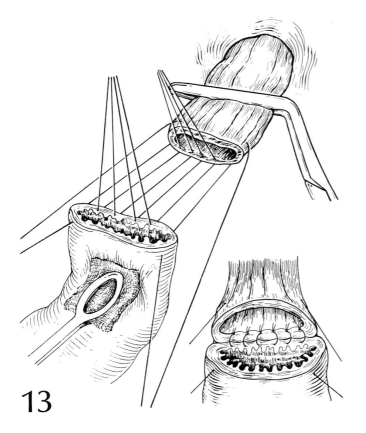

13

13 When all the sutures are in place the stay sutures on the jejunum are removed and the jejunum is pushed down the sutures with a swab mounted on a holder until the jejunum apposes the oesophagus.

The sutures are tied serially and cut. The oesophageal clamp is released and patency of the lumen confirmed.

14 The clamp may be reapplied to relieve tension during placement of the anterior row of sutures. The anterior serosubmucosal sutures are now inserted in series from jejunum to oesophagus and are held either in a series of artery forceps or in the suture-holding clamp.

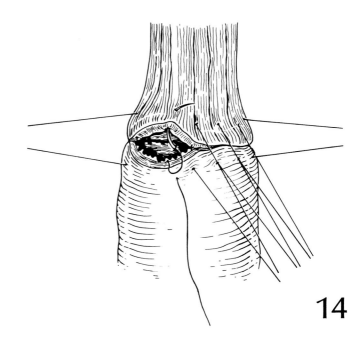

14

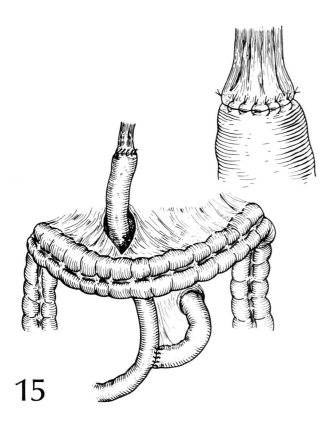

15

15 The angle sutures followed by the anterior row are tied serially and cut. There is no requirement for additional sutures and there must be no tension on the anastomosis. Drains are not used.

The end-to-side jejunojejunostomy is then made as previously described.

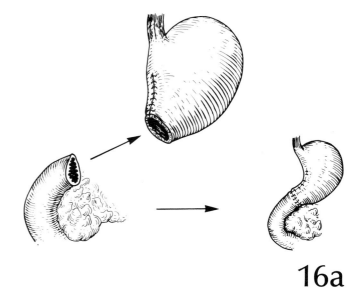

16a

RECONSTRUCTION AFTER PARTIAL GASTRECTOMY

16a–d
The options for reconstruction after partial gastrectomy are: gastroduodenal (Billroth I) (*Illustration 16a*); gastrojejunal with a Roux loop (*Illustration 16b*); gastrojejunal with a loop of jejunum (Billroth II or Pólya (*Illustration 16c*)); or interposed jejunal loop between the gastric remnant and the duodenum (*Illustration 16d*).

After partial gastrectomy, a gastroduodenal anastomosis (Billroth I) is preferred but when there is residual malignant disease in the region of the proposed anastomosis with the possibility of later recurrence and obstruction, a gastrojejunal anastomosis (Billroth II/Pólya or Roux-en-Y) is preferred. In either event restoration of continuity is facilitated if the gastric remnant is first partially closed to reconstitute a 'lesser curve'.

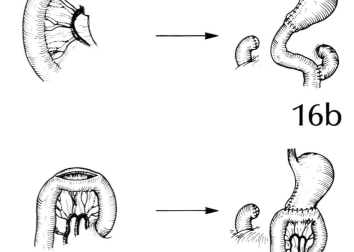

16b

16c

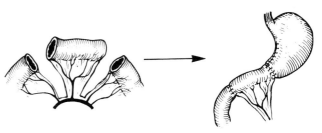

16d

Reconstitution of a 'lesser curve'

17 A pair of Schumacher clamps is placed in parallel at right angles to the greater curve of the stomach at the point of proposed division. About 4–5 cm of the stomach is incorporated and the diameter should exceed that of the duodenum for gastroduodenal anastomoses.

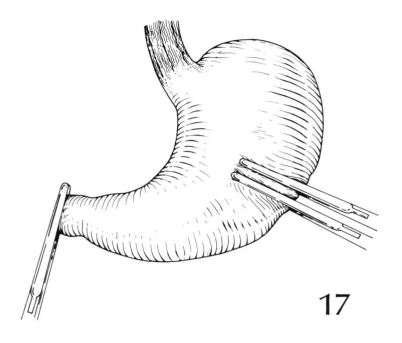

17

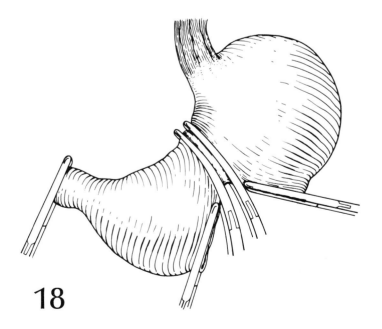

18

18 The stomach is divided between the Schumacher clamps. Two Parker–Kerr clamps are applied, extending from the tips of the Schumacher clamps across the lesser curve and angled towards the cardia. The Parker–Kerr clamps are applied with a gap of approximately 0.5 cm between them.

19 The stomach is divided distal to the Parker–Kerr clamps and the resected stomach removed.

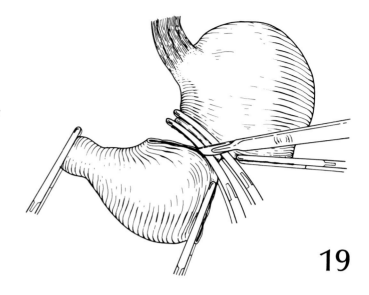

19

20 The distal Parker–Kerr clamp is released, leaving a cuff of crushed gastric tissue distal to the proximal clamp.

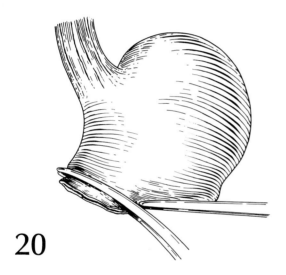

20

21 The proximal clamp is used to present the stomach for the insertion of a continuous layer of 3/0 (2-metric) all-coats polydioxanone.

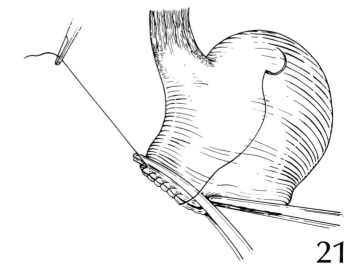

21

22 The proximal Parker–Kerr clamp is removed and the first layer of continuous polydioxanone suture buried with a second layer of continuous 3/0 (2-metric) serosubmucosal polydioxanone. Routine reconstitution of a 'lesser curve' simplifies subsequent gastroduodenal or gastrojejunal anastomosis, avoiding any valve or more complex reconstruction.

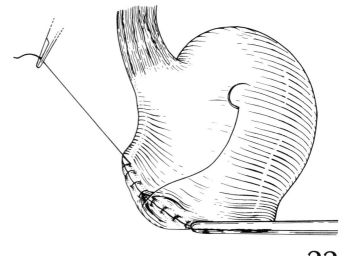

22

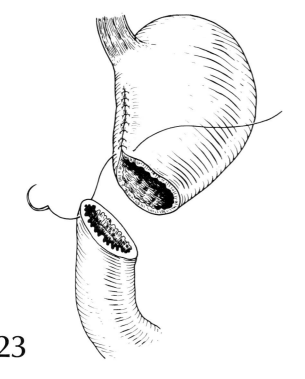

23

Gastroduodenal anastomosis

23 The most important suture in making a safe gastroduodenal anastomosis is the superior angle stitch which is inserted in the serosubmucosal plane on the anterior aspect of the stomach. This emerges near the oversewn edge of the reconstructed lesser curve and is reinserted in a similar fashion in the posterior aspect of the reconstructed lesser curve. It is then placed horizontally and serosubmucosally through the superior aspect of the divided duodenum and held in artery forceps. A similar horizontal angle suture is inserted through the greater curve aspect of the divided gastric remnant and correspondingly into the inferior border of the duodenum, and is held in artery forceps. These angle stitches are placed about 5 mm from the cut edge in each case. The divided ends of the stomach and duodenum should come together without tension but during placement of the sutures a gap of 2–3 cm should be maintained to allow accurate placement of the posterior layer.

24 The posterior row of serosubmucosal sutures is inserted serially. A mid point marking suture may be of help. The distance between the sutures is approximately 5 mm, but according to discrepancy in size this may be larger on the gastric side and smaller on the duodenum. In each case about 5 mm of tissue is incorporated. The sutures are placed serially and held by an assistant. When all have been placed they are tied and cut. The knots lie on the luminal aspect but are overlaid to a considerable extent by the mucosa.

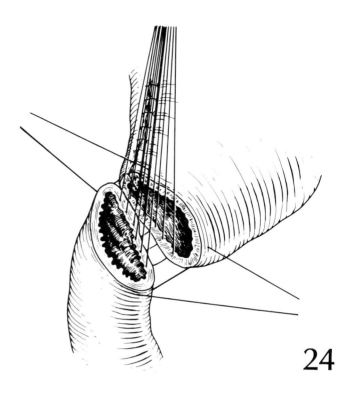

24

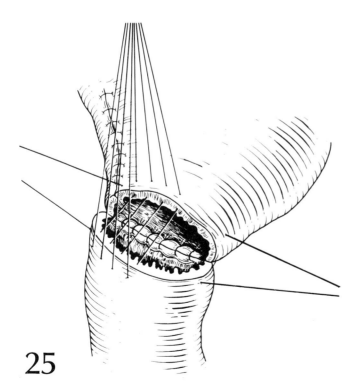

25

25 The anterior row of sutures is placed in a similar fashion in the serosubmucosal plane. A mid point marking suture is helpful in achieving accurate suture placement, particularly if the size of the lumen exceeds 3 cm. When the anterior sutures have been inserted, the angle sutures are tied and held. The anterior sutures are then tied serially and cut.

26 The angle sutures are cut and the anastomosis is complete.

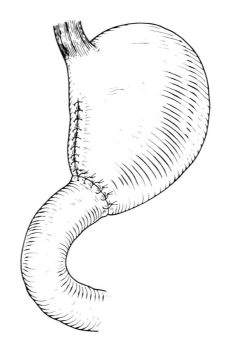

26

Gastrojejunal anastomosis with Roux loop

This is performed in the same way as a gastroduodenal anastomosis.

Gastrojejunal anastomosis to loop of jejunum (Pólya/Billroth II)

After identification of the duodenojejunal junction, a loop of proximal jejunum is brought in either a retrocolic or antecolic direction to lie in lax apposition with the distal stomach in an isoperistaltic direction.

27 An angle suture is placed through the corners of the reconstructed lesser curve as for a Billroth I anastomosis and inserted as a horizontal serosubmucosal suture through the jejunum on the antimesenteric border. A horizontal serosubmucosal angle suture is placed on the greater curve aspect of the gastric remnant and horizontally through the jejunum at the proximal end of the proposed enterotomy. A longitudinal enterotomy of 5–6 cm is made. The posterior row of interrupted serosubmucosal sutures is inserted serially, tied on the luminal aspect and cut. A mid point marking suture may be used to subdivide the anastomosis.

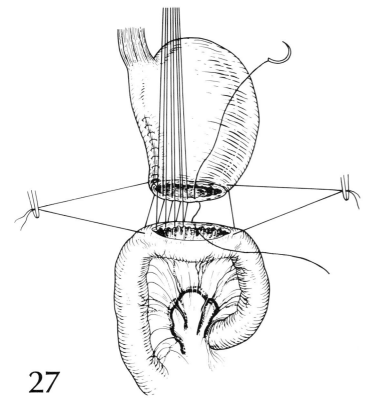

27

28 The anterior sutures are inserted serially. When the anterior sutures have been placed the angle sutures are tied and held.

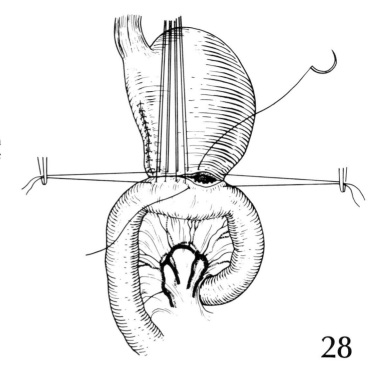

28

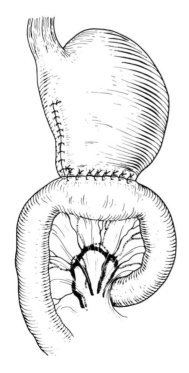

29

29 The anterior row of sutures is tied serially and cut, the angle sutures are cut and the anastomosis is complete.

Jejunal interposition

It is occasionally necessary in reconstructive gastric surgery to interpose a segment of proximal jejunum between the gastric remnant and the duodenum. The gastrojejunal anastomosis is made as shown in *Illustrations 23–26*, and the jejunoduodenal anastomosis is a straightforward end-to-end anastomosis.

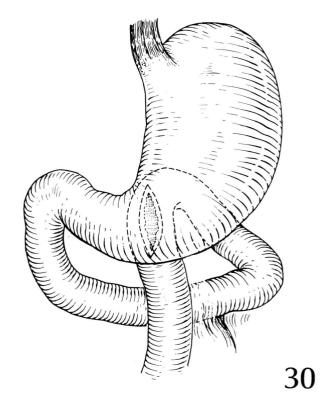

GASTROJEJUNOSTOMY

30 The anastomosis to be described is retrocolic with a vertical stoma in the gastric antrum. Accessibility together with the profuse vascularity of the stomach makes a continuous single layer technique attractive.

30

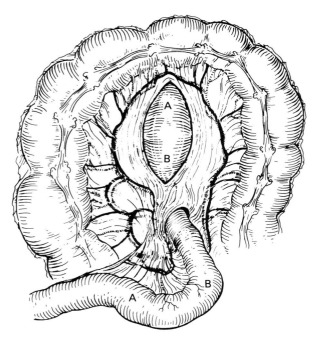

31 The greater omentum and transverse colon are raised to expose the posterior aspect of the transverse mesocolon. Both layers are incised vertically, taking care to avoid the middle colic vessels and tributaries, and to expose the posterior aspect of the gastric antrum. The greater curve is at A and the lesser at B. The alignment of the proposed anastomosis is shown by A and B on the jejunum.

31

32 The greater and lesser curves are lightly grasped with a pair of Babcock's tissue forceps and rotated to align the stomach with the proximal jejunum. The proximal jejunum is identified at the duodenojejunal flexure and a convenient segment isolated between the Babcock's forceps. The jejunum is disposed afferent end to lesser curve and should lie with laxity. The afferent loop need not be excessively short with the anastomosis close to the duodenojejunal junction.

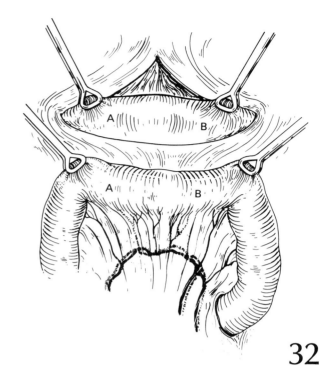

32

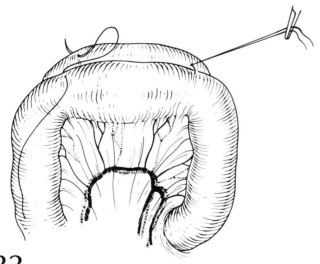

33

33 An angle suture is inserted serosubmucosally through the jejunum proximally and the posterior wall of the stomach close to the lesser curve. This is tied and held. A similar suture is inserted through the jejunum and close to the greater curve of the stomach. Strips soaked in topical antiseptic are laid round the anastomotic site.

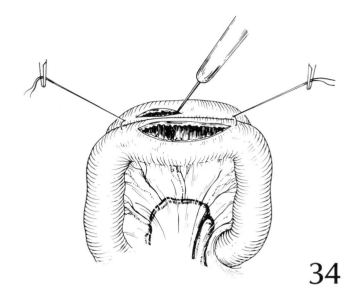

34 The jejunum and then the stomach are opened with cutting diathermy. The gastric contents are aspirated with suction, taking care to avoid contamination. Haemostasis is secured with accurate diathermy of the submucosal vessels.

34

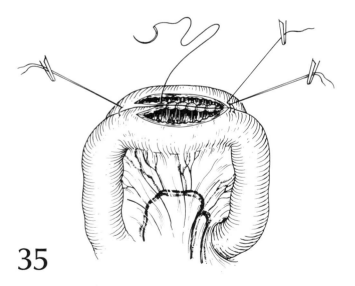

35

35 The anastomosis is started at the proximal end of the jejunotomy with a continuous 3/0 polydioxanone suture. The suture is passed from the serosal aspect of the jejunum to emerge on the gastric serosa and knotted on the outside; it is then passed through the gastric wall to emerge on the mucosal aspect. Continuous insertion then begins at approximately 5-mm intervals. The suture is place in the serosubmucosal plane on the jejunal side but may include the mucosa on the gastric side if necessary for complete haemostasis.

36 At the corner a loop of suture is held on the serosal aspect of the jejunum and the needle is passed through the stomach to emerge on the mucosal aspect. It is then passed through the jejunum from the mucosal aspect and the suture is locked at the corner by passing it through the loop on the serosal aspect.

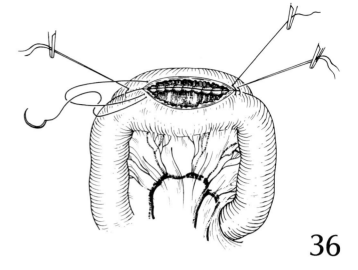

36

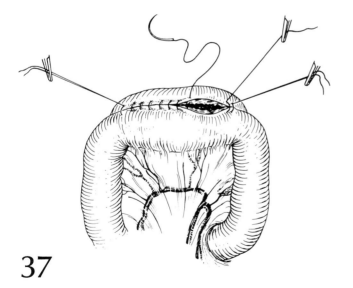

37

37 The direction of suturing is then reversed, passing back through the jejunum to the stomach on the anterior aspect of the anastomosis. Serosubmucosal placement eliminates mucosal pouting.

38 Once the final stitch has been placed the continuous suture is knotted close to its proximal end.

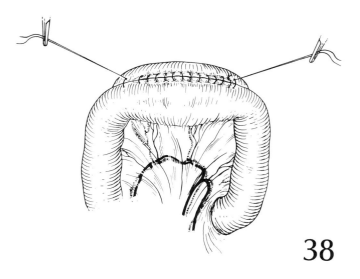

38

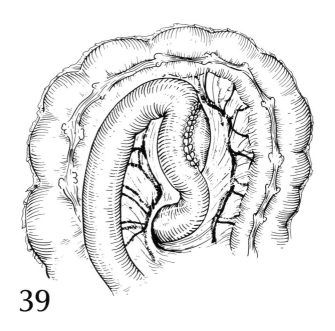

39

39 The angle sutures are cut and the stomach allowed to return to its normal position as shown in *Illustration 30*.

Postoperative care

Following total gastrectomy with oesophagojejunal anastomosis oral fluids are withheld for 7 days until a radiographic contrast study has shown an intact anastomosis. In contrast, oral fluids are commenced after 24 h following partial gastrectomy or revisional gastric surgery.

References

1. Irwin ST, Krukowski ZH, Matheson NA. Single layer anastomosis in the upper gastrointestinal tract. *Br J Surg* 1990; 77: 643–4.

2. Matheson NA, McIntosh CA, Krukowski ZH. Continuing experience with single layer appositional anastomosis in the large bowel. *Br J Surg* 1985; 72(Suppl): S104–6.

Stapling techniques for gastric anastomoses

J. L. Chassin MD
Chairman, Department of Surgery, The New York Hospital Medical Center of Queens, New York, USA

STAPLED OESOPHAGOJEJUNAL ANASTOMOSIS AFTER TOTAL GASTRECTOMY

After total gastrectomy it is essential that an oesophago-jejunal anastomosis be constructed in the Roux-en-Y fashion. If the descending limb of the jejunum between the oesophagojejunostomy and the jejunojejunostomy measures 60–70 cm, the danger of bile refluxing into the oesophagus is eliminated. Reflux of bile produces a serious and painful oesophagitis. A side-to-end oesophagojejunal anastomosis can be constructed efficiently and safely using the EEA device if proper precautions are observed. Ideally, the cut end of the oesophagus will have a diameter sufficiently large to admit a 28-mm or 31-mm diameter EEA cartridge. If a 25-mm (EEA-25) cartridge is used, the anastomosis will be too small to accommodate passage of all of the foods generally consumed by 10–15% of patients on a regular diet. Correction requires postoperative dilatation of the stricture. In most patients, gentle dilatation of the oesophagus in the operating room will permit the passage of the EEA-28 cartridge. It is dangerous to perform vigorous dilatation as this may result in an occult tear in the lining of the oesophagus and possible postoperative leakage.

Preparation of oesophagus

After digital dilatation of the lumen of the oesophagus, the diameter of the lumen is measured using the sizer. Sizers are produced with diameters of 25, 28 and 31 mm. Lubricating jelly is used to facilitate the passage of the instrument into the oesophagus. This will determine which cartridge is to be used.

Insertion of EEA device

1 A 2/0 polypropylene (Prolene) purse-string suture is inserted through the full thickness of the oesophagus, starting at the top about 3–4 mm from the cut end of the oesophagus. Bites of about 4 mm are taken, and care is taken to ensure that the mucosal layer is caught by each bite of suture material. Four guy sutures are inserted for traction at 1, 4, 7 and 10 o'clock, and a clamp is applied to each.

The cut end of the jejunum is gently dilated using lubricated fingertips and the EEA sizers are inserted to determine whether the lumen of the jejunum will in fact admit the selected cartridge. The anvil of the EEA cartridge is then removed and lubrication applied to the instrument. The EEA device is passed gently into the lumen of the jejunum. When the device has been inserted about 6 cm, the wing-nut is rotated in a counterclockwise fashion so that the central rod will protrude from the cartridge and impinge on the antimesenteric border of the jejunum. When this has been confirmed by palpation, electrocautery is used to make an incision over the rod that will be just large enough to permit passage of the rod through the wall of the jejunum. A small purse-string suture of polypropylene is inserted into the jejunum close to the rod and the anvil is attached to the protruding rod. It is important to ensure that the screw fastening the anvil to the rod is tight. A serious error in construction of this anastomosis can result if the mucosa at point Y is caught by the advancing cartridge and taken to point X. If this occurs, firing the stapler will occlude the efferent limb of the jejunum and the anastomosis will be completely obstructed.

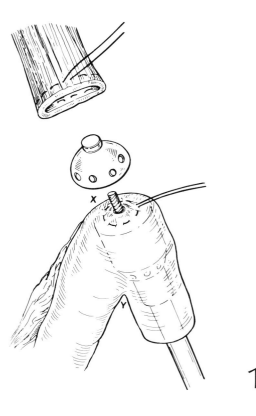

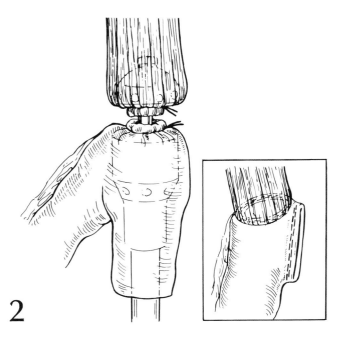

Passage of anvil into oesophagus

2 The lumen of the oesophagus is again gently dilated with lubricated fingertips. The assistant grasps the four clamps attached to the guy sutures to stabilize the oesophagus and the anvil of the EEA device is gently inserted into the oesophagus. When this has been accomplished, the oesophageal purse-string suture is tied snugly around the central rod of the EEA device and the tails of this suture are cut. The guy sutures are then removed.

Firing the EEA device

The wing-nut is turned in a clockwise direction until the space between the anvil and the cartridge has been properly closed. It is necessary to ascertain that no extraneous tissue has been trapped between the cartridge and the anvil before this closure, after which the EEA device is fired. The wing-nut is then turned in a counterclockwise direction for about seven half-turns. The instrument is rotated, the anvil disengaged from the anastomosis, and the EEA device removed from the operative field.

The anvil is detached from the cartridge and the two doughnuts of tissue removed. Both doughnuts should be demonstrated to form complete rings of tissue if the stapling device has performed properly.

Checking the integrity of the anastomosis

The index finger is inserted through the open end of the jejunum, through the anastomosis and into the oesophagus. The anastomotic ring should be intact. The finger is then withdrawn just enough to allow insertion into the efferent segment of the jejunum. If the XY error described in *Illustration 1* has occurred, then entrance into the efferent segment is completely obstructed by an erroneously placed staple line. In this case, the anastomosed segment is excised and a new oesophagojejunal anastomosis is performed.

If no errors are detected by palpation, a TA 55 stapling device is applied to the blind segment of jejunum at a point about 1.5 cm proximal to the oesophagojejunostomy (*Illustration 2*). This is then closed and fired, and the surplus jejunum excised along the stapling device. The everted mucosa noted in the staple line is lightly electrocoagulated and the anastomosis inspected on all sides to detect any visible defect. An additional check of the integrity of the anastomosis can be conducted by asking the anaesthetist to inject 1–200 ml of methylene blue solution through the nasogastric tube into the oesophagus while the efferent limb of jejunum is occluded either by manual compression or a non-crushing Doyen clamp. Leakage of blue dye from the anastomosis or the stapled proximal end of jejunum may then be seen.

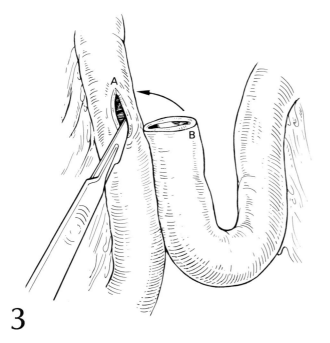

3

Construction of Roux-en-Y jejunojejunostomy

3   A point on the efferent segment of jejunum 60 cm distal to the oesophagojejunostomy is identified and a longitudinal 1.5-cm incision using either scalpel or electrocautery is made on the antimesenteric surface of the jejunum. The proximal cut end of jejunum is identified at point B and the open end of jejunum is aligned so that it points in a cephalad direction. This segment is then apposed to the antimesenteric border of the descending limb of jejunum adjacent to the incision at point A.

4 One fork of the GIA stapling device is inserted into the jejunal incision at point A (*Illustration 3*) and the other fork into the open end of the proximal jejunum. The device is closed, fired and removed.

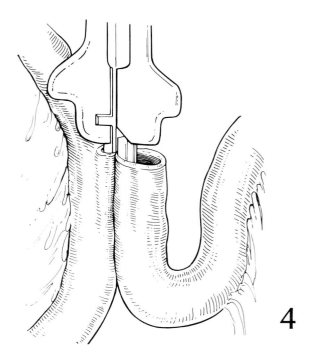

4

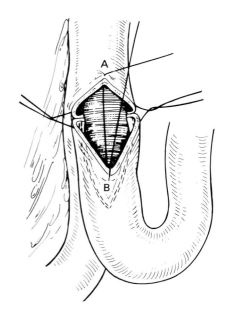

5

5 This stapling accomplishes the posterior layer of a front-to-back anastomosis between the proximal and efferent segments of jejunum. Guy sutures are placed to capture the ends of the GIA staple line at points C and D (*Illustration 6*). A third guy suture is inserted to bisect the anastomosis.

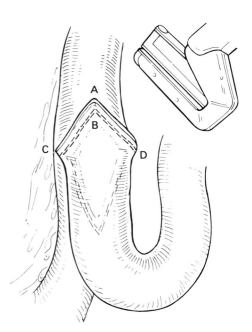

6

6 Tying this suture will approximate point A to point B. A clamp is attached to each of the three guy sutures and additional Allis' clamps are placed along the everted tissue from points A to C. A TA 55 stapler with 3.5-mm staples is then applied and this portion of the anastomosis is closed in eversion. The stapler should be placed deep to the guy sutures at points AB and C. The redundant tissue is excised but the guy suture is preserved at point AB. The stapling device is removed and the everted mucosa is lightly electrocoagulated. Several Allis clamps are applied to the everted jejunal tissue from point AB to point D. Again, the stapling device should be deep to the guy suture at point AB as well as point D. When the stapler has been properly positioned, the staples are fired and the surplus jejunal tissue is excised. The everted mucosa is lightly electrocoagulated and the stapling device removed.

All aspects of the anastomosis are inspected carefully. A large functional end-to-side anastomosis has been constructed. When properly performed this has proved to be a very effective, simple and safe anastomosis.

STAPLED GASTRO-OESOPHAGEAL ANASTOMOSIS AFTER OESOPHAGOGASTRECTOMY

A distressing long-term complication after anastomosis of the oesophagus to the gastric remnant following resection is the regurgitation into the oesophagus of bile and pancreatic secretions. This regurgitation frequently produces an ulcerative oesophagitis that is more painful even than the reflux of acid into the oesophagus. If more than half of the proximal stomach has been removed, end-to-end anastomosis of the oesophagus to a small gastric remnant is highly likely to produce a severe oesophagitis. (To avoid this complication, it may be preferable to perform a total gastrectomy with Roux-en-Y oesophagojejunostomy which will avoid reflux oesophagitis.)

If a gastric remnant is to be retained, an extensive Kocher manoeuvre is performed after lesion resection, and the head of the pancreas and proximal duodenum are elevated in a cephalad direction. The cut end of the oesophagus is brought down over the anterior surface of the gastric remnant. If an end-to-side gastro-oesophageal anastomosis can be performed at a point at least 6 cm distal to the proximal cut end of the gastric remnant, gastro-oesophageal reflux will be minimized.

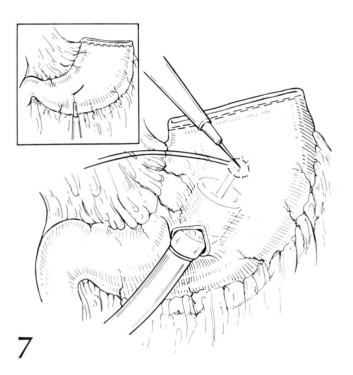

7

Construction of the EEA anastomosis

7   To insert the EEA stapling device into the gastric pouch, a 3-cm incision is required. If a Heineke–Mikulicz pyloroplasty is planned, the longitudinal incision is made across the pylorus using electrocautery at this time, and the EEA cartridge is inserted through this incision. Otherwise, electrocautery is used to make an incision of 3 cm in the anterior wall of the lower half of the gastric remnant.

The anvil is removed from the tip of the EEA device which is then inserted into the gastric incision. The wing-nut at the base of the stapling device is rotated in a counterclockwise direction so that the central rod protrudes from the cartridge. A 2/0 polypropylene purse-string suture is made in the stomach around the tip of the rod and electrocautery is used to make a stab wound directly over the central rod. The rod is pushed through this stab wound and the anvil reattached to the rod. The stab wound should be made at a point 5–6 cm distal to the proximal margin of the gastric remnant. The purse-string suture is tied around the central rod and the tails of this suture are cut.

8 A 2/0 polypropylene purse-string suture is placed in the distal end of the oesophagus. Each stitch should include the full thickness of the oesophagus, including the mucosa. The tails of this stitch are grasped with a haemostat and guy sutures are inserted just deep to the purse-string suture at 2, 5, 8 and 11 o'clock. A haemostat is attached to each of the guy sutures and the assistant positions these four sutures so that the lumen of the oesophagus is held wide open. It is helpful to dilate the oesophagus gently with lubricated Hegar dilators. Vigorous dilatation may induce tears in the mucosa. If a tear is undetected, it may contribute to a postoperative anastomotic leak.

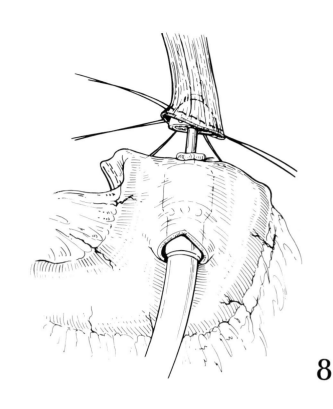

8

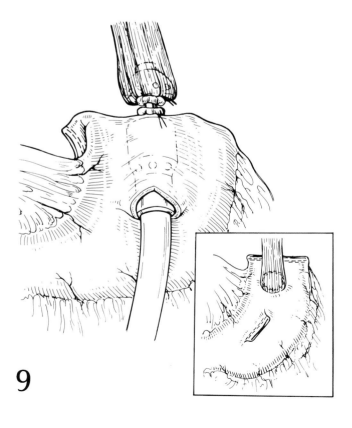

9

9 The lubricated anvil is inserted into the oesophagus, the purse-string suture tied and the guy sutures removed. The wing-nut on the stapling device is rotated so that the anvil is properly approximated to the cartridge, and the staples are fired. The wing-nut on the stapling device is then rotated to separate the anvil from the cartridge and the anvil is disengaged from the newly fashioned anastomosis. The stapling device is removed from the stomach. The two doughnuts of tissue are removed from the cartridge. If either of the doughnuts is not intact, there may be a defect in the anastomosis. If this possibility exists the anaesthetist should instil several hundred millilitres of methylene blue solution and the entire anastomosis should be observed to detect a possible leak. If there is a defect in the anastomosis, this is repaired with several sutures of 4/0 silk.

Closure of gastrotomy

Several Allis' clamps are applied to approximate the gastrotomy incision with the mucosa in eversion. A TA 55 stapler with 4.8-mm staples is placed beneath the Allis' clamps, closed and fired. The tissue protruding from the stapling device is excised using a scalpel and the everted mucosa is lightly electrocoagulated before removal of the stapling device.

In some cases this anastomosis can be expedited by using the CEEA stapling device. With the CEEA technique the anvil is detached from the cartridge and is then passed into the oesophagus. The purse-string suture is tied around the anvil and the cartridge is passed into the gastric remnant as described above. By rotating the wing-nut, a sharp spear can be made to protrude from the cartridge through the gastric wall. The anvil is then reattached to the cartridge. Otherwise, the technique is the same as described for the EEA device.

Anastomosis when the oesophagus is narrow

When the lumen of the oesophagus is too narrow to permit the passage of anything but an EEA-25 cartridge, the method of choice of constructing a gastro-oesophageal anastomosis is the GIA technique, as described below. Using this technique, a large anastomosis can be constructed in spite of the smaller lumen of the oesophagus. When a 25-mm cartridge is used, a significant number of patients will require postoperative dilatation of stricture.

Gastro-oesophageal anastomosis using the GIA technique[1]

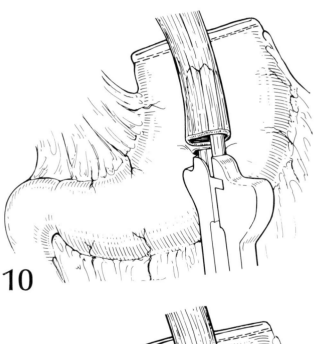

10 Successful use of the GIA technique for gastro-oesophageal anastomosis requires that the distal end of the oesophagus reaches a point at least 6 cm caudal to the cephalad margin of the gastric remnant. A longitudinal incision of 1.5 cm is made in the anterior wall of the stomach just behind the distal margin of the oesophagus using electrocautery. The GIA stapling device is inserted for a distance of about 3.5 cm, with one fork in the gastric remnant and the other in the open lumen of the oesophagus. The device is locked and the staples fired. This manoeuvre accomplishes anastomosis between the back of the oesophagus and the front of the gastric remnant.

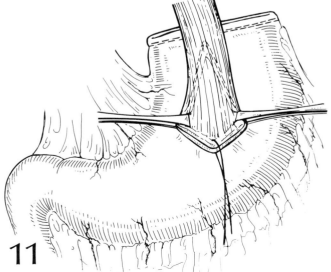

11 The right and left ends of the GIA staple line are grasped in Allis' clamps. The oesophagus and stomach are bisected midway between the two Allis' clamps with a 4/0 guy suture. The remaining defect between the oesophagus and stomach is then closed by triangulation with two applications of a TA 55 stapling device as now described.

12 Additional Allis' clamps are applied between the left Allis' clamp and the guy suture to approximate the oesophagus and stomach in eversion. A TA 55 stapling device is placed just deep to the Allis' clamp and the guy suture, closed and fired.

The redundant tissue protruding from the stapler is excised with Mayo scissors, but the guy suture is not cut. The everted mucosa is lightly electrocoagulated.

Additional Allis' clamps are applied to close the remaining defect between the stomach and the oesophagus. A TA 55 stapler is placed deep to the guy suture and the Allis' clamps. The stapling device is then fired and the protruding tissue excised with Mayo scissors together with the guy suture. The everted mucosa is lightly electrocoagulated and the stapling device removed.

Staples of 4.8 mm are used for these anastomoses unless the thickness of the stomach and oesophagus are significantly less than average.

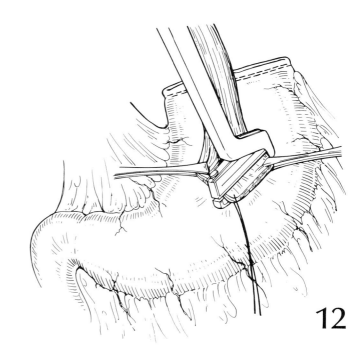

12

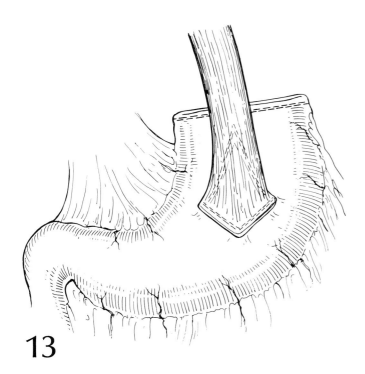

13

13 The completed back-to-front gastro-oesophageal anastomosis is checked for integrity by injection of several hundred millilitres of methylene blue solution into the stomach through the nasogastric tube.

After oesophagogastrectomy, 15% of patients experience persistent difficulty in gastric emptying, so most surgeons perform some type of drainage procedure. The author prefers a pyloromyotomy.

STAPLED GASTROJEJUNOSTOMY AFTER BILLROTH II GASTRECTOMY

Resection of stomach

14 The omentum is detached from the greater curvature of the stomach as described in the chapters on pp. 178–188 and 436–449. The desired point of transection of the stomach is determined, ensuring that the nasogastric tube is retracted by the anaesthetist above the line of transection. A Payr clamp is applied across the body of the stomach, and a TA90 stapler 1 cm cephalad to the Payr clamp. Using 4.8-mm staples, the stapler is closed and fired. The stomach is then incised flush with the staples and the stapler is removed. The everted gastric mucosa is lightly electrocoagulated.

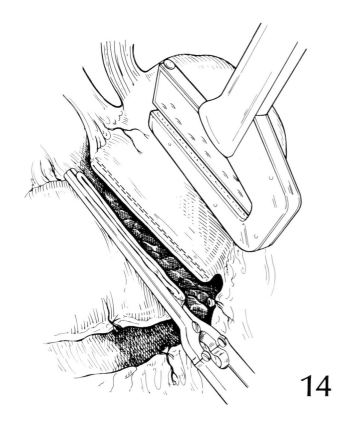

14

Duodenal closure

15 After dissection of the stomach and duodenum off the pancreas for a distance of 2–3 cm beyond the pylorus, a TA 55 stapler with 4.8-mm staples is applied to the duodenum beyond the pylorus. Although stapling a duodenum which is mildly or moderately thickened is a safe procedure, in some patients with chronic ulcer disease the duodenum is remarkably thickened, to the extent that a stapler will devitalize the tissue. In such rare cases, stapling is contraindicated. When the stapler has been applied and fired, a straight clamp is placed across the proximal duodenum or pylorus and the duodenum divided flush with the stapler. The stapler is then removed and the everted mucosa lightly electrocoagulated. It is not necessary to invert the staple line with a layer of sutures.

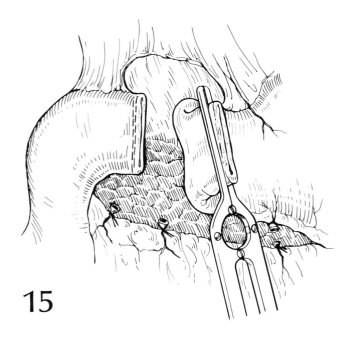

15

Stapled gastrojejunostomy

A 1-cm transverse stab wound is made with the electrocoagulator on the posterior surface of the gastric pouch 3 cm proximal to the gastric staple line. A second 1-cm stab wound is then made on the antimesenteric border of the jejunum.

16 The GIA stapler is inserted with one fork in the gastric stab wound and the other in the jejunal stab wound. The stapler is locked and a 4/0 atraumatic silk suture is inserted between the stomach and jejunum just beyond the tip of the stapling device. The stapler is fired. This will produce a side-to-side anastomosis between the gastric pouch and the jejunum about 5 cm in diameter. The stapling device is removed and the GIA staple line through the stab wound is carefully inspected. Bleeding points are controlled with careful electrocoagulation or with a 5/0 atraumatic polyglactin (Vicryl) suture. If there is diffuse bleeding along the entire staple line, the staple line can be oversewn with a continuous 5/0 polyglactin suture to achieve haemostasis. Significant bleeding is uncommon.

It is important that the anastomosis is constructed at a point no closer than 3 cm from the distal termination of the gastric pouch, otherwise the blood supply of a thin strip of stomach between the anastomosis and the gastric staple line will be inadequate.

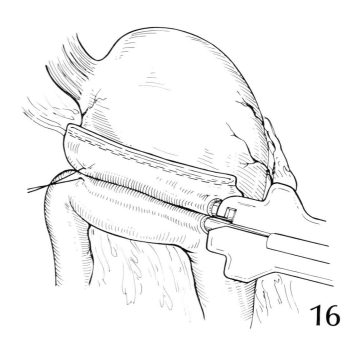

16

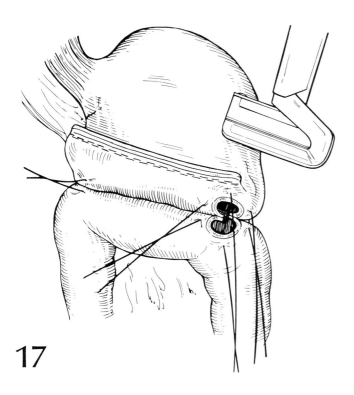

17

Closure of stab wound

17 The stab wound between the stomach and jejunum is closed with a TA 55 stapler, usually with 3.5-mm staples. To expedite this step it is necessary to identify both ends of the GIA staple line and to capture them either with silk stitches or Allis' clamps. One or two stitches or Allis' clamps are inserted to close the remaining defect with the mucosa in eversion. The TA 55 stapler is applied beneath either the guy sutures or the Allis' clamps, closed and fired. Redundant tissue protruding from the stapler is excised and the everted mucosa is lightly electrocoagulated. The stapling device is removed.

STAPLED HEINEKE–MIKULICZ PYLOROPLASTY

18 A 5–6-cm longitudinal incision is made on the anterior wall of the gastroduodenal junction using electrocautery. The incision should be centred over the pyloric muscle. Guy sutures encircling the cephalad cut end of the pyloric muscle and the caudal termination of the divided pyloric sphincter are inserted, and a third guy suture is placed through the full thickness of the gastric and duodenal walls at the midpoint between the two previously placed sutures. The middle guy suture approximating stomach and duodenum is tied, and additional Allis' clamps are applied to the full thicknesses of stomach and duodenum to close the defect with the mucosa in eversion.

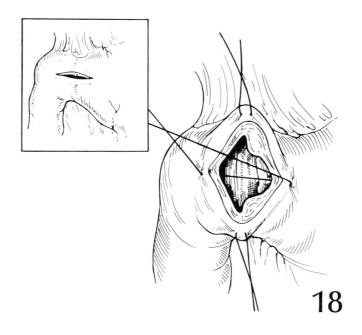

18

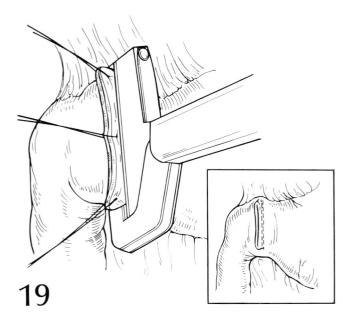

19

19 A TA 55 stapler is placed just deep to the Allis' clamps and the guy sutures. The stapler is closed and fired, and a scalpel is used to excise the redundant tissue flush with the stapler. The everted mucosa is lightly electrocoagulated and the stapling device removed.

STAPLED GASTROJEJUNOSTOMY

20 The transverse colon is elevated and the avascular portion to the left of the middle colic artery is identified. An 8–10-cm transverse incision is made through the avascular mesocolon and the posterior wall of the lower gastric antrum extracted through this incision.

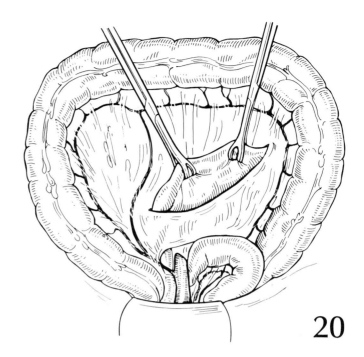

20

21 To fix the mesentery of the colon to the gastric wall throughout the circumference of the protruding stomach, 4/0 interrupted sutures are applied.

The ligament of Treitz is identified and a segment of proximal jejunum, 10–15-cm distal to this ligament, is placed adjacent to the stomach. A 1-cm longitudinal stab wound is made on the antimesenteric border of the jejunum using electrocautery, and a similar 1-cm stab wound is made through the wall of the adjacent stomach. The GIA stapling device is inserted with one fork in the stomach and the other in the jejunum. The stapling device is locked and a 4/0 silk suture is inserted to fix the stomach and jejunum near to the tip of the stapling device. The stapling device is fired, removed and the GIA staple line is inspected for bleeding.

Allis' clamps are applied to the left and right ends of the GIA staple line, along with one or two additional Allis' clamps, and the stab wound is closed with the mucosa in eversion. A TA 55 stapler is placed just deep to the Allis' clamps, the jaws of the stapler closed and the staples fired. The redundant tissue is excised flush with the stapler, and the everted mucosa is lightly electrocoagulated. The stapling device is then removed to complete construction of a large gastrojejunal anastomosis.

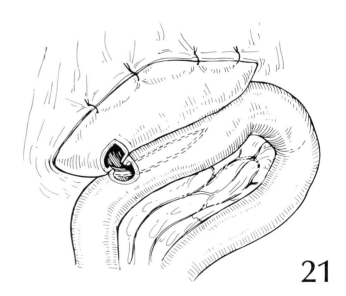

21

References

1. Chassin JL. Stapling technique for esophagogastrostomy after esophagogastric resection. *Am J Surg* 1978; 136: 399–404.

Further reading

Chassin JL. *Operative Strategy in General Surgery: An Expositive Atlas*. 2nd edn. New York: Springer-Verlag, 1993.

Illustrations by Paul Richardson

Small intestine as a replacement after oesophageal resection

P. G. Devitt FRACS, FRCS
Senior Lecturer in Surgery, Department of Surgery, Royal Adelaide Hospital, Adelaide, Australia

Principles and justification

The small intestine is rarely the first choice for interposition after oesophageal resection, but there are instances when it is not practical to use either stomach or colon. These include cases where total gastrectomy and distal oesophagectomy have been performed for lesions at the cardia or where there has been previous distal gastric resection. Similarly, colon may not be available because of previous resection or extensive diverticular disease. Stomach and colon have the advantages of mobility and length over small intestine, but small intestine has a better vascularity than colon and the patient is spared the rigours of bowel preparation.

Operations

JEJUNAL LOOP

1 The jejunum is of limited use for transposition and is only suitable after procedures such as total gastrectomy where no or only a short segment of oesophagus has been resected. No bowel or mesenteric blood vessels are divided. A suitable loop of jejunum, 15–20 cm beyond the duodenojejunal flexure, is brought up to abut against the cut end of the oesophagus. The loop may be brought up retrogradely or in antecolic fashion, whichever is the easier route and where the small intestine can lie without tension or obstruction. A single layer interrupted suture (e.g. 3/0 polydioxanone) is suitable.

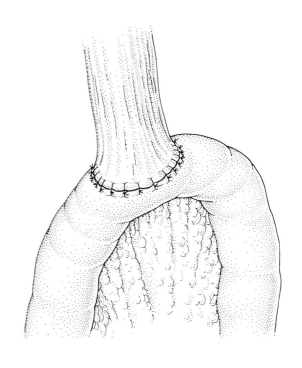

1

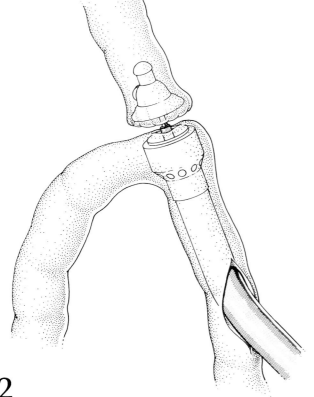

2

2 Alternatively, a stapled anastomosis may be performed, introducing the stapler through a small enterotomy in one of the jejunal limbs.

ROUX-EN-Y

Selection of a segment of small intestine

3 The length of jejunum that can be used for oesophageal replacement will depend on its vascularity and collateral blood supply. One or two vascular arcades can usually be clearly identified in the proximal jejunum and the outer arcade must be preserved when the isolated limb of bowel is fashioned.

The duodenojejunal flexure is identified and a segment of jejunum 10–15 cm distal to the flexure is held up out of the abdomen and transilluminated. The vascular tiers and their connecting vessels are carefully identified. The mesentery on both sides of the connecting vessels is divided and the vessels isolated.

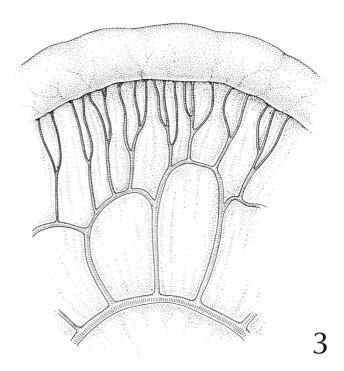

3

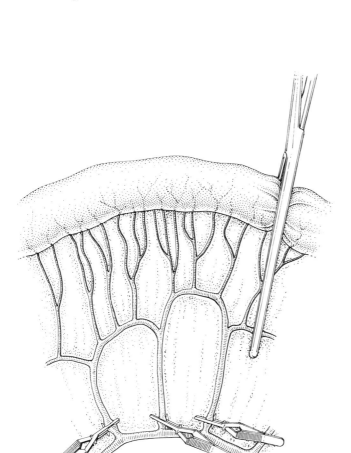

4

4 When a sufficient number (usually three or four) of the vessels have been isolated, the individual vessels are temporarily clamped to allow the viability of the proposed limb of jejunum to be assessed. At the same time a non-crushing clamp must be placed on the distal end of the segment and its adjoining mesentery to occlude the blood supply here as well.

Provided the blood supply is satisfactory, the vessels can be divided and ligated and the segment of jejunum prepared for transposition. Division of four connecting vessels should produce a segment of sufficient length to reach the clavicle without tension. The proximal end of jejunum is divided as far distal to the first isolated vascular arcade as possible. The longest distance is bridged when the transposed segment is taken up in a retrocolic fashion.

It should be remembered that the proximal end of the jejunum will be tethered by its mesentery. Provided sufficient length has been obtained, this tethering can be used to advantage when performing a stapled end-to-side anastomosis (*see Illustration 9*). If every centimetre of transposed jejunum is required and an end-to-end anastomosis is to be made, the terminal vessels in the mesentery are divided to allow the proximal end of the bowel to straighten.

Formation of anastomosis

5 The transverse colon is held up taut and an avascular area in the mesocolon found. A hole large enough to admit the jejunal segment and its length of mesentery is made. If required, the jejunum can be tunnelled behind the body of the pancreas to give better lie and more length. The divided end of the oesophagus has been held in a non-crushing right-angled clamp and a purse-string suture of 2/0 polypropylene is now placed.

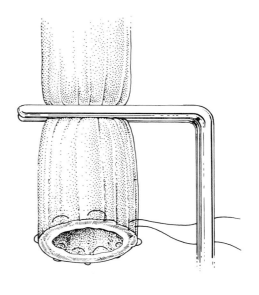

5

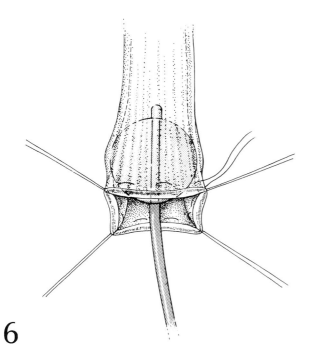

6

6 Four anchoring sutures are inserted to hold the cut end of the oesophagus open and a Foley catheter with a 30-ml balloon is introduced into the oesophagus.

7   The end of the oesophagus is frequently narrowed after the purse-string suture has been inserted and the balloon of the Foley catheter can be inflated and the oesophagus carefully dilated to allow admission of the largest diameter circular stapling device practicable. The anvil and shaft of the stapling device are introduced into the oesophagus and the purse-string suture is drawn tight and tied.

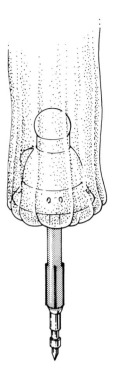

7

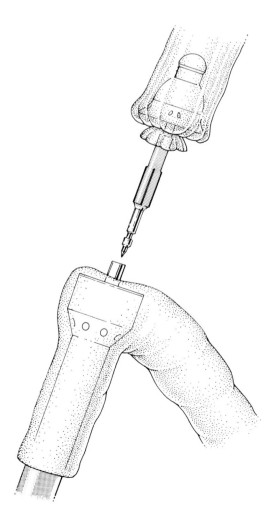

8

8   With the jejunal segment and its mesentery correctly aligned, the stapling device is introduced into the opened end of the jejunum; the point is brought out through the antimesenteric border at the apex of the segment and joined to the shaft and anvil.

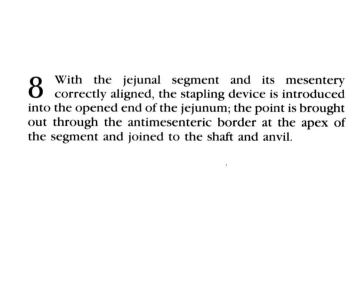

9 On completion of the anastomosis the open end of the jejunum is closed with a linear stapler. Alternatively the jejunum may be closed with a single layer of interrupted sutures.

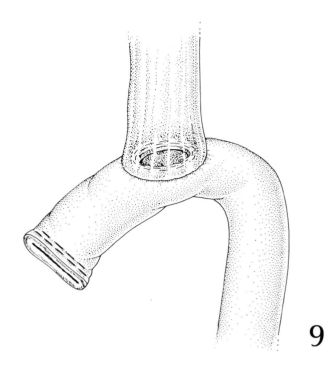

9

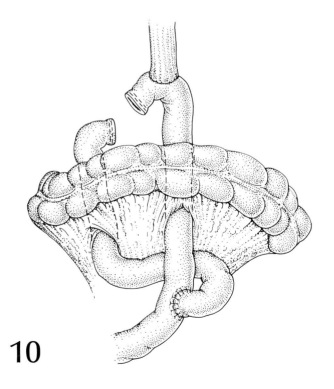

10

10 The apex of the Roux-en-Y is completed with an end-to-side anastomosis placed 40–45 cm down the isolated jejunal segment to minimize the risk of bile reflux. A single layer of interrupted sutures (e.g. 3/0 polydioxanone) provides a suitable anastomosis.

FREE JEJUNAL GRAFT

This is an ideal procedure to perform when a segment of cervical oesophagus and hypopharynx needs to be replaced. If thoracic oesophagus has to be excised, a total oesophagectomy should be undertaken and some other form of replacement, such as gastric or colonic interposition, used.

Two surgical teams are necessary. The first team undertakes the definitive surgery in the neck and prepares the field for jejunal transposition. This involves identification and preservation of the superior and inferior thyroid arteries, one of which will be used for arterial anastomosis. The venous anastomosis will be an end-to-end attachment to a tributary of the internal jugular vein, e.g. the common facial vein.

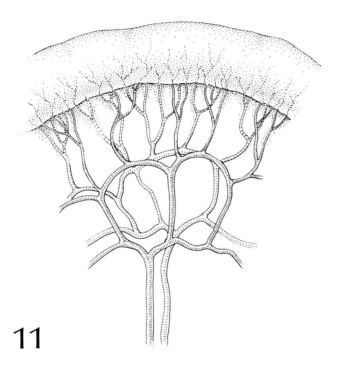

11

11 The second team prepares the abdomen, makes a small midline incision, identifies a proximal loop of jejunum and delivers it into the wound. The proximal jejunum is preferred as there are fewer vascular arcades and larger vessels. A large connecting vessel is sought and traced towards the root of the mesentery. This will be the vascular pedicle of the graft. The mesentery over the artery and vein is divided, fat is cleared away and the vessels are divided.

About 25 cm of jejunum will be required. The bowel for grafting is excised and continuity restored with single-layer interrupted sutures and an end-to-end anastomosis. The abdomen is closed in the standard manner. The graft is not heparinized to minimize the formation of haematoma.

More jejunum will have been prepared for the graft than will be required. It is important not to insert too long a segment, otherwise it will kink and obstruct. A 3–4-cm segment of jejunum will be detached from the remainder of the intestine, but left on the vascular pedicle. At the end of the operation, when the skin has been closed, this short segment will be wrapped in saline-soaked gauze and left on the wound. It can then be checked at regular intervals, when its vascularity will reflect that of the underlying graft. Provided it (and thus the underlying jejunum) remains healthy, it can be excised about 7 days after the operation.

12 The vascular anastomosis is performed first. A microvascular clamp is used to approximate the mesenteric vein to the prepared tributary of the internal jugular vein and an interrupted end-to-end anastomosis performed with 10/0 nylon. The arterial anastomosis to the thyroid artery is then performed in a similar manner.

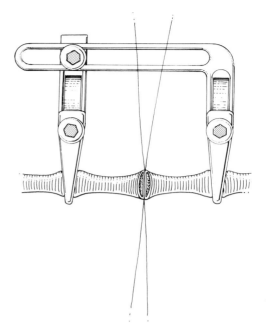

12

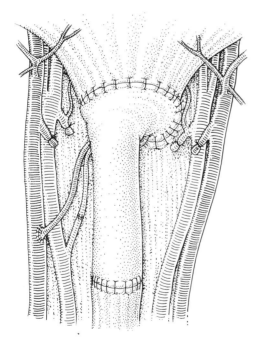

13

13 Both ends of the jejunum are now anastomosed to the digestive tract with a single layer of interrupted 3/0 polydioxanone. The proximal end of the jejunum will need to be opened along its antimesenteric border to accommodate the large defect of the base of the tongue and pharynx. The distal end of the jejunum can be anastomosed end-to-end to the stump of cervical oesophagus.

Postoperative care

Postoperative care and complications are discussed in the chapter on pp. 39–44.

Illustrations by Mary Jean McFadden

Use of colon as an oesophageal replacement

Jeffrey A. Hagen MD
Esophageal Fellow, Department of Surgery, University of Southern California School of Medicine, Los Angeles, California, USA

Scott Johnson MD
Esophageal Fellow, Department of Surgery, University of Southern California School of Medicine, Los Angeles, California, USA

Tom R. DeMeester MD
Professor and Chairman, Department of Surgery, University of Southern California School of Medicine, Los Angeles, California, USA

History

The use of long segments of colon for replacement or bypass of all or part of the thoracic oesophagus was introduced independently by Kelling[1] and Vulliet[2] in 1911. Subsequently, the interposed colon has emerged as a durable, well functioning substitute for the oesophagus. Initially it was used in patients with malignancy of the upper oesophagus. Subsequently, with refinements in technique and improved results it, rather than the stomach, has been used for an oesophageal substitute in advanced benign disease or early malignancy arising in the distal oesophagus, cardia and proximal stomach, particulary when it is expected that the replacement must function for a decade or more.

Two factors that have, over time, emerged as being crucial to the success of a colonic interposition are the reliability of the blood supply to the colonic graft and the ability of the graft to propel food effectively from the pharynx to the stomach. With careful attention to preoperative preparation and intraoperative technical detail the operation can be performed with low morbidity and mortality rates and excellent long-term function.

Overall, the operation is associated with a 5% mortality rate, often due to the run down physiological state of the patient from repeated pulmonary insults in those with reflux disease or malnutrition in those with carcinoma. With better patient selection and the use of preoperative mesenteric angiography the mortality rate has been reduced to 2%. The complication rate is relatively low with a leakage rate of 1.5% in one of the three anastomoses and a 2% rate of graft necrosis. These results have given confidence to recommend colonic interposition in patients with benign oesophageal diseases refractory to more conservative measures. This is particularly so if a vagal-sparing oesophagectomy can be performed. This allows normal gastric and bowel function after colonic interposition and provides, without doubt, the best oesophageal replacement from a functional point of view.

Principles and justification

A vagal-sparing oesophagectomy is performed by dividing the oesophagus in the neck and the gastro-oesophageal junction in the abdomen, sparing the vagal nerves. The isolated oesophagus is removed by passing a vein stripper up through the oesophagus from a small incision in the gastro-oesophageal junction, securing it to the distal portion of the divided cervical oesophagus, and invaginating the oesophagus as it is pulled through the oesophageal hiatus of the diaphragm. The vagal nerves are sheared off as the muscular wall turns in during the invagination process. The remaining tunnel is dilated with a 90 ml Foley catheter to make room for the colonic interposition. This allows the colon to be anastomosed to a fully innervated stomach. The resulting function is excellent. The procedure is applicable only to patients with benign disease who have not had their vagal nerves divided or do not have delayed gastric emptying from other causes.

More commonly the colon is anastomosed to a denervated stomach and the stomach empties slowly because of previous or concomitant vagotomy performed as part of an oesophagectomy for cancer. This situation results in the regurgitation of gastric contents back up through the interposed colon. Many of the problems ascribed to colonic interposition are the result of poor gastric emptying. Because of this the authors routinely perform a two-thirds proximal gastric resection whenever a colonic interposition is performed to a stomach that is denervated. This gives a better functional result in that the colonic interposition functions as a contracting reservoir for the retained antrum which continues its own innate 3 contractions/min, maintaining its pump function.

The most common symptom after oesophageal replacement with colon is the sensation of fullness or pressure following meals. This complaint occurs in those patients who have had a vagotomy and is exaggerated if they ingest too large an amount of food at one time. This is because of the limited reservoir capacity of the colon compared with the stomach. The complaint does not occur if the colon is attached to an innervated stomach. The symptom is often interpreted incorrectly as dysphagia, but true dysphagia is uncommon after colonic interposition and, when it occurs, is usually due to an anastomotic stricture or redundancy of the graft.

One consequence of transposing the stomach or colon into the chest to re-establish gastrointestinal continuity is the development of gastritis or colitis secondary to duodenogastric reflux. This can occur even when a pyloroplasty has not been performed. The complication results from a pressure differential that develops across the oesophageal hiatus, between the negative intrathoracic stomach or colon and the positive intra-abdominal duodenum. As a consequence, duodenal contents tend to flow into the stomach or colon. The complication is unlikely to occur after colonic interposition following a vagal-sparing oesophagectomy because the stomach and duodenum remain innervated and undisturbed in their normal abdominal location.

Indications

Clinical situations in which the colon is recommended as an oesophageal substitute are: (1) when stomach is not available; (2) when gastrointestinal continuity is re-established after a curative resection of a malignant tumour of the distal oesophagus, cardia or proximal stomach; (3) when gastrointestinal continuity is re-established using the substernal route; (4) when the oesophageal replacement must last for a decade or more; and (5) when a vagal-sparing oesophageal resection can be performed.

Contraindications

Absolute contraindications to colonic interposition are the presence of intrinsic colonic disease, such as inflammatory bowel disease, or malignancy, and inadequate arterial blood supply. In the latter patients, a segment of right colon based on the middle colic vessels can often be utilized instead of the standard left colonic segment based on the inferior mesenteric artery. Other options include the use of a free jejunal graft or the stomach, if it is available.

Relative contraindications include portal hypertension, extensive diverticular disease and multiple colonic polyps. Mild diverticulosis without extensive inflammatory changes and the presence of a few colonic polyps that can be removed before surgery do not preclude the use of the colon for interposition. Advanced age or the presence of severe cardiac or pulmonary disease are also relative contraindications. In these patients, the additional surgical dissection and operative risk is not warranted because their life expectancy makes it unlikely that the replacement must last longer than a decade.

Choice of colonic segment to be interposed

The choice of colonic segment to be used centres around the reliability of the respective vascular pedicles. In this respect the authors feel that the use of the left colon based on the left colic artery and vein, placed in an isoperistaltic fashion, is superior. In the initial report of the procedure, Kelling described an isoperistaltic left colonic transplant, while Vulliet described an antiperistaltic colonic interposition utilizing the transverse colon. Vulliet stated that the procedure was technically easier, and that the functional result was the same, since the colon does not normally exhibit peristalsis. Since that time studies have shown that the colon is not simply an inert tube, especially when challenged by a variety of stimuli; it is active in peristalsis, with a frequency that seems to increase the longer it is in place. In fact, in patients with a long-standing antiperistaltic colonic interposition, peristaltic movement of a barium bolus has been shown to proceed against gravity, towards the pharynx, resulting in choking and chronic aspiration. Consequently, an isoperistaltic interposed colonic segment should always be used.

1a, b The importance of a reliable vascular pedicle for the success of the colonic interposition cannot be overemphasized. An arteriogram of the coeliac axis and superior and inferior mesenteric arteries is of help in directing the choice of the colonic segment to be used. Experience in the authors' hospital, and that of others[3], indicates that the incidence of graft ischaemia is lowest after the use of the left colon based on the inferior mesenteric artery and vein. This technique should not be used if there are significant arteriosclerotic changes involving the origin and initial portion of the inferior mesenteric artery. In this situation the right colon can be used provided that it is of adequate length. Often the right colon cannot reach to the neck and a high intrathoracic anastomosis is required. *Illustration 1a* and *1b* are arteriograms showing a selective injection of the inferior mesenteric artery to illustrate the arterial supply to the left transverse and descending colon via the ascending branch of the left colic artery and the marginal branch (*1a*) and their venous drainage via the inferior mesenteric and superior haemorrhoidal veins (*1b*). This represents the ideal vascular supply to utilize the transverse and descending colon for oesophageal reconstruction.

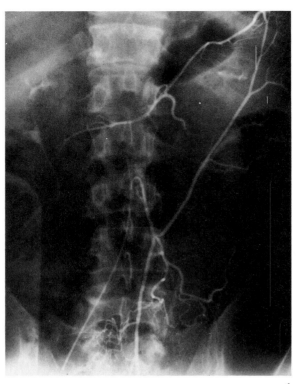

1a

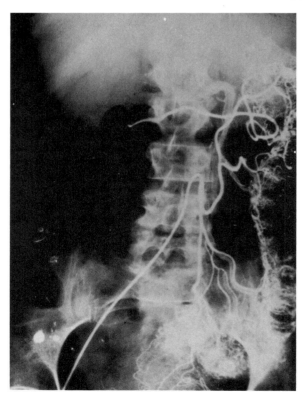

1b

Preoperative

It is advisable to assess the patient's physiological reserve before performing any procedure of this magnitude. Although valuable information can be obtained by thorough history-taking and physical examination, neither is able accurately to quantify the patient's reserve. Consequently, a more objective assessment of respiratory and cardiac reserve is necessary in all patients over the age of 50 years, or in those with a history suggestive of cardiorespiratory disease. Patients with a forced expiratory volume of less than 1.25 litres, or a resting cardiac ejection fraction less than 0.40 which drops further on exercise, are considered poor candidates for such an extensive procedure.

Colonoscopy is performed in all patients considered for colonic interposition to evaluate the state of the colonic mucosa. The presence of limited diverticular disease does not preclude the use of the colon, but extensive diverticulosis, especially if it is associated with inflammatory fibrosis, is a contraindication to the procedure. Similarly, the presence of occasional colonic polyps, whether hyperplastic or adenomatous, does not preclude the use of the colon, but extensive polyposis and the presence of malignancy is a contraindication.

The arterial anatomy of the colon is crucial to the success of the procedure, and a preoperative arteriogram is a necessity. It should include selective injections of the coeliac axis and the superior and inferior mesenteric arteries. Special attention is paid to the status of the inferior mesenteric artery, especially in older patients with atherosclerosis. In addition, the marginal artery in the region of the splenic flexure is carefully assessed, as this important arcade is absent or incomplete in 5% of patients, and the anatomy of the middle colic vessels must be defined as it is highly variable.

The patient is prepared for colonic interposition using the technique of whole gut lavage with isosmotic electrolyte solution (GoLytely) in combination with oral antibiotic administration. The patient receives broad-spectrum parenteral antibiotics before and for 3 days after the procedure. Subcutaneous heparin for deep vein thrombosis prophylaxis is started at the time of admission.

Operation

2 The colon is usually prepared through an upper midline abdominal incision. The omentum is dissected off the transverse colon, the splenic and hepatic flexures are taken down, and the ascending and descending colon are mobilized to the midline so that the whole colon from the sigmoid to the caecum is free on its mesentery. This is done carefully to prevent injury to any mesenteric vessels. By stretching the mesentery in a cephalad direction, the ascending branch of the left colic artery can easily be identified as it forms a natural pedicle ascending in the direction of the splenic flexure adjacent to the ligament of Treitz.

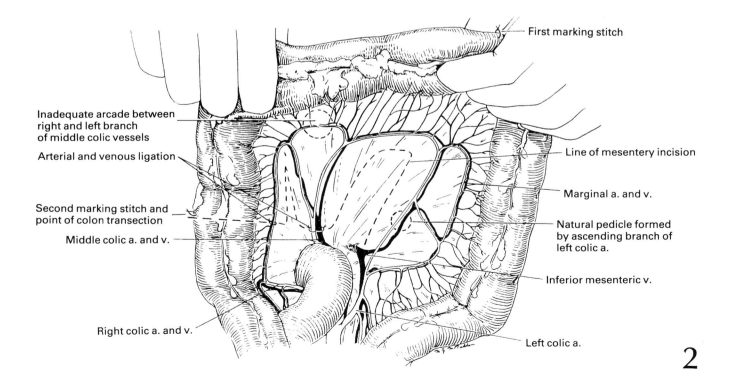

First marking stitch

Inadequate arcade between right and left branch of middle colic vessels

Arterial and venous ligation

Second marking stitch and point of colon transection

Middle colic a. and v.

Right colic a. and v.

Line of mesentery incision

Marginal a. and v.

Natural pedicle formed by ascending branch of left colic a.

Inferior mesenteric v.

Left colic a.

2

3 The length of the colonic graft is measured by tethering the colon as much as possible in a cephalad direction on the natural pedicle made by the ascending branch of the left colic artery. The apex of the colon will usually reach up to or slightly above the xiphoid. A marking stitch is placed on the antimesenteric border of the colon directly opposite the tethering artery. The distal part of the colon is usually somewhat redundant if the tethering artery is the limiting factor. The distance from this point (usually at or above the xiphoid) to the angle of the jaw is measured liberally with an umbilical tape. The same distance is then measured from the first marking stitch proximally along the transverse and ascending colon and marked with a second marking stitch. This corresponds to the proximal anastomotic site.

The second marking stitch will usually lie to the right of the right branch of the middle colic artery (*see Illustration 2*). The marginal artery and vein are ligated at the point of the second marking stitch. Because of the poorly developed peripheral arcade between the right and left branches of the middle colic artery, the middle colic artery and vein are ligated proximal to their right and left branches (*see Illustration 2*).

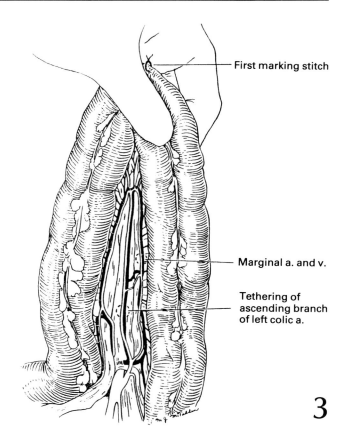

First marking stitch

Marginal a. and v.

Tethering of ascending branch of left colic a.

3

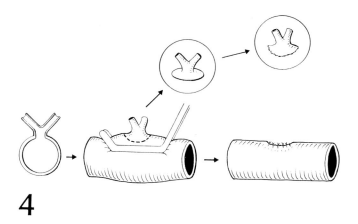

4

4 This ligation may require the excision of a button of superior mesenteric artery and vein, and the suturing together of the margins to maintain patency between the left and right branches which ensures blood flow to the most proximal portion of the graft.

Before ligation and division of any vessels it is wise to occlude them with small Bulldog clamps and to check the adequacy of blood flow to the proximal end of the graft by palpating pulses or assessing Doppler flow. The patency of the venous outflow is similarly assessed by seeking signs of venous hypertension. If the arterial inflow and venous outflow appear to be adequate the vessels may be divided, including those small end arteries and veins to the colon at the point of its transection. The transection of the colon itself is delayed until later in the operation.

The site of the proximal anastomosis is prepared in the neck. A left neck approach is preferred for the following reasons: (1) the cervical oesophagus lies slightly to the left; (2) the right recurrent laryngeal nerve lies slightly more lateral to the oesophagus than does the left nerve and is subsequently less prone to injury when encircling the oesophagus from the left; and (3) if there is an aberrant recurrent laryngeal nerve it usually occurs on the right side.

5 If the substernal route is chosen, the left half of the manubrium, the medial end of the first rib and the sternal head of the left clavicle are resected to enlarge the thoracic inlet. This is done carefully so as not to enter the pleura or destroy the internal mammary artery and vein which may be used later as a source of blood supply for a free jejunal transfer should this procedure fail. The resection is achieved by dividing the left clavicle just lateral to its sternal head by passing a Gigli saw just underneath it at the angle with the first rib. The bone is sawn as close as possible to this angle to preserve some of the costoclavicular ligament to anchor the remaining clavicle to the first rib.

If a long segment of native proximal oesophagus is available, resection of a portion of the clavicle, first rib and manubrium may not be necessary since bolus transport into the thorax is facilitated by the normal contracting proximal oesophagus. If the substernal route is chosen, a tunnel can usually be created safely using blunt dissection as long as there has not been previous scarring in the anterior mediastinum. If scarring is present, a median sternotomy may be necessary.

After the site of the proximal anastomosis has been prepared the colonic graft is re-examined to evaluate the status of its vascular supply. If there is any doubt about the adequacy of the arterial supply or venous outflow of the graft then the reconstruction is delayed. This requires moving the small bowel through an incision in the transverse mesocolon so that it lies cephalad and anterior to the transverse colon. The mobilized colon is placed underneath the small bowel and fixed to the right inferior abdominal wall so that it will not adhere to the denuded posterior peritoneal surfaces left behind by its mobilization. This surrounds the colonic graft with small bowel and makes subsequent mobilization of the colon easier. A cervical end oesophagostomy is constructed. A feeding jejunostomy is inserted to allow for continued nutritional support.

6 If the decision is taken to proceed with the colonic interposition the colon is transected with a GIA stapler at the proximal marking stitch. The distal division is delayed until later in the operation. The colon is then laid on the anterior chest wall to determine that the mesentery is not twisted.

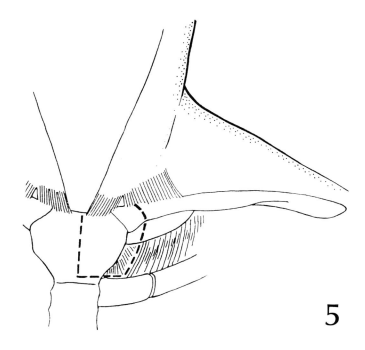

5

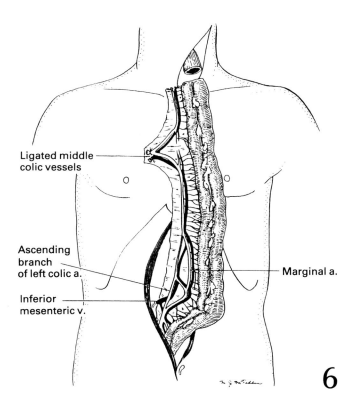

Ligated middle colic vessels

Ascending branch of left colic a.

Inferior mesenteric v.

Marginal a.

6

7 The proximal end of the graft is then sutured inside the funnel of an inverted Mousseau–Barbin tube. A plastic bowel bag is wrapped around the graft and funnel and moistened generously with water to allow atraumatic passage of the colon through a posterior or substernal tunnel. Tension is applied to the bag rather than the graft which allows it to be pulled up into the neck under minimal friction. Its course should be posterior to the stomach and through the oesophageal hiatus for posterior mediastinal grafts and through the gastrohepatic ligament into the substernal tunnel for substernal grafts.

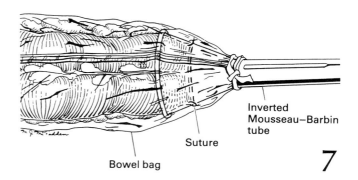

Inverted Mousseau–Barbin tube

Suture

Bowel bag

7

8a, b The proximal anastomosis is performed by division of the oesophagus at the planned level and fixation of its mucosa to the muscular layers of its wall with three or more silk sutures; this prevents retraction and aids the anastomosis. The staple line of the proximal colon is excised and the oesophagocolic anastomosis is peformed using a single layer technique with permanent 4/0 monofilament interrupted sutures. All knots are tied on the inside except for the final anterior four or five stitches which are placed using a modified Gambee technique.

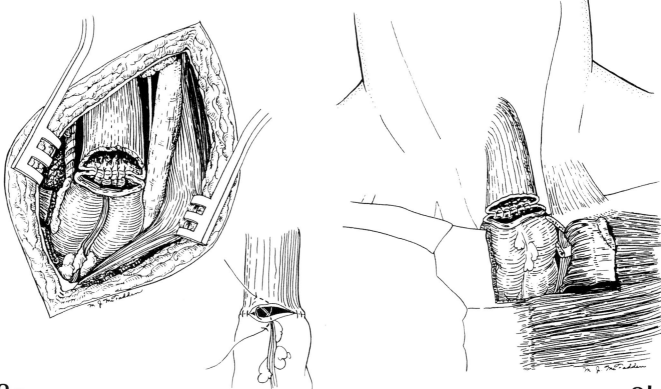

8a

8b

9 The colon is placed on gentle stretch to prevent redundancy but not so much that excessive force is placed on the anastomosis. It is then anchored in its straightened position by sutures to the left crural margin of the hiatus or the left margin of the opening in the diaphragm into the substernal tunnel. This is done since the straighter the colon, the better its postoperative function. The colon is not sutured circumferentially around the hiatus of the diaphragm opening because of the tendency to bowstring the colon transversely and produce a functional obstruction. It is important to avoid kinking the vessels to the colonic graft on the edge of the diaphragm at the entry into the substernal tunnel when using the substernal route. This may require a 2–3-cm longitudinal incision into the pericardium above and below the edge, with closure in a transverse plane similar to a Heineke–Mikulicz pyloroplasty. This converts the acute angle formed by the diaphragm and pericardium into a gentle rounded one.

Left crus of oesophageal hiatus

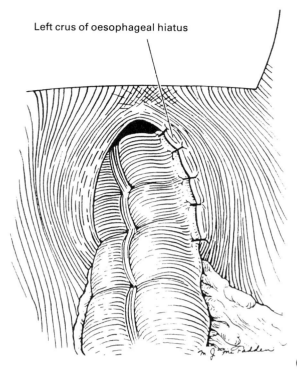

9

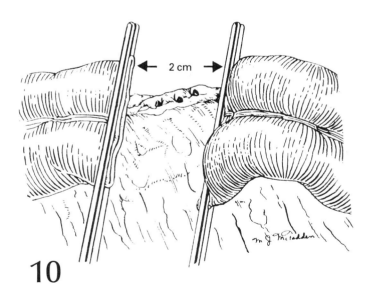

10

10 The distal end of the colonic graft is then transected 10 cm below the diaphragmatic opening. At the site of division the colon is freed from its mesentery for a distance of 2 cm along its mesenteric border by dividing the small end vessels while taking care not to injure the marginal artery. The colon is transected without dividing the mesentery other than just along its mesenteric border. This preserves additional blood supply from the marginal artery via the sigmoid arteries and venous drainage through the haemorrhoidal and sigmoid veins.

11 If the stomach has been denervated by a concomitant or previous vagotomy a proximal two-thirds gastrectomy is performed. The distal end of the colonic graft is anastomosed to the remaining one-third of the stomach. In this situation the loss of the gastric reservoir is replaced by the interposed colon. If the vagotomized proximal stomach is retained, gastric atony, delayed gastric emptying and excessive regurgitation may occur. The anastomosis is performed in a double-layer fashion using interrupted 3/0 silk sutures. A pyloromyotomy should be performed. Colonic continuity is re-established by bringing the previously mobilized right colon over to the distal end of the divided colonic graft and performing an end-to-end double-layer anastomosis using interrupted 3/0 silk sutures. When complete, the colocolic and the gastro-colic anastomoses lie in close proximity to each other.

It should be emphasized again that the mesentery of the descending and sigmoid colon is not divided. This preserves as much arterial supply and venous drainage to the colonic graft as possible via the sigmoid arteries and haemorrhoidal veins. The mesentery of the right colon is sutured to that of the descending colon to avoid internal hernia. An intramural feeding jejunostomy tube is routinely inserted 25 cm distal to the ligament of Treitz. This allows for early postoperative nutrition which can be tapered off as adequate oral intake is resumed.

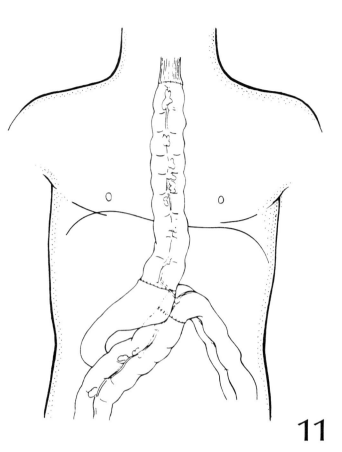

11

12a–c If a vagal sparing oesophagectomy is possible the stomach is preserved and the distal end of the colonic graft is anastomosed to the posterior surface of the stomach at a point one-third the distance between the tip of the fundus and the pylorus. The anastomosis is performed using a GIA stapler by inserting one staple head through a small gastrotomy in the posterior wall of the stomach and the other through a small colotomy in the antimesenteric wall of the colonic graft. The stapler is closed, bringing the colonic and gastric walls together, and fixed, creating a longitudinal anastomosis between the stomach and colon.

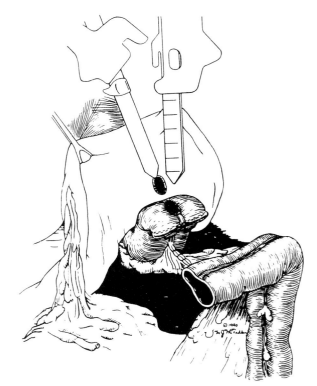

12a

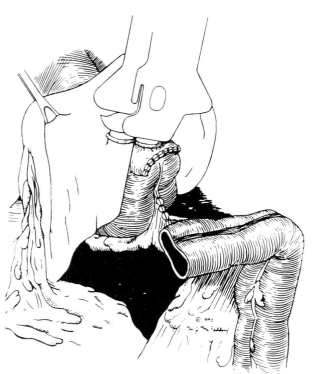

12b

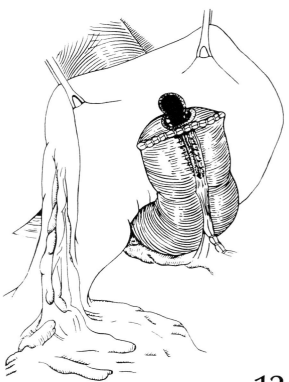

12c

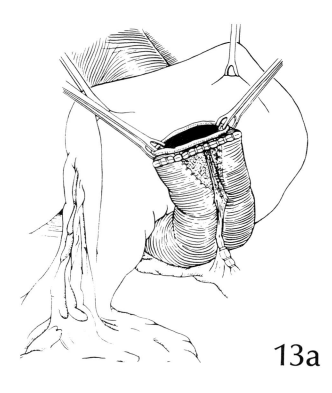

13a

13a, b The stapled anastomosis is spread apart laterally forming a triangular-shaped opening. The free edge of the stomach and colon forming one side of the triangle are joined together with a T60 stapler, forming a triangular anastomosis.

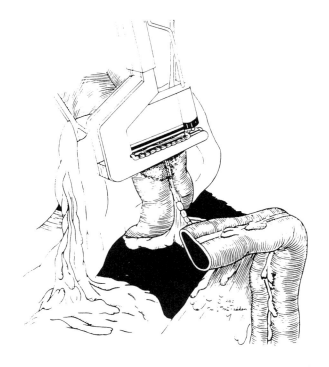

13b

14 Colonic continuity is re-established with an end-to-end colocolostomy as previously described.

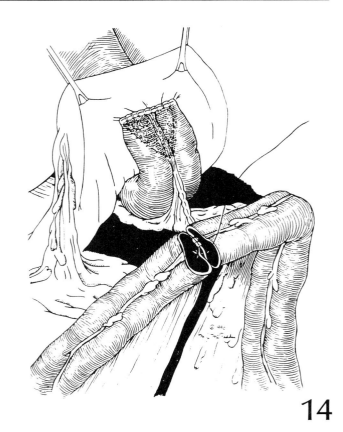

14

15 When the procedure is complete, the interposed colon re-establishes gastrointestinal continuity between the cervical oesophagus and the vagally innervated stomach. This type of reconstruction is particularly suited for oesophagectomies performed for advanced achalasia, benign stricture that cannot be dilated, or an oesophagus destroyed by caustic agents.

In patients with caustic injuries, special consideration is given to the site of the proximal anastomosis. If the cervical oesophagus has been destroyed and a pyriform sinus remains open, the anastomosis can be made to the lateral hypopharynx through an anterior suprahyoid approach as advocated by Huy and Celerier[4]. When there is scarring of the hypopharynx and loss of both pyriform sinuses, an extensive pharyngoplasty is required, as advocated by Popovici[5]. Preservation of the larynx in this situation is a challenging problem and reconstruction in these patients should be staged. The first stage consists of performing a tracheostomy to maintain an adequate airway during the reconstruction, a feeding jejunostomy to deliver adequate nutrition, transposition of the left colon to the cervical region through the posterior mediastinum or substernal space, and anastomosis of the interposed colon to the posterior stomach if the vagus nerves are intact. If there has been a previous or concomitant vagotomy a proximal two-thirds gastrectomy is performed and the interposed colon is anastomosed to the distal third of the stomach. The proximal anastomosis is not performed. A minimum of 90 days is allowed to pass before further reconstruction to allow for resolution of neck and graft oedema. The second stage is pharyngocolic anastomosis. This almost always requires partial resection of the hyoid and thyroid cartilages to perform the anastomoses. Recovery of swallowing ability takes time even in patients in whom the operation is technically successful.

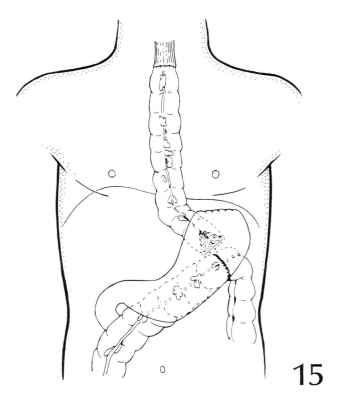

15

Postoperative care

The patient is admitted to the intensive care unit immediately after the procedure. Arterial and central venous pressures are monitored. Swan–Ganz catheters are used as indicated. Fluid is administered liberally because of the propensity for 'third space' losses after a procedure of this magnitude. Colloid solutions are preferable if the serum albumin level is low, otherwise lactated Ringer's solution is used. Hypovolaemia and hypotension must be avoided to prevent intense vasoconstriction of the gut which can result in ischaemic injury to the colonic graft.

The patient is intubated during the initial recovery phase because of the magnitude of the dissection and the length of the procedure. Further, the interruption of lymphatic drainage, especially following resection of an oesophageal cancer, results in interstitial pulmonary oedema, hypoxia and loss of pulmonary compliance. The tube is usually removed on the third day after surgery when patients are haemodynamically stable, alert and capable of protecting their airway from the possibility of aspiration.

A nasogastric tube is placed during the operation, and is maintained on suction afterwards until gastrointestinal function returns. This usually occurs on the sixth or seventh day after operation, at which time a video-oesophagogram is obtained to assess the function of the colonic graft. If this is satisfactory, oral feeding may commence. Before this, nutrition is provided by a jejunostomy tube placed during the procedure. On resumption of oral intake, supplemental jejunostomy feedings are required until the colonic graft function improves sufficiently to allow full nutritional requirements to be taken orally.

Complications

The development of colonic graft ischaemia is the most dramatic and difficult complication to diagnose after a procedure of this magnitude. Fortunately this complication is a rare occurrence in most recent series. Ischaemia may result from inadequate arterial inflow or venous outflow, but this is unusual today with proper preoperative and intraoperative assessment of flow. Other causes are excessive traction on the mesentery, or twisting and kinking of the pedicle. These problems can be prevented by strict attention to detail during the procedure. More commonly this complication results from hypoperfusion of the graft because of inadequate fluid replacement or cardiac arrhythmia, both of which can cause intense vasoconstriction of the splanchnic circulation in the presence of normal central haemodynamic parameters.

It is important that graft ischaemia is detected before the development of septic complications. This can be quite difficult as the signs and symptoms are not specific. The authors have come to rely on the presence of an unexplained base deficit and/or increased lactate level as an indicator of colonic ischaemia. Signs of sepsis, such as leucocytosis, fever, tachypnoea, tachycardia and elevation of the serum bilirubin usually occur later. To confirm the diagnosis the mucosa of the colonic graft is visualized using bedside endoscopy. The presence of a greenish or brownish mucus that does not easily wash off the mucosal surface is an early sign of mucosal ischaemia. Serial endoscopic examinations are required as the early findings are often very subtle. An infusion of low-dose dopamine, 3 μg/min, can be beneficial when the cause is splanchnic vasoconstriction.

If systemic sepsis occurs, the segment of ischaemic colon must be removed and the mediastinum drained. A cervical oesophagostomy is performed, retaining as much of the oesophagus as possible. The site of anastomosis to the stomach is closed. If not already present, a jejunostomy tube is placed for nutritional support. Reconstruction is accomplished as a separate procedure 90 days later.

Anastomotic leakage occurs in approximately 2% of patients undergoing oesophageal replacement by colonic interposition[6]. The aetiology in most situations is inadequate blood supply to the terminal portion of the graft or technical errors in the performance of the anastomosis. Leaks occur most commonly at the oesophagocolic anastomosis and most can be managed conservatively. This complication usually presents between 7 and 12 days after operation with signs of infection or drainage at the cervical wound. Occasionally it remains asymptomatic and is discovered when an oesophagogram is performed on the seventh day after surgery. Leakage is almost always managed effectively by establishing adequate drainage and withholding oral feeding for 2–3 weeks. The patient can usually be discharged on jejunostomy feedings with daily cervical wound care.

The second most common site for an anastomotic leak is the colocolic anastomosis. This complication presents in a manner identical to intra-abdominal anastomotic leak, including sepsis, peritonitis, abscess formation and fistulization. Aetiology is most commonly technical misadventure. However, in patients in whom the artery is divided proximal to the right branch of the middle colic vessels, ischaemia may play a role because of inadequate collateral flow from the right colic vessels. This complication usually responds to drainage and rarely requires a proximal diversion colostomy.

The cologastric anastomosis is least likely to leak. To prevent this complication, care should be taken to preserve the circulation to the remaining stomach during its mobilization. Patients with this complication may present with abdominal findings similar to those with colonic anastomotic leaks. The leak almost always heals with percutaneous drainage of the associated abscess.

Stricturing of any anastomosis is extremely uncommon but may occur at the oesophagocolic anastomosis if there has been previous radiation or leakage.

In a few patients, ulceration of the colon may result from reflux of bile. If the ulcer persists, a bile diversion procedure may be necessary.

Outcome

Patient satisfaction with the long-term results of the procedure is impressive. Of our patients, 82% consider themselves to be cured by the procedure, and the remainder consider themselves to be improved. Patients have been able to maintain their weight at or above their preoperative level. Detailed studies on the function of the colonic graft have shown that patients tend to eat smaller meals more slowly than normal subjects, that solids empty better when mixed with fluids, and that liquids empty better when they are acidic.

Acknowledgements

The illustrations in this chapter have been reproduced with permission from Professor T. R. DeMeester, the copyright holder.

References

1. Kelling G. Oesophagoplastik mit Hilfe des Querkolon. *Zentralb Chir* 1911; 38: 1209–12.

2. Vulliet H. De l'oesophagoplastie et de ses diverses modifications. *Semaine Med* 1911; 31: 529–30.

3. Wilkins EW Jr. Long-segment colon substitution for the esophagus. *Ann Surg* 1980; 192: 722–5.

4. Huy PTB, Celerier M. Management of severe caustic stenosis of the hypopharynx and esophagus by ileocolic transposition via suprahyoid or transglottic approach. *Ann Surg* 1988; 207: 439–45.

5. Popovici Z. Pharyngeal–oesophageal reconstruction with laryngeal preservation following severe caustic injury to the pharynx and oesophagus. In: Hennessy TPJ and Cuschieri A, eds. *Surgery of the Oesophagus*. 2nd edn. Oxford: Butterworth–Heinemann, 1992: 328–49.

6. DeMeester TR, Johansson KE, Franze I *et al*. Indications, surgical technique, and long-term functional results of colon interposition or bypass. *Ann Surg* 1988; 208: 460–74.

Use of the stomach as an oesophageal substitute

Arnulf H. Hölscher MD
Assistant Professor of Surgery, Department of Surgery, Technical University of Munich, Munich, Germany

J. Rüdiger Siewert MD
Professor of Surgery, Chairman of the Department of Surgery, Technical University of Munich, Munich, Germany

History

The use of the stomach as an oesophageal substitute was introduced by Kirschner in 1920 as a non-resectional operative bypass. His operation consisted of skeletonization of the greater curvature of the stomach, and the mobilized stomach was then brought subcutaneously up to the divided cervical oesophagus. The application of this procedure using either the orthotopic or the retrosternal route after oesophagectomy and the standardization of this method was largely due to the work of Ong, Nakayama and Akiyama[1].

Principles and justification

The reconstruction of intestinal transit after oesophagectomy is normally made using stomach or colon. The small bowel is used much less frequently for complete substitution of the oesophagus. Small bowel interposition does have a place, however, for partial oesophageal replacement of both proximal and distal oesophagus.

Gastric interposition is the simplest form of oesophageal replacement[2]. Furthermore, as it guarantees good long-term functional results[3], it has become the method of first choice as an oesophageal substitute, especially after oesophagectomy for cancer[4]. It is only when the stomach is not available because of previous operations or in benign oesophageal diseases that colonic interposition is used.

An important question to be answered in planning an oesophageal replacement is where to site the oesophago-enteral anastomosis. In the authors' experience a cervical anastomosis has proved best. If intrathoracic anastomoses are performed they should be carried out near the apex of the pleura. Anastomotic leakage is less likely to occur with intrathoracic anastomosis than with cervical anastomosis but the consequences of such a leak are much more serious[5]. With regard to oncological radicality (remaining oesophagus) and long-term results, both anastomoses are similar.

Finally, the site for the oesophageal substitute has to be chosen. Antesternal subcutaneous placement is usually not indicated[4]. This leaves the posterior and anterior mediastinal routes available. When a tumour has invaded outside the wall of the oesophagus (T3 or T4) the authors believe that reconstruction in the posterior mediastinum should be avoided to overcome the possibility of local recurrence and to keep the posterior mediastinum free for postoperative radiotherapy. For these reasons, the oesophageal substitute should be placed retrosternally in the anterior mediastinum.

When the cancer is localized to the oesophageal wall (T1 or T2) or the case is one of benign oesophageal disease, the interposition of the stomach should be performed in the posterior mediastinum. Swallowing, at least in the early postoperative phase, is more normal when the interposition is in the posterior mediastinum. It should also be noted that the distance through the posterior mediastinum is the shortest[6].

Preoperative

The stomach may be used as an oesophageal substitute only if it has not previously been operated on: following gastric resections the length will be insufficient and after vagotomy procedures the vascularization is doubtful. If lesser procedures (such as suturing of a bleeding ulcer or closure of a perforation) have been performed, then a transposition of the stomach may be possible but the vascularity should be checked at the beginning of the operation. A preoperative gastroscopy should be carried out to exclude any mucosal pathology and to confirm the borders of the oesophageal tumour. If the cancer is infiltrating the cardia or the subcardial area, the safety margin between the lower edge of the tumour and the resection line of the gastric tube may not be sufficient. Lymph node metastases to the lesser curvature (compartment I according to the classification in gastric cancer) and the coeliac trunk (compartment II) should be detected by preoperative endoscopic ultrasonography[2].

In all cases the colon should be prepared by bowel lavage and colonoscopy so that it may be used if the stomach should prove unusable.

Anaesthesia

The type of anaesthesia used depends more on the type of oesophagectomy than on the method of reconstruction (see the chapter on pp. 280–291). If an intrathoracic anastomosis is to be performed, a double-lumen endotracheal tube should be used.

Anatomical points

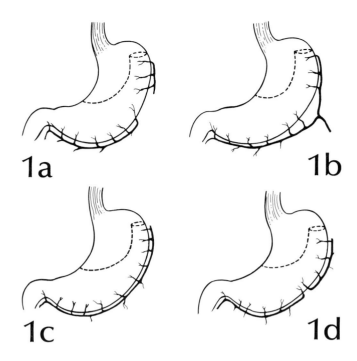

1a   1b
1c   1d

1a–d A knowledge of the arterial blood supply of the stomach is essential for its use as an oesophageal substitute. The arterial supply of the stomach originates from the coeliac trunk. This vessel has a short stem which immediately divides into three branches. The left gastric artery runs in a cranial ventral direction, covered by the peritoneum of the posterior wall of the lesser sac. Subcardially it turns to the lesser curvature in an aboral direction where it supplies the anterior and posterior gastric wall by small branches. The left gastric artery has anastomoses with the right gastric artery, which originates from the common hepatic artery and approaches from the region of the pylorus. By these means, an arterial ring along the lesser curvature is completed with its strongest inflow being from the left gastric artery.

The second vessel of the coeliac trunk is the splenic artery, which runs along the upper border of the pancreas behind the posterior wall of the omental bursa to the hilum of the spleen. At the splenic hilum the short gastric vessels originate; they proceed to the fundus and the cranial third of the greater curvature of the stomach. The left gastroepiploic artery arises from the splenic artery and runs through the gastrocolic ligament parallel to the greater curvature of the stomach in a caudad direction. This artery gives gastric branches to both walls of the stomach and epiploic branches to the greater omentum. It anastomoses with the right gastroepiploic artery, which comes from the region of the pylorus. Thus the greater curvature also has a vascular ring, with its strongest supply being from the right gastroepiploic artery. This artery has a number of anatomical variations, which may be relevant to gastric interposition.

The third vessel of the coeliac trunk, the common hepatic artery, turns to the right, in the direction of the hepatoduodenal ligament of the small omentum. There it divides into the hepatic and gastroduodenal arteries. The hepatic artery runs through the hepatoduodenal ligament to the liver and usually gives rise to the right gastric artery, which proceeds to the lesser curvature of the stomach. The right gastric artery may also originate from the gastroduodenal artery. The gastroduodenal artery runs posterior to the superior part of the duodenum distal to the pylorus and comes out caudad to the duodenum where it divides into the right gastroepiploic and superior pancreaticoduodenal arteries. All gastric arteries anastomose between themselves directly or indirectly by intramural or extramural branches. Therefore, the ligation of two or even three gastric arteries preserves the blood supply of the stomach under normal circumstances.

The veins of the stomach lead the blood to the portal vein. With only minor exceptions they correspond in their course to the four gastric arteries. From the gastric fundus the short gastric veins run through the gastrosplenic ligament to the splenic vein. The left gastroepiploic vein from the greater curvature also proceeds in this direction to the left side. It reaches the splenic vein through the gastrosplenic ligament. The right gastroepiploic vein accompanies its artery to the area of the pylorus. At this point, the vein turns in a posterior direction and flows into the superior mesenteric vein. At the lesser curvature, a venous arch runs along both arteries (coronary or left gastric vein). This vein flows near the right gastric artery into the portal vein or splenic vein within the hepatoduodenal ligament. At the cardia, the venous arch follows the left gastric artery up to the area of the coeliac trunk.

Operation

Position of patient

2 The patient lies in a supine position with the head turned to the right in order to provide a free approach to the left side of the neck. A rolled up towel or a sandbag is placed behind the shoulders to facilitate the approach to the anterior mediastinum, and under the lumbar region to facilitate access to the stomach.

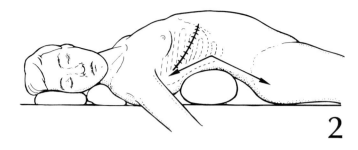

2

Incision

3 The abdomen is opened by a transverse incision extended by an upper midline incision in the direction of the xiphoid process. This ensures a good view of the epigastric area.

3

Preparation of the stomach

Skeletonization of the stomach begins along the greater curvature outside the gastroepiploic arch. It is performed stepwise in the direction of the fundus. Although the supply to the stomach from the right gastroepiploic artery shows variations (as shown in *Illustration 1*), it is sufficient in nearly all cases to guarantee a blood supply to the gastric tube. After dividing the left gastroepiploic artery the preparation of the upper third of the gastric fundus may be performed close to the stomach wall.

4 In an aborad direction the preparation must be done very carefully outside the gastroepiploic arch to the origin of the right gastroepiploic artery from the gastroduodenal artery.

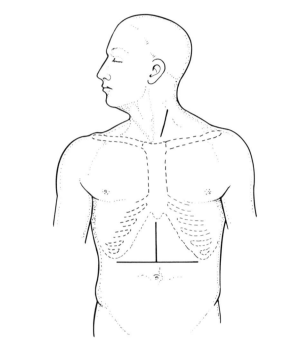

4

5 It is also important to maintain the venous drainage via the right gastroepiploic vein.

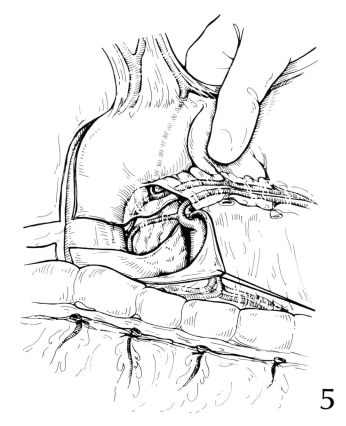

5

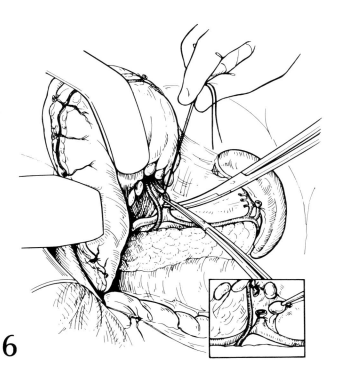

6

Lymph node dissection

The gastroduodenal artery is dissected immediately distal to the pylorus. This allows the common hepatic artery to be easily identified. Dissection proceeds in a medial direction in order to preserve the origin of the right gastric artery from the common hepatic artery. The right gastric artery may aid the vascularization of the gastric tube, and it should be spared if possible.

6 The lymph nodes are dissected in a manner similar to that which is carried out in gastric cancer, which means that all lymph nodes along the common hepatic artery, the coeliac trunk and the medial part of the splenic artery are dissected and taken with the specimen. The ligation of the left gastric artery is performed near its trunk of origin.

After dissecting the lesser omentum the oesophagus, which has previously been dissected by a transthoracic or transmediastinal approach, is pulled out of the oesophageal hiatus for the final preparation of the gastric tube.

Formation of the gastric tube

7   Akiyama[1] recommends that the highest point of the stomach should be marked by two stay sutures. This point is located quite a long way to the left of the cardia. The skeletonization of the lesser curvature involves about two-thirds of the lesser curvature, which means it starts distal to the third or fourth branch of the left gastric artery, at the region of the 'crow's foot' and continues close to the gastric wall in the direction of the cardia.

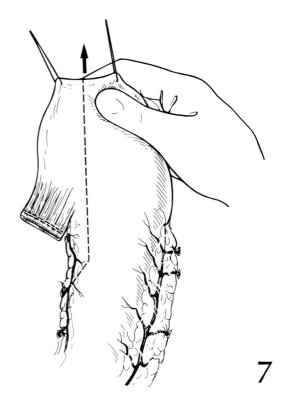

7

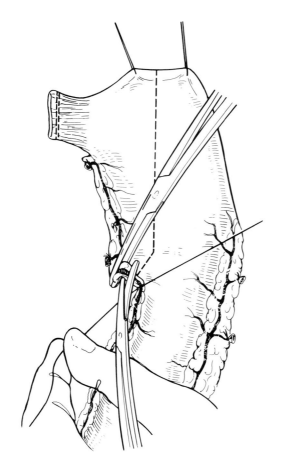

8

8   The lesser omentum should be divided in this area and the vascular arcade suture ligated. The stomach now can be cut in an oblique direction between the distal point of skeletonization and the highest point of the gastric fundus (interrupted line in *Illustrations* 7 and *8*). This means about half of the gastric fundus including the lymphatic drainage along the left gastric artery (compartment I) is removed. The resulting gastric tube has a width of 3–4 cm.

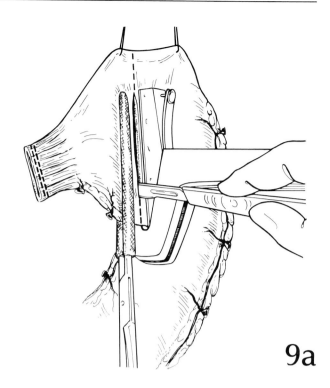

9a–c Before the stomach is finally cut along this line the gastric fundus should be opened near the cardia and a pair of long forceps inserted in order to carry out an intraluminal pyloric dilatation. This helps to avoid early postoperative pylorospasm. The best way to divide the stomach is to use a linear stapler (TA 90). Two applications of this stapler are usually required in order to close the quite long resection line.

9a

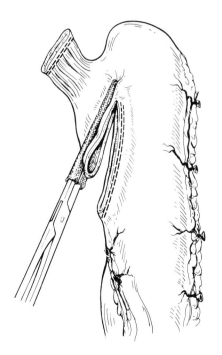

9b

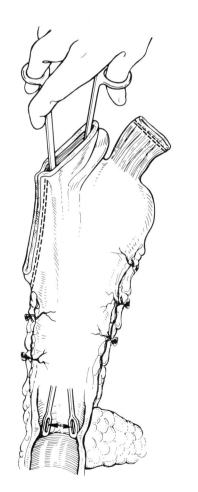

9c

10 If the stomach appears too short for elevation to the neck, cutting the seromuscular layer with a scalpel and then closing the mucosa by stapler results in greater elasticity of the gastric tube.

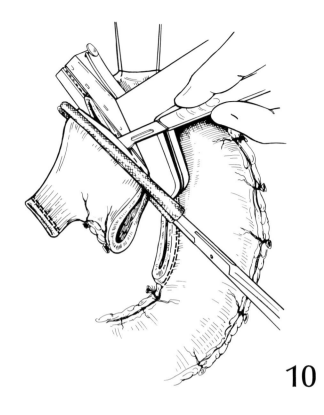

10

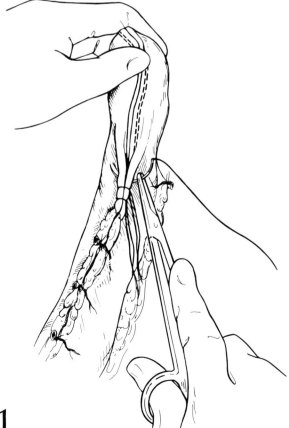

11

11 If additional suturing of the staple line is undertaken it is best to use interrupted rather than running sutures to avoid shortening of the tube by a 'purse-string' effect.

Interposition of the whole stomach

It is possible to use the whole stomach, rather than a gastric tube, as the oesophageal interposition. This can only be performed if the tumour is not infiltrating the gastro-oesophageal junction. The skeletonization should start at the same point and in the same manner as for the formation of the gastric tube. However, it is continued along the lesser curvature up to the cardia.

12 The staple line (using a TA 55 stapler) is then placed directly below the cardia to preserve the whole gastric fundus.

Pyloric dilatation is not performed because it would mean an additional incision in the preserved stomach. Fortunately this dilatation is not absolutely necessary[3,4].

The advantage of using the whole stomach as the oesophageal substitute is that the gastro-oesophageal anastomosis does not include the tangential staple line at the highest point of the gastric fundus. This may avoid a 'locus minoris resistentiae' of such an anastomosis.

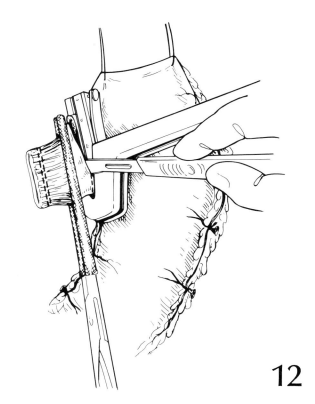

12

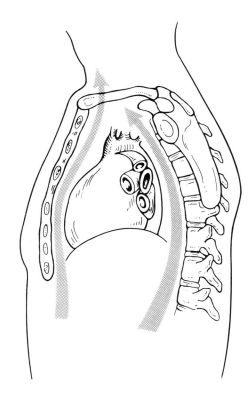

13

Duodenal mobilization

An essential prerequisite for a tension-free stomach interposition is a careful and extensive duodenal mobilization. This Kocher manoeuvre is performed in the usual way from the right side and should be continued until the vena cava and the aorta up to the superior mesenteric artery are freed. This means that the duodenum and the head of the pancreas are quite mobile.

Another important step is to separate the right colonic flexure from the head of the pancreas and the duodenum. This mobilization should be performed up to the middle colic vein. After this manoeuvre the pylorus can easily be moved up to the oesophageal hiatus or even higher.

Preparation of the tunnel for the interposition

13 If the interposition is to be placed in the posterior mediastinum, some form of tape or Penrose tubing must be drawn down as the oesophagus is removed. This is attached to the stomach so that the gastric tube can be pulled upwards without further preparation, in the bed of the former oesophagus. If it is planned for the interposition to be placed in the anterior mediastinum, a retrosternal tunnel is prepared by blunt dissection.

14 This blunt dissection can be performed with the help of a swab in sponge-holding forceps. It is essential to limit this preparation strictly to the midline and always with contact to the posterior part of the sternum. Once the sponge-holding forceps has reached the cervical incision, the channel is dilated in a stepwise fashion so that the interposition can be accommodated without compression.

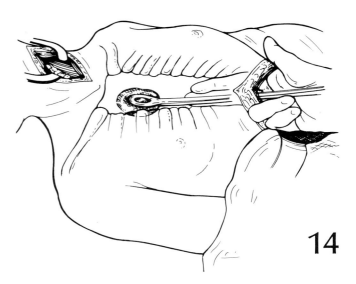

14

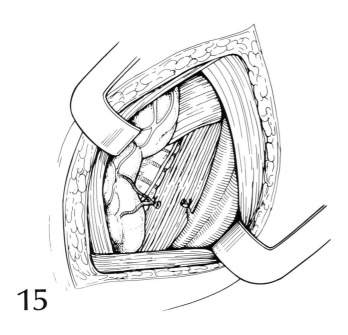

15

Elevation of the stomach and cervical anastomosis

15 While the abdominal team is operating another team starts the cervical part of the operation using a left lateral incision along the sternocleido-mastoid muscle. The omohyoid muscle and the inferior thyroid artery are ligated and divided, the left thyroid lobe is mobilized and the recurrent laryngeal nerve is dissected and preserved.

Following transthoracic oesophagectomy it is usually easy to mobilize the oesophageal remnant and extract it from the posterior mediastinum. It is important to extend the preparation of the oesophagus in the direction of the hypopharynx until it is completely free so that the oesophagus passes directly to the anasto-mosis without kinking.

If the interposition is placed in the anterior mediasti-num, the retrosternal space must also be opened from the cervical incision in order to complete the tunnel from the abdominal and cervical directions. It is a good idea to place the stomach in a plastic bag when drawing it through the tunnel in order to avoid any trauma to the organ. This part of the operation is facilitated by placing a tube via the cervical incision through the anterior or posterior mediastinum.

16 The stomach is then sutured to the lower tip of the tube. The stomach can be slowly pulled through the mediastinum in an upwards direction. It is important to push the stomach upwards from the abdomen as well.

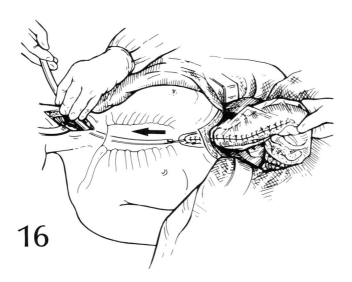

16

17a–c The gastric interposition usually has sufficient (and sometimes even excessive) length and reaches the neck without tension. Often the cervical oesophageal stump overlaps the gastric tube, and an additional resection of the stomach can be performed. The vascularization of the top of the fundus is unreliable and should be resected. The anastomosis with the cervical oesophagus is performed in the upper part of the gastric corpus. The anastomosis is usually located just above the clavicle. Before the anastomosis is performed, the back wall of the stomach is fixed to the neck by two or three sutures. The back wall of the anastomosis is constructed using interrupted sutures which emerge between the mucosa and muscularis; the anterior wall is completed using all-layer interrupted sutures.

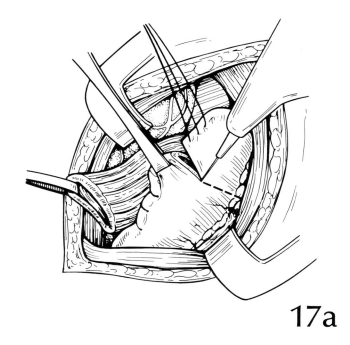

17a

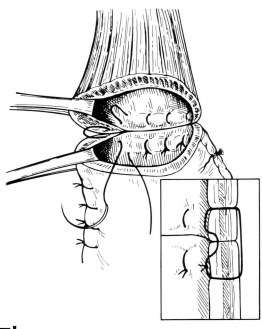

17b

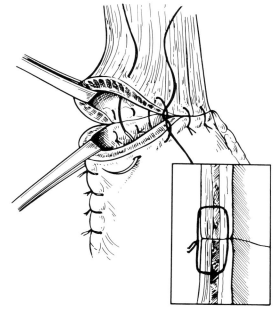

17c

18 The anastomosis is splinted by a transnasal gastric tube in order to guarantee postoperative decompression of the stomach. The wound is closed by subcutaneous and skin sutures.

As an alternative the cervical anastomosis can be performed using a stapling technique (see chapter on pp. 84–87). The detachable head of the EEA stapler is introduced into the oesophageal stump, which is closed around the mandrel by a purse-string suture. The most appropriate size of stapler is usually size 28: smaller staplers tend to induce postoperative anastomotic stenosis. It is recommended that the specially designed shorter head of the EEA stapler is used for introduction into the cervical oesophagus because it can more easily be placed into the oesophageal stump. The stapler is inserted through an incision at the top of the stomach and the central spike is driven out 5–7 cm aborad through the stomach front wall. After turning the stapler in the direction of the oesophageal remnant the central pin is connected with the mandrel, the stapler is closed, fired and removed. The site of introduction in the stomach is closed using a TA 55 linear stapler.

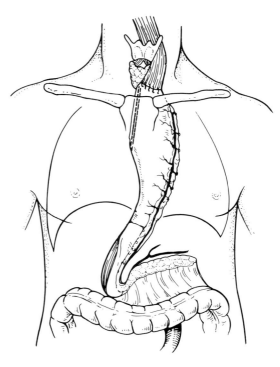

18

Elevation of the stomach and intrathoracic anastomosis

If an intrathoracic anastomosis is planned it should be performed towards the apex of the pleura. It is important for the postoperative long-term results that the stomach is completely transferrred into the thorax[3]. This means that the preparation of the stomach is identical to the preparation for an abdominocervical interposition. When the preparation of the stomach has been finished, the gastric tube is pushed through the oesophageal hiatus into the posterior mediastinum and the right pleural cavity. The abdominal approach is temporarily closed and the patient is turned for a right thoracic approach to the oesophagus. The anastomosis is now performed directly between the oesophageal stump and the stomach, either end-to-end or as an implantation of the oesophageal remnant on the front wall of the stomach. The suture technique (by hand or by stapler) should be the same as described for the cervical anastomosis. If the gastric tube is long enough to preserve a blind oral part of the stomach above the anastomosis, then this can be used to cover the front wall suture line of the oesophagogastrostomy.

A disadvantage of an intrathoracic anastomosis is that the gastric tube has to be positioned in the posterior mediastinum. This may be a problem if an advanced tumour has been resected and if a postoperative recurrence occurs or postoperative radiation of the former site of the oesophagus is planned.

Drainage

The cervical anastomosis is drained by a Penrose or other soft drain. Another option is to leave the lower part of the cervical incision open and put in a dressing impregnated with povidone-iodine. In an intrathoracic anastomosis the pleural cavity is drained by two tube drains.

Finishing the abdominal operation

After completing the gastro-oesophageal anastomosis in the neck or the thorax the abdominal operation should be completed. The operative field is checked for haemostasis. Drainage of the peritoneal cavity is not necessary. When the gastric interposition is positioned well, the pylorus should be located in the area of the diaphragm. The abdomen is closed in layers.

Postoperative care

Postoperative care should follow the course described for gastro-oesophagectomy for adenocarcinoma of the cardia on pp. 280–291.

Complications

The most common complication of gastric interposition is leakage from the cervical anastomosis. In the authors' experience this complication is unlikely if the gastric tube is elevated as proximally as possible so that the end-to-end anastomosis is performed in a well vascularized area of the stomach. Other kinds of cervical anastomoses cannot be recommended, as often the gastric part orad to the anastomosis develops necrosis.

If leakage does develop a salivary fistula results which usually heals without complications providing sufficient external drainage is present. If there is insufficient drainage a phlegmon in the cervical soft tissue may develop. Therefore, whenever a fever of unknown origin develops postoperatively the cervical anastomosis should be checked. This can be performed radiologically using contrast medium, but sometimes it is safer to check the anastomosis directly by opening the cervical incision.

If leakage has occurred open treatment of the cervical wound is appropriate. The leakage can be stented by a T-tube drain to avoid long-term application of a nasogastric tube. Early and adequate external drainage of a cervical leak is necessary to avoid spread of infection into the mediastinum.

More major (or even complete) necrosis of the interposed stomach is extremely rare as the gastric tube usually has a very good blood supply. Very occasionally postoperative pylorospasm may occur leading to clinically relevant delay in gastric emptying. Such a situation can easily be treated by a careful endoscopic dilatation of the pylorus. Gastric dilatation as a consequence of postoperative paralysis is extremely rare after gastric tube formation by this technique. A dislocation of the interposed stomach from the mediastinum into one of the pleural cavities is also very rare. If the stomach is shown to be distended with air on postoperative thoracic radiography, temporary placement of a nasogastric tube is suggested. This avoids compression of mediastinal organs and also avoids aspiration.

The most important long-term complication is the development of an anastomotic stricture. This is usually caused by scarring as a result of anastomotic vascular insufficiency, but use of too small a stapler could also cause dysphagia from anastomotic stenosis. In either case the problem can be solved by endoscopic dilatation. If it has no lasting effect, resection of the stenosis and reanastomosis is recommended.

Outcome

Functional studies of patients with intrathoracic stomach as oesophageal replacement have shown good long-term results[3, 4]. Despite a persistent acid secretion of the vagotomized thoracic stomach, no pathological gastro-oesophageal reflux or oesophagitis were found proximal to the cervical anastomosis. Gastric biopsies mostly reveal mild gastritis of the antral mucosa, and metaplasia is rare. The intrathoracic stomach needs no drainage to facilitate emptying. Postoperative reflux oesophagitis is prevented by complete intrathoracic stomach transposition with cervical oesophagogastro-stomy.

In young patients with benign oesophageal diseases requiring an oesophagectomy the authors prefer to use the colon as an oesophageal substitute in order to preserve the gastric reservoir.

References

1. Akiyama H. Surgery for carcinoma of the esophagus. *Curr Probl Surg* 1980; 17: 53–120.

2. Siewert JR, Hölscher AH. Eingriffe beim Ösophaguscarcinom. In: Siewert JR, ed. *Chirurgie des Abdomens 2. Ösophagus, Magen und Duodenum. Chirurgische Operationslehre Band IV*. München: Urban and Schwarzenberg, 1989: 15–54.

3. Hölscher AH, Voit H, Buttermann G, Siewert JR. Function of the intrathoracic stomach as esophageal replacement. *World J Surg* 1988; 12: 835–44.

4. Siewert JR, Hölscher AH. *Diseases of the Esophagus*. Berlin: Springer, 1988.

5. Chasseray VM, Kiroff GK, Buard JL, Launois B. Cervical or thoracic anastomosis for esophagectomy for carcinoma. *Surg Gynecol Obstet* 1989; 169: 55–62.

6. Ngan SY, Wong J. Lengths of different routes for esophageal replacement. *J Thorac Cardiovasc Surg* 1986; 91: 790–2.

Pouches as gastric substitutes

Christian Herfarth MD
Professor and Head, Department of Surgery, University of Heidelberg, Heidelberg, Germany

Klaus Buhl MD
Department of Surgery, University of Heidelberg, Heidelberg, Germany

Several sequelae occur as a consequence of gastric resection, whether it is a total or a subtotal gastrectomy. In contrast to the biochemical functions of the stomach such as the production of intrinsic factor or gastric acid, it is possible to restore mechanical tasks such as the reservoir capacity to improve problems due to malnutrition and to prevent reflux of duodenal contents into the oesophagus.

1 More than 60 different and, to some extent, very complex methods have been described for the restoration of the alimentary tract since Carl Schlatter successfully performed the first total gastrectomy in man in 1897 with a reconstruction by simple end-to-side oesophagojejunostomy. Various problems encountered after total gastrectomy soon became obvious. Postoperative syndromes included reflux of duodenal contents and malnutrition. This was almost inevitable when reconstruction techniques such as simple oesophagojejunostomy (Schlatter) or end-to-end oesophagoduodenostomy (Harvie, Brigham) were applied. First attempts to avoid reflux by suturing the afferent loop to the diaphragm (Herczel, Moynihan) were ineffective, as was side-to-side jejunojejunostomy (Schloffer). This problem was solved by using interpositions of longer sections of bowel (Longmire, Gütge-mann) or by having the duodenal contents entering the jejunum more than 40 cm aboral to the oesophago-jejunostomy (Roux-en-Y).

In 1922 Hoffmann proposed a pouch made up by a wide side-to-side anastomosis between the limbs of the first jejunal loop in order to improve malnutrition. This idea was first realized by Steinberg and Engel in 1949. The interposition of the right hemicolon (Hunnicutt) and the formation of double-lumen pouches both had the same goal, which was to form a reservoir. The duodenum may be excluded by means of a Roux-en-Y procedure (Hunt, Rodino) or kept in stream (Hunt, Soupault). Various modifications have been described (Mikkelsen, Riva, Poth, Knöfler) and pouches have been constructed of three jejunal limbs (Hays, Tolley) to increase food capacity. These modifications have not achieved general acceptance because of their complicated technique. Furthermore, there has been no evidence that they further improve the clinical results.

Some special efforts were undertaken to reduce the risk of leakage at the oesophageal anastomosis, e.g. the invagination of the oesophagus (Coenen) as well as protection with peritoneal flaps (Lahey) or parts of small bowel (Hilarowicz, Graham, Hollenbach). Jejunoplications have also been performed to reconstruct the antireflux function of the distal oesophagus (Siewert, Schreiber, Herfarth).

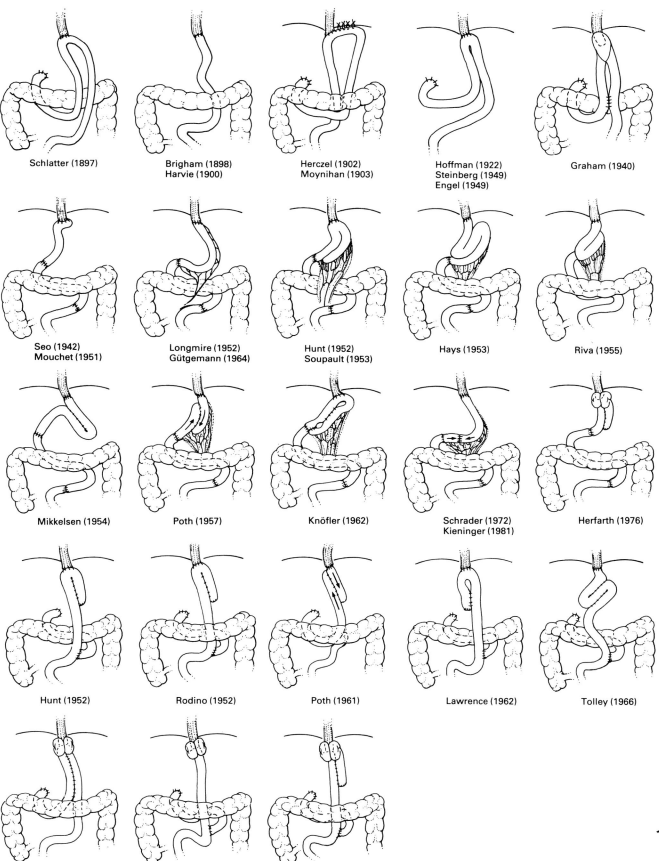

Schlatter (1897)

Brigham (1898)
Harvie (1900)

Herczel (1902)
Moynihan (1903)

Hoffman (1922)
Steinberg (1949)
Engel (1949)

Graham (1940)

Seo (1942)
Mouchet (1951)

Longmire (1952)
Gütgemann (1964)

Hunt (1952)
Soupault (1953)

Hays (1953)

Riva (1955)

Mikkelsen (1954)

Poth (1957)

Knöfler (1962)

Schrader (1972)
Kieninger (1981)

Herfarth (1976)

Hunt (1952)

Rodino (1952)

Poth (1961)

Lawrence (1962)

Tolley (1966)

Siewert (1973)

Schreiber (1975)

Herfath (1976)

1

Principles and justifications

Gastric reconstruction is generally required for patients who have undergone total gastrectomy for carcinoma, sarcoma, lymphoma, Zollinger–Ellison syndrome, gastric polyposis or Ménétrièr's disease. Occasionally a pouch reconstruction may be necessary after subtotal gastrectomy to enlarge a small gastric remnant, when conservative treatment of the dumping syndrome has failed.

An individual's prognosis should be considered in selecting the most appropriate gastric substitute. However, depending on the general condition of the patient, the authors feel that gastric reconstructions are worthwhile even if lengthy survival cannot be anticipated because they enable patients to adapt more quickly to their agastric condition. A gastric substitute provides an adequate reservoir capacity, and even patients with a short life expectancy are given the opportunity for improved nutrition.

Two types of procedure are available for bridging the gap left by total gastrectomy: (1) a Billroth I type of reconstruction which maintains duodenal passage of nutrients, and (2) a Billroth II type which excludes duodenal transit (*Illustration 1*). Although it seems reasonable to expect a dissociation of digestive processes with duodenal exclusion, to date no adverse effects have been demonstrated. On the contrary, humoral regulation systems integrated in the upper jejunum appear able to assume the most important integrative functions. Disturbances of carbohydrate metabolism due to alterations of insulin secretions are well known, but they produce only minor clinical effects.

With improvement in nutritional capacity and avoidance of reflux oesophagitis, it is anticipated that the classic sequelae of total gastrectomy such as severe steatorrhoea, hypoproteinaemia and dysproteinaemia, iron deficiency anaemia and alterations in calcium metabolism will be minimized. Vitamin B_{12} replacement remains the only requirement for such patients.

Preoperative

Preoperative assessment and preparation of the patient and anaesthesia have been considered in the chapter on pp. 39–44.

Operations

2 Important prerequisites for the construction of a gastric reservoir are a constant exposure of the operative field and the oesophagus (the authors use a self-retaining retractor and costal arch retractor). It is, of course, important to have an adequate blood supply at the prospective resection lines. If adequate tension-free exposure cannot be obtained, the hiatus should be incised anteriorly, avoiding injury to the blood vessels supplying the diaphragm. As an alternative, a combined abdominothoracic approach with division of the left costal arch can be used.

Haemostasis must be checked meticulously after gastrectomy, lymphadenectomy and other resective parts of the operation. The end of the oesophagus is held with two traction sutures or with a soft right-angled clamp (e.g. Satinsky clamp). Alternatively, the gastric specimen can be left attached proximally and used to apply traction to the oesophagus. In the latter case it is important to occlude the aboral end of the oesophagus with a right-angled clamp after cleaning it with cytotoxic solutions (e.g. Sublimat) to prevent reflux of tumour material from the stomach into the anastomotic area (danger of implantation metastases).

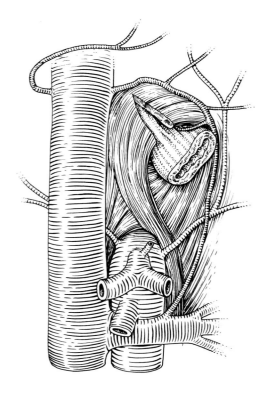

2

Jejunal preparation

3 To identify an appropriate jejunal segment the vascular anatomy of the mesentery must be visualized to ensure the most radial dissection possible for traction-free mobilization of the corresponding bowel segment. Transillumination of the mesentery helps this manoeuvre even when the mesentery is adipose. The jejunum is transected about 30 cm distal to the ligament of Treitz by staples and the row of staples can be secured further by a continuous seromuscular suture. The afferent loop is temporarily closed, for example, by a Murphy clamp and covered during this part of the operation.

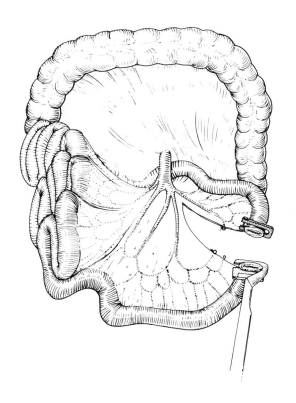

3

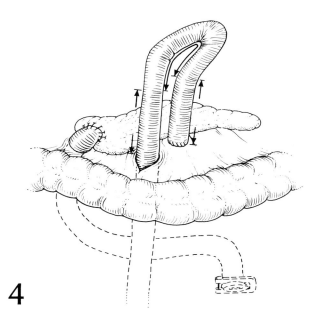

4

Transposition of the jejunum

4 The pouch is constructed in the upper abdomen. The isolated loop is transposed upward through an incision in an avascular zone of the transverse mesocolon. A 50-cm long loop of jejunum is used for construction of the pouch; 15–17 cm on each side are used for the pouch itself, and the central sector is preserved for a jejunoplication.

JEJUNOJEJUNOSTOMY

Posterior wall

5   The construction of the pouch starts by fixing the two limbs at each end with traction sutures. A wide side-to-side jejunojejunostomy is then performed, beginning with the posterior wall, which will consist of two rows of sutures. During this period the mesentery pedicle is clamped. A continuous seromuscular suture (3/0 absorbable material) joins the two limbs, which are then incised for a distance of about 15 cm lengthwise bilaterally.

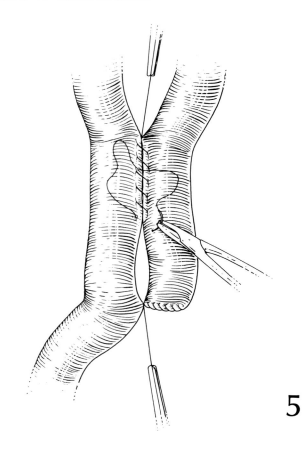

5

6   The posterior wall anastomosis is completed with a continuous all-coats interlocking suture for haemostasis.

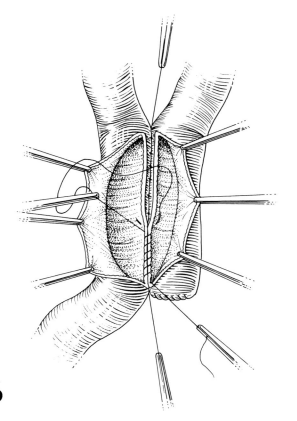

6

7 The corner sutures are brought out over the corners and the anterior and posterior walls are joined.

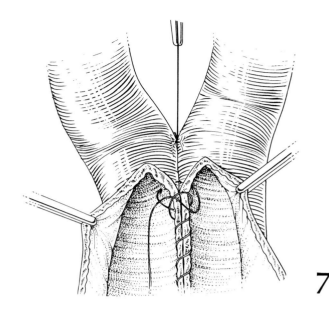

7

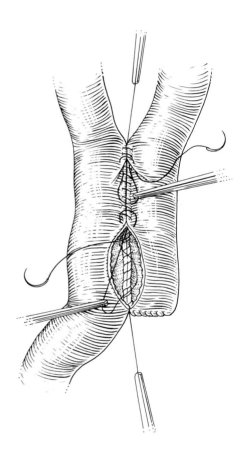

8

Anterior wall

8 The first row of the anterior wall is sutured with a continuous all-coats inverting suture which is then covered with a second row of a continuous seromuscular suture.

Stapled jejunojejunostomy

9 Alternatively, the pouch can be constructed using staples. A GIA 90 stapler is introduced twice over small incisions aborally with traction sutures being applied at each end. The incisions are closed with interrupted sutures (4/0 absorbable material) to avoid stenoses of the efferent loop.

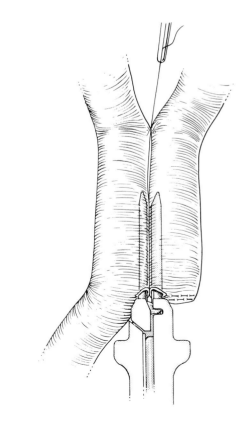

9

OESOPHAGOJEJUNOSTOMY

10 The pouch is anastomosed end-to-side to the oesophagus at the site between the efferent limb and the unsutured jejunal loop above the enteroenterostomy. At this point the anterior jejunal wall is opened for a distance of 2.5 cm with a slightly S-shaped enterotomy. First corner sutures are placed by all-coats stitches (3/0 absorbable material).

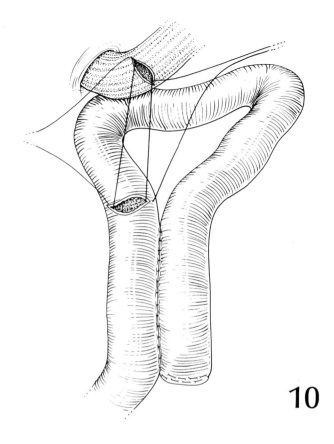

10

Posterior wall

11 The sutures of the posterior wall are applied as all-coats back stitches which coapt the mucosal surface. The distance between the single stitches should be about 0.5 cm and at least 1.0 cm of the jejunal and oesophageal wall should be enclosed on each side to ensure sound anchoring of the sutures.

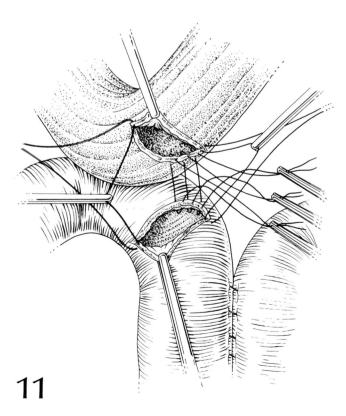

11

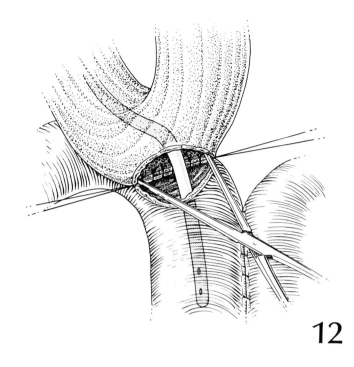

12 The jejunal and oesophageal site are approximated carefully over the taut threads and the sutures are tied. A gastric tube is then pulled from the oesophagus and its tip is placed in the pouch for further drainage.

12

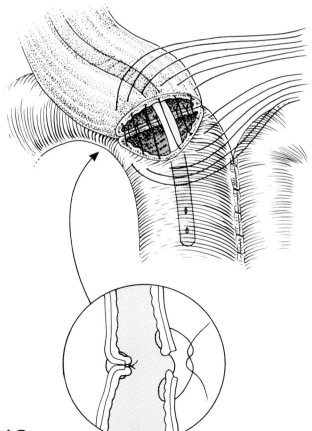

Anterior wall

13 After complete transection of the oesophagus interrupted sutures for closure of the anterior wall are placed in a manner similar to that of the posterior wall except that they are knotted on the outside.

13

Stapled oesophagojejunostomy

14 Alternatively, the end-to-side oesophagojejunostomy may be performed using staples. After a purse-string suture has been applied to the oesophageal resection line, the head of a CEEA 25 stapler is inserted into the lumen of the oesophagus and its body is brought into the pouch over the reopened end at its afferent loop. Its tip perforates the anterior wall of the efferent loop about 1.5 cm above the enteroenterostomy and is then closed. This technique is especially useful when the oesophagojejunostomy has to be performed transhiatally above the level of the diaphragm.

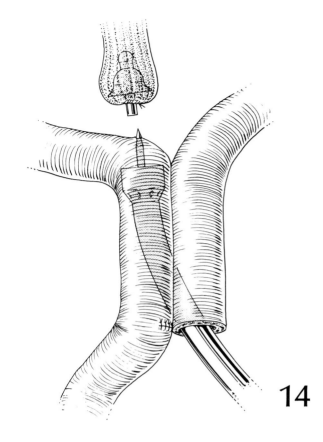

14

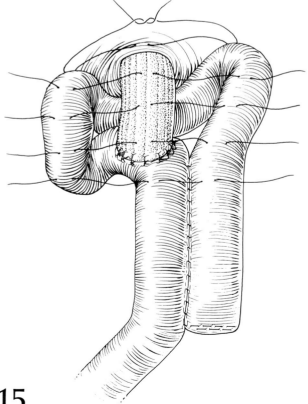

15

JEJUNOPLICATION

15 The free loop is positioned behind the anastomoses, wrapped around the oesophagus and fixed with seromuscular sutures which take bites of the oesophageal muscle (the last suture pierces the seromuscularis of the pouch).

Roux-en-Y anastomosis

16 The afferent loop of the jejunum (attached to the duodenum) which was temporarily closed with, for example, a Murphy clamp is anastomosed end-to-side to the efferent loop 30–40 cm distal to the pouch with 4/0 absorbable sutures to prevent reflux of duodenal contents. The incision in the mesocolon is closed and sutured to the inferior part of the pouch, making sure it does not press on the pouch.

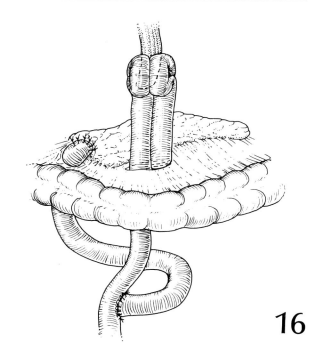

16

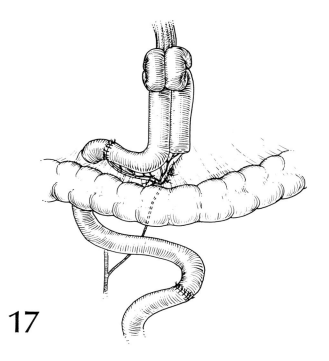

17

Pouch with orthograde duodenal transit

17 Alternatively it is possible to re-establish orthograde duodenal transit by constructing an end-to-end anastomosis between the duodenal resection line and the distal efferent loop of jejunum.

Postoperative care

Postoperative care in general has been described in the chapter on pp. 39–44. Patients are placed on total parenteral nutrition for 7–10 days. The nasogastric tube is usually removed after 7 days when leakage of the anastomosis has been excluded by radiological examination of the gastrointestinal tract using a water-soluble contrast medium. Enteral feeding is started cautiously, and in the first months patients take in numerous (6–8) small meals daily until the reservoir capacity of the pouch increases and they are able to eat adequate quantities. Dietetic consultations during this time are very helpful.

Outcome

Severe heartburn due to reflux of duodenal contents, dumping syndrome, and the sequelae of malnutrition and malabsorption impair the patient's wellbeing, capacity to work and quality of life. As a result of these symptoms the nutritional status of patients undergoing total gastrectomy can be reduced significantly.

Follow-up examinations of gastric pouches at several centres including that of the authors have shown that pouch reconstruction generally has a favourable outcome. Reflux oesophagitis is avoided by the Roux-en-Y reconstruction and the effects of the jejunoplication. Because of the increased reservoir capacity of the pouch, patients are able to eat sufficient quantities earlier and their bodyweight exceeds individual optimal weights more frequently than after simple reconstruction methods. Incompatibilities with certain foods as well as the dumping syndrome occur only infrequently. Anaemia does not occur providing vitamin B_{12} is given regularly (500–1000 µg every 6 weeks).

Further reading

Buhl K, Schlag P, Herfarth C. Quality of life and functional results following different types of resection for gastric carcinoma. *Eur J Surg Oncol* 1990; 16: 404–9.

Herfarth C. Gastric reconstruction. In: Becker HD, Herfarth C, Lierse W, Schreiber HW, eds. *Surgery of the Stomach*. Berlin, Heidelberg, New York: Springer, 1988: 130–59.

Herfarth C, Schlag P, Buhl K. Surgical procedures for gastric substitution. *World J Surg* 1987; 11: 689–98.

Troidl H, Kusche J, Vestweber KH, Eypasch E, Maul U. Pouch versus esophagojejunostomy after total gastrectomy: a randomized clinical trial. *World J Surg* 1987; 11: 699–712.

Extra-anatomical reconstruction of the resected oesophagus

André Duranceau MD
Professor of Surgery, Department of Surgery, University of Montréal, Division of Thoracic Surgery, Hôtel-Dieu de Montréal, Montréal, Québec, Canada

Principles and justification

Following resection or exclusion of the oesophagus, it may be necessary to reconstitute upper digestive continuity away from the normal anatomical oesophageal route. Extra-anatomical reconstruction in patients with cancer avoids the problem of local recurrence leading to obstruction of the interposed organ.

1 The substernal route is the preferred extra-anatomical reconstruction in the author's institution. Subcutaneous positioning of the transplanted stomach, colon, or jejunum can also be undertaken, but it has the disadvantage of being a longer route to reach the cervical oesophagus. The left or right prehilar positioning of the transplanted organ may also be considered in order to bypass a previously used anterior mediastinum, but again with the disadvantage of a longer distance to reach the cervical oesophagus. Extrathoracic alimentary continuity is also possible by the use of a tube to bridge from an oesophagostomy to either a large tube gastrostomy or jejunostomy.

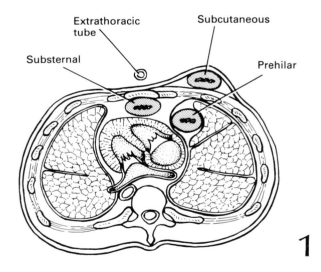

1

Preoperative

Whenever an oesophagectomy is planned both stomach and colon are prepared to allow either to be used as the replacement organ as necessary.

Colon preparation is achieved by the administration of 4 litres of a polyethylene glycol solution (GoLytely) the afternoon before the operation. Ringer's lactate or physiological saline is administered intravenously for 12 h before the operation in order to balance liquid losses during preparation.

Prophylactic antibiotics are administered in order to cover both the aerobic and anaerobic flora found in the oesophagus. A first-generation cephalosporin with metronidazole (Flagyl), 500 mg, or clindamycin, 600 mg, are administered before the start of the operation and at regular intervals for a maximum of four doses.

Heparin, 5000 units, is given subcutaneously the morning of the operation and administered every 12 h until the patient is fully ambulatory.

Operations

USE OF THE ANTERIOR MEDIASTINUM

Position of patient

The patient is placed in the dorsal decubitus position, with the arms along the sides. The head is hyper-extended and turned toward the right. Draping is such that access to the anterior chest to the level of both anterior axillary lines is provided.

2 A midline epigastric incision is completed first. It extends proximally over the distal sternum and the xiphoid process is removed. Distally the incision is completed with a left paraumbilical extension.

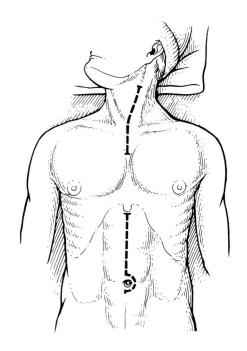

2

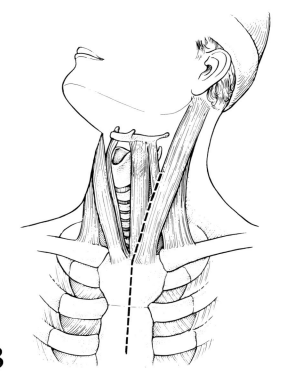

3

3 The cervical incision extends from midway along the anterior border of the sternocleidomastoid muscle to the sternal notch and then presternally to the level of the third rib.

The sternocleidomastoid muscle is freed from its insertion on the sternum, manubrium and clavicle. The pectoralis muscle is also freed from its sternal attachments to the level of the third rib cartilage. The muscles are retracted laterally.

4 In order to prepare a tunnel in the anterior mediastinum, a significant enlargement of the thoracic inlet is required. To achieve this, a proximal sternotomy is made to the level between the second and third rib. The manubrium is sectioned laterally immediately over the head of the second rib. A Gigli saw is then positioned lateral to the posterior prominence of the head of the clavicle and brought out parasternally at the level of the transverse sternal section. The whole junction of manubrium, medial clavicle and first rib is then removed, allowing the hand to pass freely between the anterior mediastinal structures and the neck.

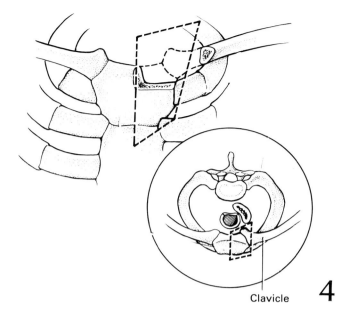

Clavicle

4

5 In the neck all the prethyroid muscles are sectioned along the axis of the incision and the deep cervical fascia is opened proximal and distal to the inferior thyroid artery. If possible, this artery is preserved in order to maximize blood supply to the cervical oesophagus. The proximal anterior mediastinum is exposed and all mediastinal muscle extensions from the prethyroid muscles are divided. The innominate vein is identified: it is the most anterior mediastinal structure at the thoracic inlet.

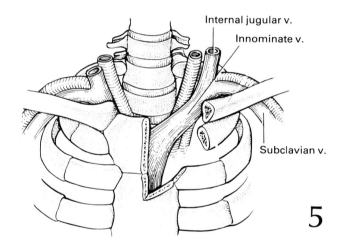

Internal jugular v.

Innominate v.

Subclavian v.

5

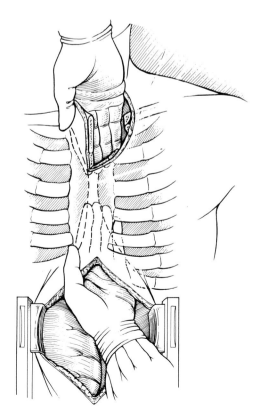

6

6 The substernal tunnel is completed using the cervical and abdominal incisions simultaneously. Through the abdominal incision, the midline diaphragmatic insertions are freed bluntly just behind the distal sternum in order to allow free passage of a hand and forearm immediately posterior to the sternum. The pleura should be displaced toward the right and left chest, but it is easy to enter it. Both hands should reach freely and widely behind the sternum.

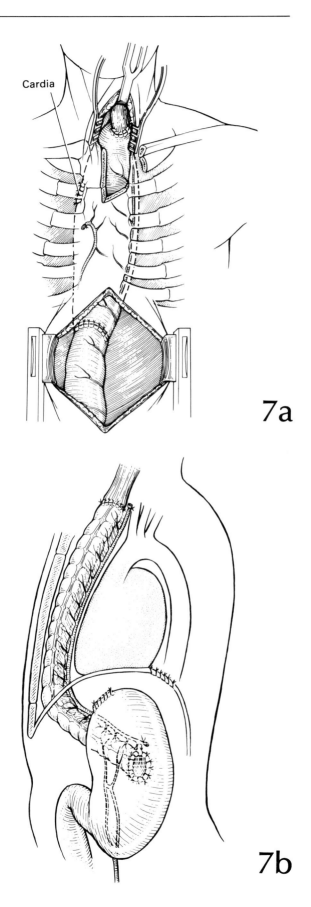

7a, b The stomach or colon is fed through this wide tunnel with maximum attention being paid to protection of the vascular supply of the organ during manipulation. The interposed organ is put into a clear polythene arthroscopy bag and the proximal tip of the bag attached to a Foley catheter. With suction applied to the catheter the bag is pulled through the mediastinum, delivering stomach or colon to the cervical location without fear of it being retained or damaged by a mediastinal structure.

PREHILAR ROUTE

If the anatomical route is not available and the transplanted organ is placed in the chest cavity, it is put in a prehilar position (*see Illustration 1*). The pleura is usually sealed against the 'unusable' anterior mediastinum. Distally, taking down of the diaphragmatic insertion is carried out more laterally than for the substernal tunnel position.

When the anterior prehilar approach is used, removal of the junction of sternum, mid-clavicle and first rib may still afford an easier access to the remaining cervical oesophagus.

SUBCUTANEOUS ROUTE

A tunnel for the subcutaneous route (*see Illustration 1*) is made immediately anterior to the pectoralis major muscle, freeing enough space for the interposed organ. It is essential to avoid compression on the replacement tube in order to protect the arterial supply and the venous drainage. When using this route it is helpful to have a long proximal oesophageal stump, as this allows an easy anastomosis to be made in a left parasternal position.

PRETHORACIC TUBING

8 If the patient has a terminal oesophagostomy with a gastrostomy and/or a jejunostomy, tubes of the Pezzer type or as devised by Akiyama can be installed between the oesophagostomy and the distal stoma. In those patients where reconstruction is not possible, the use of these external tubes can be valuable to provide relatively normal food ingestion.

Postoperative care

All patients undergoing oesophageal reconstruction are observed in an intensive care facility in the immediate postoperative period as previously discussed on pp. 39–44. The author routinely inserts chest tubes in the right and left chest cavities for substernal bypass. These are removed when no significant drainage is observed.

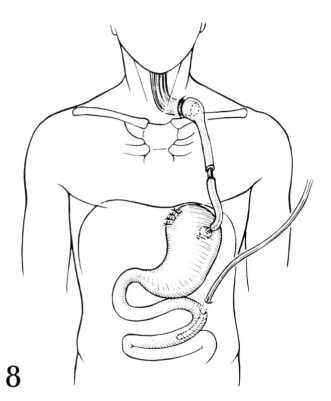

8

Surgical anatomy of the cervical oesophagus

Glyn G. Jamieson FRACS, FACS
Dorothy Mortlock Professor of Surgery, University of Adelaide, Department of Surgery, Royal Adelaide Hospital, Adelaide, Australia

The cervical oesophagus lies behind the lower part of the larynx and trachea. The first 2–3 cm of the oesophagus lies behind the larynx and is not easily separable from it, so that a 'total' oesophagectomy nearly always leaves behind about 2 cm of the proximal oesophagus.

1 Laterally, the cervical oesophagus is separated from the lobes of the thyroid gland by the deep cervical fascia, under which also lie the inferior thyroid arteries emerging from behind the carotid sheaths. The recurrent laryngeal nerves lie in the tracheo-oesophageal grooves in about 50% of cases (white dot). In about 10% of cases the nerves are more posterior as a direct lateral relation of the oesophagus (black dot). In the remainder of cases they lie more anteriorly as a direct lateral relation of the trachea (black dot).

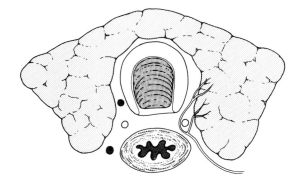

1

Posteriorly, the oesophagus lies on the vertebral bodies and the longus colli muscles which lie along the lateral sides of the anterior part of the vertebral bodies. The oesophagus is separated from these structures by the prevertebral fascia.

The thoracic duct lies to the left of the oesophagus in the region of the thoracic inlet. More proximally, it passes laterally behind the carotid sheath and out of the field.

2 The inferior constrictor muscle of the pharynx arises from the cricoid cartilage and the thyroid cartilage and sweeps upwards and backwards to insert in the midline raphe with its fellow of the opposite side. Morphologically, there is no distinction between any of the muscle fibres of the inferior constrictor, or indeed between the lower fibres of inferior constrictor and the circular oesophageal muscle, except for a small area anteriorly where the inferior constrictor arises from the cricoid cartilage (known in some texts as the Killian–Jamieson area). Nevertheless, the lowermost fibres of the inferior constrictor differ physiologically from the fibres both distal and proximal in being maintained in tonic contraction. Physiologically this is the upper oesophageal sphincter and morphologically it corresponds best with the part of the inferior constrictor arising from the cricoid cartilage and thus called cricopharyngeus. This part may have a different nerve supply from the rest of the muscle, via the recurrent laryngeal nerve. The remainder of the muscle arises from a tendinous arch over the cricothyroid muscle and the oblique line on the thyroid cartilage, and so it is sometimes called thyropharyngeus to distinguish it from the cricopharyngeus. The thyropharyngeus obtains its nerve supply through the pharyngeal plexus.

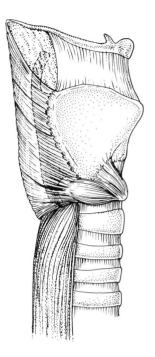

2

The digestive tube cannot be removed proximal to the cricoid cartilage without entering the pharynx. It may sometimes be necessary to make an anastomosis between the pharynx and the stomach or colon. To do this it is best to make an incision as posterior as possible in order to avoid damaging or constricting the arytenoid muscles and other muscles of the laryngeal inlet. Posteriorly, the incision (theoretically) can be taken as high as the base of the skull.

A diverticulum from the pharynx is sometimes found protruding posteriorly immediately proximal to the cricopharyngeus muscle. The primary defect in patients with pharyngeal diverticulum is an inability of the cricopharyngeus to open adequately. This is related to fibrosis affecting the muscular fibres. In order to squeeze food through the constriction, high pressures are generated in the pharynx, and the mucosa bulges immediately proximal to the fibrotic muscle. Why the mucosa tends to bulge posteriorly and to the left is unknown, but obviously this is the weakest point of the general area.

In removing a symptomatic diverticulum, it makes sense to divide the narrowed zone of muscle (crico-pharyngeal myotomy). Division of this muscle is also sometimes undertaken for other conditions. Because there is no dividing line between the muscle fibres above and below the cricopharyngeus to carry out a myotomy, it is usual to mobilize the upper oesophagus and divide from a point 2 or 3 cm down the oesophagus upwards for 4–5 cm. The pharynx above can be recognized because its wall tends to balloon more than the oesophagus. Landmarks for the level of the cricopharyngeus are the point where the inferior belly of omohyoid crosses the viscera, the cricoid cartilage, and the inferior horn of the thyroid cartilage which is almost level with the most distal fibres of origin of cricopharyngeus. When a pharyngeal pouch is present, the cricopharyngeus indents its neck considerably and it is important to be sure that all muscle and fibrous tissue fibres are divided when dissecting the pouch free. The mucosa bulges without restriction from oesophagus to the neck of the sac when complete division has been achieved. As the pouch tends to arise posteriorly, it is usual to undertake the myotomy towards the midline posteriorly, although a more lateral myotomy may well achieve the same effect.

Recurrent laryngeal nerves

The right recurrent laryngeal nerve arises from the right vagus and passes around the right subclavian artery to pass upwards approximately in the tracheo-oesophageal groove. It disappears from view beneath the inferior constrictor muscle of the pharynx behind the inferior cornu of the thyroid cartilage.

The left recurrent nerve passes from lateral to medial under the arch of the aorta but thereafter its course is similar to the right nerve.

Although the nerve lies in the tracheo-oesophageal groove in about 50% of cases, in the remainder it lies either further laterally or more anteriorly alongside the trachea and occasionally more posteriorly alongside the oesophagus. Occasionally it even traverses the substance of the thyroid gland.

There is perhaps only one essential fact to know in regard to the relationship of the recurrent laryngeal nerve to the inferior thyroid artery and that is that the two always have a very close relationship (except in the rare case where the nerve is not recurrent). The most usual relationship is for the nerve to pass between the two branches of the inferior thyroid artery, but it may pass in front of or behind the artery, and the relationship frequently differs on the two sides. Providing the inferior thyroid artery is divided laterally, near its point of emergence from behind the carotid artery, then the recurrent laryngeal nerve should not be endangered by the division.

Mobilization of the cervical oesophagus

The cervical oesophagus can be approached through an incision in the right or left side of the neck. Because the oesophagus tends to lie to the left of the midline, the left side is often chosen, although in practical terms there is little difference between the two sides.

An incision is made along the anterior border of sternomastoid from the sternal notch below to a few centimetres below the ear lobe above, and the incision is deepened through the subcutaneous tissues and platysma.

A branch of the cervical cutaneous nerve is usually seen in the upper part of the incision and should be preserved if possible. The omohyoid muscle is divided; it usually contains a moderate sized blood vessel within its substance which requires ligature or cautery. The prethyroid muscles and their investing fascia are also divided to expose the carotid sheath. This is retracted laterally and the middle thyroid veins are divided and the inferior thyroid artery is sought. Although it can be divided with apparent impunity, it is one of the major arteries supplying the cervical oesophagus. It is probably sensible practice to preserve it, if practicable, and it usually is.

Whether the recurrent laryngeal nerve should be sought and dissected free is a moot point. Such an approach is often followed by nerve dysfunction and, although usually only temporary, it may deprive the patient of the ability to cough normally during the vital early postoperative period. The nerve can usually be seen or palpated along its course and it is the author's practice to keep the dissection very close to the oesophageal wall without identifying the nerve, and separate the oesophagus from its investing fibroalveolar attachments by a mixture of sharp and blunt dissection.

Anteriorly and proximally, it is not easy to be sure where the oesophagus commences. The inferior cornu of the thyroid cartilage can usually be palpated and is a useful landmark for the commencement of the oesophagus. Difficulty may be encountered in mobilizing the anterior 2 cm, and as the blood supply enters here it is better to leave this part of the cervical oesophagus undissected.

Using a dissecting swab it is not difficult to mobilize the oesophagus by blunt dissection well down into the superior mediastinum.

The right side of the oesophagus is not always easy to determine, but with judicious retraction and a curved clamp it can usually be dissected free under direct vision.

Illustrations by Paul Richardson

Cricopharyngeal myotomy and excision of a pharyngo-oesophageal diverticulum

Glyn G. Jamieson FRACS, FACS
Dorothy Mortlock Professor of Surgery, University of Adelaide, Department of Surgery, Royal Adelaide Hospital, Adelaide, Australia

André Duranceau MD
Professor of Surgery, Department of Surgery, University of Montréal, Division of Thoracic Surgery, Hôtel-Dieu de Montréal, Montréal, Québec, Canada

It has now been established that Zenker's diverticula form because of an inability of the cricopharyngeus to open adequately during swallowing. It is thus rational to divide the cricopharyngeus muscle when treating a patient with Zenker's diverticulum. If the diverticulum is small (less than 2 cm in diameter) nothing further need be done. If the diverticulum is slightly larger (2–4 cm) then the diverticulum is suspended upside down after performing the cricopharyngeal myotomy. If the diverticulum is larger than 4 cm in diameter, it is best to remove it after performing a cricopharyngeal myotomy.

Operation

Position of patient

The patient is placed in a supine position with a small pillow under the shoulders. The head is supported on a doughnut type pillow and is hyperextended and turned to the right. If the patient has a thin neck, the thyroid cartilage and the cricoid cartilage below it can often be clearly felt.

Incision

1 An incision is made along the anteromedial border of the left sternomastoid muscle from a few centimetres below the ear lobe to a point just above the sternal notch. Subcutaneous tissues and the platysma are divided.

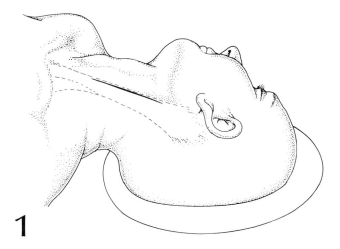

1

2 A branch of the cervical cutaneous nerve may be seen in the upper third of the field. It should be protected if practicable because its division causes dysaesthesia in the submandibular skin.

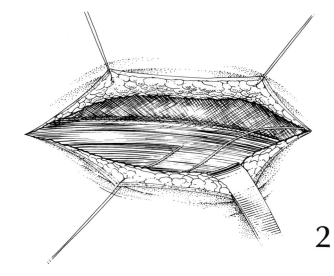

3 The sternomastoid muscle is freed by sharp dissection from the underlying vascular structure. The omohyoid muscle and the prethyroid muscles are cut to expose the jugular vein, the carotid artery and the thyroid gland.

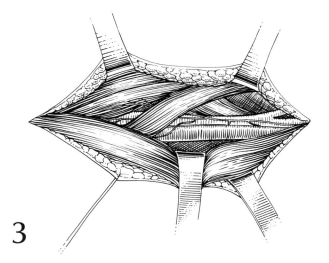

4 The middle thyroid vein, when present, is divided. This allows the thyroid to be retracted towards the midline which places the deep cervical fascia under tension. It is necessary to open this fascia formally in the line of the incision, after which the inferior thyroid artery is sought and isolated. To protect the recurrent laryngeal nerve, the artery is divided far laterally where it emerges from behind the carotid sheath.

After ligation of the inferior thyroid artery, the pharynx and oesophagus are easily dissected free from the prevertebral fascia. The recurrent laryngeal nerve may be identified in the groove between the trachea and the oesophagus.

A 36-Fr mercury bougie is passed into the oesophagus for use as a stent. This can be passed early in the operation when a cricopharyngeal myotomy alone is being undertaken. However, if it is used with diverticulum excision it should not be passed until the surgeon can be sure that the bougie does not enter the diverticulum.

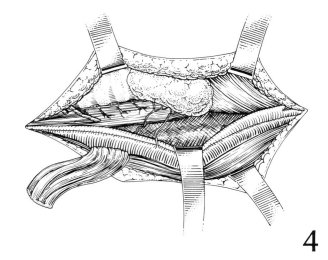

5 The pharyngo-oesophageal junction can be recognized by palpating the cricoid cartilage and noting the change from the capacious pharyngeal wall (which may contain adipose tissue) to the smaller diameter of the oesophagus. Other landmarks for the level of cricopharyngeus are the level of crossing of the inferior belly of the omohyoid muscle and the tip of the inferior horn of the thyroid cartilage, which is often easily palpable. The assistant retracts the whole larynx and pharynx anteriorly and rotates it at the same time to expose the midline posteriorly.

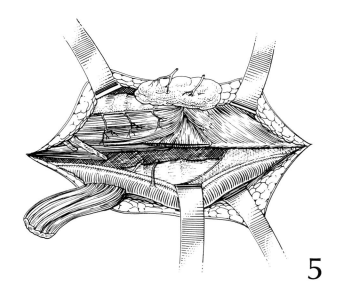

5

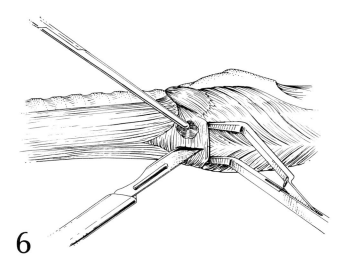

6

6 If a myotomy alone is to be performed, the procedure is as follows. The surgeon takes a scalpel with no. 15 blade. A right-handed surgeon uses an instrument with a dissector swab in the left hand to produce lateral traction on the muscle while gently cutting with the scalpel in the right hand. Myotomy is begun on the oesophagus and proceeds proximally. The mucosa is recognized by its slightly bluer colour compared with muscle and by the submucous plexus of vessels that overlies it. Meticulous haemostasis is essential and is achieved by judiciously using very low intensity or bipolar diathermy. The muscle fibres at the cricopharyngeal junction tend to be thicker than oesophageal musculature. The pharyngeal muscle may be atrophic or infiltrated with adipose tissue. If the myotomy incision is taken too deeply, then the submucous venous plexus may be cut, causing troublesome bleeding, and this requires fine silk sutures to restore haemostasis.

7 If a large diverticulum is present, it is easy to see it as bulging tissue attached laterally to the upper oesophagus. This tissue is grasped with atraumatic forceps and the layers of fascial condensation around it are dissected from the sac. It is not always easy to know when the sac has been adequately defined, and the most difficult area to define is the neck. On the one hand, proximally the neck blends imperceptibly with the pharynx above, and on the other it is difficult to know when adequate distal dissection has taken place in the region of the cricopharyngeus.

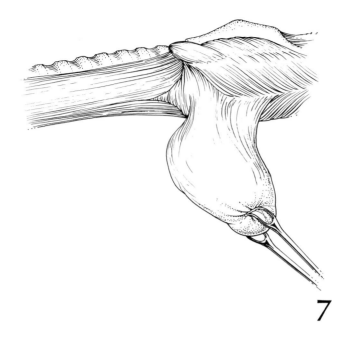

7

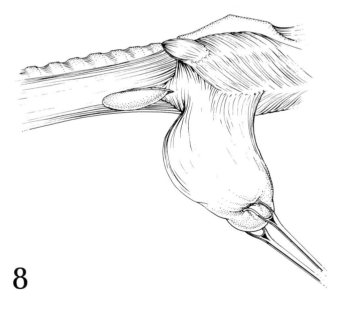

8

8 In order to be certain that all the muscle tissue of cricopharyngeus is divided, the myotomy should be begun on the oesophagus and progressed proximally, making sure that the mucosa bulges through the myotomy in continuity with the mucosa of the sac. A strip of muscle approximately 1 cm wide is removed from the proximal 2 cm of the oesophagus and dissection proceeds upwards onto the sac itself. Oesophageal muscle and the cricopharyngeal muscle here are much thinner than oesophageal muscle lower down on the oesophagus, and so great care is required in performing the myotomy. A mosquito forceps can prove useful in developing a plane deep to the oesophageal muscle and it proves easiest to commence the oesophageal myotomy with the forceps pointing distally.

9 Once the plane is established, the direction is reversed with proximal dissection onto the neck of the sac. It is only by dividing all of the muscle that an adequate myotomy can be accomplished.

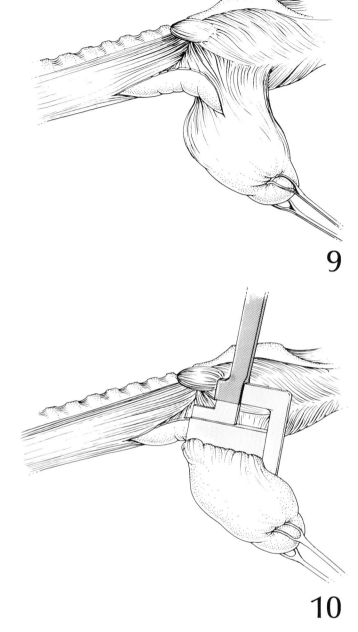

9

10 When the dissection has been completed, a Babcock clamp is placed to hold the sac out and a 32-Fr bougie can be placed in the oesophagus if it has not already been positioned. A transverse stapler with 3.5 mm staples is applied across the sac, and it is probably better to err on the side of leaving too much rather than too little mucosa. The stapler is fired and the sac is cut away. It is not necessary to repair the muscle over the staple line, although some surgeons do. Indeed, it may be best not to repair the muscle in case the area is narrowed.

If the sac is of the order of 2–4 cm in its largest diameter, it can simply be upended after it has been dissected free, and sutured either to the retropharyngeal fascia or to the anterior spinal ligament. No drains are used, nor is a nasogastric tube necessary.

10

Postoperative care

The patient is commenced on fluid on the following day and a liquid diet on day 2. Fit patients can be discharged once they have resumed a normal diet, usually three days after surgery. However, patients undergoing a cricopharyngeal myotomy alone often have neural or vascular disease of some type and so resumption of feeding may be a slower process. Similarly, some patients undergoing diverticulectomy are very elderly and discharge may be delayed for medical reasons. Very occasionally patients develop a leak from the operative site. This manifests itself at any time from the first postoperative day. It may cause surgical emphysema, a wound infection or a salivary fistula, or any combination of these three. It is best treated as for other oesophageal leaks (*see* chapter on pp. 39–44), i.e. essentially nil by mouth and antibiotics until healing is demonstrated by a contrast swallow. Not only is such leakage uncommon, but it nearly always runs a 'benign' course in this condition.

Illustrations by Antoine Barnaud

Abdominal and right thoracic subtotal oesophagectomy

Bernard Launois MD, FACS
Professor, Digestive and Transplantation Surgery, Hôpital Pontchaillou, Rennes, France

Guy J. Maddern PhD, MS, FRACS
Jepson Professor of Surgery, University of Adelaide, The Queen Elizabeth Hospital, Adelaide, Australia

History

Before 1946, the only widely practised approach to the thoracic oesophagus had been described by Sweet[1] using a left-sided thoracotomy. Although this operation permitted relatively good access to the lower third of the oesophagus, cancers of the middle and upper third of the oesophagus were dissected with greater difficulty because of the overlying aortic arch. In 1946 Lewis described the abdominal and right thoracic approach[2] for subtotal oesophagectomy. This operation was adopted by Tanner in the UK[3] (Lewis–Tanner operation) and by Santy[4] in France (Lewis–Santy operation), and has remained the favoured operation for an abdominal and right thoracic subtotal oesophagectomy.

Operations

ABDOMINAL APPROACH

The operation is usually commenced with the abdominal approach which enables the assessment of liver metastases, the involvement of draining lymph nodes and the performance of gastrolysis.

Incision

1a, b A midline incision is used, with the approach to the hiatus being facilitated by a substernal retractor. This provides improved access to the intra-abdominal oesophagus.

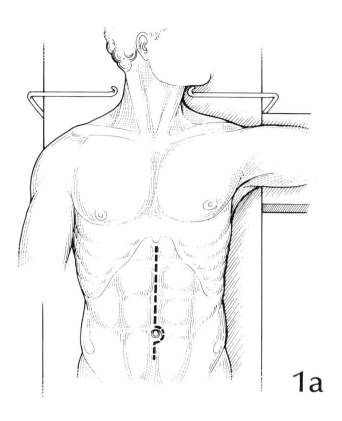

1a

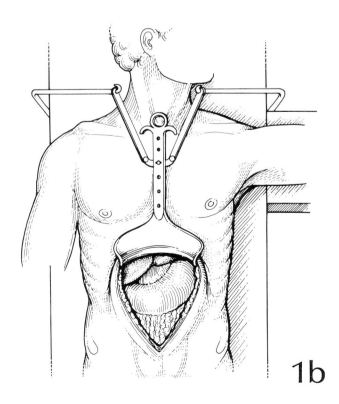

1b

2a, b

The first step is to tie and divide the vessels of the gastrocolic ligament and the short gastric vessels. It is important during the mobilization of the greater curve of the stomach to identify and preserve the right gastroepiploic vessels. The abdominal oesophagus is dissected next. The left triangular ligament of the liver is divided and the left lobe retracted to the right to reveal the oesophageal hiatus. This should be dissected with scissors under direct vision after dividing the peritoneum in front of the oesophagus. By opening the tissues to the left and right of the oesophagus a curved clamp can be introduced and a tape passed around the oesophagus. The tape can then be used to provide traction on the abdominal oesophagus which aids in the ligation and division of the remaining short gastric vessels.

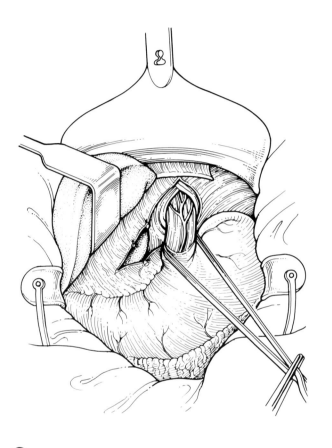

2a

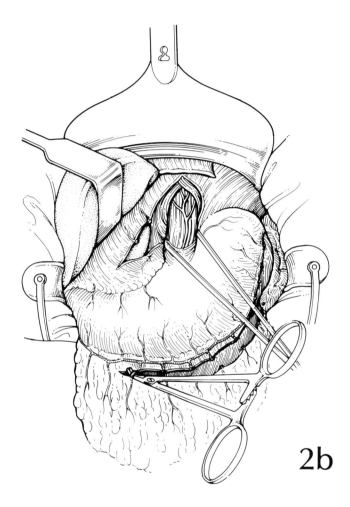

2b

3 From inside the lesser sac, with the mobilized greater curve of the stomach held upward and to the right, the left gastric vascular pedicle and its associated lymph nodes are dissected. The left gastric vein and artery are individually identified, ligated and divided.

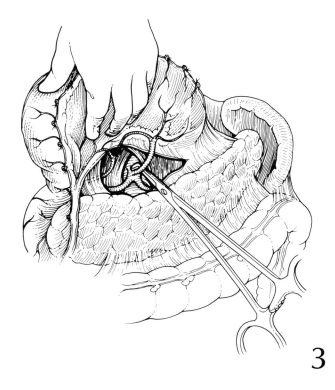

3

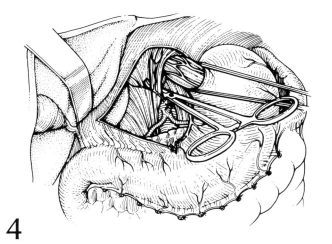

4

4 The lesser omentum is then ligated and divided from the hiatus down to the pylorus. Mobilization of the duodenum (Kocher manoeuvre) is not routinely performed for this operation but can be undertaken if increased gastric mobility is required.

A pyloroplasty or a pyloroclasia is performed to help prevent delay in gastric emptying, which sometimes occurs after this procedure. Pyloroclasia is usually performed using the thumb and middle finger as dilators which pass through the pylorus by invaginating the gastric or duodenal wall to disrupt the sphincteric mechanism.

The right crus is divided and the hiatus opened. The intra-abdominal oesophagus is then freed from all its hiatal attachments by a combination of blunt and sharp dissection.

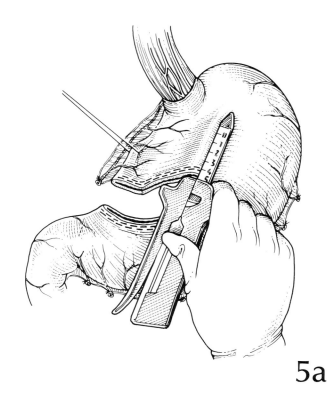

5a

5a, b A gastric tube can be constructed at this stage, although this can be delayed until the thoracic part of the operation. The gastric tube is constructed from below the 'crow's foot' on the antrum of the stomach up to the hiatus. This is most readily performed by using a surgical stapler (e.g. GIA) and leaving the last 5 cm at the cardia unstapled until the oesophagus and stomach have been successfully mobilized and delivered into the chest. The danger of completing the gastric tube at this stage is that, should the oesophageal cancer prove unresectable, then a complete obstruction has been created unnecessarily. The staple line is oversewn to ensure haemostasis and minimize the possibility of a leak.

A feeding jejunostomy can now be inserted to facilitate postoperative enteric nutrition.

Wound closure

A closed suction drain is placed behind the stomach up to the hiatus and the abdomen is closed.

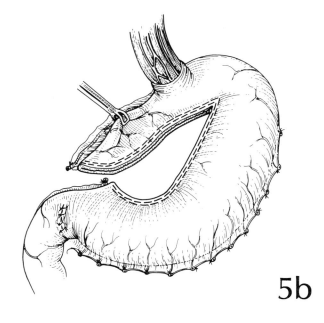

5b

THORACIC APPROACH

Position of patient

6 The patient is placed on the left side with a sandbag under the left ribs. Great care should be taken to ensure not only that the patient is well supported and secured, but that no unsupported pressure points exist. The right arm is most conveniently strapped to a padded overhead rail.

Incision

There are two possible thoracic incisions, one using a rib resection and the other passing through the intercostal space. The authors have found an unacceptable incidence of paradoxical respiration after rib resection and now recommend an intercostal approach through either the sixth intercostal space for lower third cancers or the fifth intercostal space for cancers of the middle and upper third. Gradual increase in the rib retraction at intervals during the procedure can produce adequate retraction without rib fracture even in elderly patients. The scapula, once freed from its muscular attachments inferiorly, should be retracted upwards. At this stage it is possible to confirm the location of the ribs by counting from the second rib, felt at the apex of the thorax, down to the desired interspace. The periosteum of the rib is lifted with a periosteal elevator and the intercostal space opened on the lower border of the rib. The pleura is then opened.

A Finochietto or Lortat–Jacob retractor is positioned and gently opened. Any pleural attachments are freed, and the lung mobilized to the hilus. The lung is retracted forwards and collapsed. It can be held in this position by fixing a broad blade attached to the rib retractor.

7 The right pulmonary triangular ligament is divided close to the posterior edge of the inferior lobe of the right lung, up to the right inferior pulmonary vein.

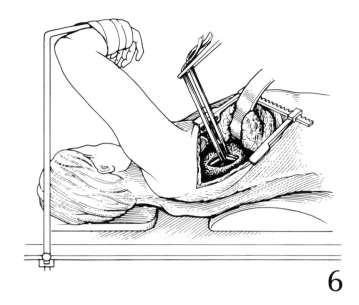

6

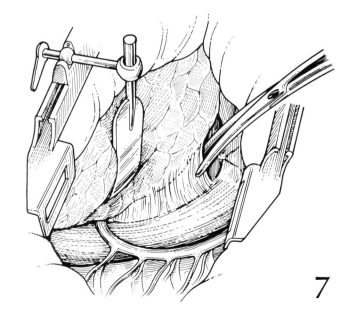

7

8 Scissors are introduced vertically between the pericardium and the posterior mediastinum. Opening the scissors reveals a plane close to the pericardium, and it is then possible to dissect upwards along this plane.

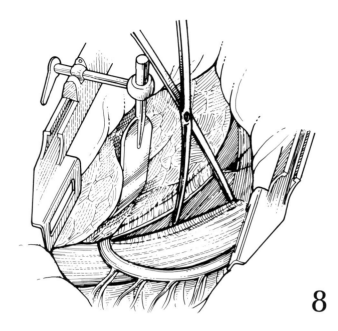

8

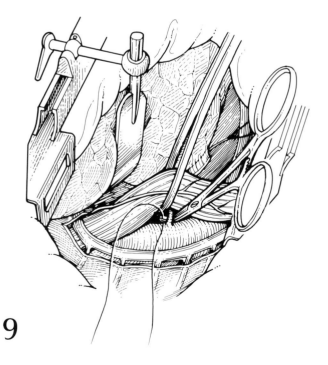

9

9 The fingers of the left hand can palpate the posterior aspect of the oesophagus and retract it from the posterior mediastinum. The pleura is then opened along the vertebral column. The scissors are opened horizontally, exposing the oesophageal arteries which are tied and divided.

10 The azygous vein is identified and ligated in continuity or transfixed and then divided.

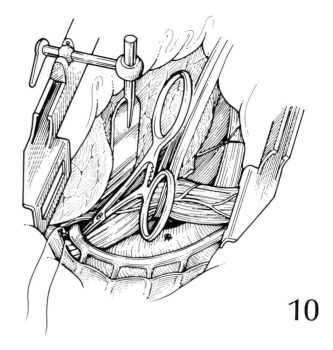

10

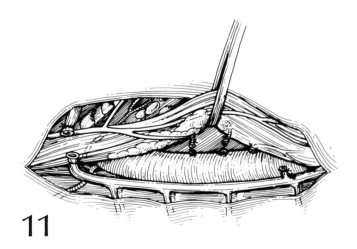

11

11 The oesophagus is mobilized above and below the tumour and tapes are passed around it to aid in retraction during the tumour dissection.

12 The oesophagus and tumour are now dissected from the surrounding structures, including the pericardium, the right and left main bronchi and the aorta. While it is desirable not to open into the tumour during the dissection, this is a preferable option to an unexpected aortic or bronchial laceration.

Difficulty in this dissection can occur at the pericardium, the trachea and/or the aorta. Extension of dissection into the pericardium is not a contraindication to resection, as a portion of pericardium can be excised safely. The pericardium is opened in front of the adhesions and then divided around the margin of the tumour. Dissection is almost never extended into the right inferior pulmonary vein.

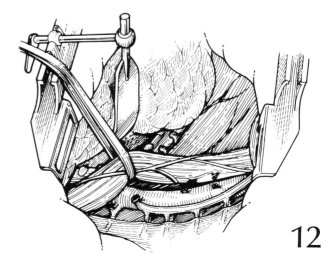

12

13 The aorta is sometimes involved by neoplastic spread. The technique used to free the cancer in these circumstances is to dissect between the intima and the adventitia of the aorta. It is important, however, to return outside the adventitia once the tumour is freed. The large oesophageal artery that arises from the aortic arch is best ligated and divided. Sometimes the artery is involved in the tumour. Ligation is not then possible, and the artery must be oversewn after the tumour is resected.

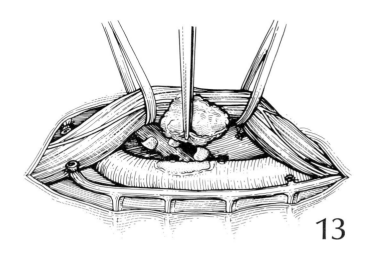

13

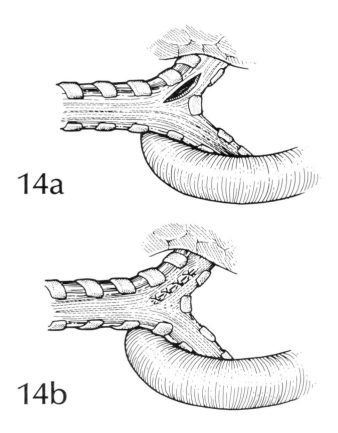

14a

14b

14a, b In some cases the most difficult part of the dissection is to detach the tumour from the trachea and the bronchus. When the neoplastic process involves the cartilaginous rings or the carina, there is little risk of opening the respiratory tree. However, when the membranous portion is involved, dissection is trickier. It is usually possible to find a plane between the trachea and a thin membrane covering it. This dissection should be directed to cutting only the neoplastic adhesions, otherwise a tracheal tear can occur. If such a tear appears, it is possible to repair it with interrupted stitches of 5/0 polypropylene (Prolene). This is relatively straightforward and usually successful.

15 The thoracic duct is found in the groove between the oesophagus and the vertebral bodies. It is important to ligate at least its inferior portion if a subsequent chylothorax is to be avoided.

Once the oesophagus and cancer are fully mobilized the stomach is delivered into the chest. Care should be taken to maintain the correct orientation and to avoid possible twists. The nasogastric tube is withdrawn into the cervical oesophagus.

A gastric tube can be formed at this stage either by using a GIA stapler or with a TA 90, which is easily manipulated in the thorax, leaving the last 5 cm at the cardia unstapled.

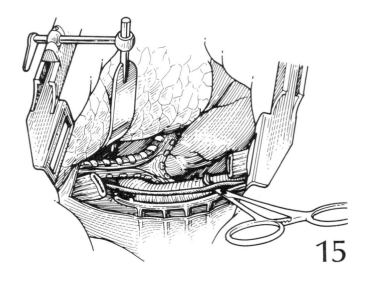

15

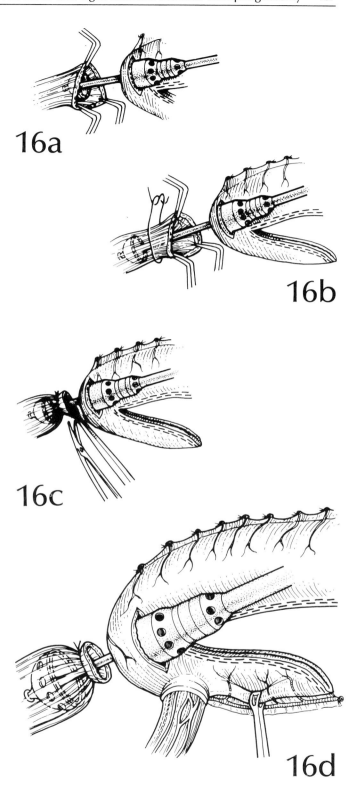

16a

16b

16c

16d

16a–d The proximal portion of oesophagus is grasped with a Satinsky clamp and divided below. Two methods can be used to tie a purse-string to the anvil of the stapler. The first is to place a tie around the anvil rod after it has been introduced into the oesophagus. This is done by placing three clamps on the oesophageal wall to hold open the lumen of the oesophagus and then the anvil is introduced into the lumen and a ligature is tied 'en masse' around the entire oesophageal wall[5]. Excess oesophagus distal to the ligature is then trimmed off. The second method is to place an over and over purse-string suture in the oesophageal stump (see chapter on pp. 79–83).

A gastrotomy is made below the apex of the gastric tube. Often it is convenient to make the gastrotomy in the portion of the stomach destined to be removed. The stapling device is introduced through the gastrotomy, into and through the stomach, the anvil is attached and secured and the anastomosis is performed by fitting the stapler.

17 The remaining stomach is removed with the gastrotomy by stapling the remaining section of the tube and the staple lines are then oversewn. The nasogastric tube is passed down into the stomach and the thoracic drain inserted. The chest is then closed.

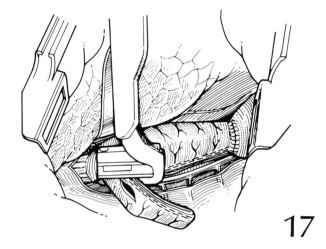

17

Postoperative care

A nasogastric tube is positioned below the anastomosis under visual control during thoracotomy and the thoracotomy is closed around a thoracic drain placed at the base of the thorax. Another drain is located at the apex in case of air leakage. The patient is then transferred to the intensive care unit and is intubated and ventilated for 24 h or more until the blood gases are satisfactory. The patient is then moved to the surgical ward. The drain is taken out after 3 or 4 days when there is less than 150 ml of clear effusion. Feeding by the jejunostomy is started as soon as bowel activity commences. The nasogastric tube is usually taken out after 7 days. Oral feeding is then progressively reinstated.

In case of an anastomotic leakage feeding is only performed via the jejunostomy and the anastomosis is not checked by a Gastrografin meal. If there is a suspicion of leakage (fever), the authors prefer to cease oral feeding and feed the patient by the jejunostomy.

References

1. Sweet RH. Surgical management of carcinoma of the midthoracic esophagus. *N Engl J Med* 1945; 223: 1–7.

2. Lewis I. The surgical treatment of carcinoma of the oesophagus with special reference to a new operation for growths of the middle third. *Br J Surg* 1946; 34: 18–31.

3. Tanner NC. The present position of carcinoma of the oesophagus. *Postgrad Med J* 1947; 23: 109–39.

4. Santy P, Mouchet A. Traitement chirurgical du cancer de l'oesophage thoracique. *J Chir* 1947; 63: 505–26.

5. Campion JP, Grossetti D, Launois B. Circular anastomosis stapler *Arch Surg* 1984; 119: 232–3.

Left thoracic subtotal oesophagectomy

H. Matthews FRCS
Consultant Thoracic Surgeon, Regional Department of Thoracic Surgery, East Birmingham Hospital,
Birmingham, and Professor of Surgery, Department of Biological Sciences, University of Warwick, UK

Principles and justification

Indications

This operation provides a means for resecting the whole thoracic oesophagus through a sequential two-part approach, with anastomosis of the oesophagus to the fundus of the stomach in the neck, from the left side. The principal indication for this approach is resection of tumours of the thoracic oesophagus and cardia[1], but it is also applicable to resection of benign oesophageal strictures or the severely disrupted oesophagus[2]. The main advantages of this method of subtotal oesophagectomy are: that it permits exploration of the tumour as the first part of the operation; that it is quicker and simpler than a right-sided three-part approach, i.e. laparotomy, right thoracotomy and right neck incision; and that it permits dissection of the tumour and its lymphatic or other extensions under direct vision.

Since 1980 this has been the method of choice for oesophageal resection at East Birmingham Hospital and has been used in 90% of all oesophageal resections for carcinoma.

Contraindications

The only contraindications to this approach are when a tumour is located at or above the aortic arch (judged by barium swallow and not endoscopy) and when the upper part of the stomach is involved by tumour and there is insufficient stomach to reach to the neck.

Preoperative

Assessment

Investigations before operation are designed to assess the patient's fitness for operation and to determine whether there is spread of the tumour beyond the limits of surgical resection. Routine investigations include haematological and biochemical tests and measurement of renal and hepatic function. Cardiac status is assessed by chest radiography, electrocardiography and additional tests if indicated. Respiratory assessment includes routine spirometry, with full tests of respiratory function and blood gases if significant abnormalities are found.

Possible spread of the tumour is investigated by barium swallow, oesophagoscopy and biopsy, computed tomography and/or ultrasonography in all cases, with bronchoscopy, indirect laryngoscopy, lymph node biopsy, cytology of effusions and other tests as indicated by symptoms or the findings on physical examination.

Preparation

Smoking is stopped for at least 1 week before the operation, and all patients are instructed by an experienced respiratory physiotherapist in the breathing and coughing techniques that will be required after operation and in the use of incentive spirometry.

Operation

Anaesthesia and positioning are as described in the chapter on pp. 56–60.

Left thoracolaparotomy

1 With the patient in the right lateral position, an oblique lateral incision is made starting in the left hypochondrium and continuing over the costal margin and along the line of the seventh rib to the angle of the rib posteriorly.

The superficial muscles are divided, and the pleura is opened along the upper border of the seventh rib using diathermy. The costal margin is cut cleanly with a scalpel and the diaphragm is divided peripherally for approximately 15 cm close to its origin on the ribs, leaving the phrenic nerve undamaged.

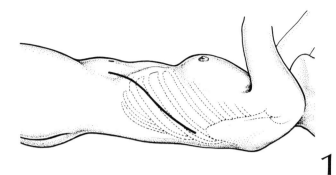

1

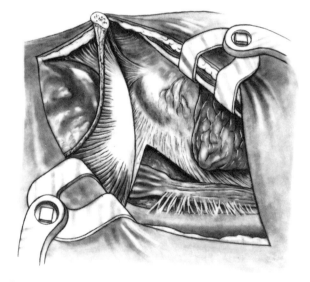

2

2 The peritoneum is opened in the line of the main incision, from the centre of the abdominal edge of the diaphragmatic incision to the edge of the rectus sheath, giving a T-shaped exposure which provides excellent access to the upper abdominal organs.

Before any further dissection is undertaken, the oesophagus, retroperitoneum and liver are examined to confirm that the tumour is resectable, and the stomach inspected to make sure that it is free of disease and suitable for taking up to the neck.

Mobilization of thoracic oesophagus

3   Assuming that resection is possible, the thoracic oesophagus and tumour are mobilized from the oesophageal hiatus upwards, into the root of the neck. The oesophagus is freed from behind the aortic arch by blunt dissection in the plane between the oesophageal muscle and the adjacent connective tissue, commencing at a level below the origin of the recurrent laryngeal nerve from the left vagus. A finger is passed behind the aortic arch so that its tip appears beneath the mediastinal pleura above the arch. This pleura is opened and a tape is passed around the oesophagus above the aortic arch. This facilitates mobilization of the upper oesophagus into the root of the neck, the level of which is identified by palpation of the inner border of the first rib.

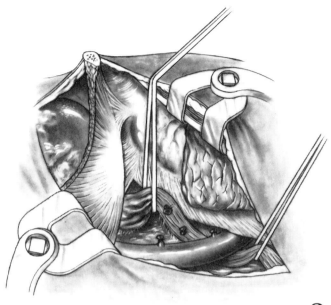

3

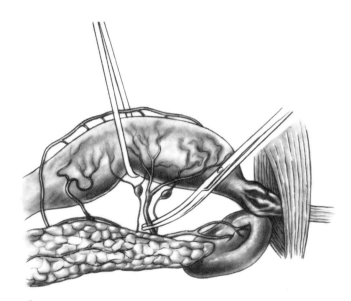

4

Mobilization of stomach

4   The gastro-oesophageal junction and stomach are fully mobilized, dividing the pleura and peritoneum at the oesophageal hiatus, the short gastric vessels and the left and right gastric arteries. The right gastro-epiploic artery and vein are meticulously preserved as the viability of the whole of the stomach depends on these vessels. Splenectomy is not routinely performed.

Division of oesophagus

5 When the oesophagus and stomach are fully mobilized, two strong transfixion sutures are placed through the oesophagus below the aortic arch (either above or below the tumour according to its location) and the oesophagus is divided transversely between the sutures. The lower oesophagus is then brought down through the hiatus, and the lower oesophagus and stomach are lifted out of the wound. The fat glands along the lesser curve and left gastric artery are excised, and the gastro-oesophageal junction is cleaned.

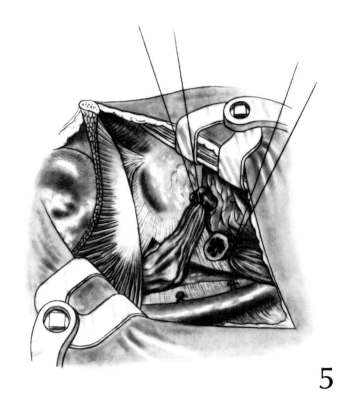

5

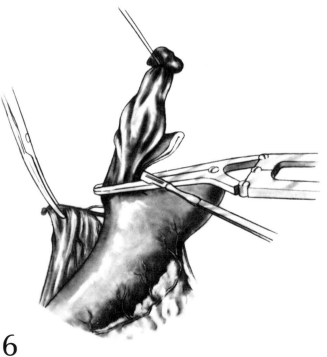

6

Division and closure of stomach

6 A Payr's crushing clamp is placed tangentially below the gastro-oesophageal junction in a position to give good clearance of the tumour, and the lower oesophagus is excised. This line of section is then closed and invaginated in two layers, with continuous synthetic absorbable sutures.

Pyloromyotomy

7 To facilitate gastric drainage and the early resumption of oral intake, a longitudinal pyloromyotomy is performed posteriorly using a pair of Pott's scissors, without opening the gastroduodenal mucosa.

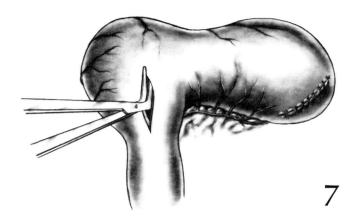

7

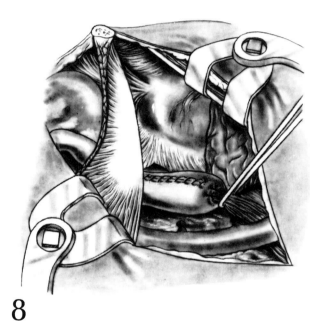

8

Positioning of stomach in the chest

8 The stomach is then taken up through the oesophageal hiatus, and the stump of the oesophagus is sutured securely to the fundus of the stomach at the point which will later be used for the anastomosis.

9 The oesophagus and stomach are then passed medial to the aorta, so that a 'bubble' of fundus lies in the apex of the left chest. Haemostasis in the thorax and abdomen is secured, and the left lung is re-expanded before closure of the incision.

Closure

Closure and drainage are undertaken as described in the chapter on pp. 56–60, with the addition of closure of the diaphragm and the layers of the abdominal wall. As the ribs are approximated the lower edge of the divided costal margin should be positioned to lie over and outside the upper edge of the costal margin to prevent discomfort and crepitus.

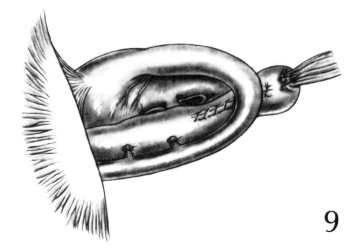

9

Left neck incision

10 When the thoracoabdominal incision has been closed the patient is placed in the supine position and the double-lumen endotracheal tube is removed. A single-lumen tube is inserted to facilitate exposure in the neck. An oblique incision 10 cm long is made along the anterior border of the left sternocleido-mastoid muscle.

The omohyoid muscle is divided together with the middle thyroid vein and the inferior thyroid artery if these are in the way of the exposure. The carotid artery and jugular vessels are retracted laterally, and the trachea is retracted medially to expose the already mobilized oesophagus. The oesophagus and fundus of the stomach are delivered through the wound and disconnected, the stomach being held with a pair of Duval forceps to prevent it slipping back into the chest.

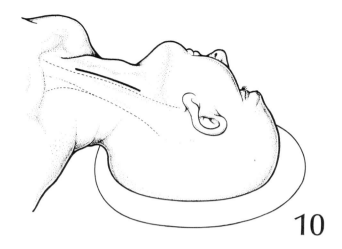

10

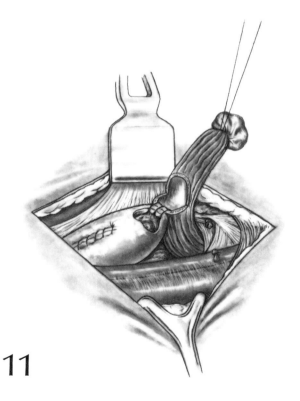

11

Cervical anastomosis

11 A small stoma is cut in the fundus of the stomach and in the oesophagus, and an end-to-end anastomosis is performed between the two organs, using one layer of continuous synthetic absorbable suture. The fundus of the stomach is then returned to the chest so that the completed anastomosis lies comfortably in the lower part of the incision and the neck is closed in layers with synthetic absorbable sutures, without drainage.

Postoperative care

This is kept as simple as possible. Nasogastric tubes and artificial ventilation are not used routinely, and intravenous fluids are limited to 5% dextrose, 2 litres/24 h, plus blood volume replacement as necessary. Oral fluids are commenced on the second day with 30 ml water every hour, followed by 60 ml on the third day, when the chest drain is removed, and 90 ml on the fourth day, when the intravenous infusion is discontinued. Feeding then progresses gradually to semisolid and solid diets, and a routine barium swallow is obtained before discharge, which is usually on the tenth postoperative day.

Complications

Complications relating to the wound have already been described in the chapter on pp. 56–60. Complications relating to the reconstruction should be uncommon, but include leaks and occasionally complete disruption.

With anastomosis in the neck, leaks can usually be treated successfully conservatively, with no oral intake, intravenous fluids and nutrition, drainage of the neck or upper chest as appropriate, and antibiotics. A complete disruption (which is usually due to ischaemia) requires immediate reoperation, with trimming and closure of the stomach, which is returned to the abdomen with a feeding gastrostomy. The cervical oesophagus is then brought out as a terminal oesophagostomy, and a second reconstruction is performed later using substernal colon.

Late complications are uncommon, but include anastomotic stricture or recurrence, which are treated by dilatation, intubation, or radiotherapy as appropriate.

References

1. Matthews HR, Steel A. Left-sided subtotal oesophagectomy for carcinoma. *Br J Surg* 1987; 74: 1115–17.

2. Matthews HR, Mitchell IM, McGuigan JA. Emergency subtotal oesophagectomy. *Br J Surg* 1989; 76: 918–20.

Transhiatal oesophagectomy

Mark B. Orringer MD, FACS
Professor and Head, Section of Thoracic Surgery, University of Michigan Medical Center, Ann Arbor, Michigan, USA

History

The feasibility of removing the oesophagus from the posterior mediastinum using an instrument similar to a vein stripper was suggested by the German anatomist Denk in 1913. In 1936, the British surgeon Grey-Turner resected the oesophagus for carcinoma through abdominal and cervical incisions. Later restoration of swallowing was achieved with an antethoracic skin tube. This, and subsequent early reports of transhiatal (or blunt) oesophagectomy in which the oesophagus was resected through abdominal and cervical incisions without the need for thoracotomy, occurred before the availability of endotracheal anaesthesia permitted safe transthoracic operations. As endotracheal anaesthesia became widely available, however, the technique was all but abandoned. It was still used at times to resect a *normal* thoracic oesophagus concomitantly with laryngopharyngectomy for pharyngeal or cervical oesophageal carcinoma, the stomach being used to restore continuity of the alimentary tract. In the 1970s several authors reported the use of transhiatal oesophageal resection for diseases of the intrathoracic oesophagus. Orringer and associates repopularized the technique[1], and during the past 15 years numerous reports have established that transhiatal oesophagectomy is a safe alternative to traditional transthoracic oesophageal resection[2]. Based upon a personal experience with more than 600 patients the author believes that there is seldom an indication for opening the thorax in patients requiring oesophageal resection for either benign or malignant disease.

Principles and justification

The leading causes of morbidity and mortality after standard transthoracic oesophagectomy and oesophageal reconstruction are pulmonary complications and mediastinitis. Pulmonary complications may result from a combined thoracoabdominal operation in a debilitated patient whose nutritional and pulmonary status have been compromised by impaired swallowing.

Mediastinitis may follow disruption of an intrathoracic oesophageal anastomosis. The technique of transhiatal oesophagectomy reduces the physiological insult to the patient by avoiding the need for thoracotomy, and cervical oesophagogastric anastomotic leak is managed by simple drainage and establishment of a salivary fistula.

The experience in the author's unit with hundreds of patients undergoing this procedure has demonstrated that with appropriate mobilization, the stomach will reach to the neck in virtually every patient. The advantages of performing total thoracic oesophagectomy and cervical oesophagogastric anastomosis in patients requiring oesophageal resection are as follows:

1. In patients with cancer, regardless of the level of the oesophageal tumour, the maximum vertical surgical margin possible is obtained, minimizing suture line tumour recurrence.
2. Postoperative death from mediastinitis and sepsis resulting from anastomotic disruption is virtually eliminated.
3. Clinically significant gastro-oesophageal reflux seldom occurs[3], in contrast to its frequent occurrence when intrathoracic oesophagogastric anastomosis is performed.

Virtually every patient requiring an oesophagectomy for either benign or malignant disease is regarded as a potential candidate for transhiatal oesophagectomy. In patients with an upper or middle third oesophageal carcinoma, bronchoscopy is performed routinely as part of the preoperative assessment. Endoscopic evidence of tracheobronchial invasion by the oesophageal tumour is an absolute contraindication to transhiatal oesophagectomy. Because of the dismal prognosis of patients with oesophageal carcinoma and distant metastatic (stage IV) disease, oesophagectomy is not undertaken in patients with metastases to the liver, supraclavicular lymph nodes or other distant sites proven by biopsy. Computed tomography (CT) is extremely important in the diagnosis of pulmonary, hepatic or other distant intra-abdominal nodal metastases, but a tissue confirmation with fine needle aspiration is generally required before oesophageal resection is denied. While CT scanning may show contiguity of the oesophageal tumour and the adjacent aorta, prevertebral fascia or tracheobronchial tree, it is not a reliable indicator of resectability as actual invasion of these contiguous structures may not be present.

Transhiatal oesophagectomy is feasible even in patients with perioesophageal fibrosis from previous oesophageal operations, corrosive injuries or radiation therapy. However, if significant perioesophageal adhesions are discovered upon palpation of the oesophagus through the diaphragmatic hiatus, the surgeon should be prepared to convert to a transthoracic approach. This is especially so in patients who have undergone previous oesophagomyotomy for either achalasia or oesophageal spasm in whom adherence between the oesophageal submucosa and adjacent aorta may predispose to disastrous intraoperative bleeding during attempted blunt dissection of the oesophagus. In every patient undergoing transhiatal oesophagectomy, the single most important contraindication to proceeding is the surgeon's assessment that there is excessive fixation of the oesophagus to adjacent tissues such as the membranous trachea or the aorta.

Transhiatal oesophagectomy has been criticized for ignoring two basic principles of surgery: adequate exposure and haemostasis. As the surgeon gains experience with this technique, however, and particularly when aided by narrow deep retractors within the diaphragmatic hiatus, more and more of the dissection is performed under direct vision (clamping, dividing and ligating the perioesophageal attachments), and less as a blunt or blind procedure. Intraoperative blood loss generally averages between 500 and 1000 ml, and most patients are no longer transfused. An additional controversy surrounds the appropriateness of transhiatal oesophagectomy as a 'cancer operation' since the procedure precludes a complete mediastinal lymph node dissection and therefore accurate staging. From a practical standpoint, however, removal of abdominal lymph nodes and low paraoesophageal lymph nodes is readily achieved, and subcarinal lymph nodes are generally accessible for staging as well. Since the overall survival of patients undergoing transhiatal oesophagectomy for carcinoma is similar to that reported after standard transthoracic resections, it is difficult to argue that the method of oesophageal resection determines survival in patients with carcinoma. The additional advantage to the abdominal approach is that it not only provides adequate exposure for oesophagectomy but also permits exposure of all portions of the gastrointestinal tract used for oesophageal substitution; if, for any reason, the stomach is found unsuitable, any portion of the colon can readily be mobilized.

Preoperative assessment and preparation

The initial history and physical examination of patients with oesophageal carcinoma is extremely important. The presence of supraclavicular lymphadenopathy merits fine needle aspiration, which, if positive for metastatic cancer, precludes oesophagectomy. Stigmata of advanced liver disease and particularly cirrhosis are indicative of markedly increased operative risk that generally precludes oesophagectomy. Liver nodularity on physical examination warrants assessment to rule out metastatic disease. The chest radiograph provides important clues as to the degree of associated chronic lung disease or pulmonary metastases. Barium swallow examination is extremely important in assessing the length of the tumour, its proximity to the aorta and carina, and distortion of the axis of the oesophagus by the tumour which suggests local extra-oesophageal spread. Staging chest and abdominal CT scans are now a standard part of the preoperative assessment as only patients with localized tumours or those extending no further than regional lymph nodes are considered as candidates for oesophagectomy. As indicated previously, preoperative bronchoscopy to rule out the presence of tracheobronchial invasion is required for cancers of the upper and middle third of the oesophagus.

Few, if any, of our patients are admitted to the hospital before the day of planned oesophagectomy, and most preoperative preparation is carried out on an outpatient basis. Strict abstinence from cigarette smoking for a minimum of 2 weeks before planned oesophagectomy is an absolute requirement in this unit. Vigorous pulmonary physiotherapy, including deep breathing exercises and incentive inspirometry, is administered for up to 14 days. Patients are instructed to walk 2–3 miles a day when possible. In patients with marked weight loss and dehydration secondary to the oesophageal obstruction, a nasogastric feeding tube is inserted, if necessary using fluoroscopic control or dilatation of the malignant obstruction at oesophagoscopy. Sufficient tube feedings are then administered at home by the patients and their family to provide between 2000 and 3000 calories per day. In the past, because of the invariable intravascular blood volume depletion in patients with high-grade oesophageal obstruction, 1 unit blood was transfused before operation for every 4.5 kg of weight lost. However, in this current era of AIDS and concern about blood transfusions, rehydration is given primarily through the nasogastric feeding tube and hexastarch preparations are used for intravascular volume enhancement during surgery, generally completely avoiding the need for blood transfusion. Preoperative dental consultation should be undertaken to repair or remove carious teeth, as poor oral hygiene can be a factor in the severity of infection associated with a cervical anastomotic leak. Finally, in patients with gastric scarring and shortening resulting from previous ulceration or caustic ingestion and those with a history of previous antireflux procedures in whom the mobilized stomach may not be suitable as an oesophageal substitute, a barium enema should be obtained to assess the suitability of the colon as an oesophageal substitute, and the colon prepared in the event that a colonic interposition is needed.

Anaesthesia

Two large-bore peripheral intravenous catheters are used routinely to permit rapid volume replacement in the event of unexpected intraoperative bleeding. It is seldom necessary to monitor central venous pressure, but if this is required the right neck should be used and the operative field on the left neck avoided. A radial artery catheter is inserted to detect hypotension which may occur when the surgeon's hand is inserted into the posterior mediastinum during the transhiatal dissection. This arterial catheter should be sutured into place and protected by padding. The patient's arms are then padded and placed at the sides to provide the surgeon access to the neck, chest and abdomen.

Endotracheal intubation with a standard unshortened endotracheal tube is used so that, in the event of a posterior membranous tracheal tear during the transhiatal dissection, the tube can be guided down the left mainstem bronchus to allow one-lung anaesthesia and repair of the injury. Close co-operation between the anaesthetist and the surgeon is mandatory to avoid prolonged hypotension during the oesophagectomy. As the transhiatal dissection is commenced, the inhalation anaesthetic agents are usually discontinued and inspired oxygen concentration increased to minimize the effects of transient hypotension which is not uncommon. The patient may be given long-acting muscle relaxants during the procedure, since postoperative mechanical ventilation the night of the operation is routine. The bladder is catheterized and urinary output is monitored during the operation.

Operation

The patient is positioned supine with the head turned toward the right on a soft ring, and the neck is extended by a small folded sheet placed beneath the scapulae. The operative field extends from the mandibles to the pubis and anterior to both midaxillary lines. The arms are padded and placed at the patient's sides. If there is unusual concern that a transthoracic exposure may be required for the oesophagectomy (for example, a patient with an upper or middle third oesophageal tumour or a history of previous oesophagomyotomy), the right side may be elevated on a folded blanket, the right arm bent with the hand placed in the small of the back, and the operating table rolled toward the right side to flatten it and provide exposure for a standard upper midline abdominal incision. If necessary, a right anterolateral thoracotomy can be performed, the lung deflated, and the oesophagectomy performed under direct vision. The author, however, generally utilizes a standard endotracheal tube with the patient in the supine position as described above, preferring to reposition the patient for a posterolateral thoracotomy in the event that a transthoracic approach is required. A self-retaining table-mounted upper abdominal retractor is utilized to facilitate exposure of the upper abdomen and hiatus. Transhiatal oesophagectomy and cervical oesophagogastric anastomosis are performed in three separate phases: the abdominal, the mediastinal and the cervical phases.

ABDOMINAL PHASE

1a, b The abdominal portion of the operation is performed through a midline supraumbilical incision.

After exploring the abdomen to exclude metastases which would preclude resection, the triangular ligament is divided with electrocautery, and the liver is padded and retracted to the right to allow exposure of the diaphragmatic hiatus. The stomach is assessed for its suitability as an oesophageal replacement. Extensive gastric scarring and shortening from previous ulcer disease or the sequelae of caustic ingestion preclude use of the entire stomach for oesophageal replacement, and in such cases the colon, which has been prepared before surgery, is mobilized. As a general rule, the oesophagectomy is not carried out until a viable conduit for replacement has been mobilized.

Gastric mobilization is begun by gently retracting the greater omentum downward and away from the stomach to facilitate identification of the gastroepiploic vessels. The course of the right gastroepiploic artery from the pyloroduodenal area to the mid greater curvature, where it generally terminates as it enters the stomach or divides into smaller branches which anastomose with the left gastroepiploic artery, is identified. The lesser sac is entered through an avascular area of the omentum, opposite the point of convergence of the right and left gastroepiploic vessels at the midportion of the greater curvature of the stomach. The left gastroepiploic and short gastric vessels are divided and ligated along the high greater curvature of the stomach initially, avoiding injury to the spleen as well as gastric necrosis from ligation of these vessels too near the gastric wall. The omentum is then separated from the lower half of the greater curvature of the stomach, applying clamps at least 2 cm below the right gastroepiploic artery to ensure that this vessel is not injured during gastric mobilization.

Once mobilization of the omentum from the stomach has been completed, attention is directed to the lesser curvature. The filmy gastrohepatic omentum is incised, and the left gastric vein is identified, divided and ligated. The left gastric artery is divided and ligated at its origin from the coeliac trunk, resecting mobile lymph nodes with the stomach. However, extensive lymphadenopathy in this area generally indicates incurable disease, and overaggressive attempts to resect the nodes may result in catastrophic haemorrhage. In such a situation, it is best to leave some of the involved lymph nodes behind. The right gastric artery is carefully identified and protected during mobilization of the lesser curvature of the stomach.

Peritoneum overlying the gastro-oesophageal junction is next incised and the gastro-oesophageal junction is encircled with a rubber drain. As the drain is retracted downward by one hand, thereby tensing the oesophagus, the other hand is inserted through the diaphragmatic hiatus, and blunt, gentle mobilization of the lower

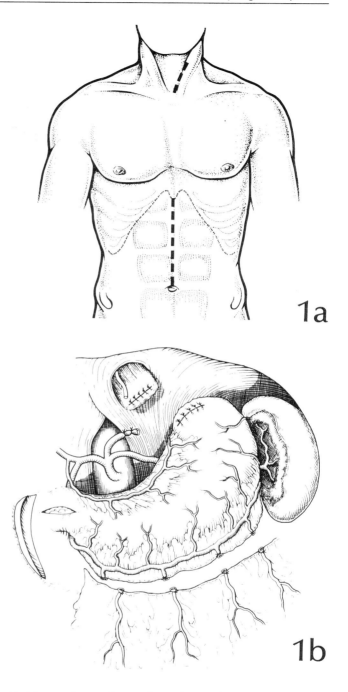

1a

1b

5–10 cm of oesophagus from the mediastinum is carried out. Mobility of the oesophagus within the posterior mediastinum is now assessed through the diaphragmatic hiatus by grasping the oesophagus (and its contained tumour, if present) and moving it from side to side to determine if there is fixation to the prevertebral fascia, aorta or adjacent mediastinal tissues. If this assessment indicates that the oesophagus is mobile and that a transhiatal resection will therefore be possible, the mediastinal dissection is discontinued for the time being. Care is taken to minimize direct traction on the stomach which may injure it.

After gastric mobilization has been completed, a generous Kocher manoeuvre is carried out to gain maximum upward reach of the mobilized stomach. Sufficient mobilization has been achieved when the pylorus can be grasped and moved from its usual position in the right upper quadrant of the abdomen to a point aligned with the xiphoid process in the midline. Because of the possibility of delayed gastric emptying after the vagotomy which accompanies the oesophagectomy, a pyloromyotomy is next performed. The pyloromyotomy extends from 1.5 cm on the stomach through the pylorus and onto the duodenum for 0.5–1 cm. The author prefers to use the cutting current of a needle-tipped electrocautery and a fine-tipped vascular mosquito clamp to dissect the gastric and duodenal muscle away from the underlying submucosa when performing the pyloromyotomy. The site of the pyloromyotomy is marked with metal clips for future radiographic localization. If the gastric or duodenal submucosa is entered during the pyloromyotomy, the hole is closed with several simple 5/0 polypropylene interrupted sutures, and the pyloromyotomy site covered with adjacent omentum sutured in place with interrupted fine sutures. A 14-Fr rubber jejunostomy feeding tube is then inserted 10–15 cm distal to the ligament of Treitz and is secured in place with a Witzel manoeuvre. The jejunostomy tube emerging from the abdomen is then covered with a towel but is not brought out through the abdominal wall until the transhiatal oesophagectomy is completed.

CERVICAL PHASE

A 5-cm long oblique cervical incision parallel to the anterior border of the left sternocleidomastoid muscle is performed (*see Illustration 1*). This incision is kept short intentionally, extending inferiorly no further than the suprasternal notch, and is centred on the cricoid cartilage, the origin of the upper oesophageal sphincter and the beginning of the cervical oesophagus. The platysma and omohyoid fascial layers are incised, and, using narrow thyroid retractors, the sternocleidomastoid muscle and carotid sheath and its contents are gently retracted laterally. The larynx and trachea are retracted medially using *only* the fingers of the first assistant or surgeon, and no metal retractor is placed against the tracheo-oesophageal groove so that the chance of recurrent laryngeal nerve injury is minimized. The middle thyroid vein and/or inferior thyroid artery may be divided and ligated as necessary. The dissection is carried directly posterior to the prevertebral fascia, which is followed bluntly with the index finger into the superior mediastinum. The plane between the trachea and oesophagus is developed by sharp dissection, keeping as posterior to the tracheo-oesophageal groove as possible to avoid injury to the recurrent laryngeal nerve. The cervical oesophagus is bluntly mobilized from adjacent tissues circumferentially, being particu-

larly careful not to injure the posterior membranous trachea, and is encircled with a rubber drain. With upward traction on this drain, blunt dissection of the upper oesophagus from the superior mediastinum is carried out, dissecting in the midline and keeping the fingers against the oesophagus at all times. The upper thoracic oesophagus is generally mobilized almost to the level of the carina through this approach.

MEDIASTINAL (TRANSHIATAL) DISSECTION

2 Attention is now redirected to the abdomen and transhiatal dissection of the oesophagus is initiated. This dissection is carried out in an orderly sequential fashion, mobilizing the posterior aspect of the oesophagus first, then the anterior surface, and finally the lateral attachments. With the left hand retracting the oesophagus downward using the rubber drain encircling the gastro-oesophageal junction, the right hand is inserted behind the oesophagus through the diaphragmatic hiatus, which is progressively dilated one finger at a time, until the entire hand and forearm can be inserted into the posterior mediastinum.

A surgeon whose glove size is larger than a size 7 may have difficulty unless the lateral crus of the hiatus is incised, but this is not routine. Transhiatal oesophagectomy should be performed as a midline dissection, with the volar aspect of the fingers closely applied to the oesophagus to minimize the chance of entry into the pleural cavities or of injury to the tracheobronchial tree, particularly in the region of the carina.

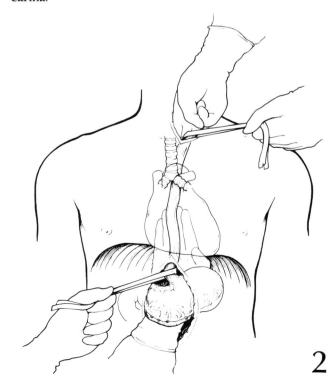

2

3   With the hand inserted through the diaphragmatic hiatus posterior to the oesophagus, blunt dissection of the oesophagus from the posterior mediastinum may be facilitated by a small gauze square held in sponge forceps and introduced through the cervical incision into the superior mediastinum posterior to the oesophagus. This sponge stick is guided along the prevertebral fascia and into the inferior mediastinum, gently sweeping away perioesophageal attachments as it is advanced. When this sponge stick can be felt by the hand inserted in the abdomen, the final filmy attachments separating the sponge from the finger tips are gently avulsed, and mobilization of the posterior oesophagus from the prevertebral fascia is completed.

During this and subsequent portions of the transhiatal oesophagectomy, careful continual monitoring of intra-arterial blood pressure is necessary to avoid prolonged hypotension which can result from cardiac displacement. After removing the sponge stick and hand from the posterior mediastinum, a 28-Fr Argyle Saratoga sump catheter is inserted through the neck wound into the posterior mediastinum, and blood is evacuated with suction.

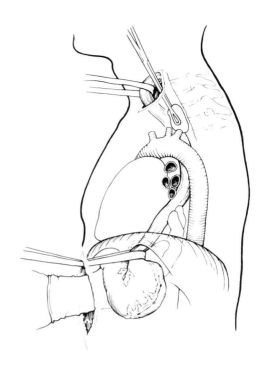

3

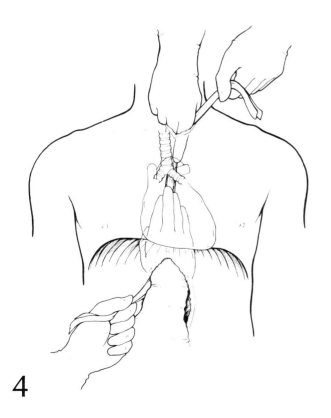

4

4   The anterior oesophageal dissection is next begun by retracting the rubber drain encircling the gastro-oesophageal junction downward with one hand and inserting the other hand palm down against the oesophagus and advancing it into the mediastinum. As the fingers are advanced into the mediastinum, attachments between the oesophagus and the posterior aspect of the pericardium and carina are gently avulsed.

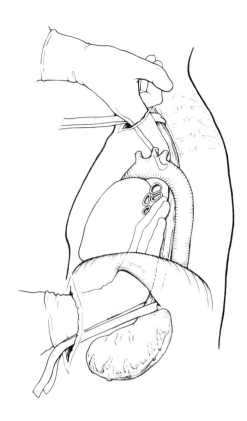

5 It is important during the anterior oesophageal mobilization to keep the hand as far posterior as possible to minimize cardiac displacement and hypotention. The characteristically filmy fibroareolar attachments posterior to the trachea are bluntly divided by simultaneous dissection through the abdominal and cervical incisions along the anterior surface of the oesophagus.

With the anterior and posterior oesophageal mobilization now completed, the lateral oesophageal attachments still remain to be divided. Upward traction on the rubber drain encircling the cervical oesophagus is once again delivered, and as the oesophagus is elevated into the neck wound from the superior mediastinum, accessible lateral attachments are swept away by the index finger applied closely to the oesophagus. In this fashion, approximately 5–8 cm of upper thoracic oesophagus are circumferentially mobilized. The upper oesophagus is then permitted to retract back into the mediastinum.

5

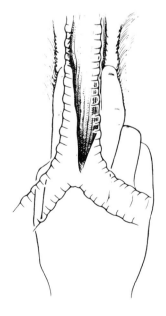

6

6 Traction on the rubber drain encircling the gastro-oesophageal junction is then applied, and the opposite hand is inserted palm downward through the diaphragmatic hiatus along the anterior surface of the oesophagus and is advanced upward into the superior mediastinum behind the trachea. The portion of upper oesophagus which was circumferentially mobilized can be identified with the fingertips. Once the intact lateral attachments are palpated, the oesophagus is trapped against the prevertebral fascia by the index and middle fingers, and a gentle downward raking motion of the hand avulses the remainder of the filmy perioesophageal attachments.

7 Sizeable vagal branches may be palpated along the middle and distal oesophagus at this point, and by placement of narrow deep retractors into the diaphragmatic hiatus, their identification, division and ligation using long right-angled clamps is possible. At times, finger fracture between the index finger and thumb of subcarinal or subaortic perioesophageal adhesions may be required.

8a–c Alternatively, access to the upper thoracic oesophagus may be facilitated by a partial upper sternal split, thereby permitting division of the remaining perioesophageal attachments under direct vision[4].

Once the entire intrathoracic oesophagus is mobile, an 8–10-cm length is delivered into the cervical wound, where a GIA surgical stapler is applied, a rubber drain is sutured to the oesophagus distal to the stapler, and the knife assembly of the stapler is advanced, thereby dividing the oesophagus. A haemostat is applied to the opposite end of the rubber drain, and the stapler is removed from the field. The stomach is then drawn out of the abdomen along with the thoracic oesophagus and the attached rubber drain which has been sutured to it. The abdominal end of the drain is clamped with a haemostat and then separated from the oesophagus so that the transmediastinal rubber drain now has a haemostat at either end. This drain is used subsequently to guide the mobilized stomach into the posterior mediastinum.

As soon as the oesophagus has been delivered from the posterior mediastinum, narrow deep retractors are inserted into the diaphragmatic hiatus so that the posterior mediastinum can be inspected for bleeding and the mediastinal pleura for lateral rents that indicate the need for a chest tube. Blood is again evacuated from the posterior mediastinum using the Argyle Saratoga sump catheter inserted through the cervical wound. A 32-Fr chest tube is inserted into the appropriate pleural cavity if entry has occurred during the oesophagectomy. A large abdominal pack is then placed in the posterior mediastinum through the diaphragmatic hiatus to tamponade any vascular oozing. Attention is then turned toward preparing the stomach for its transposition into the chest. The stomach and attached oesophagus are placed on the anterior abdominal wall and the point along the high greater curvature which will reach most cephalad to the neck is identified and held by the assistant with a moist pack. The lesser curvature of the stomach is then cleared of fat by dividing the vessels and fat between clamps at the level of the second vascular arcade from the cardia.

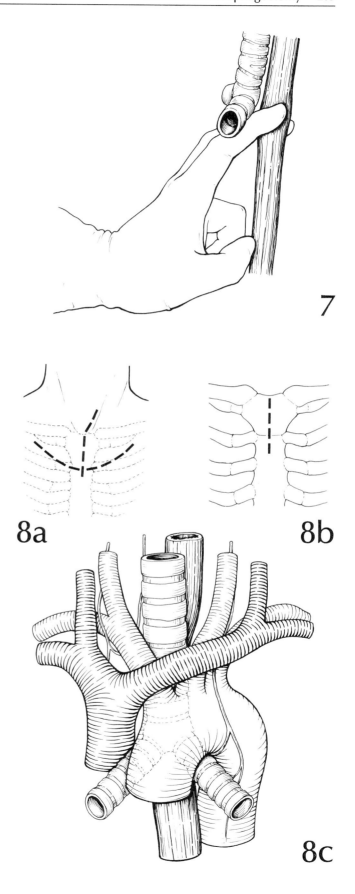

9 The GIA stapler with a 5-cm long cartridge is then applied beginning at this point. Each time the stapler is removed, traction is applied to the gastric fundus to allow the stomach to be straightened progressively, thereby maximizing its cephalad reach. The GIA stapler is applied on average three or four times.

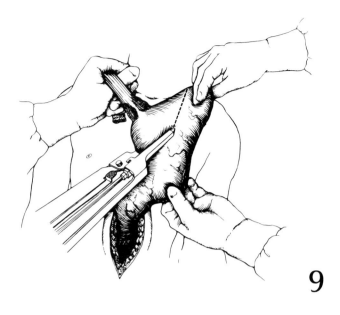

9

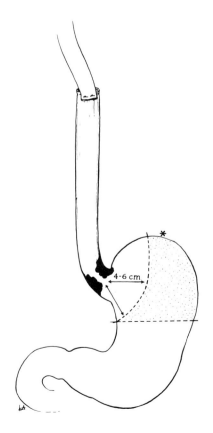

10

10 Once the partial proximal gastrectomy has been completed, the oesophagus and attached proximal stomach are removed from the field, and the gastric staple suture line is oversewn with a running 4/0 polypropylene Lembert stitch. This same technique is utilized when resecting carcinomas localized to the cardia and proximal stomach. Rather than carry out a traditional proximal hemigastrectomy which wastes valuable stomach (stippled area) that can be used for oesophageal replacement and commits the surgeon to an intrathoracic oesophageal anastomosis, the stomach is divided as described above 4–6 cm distal to the palpable tumour, thereby preserving the greater curvature and that point along the gastric fundus which reaches to the neck (*). This narrowed gastric tube functions well as an oesophageal substitute.

Attention is now redirected to the diaphragmatic hiatus. The previously placed pack is removed and, using the narrow deep retractors placed into the hiatus, a last inspection is made for any bleeding which can be controlled under direct vision through the diaphragmatic hiatus. Again, the 28-Fr Argyle Saratoga sump inserted through the neck wound provides a dry field as the posterior mediastinum is inspected through the hiatus. To ensure an adequate posterior mediastinal tunnel for the stomach, the entire hand and forearm of the surgeon are inserted through the diaphragmatic oesophageal hiatus and advanced through the posterior mediastinum until three or four fingers are visible in the cervical incision. During this procedure, the blood pressure must be watched carefully.

11 The stomach is then again delivered on to the anterior chest wall, and that point along the gastric fundus which will extend most cephalad is identified.

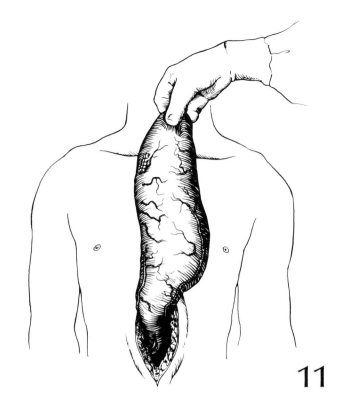

11

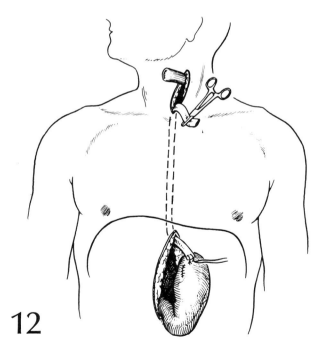

12

12 The abdominal end of the transmediastinal rubber drain is sutured to the gastric fundus at this site with two 3/0 cardiovascular sutures. The suture closer to the lesser curvature is cut short and that nearest the greater curvature is cut long to ensure that the stomach is not twisted during its mobilization through the posterior mediastinum. The stomach is carefully positioned through the diaphragmatic hiatus and into the posterior mediastinum by a combination of gentle traction of the cervical end of the rubber drain and guidance through the abdominal incision.

As the fundus appears in the cervical incision, it is gently grasped and pulled into the wound while a hand inserted into the mediastinum from the abdomen continually pushes the stomach upward beneath the aortic arch. This hand should also be used to ascertain that the stomach has not been twisted during its positioning in the chest. When the stomach has been brought through the posterior mediastinum without torsion, the sutures used to secure the rubber drain to the gastric fundus in the abdomen are orientated correctly in the neck, the long suture being nearest the patient's left side along the greater curvature and the short suture medial along the lesser curvature.

13 The anterior surface of the stomach may also be palpated simultaneously through the hiatus and the neck incision to be certain that no inadvertent twist has occurred. The gastric fundus, now in the neck, should reach several centimetres behind the divided remaining cervical oesophagus. In the abdomen, the pylorus comes to rest within 2–3 cm of the diaphragmatic hiatus.

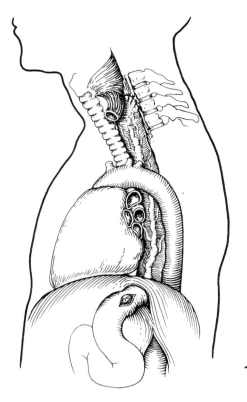

13

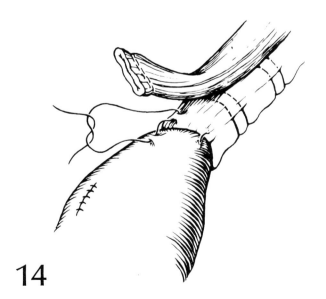

14

14 The gastric fundus is then sutured to the prevertebral fascia behind the divided cervical oesophagus with two 3/0 polypropylene sutures. These sutures anchor the stomach in the neck so that the subsequent cervical gastro-oesophageal anastomosis performed on the anterior surface of the fundus will be under no tension.

To avoid contamination of the abdomen by intraoral contents, the cervical gastro-oesophageal anastomosis is not begun until the abdominal incision is closed completely and excluded from the field. Before closing the abdomen, however, a final inspection for bleeding, particularly in the area of the spleen, is made. The diaphragmatic hiatus is narrowed with two or three no. 1 silk sutures so as to admit three fingers along the side of the stomach easily. The edge of the diaphragmatic hiatus is tacked to the adjacent anterior gastric wall with two or three 3/0 silk sutures to prevent intrathoracic herniation of bowel. The pyloromyotomy is covered by adjacent omentum, and the previously retracted left hepatic lobe is returned to its normal position. The feeding jejunostomy tube is then brought out through a left upper quadrant stab wound, and the jejunum is fixed to the anterior abdominal wall with several interrupted sutures. The abdominal incision is then closed and isolated from the field by covering it with a sterile towel and sheet. Attention is now redirected to the neck where the cervical gastro-oesophageal anastomosis is performed.

CERVICAL GASTRO-OESOPHAGEAL ANASTOMOSIS

15a–c The end of the divided upper oeso-phagus is elevated out of the neck wound and retracted superiorly. A Babcock clamp is used to elevate the anterior gastric wall from the level of the suprasternal notch (*Illustration 15a*), and a 3/0 silk seromuscular traction suture is placed in the anterior gastric wall to maintain exposure during construction of the anastomosis (*Illustration 15b*). The site for the anastomosis is selected approximately 3–4 cm below the point at which the stomach has been sutured to the prevertebral fascia on the anterior gastric wall (*Illustration 15c*), and either a 2.5-cm long vertical gastrotomy is made or a 2-cm button of the anterior gastric wall is excised using the needle tipped electrocautery.

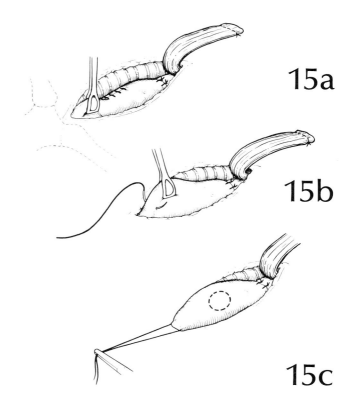

15a

15b

15c

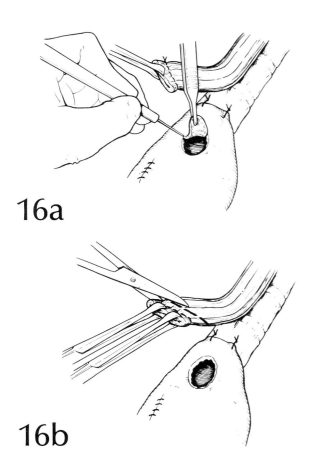

16a

16b

16a, b The length of oesophagus required for construction of a tension-free anasto-mosis must be carefully estimated and the cervical oesophagus must not be shortened excessively, since once the traction suture is removed, allowing the stomach to retract back into the superior mediastinum, additional oesophageal length is needed. The previously placed oesophageal staple suture line is amputated, bevelling the end of the oesophagus so that the anterior edge of the remaining oesophagus is 1–1.5 cm longer than the posterior edge.

17a–d The anastomosis is divided into quadrants, and interrupted 4/0 polyglycolic acid suture is used to construct the posterior quadrants, starting at the midpoints of the posterior half of the oesophageal circumference and the upper half of the gastric opening. Sutures are placed 3 mm apart, and the untied ends are fixed sequentially to the drapes with haemostats. As each suture is placed, it passes obliquely through the oesophageal wall 4–5 mm from the cut edge of the muscle and 2 mm from the mucosal edge. Six to seven sutures per quadrant are generally used. Once all of the two posterior quadrant sutures have been placed, the sutures are tied sequentially with the knots on the inside, thereby inverting the anastomosis. The sutures are tied from lateral to medial, cutting all of the sutures except the two corner stitches.

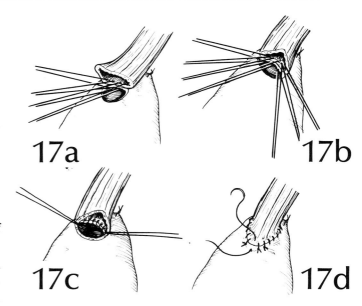

17a 17b 17c 17d

A 46-Fr tapered Maloney dilator is then inserted by the anaesthetist through the mouth and across the anastomosis into the intrathoracic stomach for several inches. The previously placed traction suture on the anterior wall of the stomach is released. Both anterior quadrants of the anastomosis are then completed with a dilator in place with sutures alternating from one side to the other. All knots are again tied on the inside until it is estimated that there is room for all except three or four additional sutures. For these last sutures, inverting far-near, near-far, outside-in, inside-out (Gambee) sutures are used. A second row of interrupted sutures may be used to reinforce the anterior half of the suture line, but this has not been done routinely. After removal of the dilator and placement of a nasogastric tube for postoperative gastric decompression, either side of the anastomosis is marked with silver clips for future radiographic evaluation, and the wound is reapproximated loosely with interrupted absorbable sutures over a 0.6-cm rubber drain placed to the depths of the wound near the anastomosis. It is rarely necessary to use more than five or six sutures to close the neck wound. Before leaving the operating room, a portable chest radiograph is obtained to rule out an unrecognized haemothorax or pneumothorax or large mediastinal haematoma, and to verify the position of the nasogastric, chest and endotracheal tubes.

Intraoperative complications associated with transhiatal oesophagectomy include: entry into one or both pleural cavities during the transhiatal dissection; disruption of the tracheobronchial tree; and haemorrhage. As indicated above, the mediastinal pleurae are inspected after removal of the oesophagus from the posterior mediastinum, and if pleural entry has occurred, a chest tube is inserted and connected to suction before the stomach is positioned in the posterior mediastinum. Tracheal tears during transhiatal oesophagectomy are generally small and linear, and involve the posterior membranous trachea. They are heralded by a rush of air from the ventilator felt either through the diaphragmatic hiatus or the neck wound during the transhiatal dissection. If the air leak is sizeable, the endotracheal

tube balloon should be deflated, and the tip of the endotracheal tube guided into the left mainstem bronchus by the hand inserted through the diaphragmatic hiatus. One-lung ventilation may then be achieved in a more controlled fashion. Addition of a partial upper sternal split may provide increased exposure of the membranous trachea to allow direct repair. Before beginning tracheal repair, however, if possible, the transhiatal oesophagectomy should be completed to improve exposure of the posterior membranous trachea. Larger tears may necessitate a right thoracotomy and direct suture closure. Major intraoperative haemorrhage should not occur during transhiatal oesophagectomy if proper patient selection is used and attempts to resect the oesophagus which is fixed to adjacent structures by tumour or fibrosis are abandoned. Should untoward bleeding occur during the transhiatal dissection, the 28-Fr Argyle Saratoga sump catheter inserted through the neck incision is used to evacuate the posterior mediastinum as the anterior surface of the aorta is inspected and direct control of the bleeding obtained. If haemostasis is not possible using this technique, the posterior mediastinum should be packed with large laparotomy pads and several minutes allowed to elapse before again inspecting the mediastinum. If bleeding resumes, the pack should be reinserted, the abdomen quickly closed, and the patient repositioned and turned to the appropriate side for a thoracotomy, left if the intraoperative bleeding occurred during dissection of the lower third of the oesophagus, and right if the bleeding occurred during dissection of the middle or upper thoracic oesophagus.

Intraoperative recurrent laryngeal nerve injury should not occur if care is taken to avoid injury to the recurrent laryngeal nerve in the tracheo-oesophageal groove. No metal retractors should be placed against the trachea during the cervical portions of the operation to prevent this complication.

Postoperative care

Regardless of how uncomplicated the operative procedure has been, endotracheal intubation and mechanical ventilatory assistance are continued during the afternoon and evening of the operation. The rationale for this is threefold: first, some patients develop a traumatic bronchorrhoea after transhiatal oesophagectomy and vigorous dissection of the oesophagus from the tracheobronchial tree; second, if inadvertent recurrent laryngeal nerve injury has occurred, impaired swallowing and aspiration in the not fully conscious but extubated patient may occur; and third, acute intrathoracic gastric dilatation with massive secondary regurgitation and aspiration may occur if for any reason the nasogastric tube should not be functioning and the patient's cough reflex has not fully returned. In almost every case, removal of the endotracheal tube early the morning after transhiatal oesophagectomy is possible.

Because of the routine preoperative emphasis upon use of the incentive inspirometer to facilitate postoperative pulmonary hygiene, resumption of use of the inspirometer is begun as soon as the endotracheal tube is removed. Ambulation is begun the day after operation, several hours after the endotracheal tube has been removed. Since transhiatal oesophagectomy is basically an upper abdominal procedure requiring little manipulation of the intestines or the root of the mesentery, postoperative ileus beyond 24–48 h is unusual, and 5% dextrose and water through the jejunostomy feeding tube may begin at a rate of 30 ml/h on the second or third postoperative day. If this rate is tolerated for 12 h, the volume is increased to 60 ml/h, and half strength jejunostomy tube feedings are begun the next day followed by full strength the next. The nasogastric tube is typically removed by the second or third postoperative day when nasogastric tube drainage is less than 100 ml per 8-h nursing shift. The arterial catheter is removed the day after operation once the endotracheal tube has been removed, the intravenous catheters once jejunostomy feedings are tolerated, the cervical wound drain on the second or third postoperative day, and the nasogastric tube once the patient is tolerating jejunostomy feedings. Once the patient has demonstrated the ability to tolerate no nasogastric tube for 24 h, oral intake is progressively advanced from a liquid to a pureed diet during the first postoperative week. A barium swallow examination is obtained on the tenth postoperative day when anastomotic healing is generally assured. Oral intake should not be withheld until this study is obtained, since the patient is swallowing saliva from the moment he emerges from general anaesthesia, and it is unrealistic to think that nothing is going across the anastomosis because of the presence of a nasogastric tube. As oral intake is advanced, the rate of jejunostomy tube feedings may be progressively decreased and eventually delivered only at night so as to not interfere with the patient's appetite

during the day. Complaints of postvagotomy dumping (varying degrees of cramping and diarrhoea) typically respond to an appropriate antidumping diet, avoiding overdistension of the stomach by minimizing the amount of liquid consumed with meals, and antispasmodics such as tincture of opium or diphenoxylate (Lomotil). The postoperative barium swallow should document that there is no extravasation of contrast at either the cervical gastro-oesophageal anastomosis or the pyloromyotomy (both areas marked by silver clips) and that there is satisfactory emptying of the intrathoracic stomach through the pyloromyotomy. Early after operation, barium often empties relatively slowly from the intrathoracic stomach, yet the patient complains of no regurgitation of swallowed food.

The patient may be discharged from hospital at any time after a satisfactory postoperative barium swallow on the tenth postoperative day. The patient is encouraged to supplement oral caloric intake with one or two cans of jejunostomy tube feedings at night at home, but this is not mandatory if the patient is eating relatively well in the hospital. When the patient returns for the initial postoperative assessment 2–4 weeks after discharge, if the feeding jejunostomy tube has not been used, it is removed by simple traction.

Early postoperative cervical dysphagia may be felt by the patient if there is anastomotic oedema. This requires no specific therapy and gradually subsides with time. However, any complaint of cervical dysphagia occurring 2–4 weeks after discharge is managed by passage of up to a 46-Fr Maloney dilator through the anastomosis on an outpatient basis. If the patient develops fever of 101°F or more 48 h after transhiatal oesophagectomy, this is presumptive evidence of an anastomotic leak until proven otherwise and is an indication for immediate contrast study of the oesophagus. A water-soluble material such as Gastrografin should be used initially to diagnose a possible leak, but if none is seen dilute barium should be utilized as this better defines the mucosal detail. If, on the other hand, the patient begins to drain swallowed liquids from the cervical wound drain site, it is obvious that a leak has occurred, and the neck wound should be opened in its entirety by removing the five or six fine sutures used to close the wound. Good mechanical cleansing of the open neck wound can be obtained by having the patient swallow water while at the same time aspirating any liquid which issues from the cervical wound. The neck wound is packed loosely with saline moistened sponges several times a day. Most cervical gastro-oesophageal anastomotic leaks will close within 2–5 days, often facilitated by passage of a 46-Fr tapered Maloney dilator which ensures that there is no associated distal obstruction (oedema or spasm).

Postoperative chylothorax may occur after transhiatal oesophagectomy and manifests as prolonged and excessive chest tube drainage (typically greater than 200–400 ml per 8-h shift). If chylothorax is suspected, administration of cream through the feeding jejunostomy tube will result in a change of the character of the chest tube drainage from serosanguineous to milky white fluid. An aggressive approach toward postoperative chylothorax in the patient who has undergone transhiatal oesophagectomy is adopted. A transthoracic approach to the thoracic duct with direct identification and suturing of the leak facilitated by cream administered through the jejunostomy tube is preferred to prolonged chest tube drainage and intravenous hyperalimentation[5].

Outcome

In the past 16 years, Orringer and associates have performed transhiatal oesophagectomy without thoracotomy in 583 patients with diseases of the intrathoracic oesophagus, 166 (28%) with benign disease and 417 (72%) with carcinoma (6% upper, 28% middle, and 68% lower third and cardia)[6]. Benign oesophageal disease included strictures (40%), neuromotor dysfunction – achalasia (24%) and oesophageal spasm (8%); recurrent gastro-oesophageal reflux (16%); acute perforation (5%); acute caustic injury (2%); and others (3%). Of the patients with benign disease, 60% had undergone at least one previous oesophageal operation. Transhiatal oesophagectomy was possible in 97% of the patients in whom it was attempted, 19 patients (13 with benign and six with carcinoma) requiring conversion to the transthoracic approach. In all but five patients, oesophageal resection and reconstruction were performed in a single operation, and the oesophageal substitute was positioned in the posterior mediastinum in the original oesophageal bed in 96%. Alimentary tract continuity was re-established using the stomach to replace the oesophagus in 553 patients (95%) and colon in 28 (5%) who had undergone previous gastric resections which precluded use of the stomach for a cervical oesophagogastric anastomosis.

The total hospital mortality rate for these 583 patients was 5% (27 deaths) and in most cases was unrelated to the technique of operation. There was one intraoperative death due to uncontrollable haemorrhage. Complications included intraoperative entry into one or both pleural cavities requiring a chest tube(s) (74%), anastomotic leak (9%), recurrent laryngeal nerve paralysis (3%), and chylothorax and tracheal laceration (less than 1% each). Reoperation for mediastinal bleeding was required within 24 h of operation in three patients. The average intraoperative blood loss was 875 ml (1023 ml for benign disease and 817 ml for carcinoma). Of the surviving patients 88% were discharged able to swallow within 3 weeks of operation, and 78% within 2 weeks. The Kaplan–Meier actuarial survival of our patients undergoing transhiatal oesophagectomy for carcinoma is similar to that reported after more traditional transthoracic oesophagectomy, the overall 2-year survival being 41% and the 5-year survival 27%. Of the patients with benign disease, long-term follow-up has indicated good or excellent functional results after a cervical gastro-oesophageal anastomosis in nearly 70%. Although approximately 44% of the patients have required one or more outpatient anastomotic dilatations within 1–3 months of operation, true anastomotic strictures have developed in only 10%. Clinically significant gastro-oesophageal reflux is unusual after cervical oesophago-gastric anastomosis and has occurred in only 3% of these patients. Our results support our contention that a thoracic incision is seldom required to resect the oesophagus for either benign or malignant disease. This procedure is safe and well tolerated if performed with care and for proper indications.

References

1. Orringer MB, Sloan H. Esophagectomy without thoracotomy. *J Thorac Cardiovasc Surg* 1978; 76: 643–54.

2. Orringer MB. Transhiatal esophagectomy without thoracotomy for carcinoma of the thoracic esophagus. *Ann Surg* 1984; 200: 282–8.

3. Orringer MB, Stirling MC. Cervical esophagogastric anastomosis for benign disease – functional results. *J Thorac Cardiovasc Surg* 1988; 96: 887–93.

4. Orringer MB. Partial median sternotomy: anterior approach to the upper thoracic esophagus. *J Thorac Cardiovasc Surg* 1984; 87: 124–9.

5. Orringer MB, Bluett M, Deeb GM. Aggressive treatment of chylothorax complicating transhiatal esophagectomy without thoracotomy. *Surgery* 1988; 104: 720–6.

6. Orringer MB, Marshall B, Stirling MC. Transhiatal esophagectomy for benign and malignant disease. *J Thorac Cardiovasc Surg* 1993; 105: 265–77.

Eversion extraction oesophagectomy

Glyn G. Jamieson FRACS, FACS
Dorothy Mortlock Professor of Surgery, University of Adelaide, Department of Surgery, Royal Adelaide Hospital, Adelaide, Australia

Eversion extraction oesophagectomy is a variation on the technique of non-thoracotomy oesophagectomy, introduced by Grey-Turner in 1931. The oesophagus is removed from the mediastinum by stripping, the technique being in all respects analogous to stripping a vein from the leg. Its feasibility is based on the fact that the blood vessels to the oesophagus branch close to its wall, so that only the very fine branches are blindly avulsed during extraction and these rapidly retract and stop bleeding.

Principles and justification

Indications

Eversion extraction has been used in China and Japan for removal of the oesophagus when a very early cancer has been discovered. In other words, it has been used when the oesophageal wall is basically normal. This is a very important prerequisite for carrying out this technique.

Diseases in which the author has used the procedure are:

1. Intramucosal cancer in columnar-lined oesophagus.
2. Megaoesophagus from achalasia.
3. Pharyngolaryngectomy with gastric pull-up.
4. Cancer of the cardia when it is elected not to open the patient's chest.
5. Cancer of the cervical oesophagus when preoperative chemoradiotherapy has led to disappearance of malignant disease.
6. Cancer of the oesophageal body when preoperative chemoradiotherapy has led to disappearance of malignant disease and a thoracotomy is thought to be contraindicated.

Operation

Incision

The abdominal and cervical approaches to the oesophagus are standard. A midline abdominal incision is used and the diaphragmatic hiatus is opened by dividing the muscle anteriorly, to accommodate the stomach later. A narrow-bladed, curved retractor is placed through the hiatus to allow visualization of the lower thoracic oesophagus, which is mobilized under direct vision.

1   No attempt is made to take this mobilization higher than is technically easy through this approach. The abdominal oesophagus is also mobilized, along with the whole of the stomach, except for retention of the right gastric and right gastro-omental (epiploic) pedicles. The stomach is then divided in a straight line at a point below the gastro-oesophageal junction, removing a portion of the lesser and greater curvatures.

The cervical oesophagus is also approached in a standard fashion. It is mobilized into the superior mediastinum under direct vision. The recurrent laryngeal nerve on the side of approach, usually the left, may be visualized and protected during this mobilization. Although the opposite recurrent laryngeal nerve is not visualized, it is protected by keeping close to the oesophageal wall during dissection.

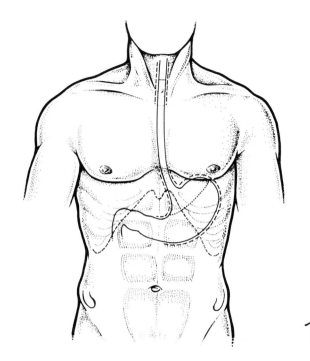

1

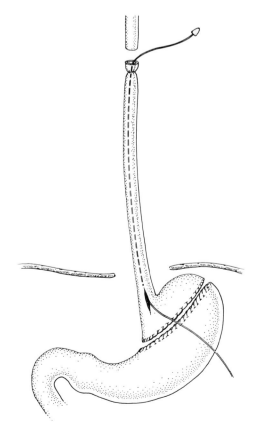

2

2   The cervical oesophagus is occluded gently with a strong silk tie, which is tied with only one throw, just distal to the point chosen for division. The oesophagus is transected proximal to this tie. An oesophagotomy is made in the abdominal oesophagus and the vein stripper is passed proximally. When it reaches the point of occlusion in the cervical oesophagus, the tie is loosened enough to allow passage of the wire and a small vein stripper head is placed in position. (The small head inverts into the oesophagus more easily than a large head.) A long tape or heavy thread is tied to the stripper head. The strong silk suture around the oesophagus is now tied down snugly, fixing the oesophagus against the stripper.

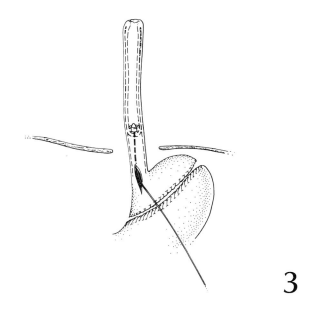

3

3 The abdominal operator exerts steady but strong traction on the stripper with one hand, while the other hand ensures that the direction of traction at the hiatus is directed craniad and caudad. Traction inverts the oesophagus and it appears everted at the hiatus. The long tape is pulled through with the oesophagus.

If any excessive resistance is encountered, blunt oesophagectomy should be reverted to, rather than risking damage to a vital structure. The abdominal end of the tape is pulled through with the oesophagus and is sutured to the highest point of the fundus of the stomach.

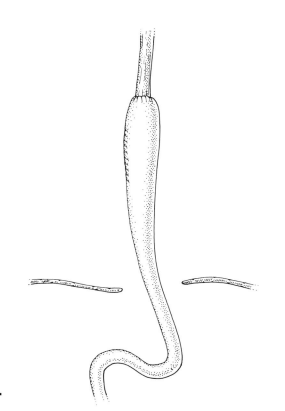

4

4 Gentle traction is exerted on the cervical end of the tape and the stomach is gently pushed up from below through the posterior mediastinum until the fundus becomes evident in the neck. A routine oesophagogastric anastomosis is then undertaken.

Outcome

This technique has been used in 24 patients. Two deaths occurred, one from a ruptured aortic aneurysm and the other from a myocardial infarction, both on the third day after operation. Excessive bleeding did not occur in any patient. Six patients had temporary paresis of a recurrent laryngeal nerve. There were four cervical anastomotic leaks which healed uneventfully. One gastric tube intramediastinal leak led to empyema requiring open drainage.

If used when there is no transmural disease of the oesophageal body, the technique is safe and can prove useful in the situations already detailed.

En bloc oesophagectomy for cancer of the distal oesophagus, cardia and proximal stomach

Jeffrey A. Hagen MD
Esophageal Fellow, Department of Surgery, University of Southern California School of Medicine, Los Angeles, California, USA

Tom R. DeMeester MD
Professor and Chairman, Department of Surgery, University of Southern California School of Medicine, Los Angeles, California, USA

History

The first successful resection of the thoracic oesophagus without re-establishing gastrointestinal continuity was performed in 1913 by Franz Torek. The patient continued to eat after surgery by placing a rubber tube between her cervical oesophagostomy and gastrostomy and lived for 13 years. The first surgeon to establish normal alimentation after oesophagectomy was Oshawa who, in 1933, performed oesophageal resection followed by oesophagogastrostomy in eight patients. Five years later Adams and Phemister reported their results with one-stage resection and intrathoracic oesophagogastrostomy.

In 1963 Logan described an *en bloc* resection for carcinoma arising in the distal third of the oesophagus and the gastric cardia. The 5-year survival rate of 16% was better than any of the other reports up to that time, but the 21% mortality rate associated with the procedure hindered widespread acceptance of the operation. Akiyama and Skinner subsequently modified the procedure, reduced the mortality rates to 1.4% and 11% respectively, and increased the 5-year survival rates to 50% and 40%, respectively. Subsequent modifications regarding the selection of patients and the extent of gastric and oesophageal resection have led to further reductions in mortality rates, while preserving the improved survival.

Principles and justification

Patients with oesophageal cancer typically present with dysphagia, a symptom which usually occurs late in the course of the disease. Consequently there is an aura of pessimism regarding cure of the disease by surgical treatment. As a result, palliation has emerged as the only reasonable therapeutic goal and more limited resections have been popularized. With this approach, cure is relegated to a chance phenomenon and the disease is considered to be systemic from the start. A criticism of this approach is that it may conceal the benefits of surgical resection in some patients by treating all patients in the same way regardless of the extent of the disease. This approach emphasizes the concept of biological determinism, i.e. that the outcome of treatment for oesophageal cancer is determined at the time of diagnosis, and that surgical treatment aimed at removing more than the primary tumour is not helpful. It also considers lymph node metastases simply to be markers of systemic disease, and that the systematic removal of involved lymph nodes is not beneficial. Based on this philosophy is the belief that the removal of the primary tumour by transhiatal oesophagectomy results in the same survival as a more extensive *en bloc* resection and that adjuvant chemotherapy should be given before surgery in an effort to increase cure rates by destroying systemic and remaining local disease.

In contrast to standard or transhiatal oesophagectomy, *en bloc* oesophagectomy removes the tumour covered on all surfaces with a layer of normal tissue, along with an extended length of foregut above and below the lesion to incorporate potential submucosal spread of tumour and involved regional lymph nodes.

To maximize these potential benefits of surgical treatment a selective approach to patients with cancer of the oesophagus is advocated. The decision to attempt to cure a patient by *en bloc* oesophagectomy depends on the location of the tumour, the patient's age and physiological fitness, and the extent of disease present. The decision can be made in most patients before surgery, but in some an intraoperative decision is required. The latter is done because of difficulties with the present staging methodology. It is based on the observation that patients with a tumour that penetrates through the oesophageal wall and metastasizes to multiple regional lymph nodes have a high probability of subclinical distant organ metastasis and poor survival.

This selective approach ensures that the extent of surgery is adequate for curative lesions. It utilizes *en bloc* resection of the oesophagus with lymph node dissection for disease suspected to be limited to the oesophageal wall with limited lymphatic spread. Patients who have transmural involvement and extensive lymphatic spread or who are physically too unfit for extensive surgery undergo simple oesophagectomy to achieve palliation of their dysphagia. An algorithm of this selective process is shown in *Figure 1*.

Cancers arising in the proximal or middle thirds of the oesophagus are not amenable to *en bloc* resection because the proximity of the oesophagus to the trachea and aorta does not allow *en bloc* resection to be performed. As a consequence, resection is performed in a similar fashion to that undertaken in patients with advanced disease, and cure is relegated to a chance phenomenon. Local lymph nodes are removed in order not to leave disease behind that can compromise the degree of palliation achieved in these patients.

En bloc resection for cure in patients over 75 years of age is unwise. The additional operative risk of this resection is not justified in the face of a relatively limited life expectancy. At this age the surgeon's goal should be to add life to years and not years to life. Regardless of how favourable the pathology of the tumour, palliative resection should be undertaken in these patients. This approach will relieve symptoms of dysphagia with less extensive surgery while still providing some possibility for cure, although the chances are small.

Oesophageal cancer is predominantly a disease of 50–70-year-old men, the same age range in which there is an increase in the prevalence of coronary artery disease. Consequently a thorough assessment of the patient's cardiovascular reserve is essential. Standard electrocardiography and clinical evaluation will often detect the presence of cardiac disease, but these techniques are not sufficient to assess cardiac reserve. More reliable information can be obtained by gated radionucleotide pool scanning. Any patient with an ejection fraction of less than 40% at rest, or a patient whose ejection fraction decreases with exercise, is a poor candidate for *en bloc* resection. In these patients, coronary arteriography may be indicated and the potential for angioplasty to improve their cardiac performance should be considered.

Similarly, routine pulmonary function testing can be used to detect the presence of significant chronic lung disease and to predict whether the patient will tolerate *en bloc* resection. In this regard, the forced expiratory volume in 1 second (FEV_1) has prognostic significance as it has been shown that a patient with an FEV_1 of less than 1.25 litres has a 40% risk of death in the next 4 years on the basis of their lung disease alone. In these patients, aggressive attempts at resection for cure are of dubious value.

The clinical staging system currently in use was adopted by the American Committee for Cancer Staging and End Results Reporting in 1983 and uses the TNM system. Clinical experience with this system has demonstrated several inadequacies. In particular, the experience in 1984 of Akiyama and that of others has shown that long-term survival is possible in patients with positive intra-abdominal nodes in specific locations. In addition, in 1985 the Japanese Committee for Registration of Oesophageal Carcinoma demonstrated that the depth of tumour invasion of the oesophageal wall is as important prognostically as the extent of nodal

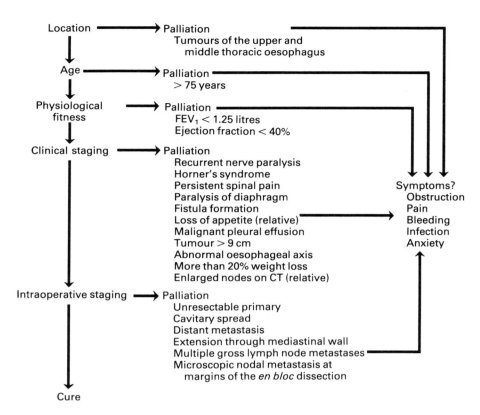

Figure 1 Algorithm of the selection process to determine whether the goal of surgery is to be cure or palliation

disease. They proposed a modified TNM system which emphasizes these prognostic indicators. The main problem of clinical staging is the difficulty in identification of lymph node metastases and the depth of wall penetration by the tumour before surgery. Computed tomography (CT) and magnetic resonance imaging (MRI) have added little to the accuracy of clinical staging, especially in patients with early lesions. Reports are now emerging that indicate that endoscopic ultrasonography may allow more accurate preoperative staging, particularly with regard to tumour wall penetration.

Clinical symptoms suggestive of an incurable advanced tumour include hoarseness because of recurrent nerve palsy, diaphragm paralysis owing to phrenic nerve palsy, fistula formation, the presence of a malignant pleural effusion and a greater than 20% loss in body weight. Special studies that suggest that surgical cure is unlikely are an overall endoscopic tumour length of 9 cm, an abnormal axis on barium upper gastrointestinal investigation, and enlarged lymph nodes on CT scan.

Because of the inaccuracy of preoperative staging, final patient selection for curative *en bloc* resection depends on intraoperative decision-making. This requires an approach which allows changing from a curative to a palliative resection if, during the course of the operation, incurable conditions are found. An algorithm for intraoperative decision-making is summarized in *Figure 2*. The procedure begins with abdominal exploration and assessment of the primary tumour and those specific nodes in the abdomen which have the same devastating effect on survival as distant metastatic disease. Reasons for abandoning the attempt at curative resection include an unresectable primary tumour due to local extension into adjacent organs, growth of the tumour through the serosa, multiple gross lymph node metastases or microscopic metastases to the lymph nodes at the margins of the resection (i.e. hepatic artery, porta hepatis, subpancreatic or periaortic nodes). In the absence of these findings, the abdomen is closed and a right posterolateral thoracotomy is performed. The extent of tumour invasion is again assessed, and if invasion of the perioesophageal tissues is present, or if distant mediastinal nodes are involved (paratracheal or superior mediastinal perioesophageal nodes), a simple oesophagectomy is performed. If neither are present, *en bloc* resection is performed.

The extent of *en bloc* resection when applied elsewhere in the gastrointestinal tract requires that the tumour be resected with a covering on all sides of a layer of normal tissue. Because of the propensity of gastrointestinal tumours to spread for long distances submucosally, long lengths of grossly normal gastrointestinal tract should be resected. Similarly, because of

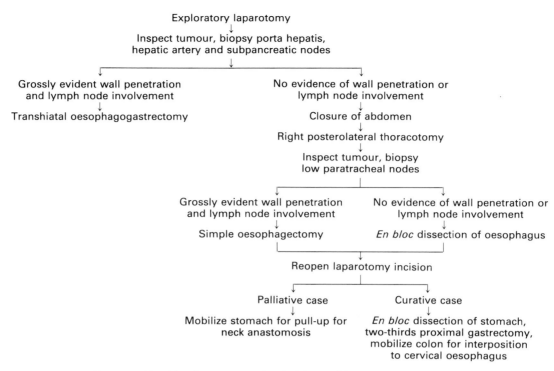

Figure 2   Algorithm for intraoperative decision-making

the propensity for relatively early lesions to spread to peritumoural lymph nodes, curative resection should include *en bloc* resection of potentially involved local and regional nodes.

Studies involving the submucosal injection of dye have revealed that the distance of longitudinal flow of lymph is six times that of transverse flow. The clinical relevance of this observation was reported by Wong when he showed that anastomotic recurrence could be prevented by obtaining a margin of at least 10 cm of normal oesophagus above the tumour. Considering that the length of the oesophagus ranges from 17 to 25 cm, this necessitates that a cervical anastomosis be performed in most patients.

Anatomical studies have shown that no barrier exists between the oesophagus and the stomach at the cardia. This is reflected clinically in the observation made by Sous and Borchard that 28% of oesophageal cancers involve the gastric cardia, and 14% of gastric cancers involve the oesophagus. Wong has shown the clinical importance of these observations in oesophageal cancer surgery by reporting that 50% of recurrences in patients who have undergone resection for cure occur in the intrathoracic stomach along the line of the gastric resection. Considering the length of the lesser curvature of the stomach, and the need for a 10-cm margin, a proximal gastrectomy greater than 50% is required if adequate margins are to be obtained. Achieving this margin often compromises the length of the stomach remaining for oesophageal replacement and necessitates

that a colonic interposition be utilized to re-establish gastrointestinal continuity.

The therapeutic benefit of *en bloc* resection of peritumoural and regional lymph nodes in continuity with the tumour has been questioned. There are, however, observations which indicate that this may be beneficial in patients with oesophageal cancer. First, cure in patients with lung cancer who have hilar nodal metastases (i.e. a tumour that also drains to mediastinal lymph nodes) is dependent on removal of the involved nodes. Secondly, patients with oesophageal cancer – like those with head and neck cancer – can die from lymph node metastases alone. Thirdly, studies involving detailed records of the location of the involved nodes removed indicate that the removal of involved peritumoural nodes is beneficial. Consequently, any attempt at curative *en bloc* resection should include resection of the peritumoural and regional nodes in continuity with the primary tumour. Several studies support this conclusion in that long-term survival of patients with involved lymph nodes has been achieved provided that they are limited in number and located in close proximity to the primary tumour. Those who believe otherwise should provide evidence of long-term survivors with involved lymph nodes that were left in place. In our experience, simple oesophagectomy in patients with early lesions, i.e. intramural tumours, with four or less involved lymph nodes is associated with significantly shorter survival time than that observed in patients with similar early lesions treated by *en bloc* resection.

Preoperative

En bloc resection requires that gastrointestinal continuity be re-established by colonic interposition. Consequently, the segment of colon to be interposed must be evaluated as discussed in the chapter on pp. 128–141. Crucial points which deserve emphasis include the status of the marginal artery in the region of the splenic flexure and the status of the origin of the inferior mesenteric artery. Anomalies of the coeliac and superior mesenteric systems are common and deserve attention. Colonoscopy should be performed to exclude the presence of mucosal disease that would preclude the use of the colon as an oesophageal substitute.

The colon is prepared by the standard technique of whole gut lavage with isosmotic electrolyte solution (GoLytely) in combination with the administration of oral antibiotics. In addition, parenteral broad-spectrum antibiotics are administered before operation and for 3 days afterwards. Patients are given subcutaneous heparin injections for prophylaxis against deep vein thrombosis. Carcinoembryonic antigen levels are obtained before surgery as they are elevated in approximately 30% of patients and can serve as a valuable marker for recurrence.

As mentioned above, the prevalence of significant cardiac and pulmonary disease is such that a thorough examination is mandatory. In addition to detecting the presence of disease, these studies will often reveal the need for specific intervention, such as coronary arteriography and possible angioplasty for coronary artery disease, or preoperative chest physiotherapy for patients with chronic obstructive pulmonary disease. All patients should be encouraged to stop smoking before surgery.

The operation is performed under general anaesthesia adminstered through a double-lumen endotracheal tube. This is replaced with a single-lumen tube for postoperative ventilation support after completion of the thoracic portion of the procedure. Pharyngeal oedema secondary to the neck dissection can make replacement of the double-lumen tube at the end of the procedure difficult. Routine haemodynamic monitoring is carried out with a central venous line and an arterial line. A pulmonary artery catheter is used as indicated.

Operation

The operation is performed through three incisions which are made in the following order: (1) upper midline laparotomy for abdominal exploration; (2) right posterolateral thoracotomy for *en bloc* dissection of the oesophagus and mediastinum, closure of the thoracotomy, repositioning of the patient in the recumbent position, and reopening of the upper abdominal midline incision for *en bloc* dissection of the stomach; and (3) left neck incision for mobilization and division of the cervical oesophagus. The dissected specimen is removed transhiatally from the thorax. Gastrointestinal continuity is re-established using interposed colon based on the left colic artery and inferior mesenteric vein, and placed isoperistaltically between the cervical oesophagus and distal stomach.

The procedure begins with an exploration of the abdomen for the presence of locally advanced disease which would preclude resection for cure. The exploration is performed through an upper midline incision. The oesophageal hiatus is examined for penetration of the tumour through the wall of the distal oesophagus or the gastric cardia. Exposure of this area is facilitated by the use of a Weinberg retractor which has been welded to the handle of a Balfour retractor. The retractor is held in place with an overarm bar, providing excellent steady exposure of the hiatus.

In the absence of local invasion, the regional lymph nodes are assessed. This requires exploration of the nodes in the porta hepatis along the hepatic artery and in the subpancreatic region by incision of the gastrohepatic omentum. If frozen section of these nodes is free of tumour and there is no distant disease in the remainder of the abdomen, the abdomen is closed, and the patient is positioned for a right posterolateral thoracotomy.

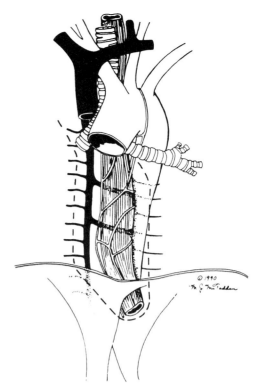

1   The right chest is opened through an incision in the seventh intercostal space above the eighth rib. The inferior pulmonary ligament is divided up to the inferior pulmonary vein, and the right lung is deflated and retracted anteriorly. The thoracic portion of the procedure entails *en bloc* removal of the thoracic oesophagus with its surrounding areolar tissue containing the low parabronchial, subcarinal, paraoesophageal and parahiatal lymph nodes, the thoracic duct, the azygos vein down to where it passes into the abdomen on the lateral surface of the vertebra, and a collar of diaphragmatic muscle around the oesophageal hiatus. The block of tissue removed is limited anteriorly by the pericardium, laterally by the right and left mediastinal pleura, and posteriorly by the intercostal arteries, aorta and anterior vertebral ligaments.

2   The thoracic dissection begins with the incision of the parietal pleura parallel to the spine. The individual branches of the azygos vein are ligated from its arch down to where it passes into the abdomen on the lateral surface of the vertebra.

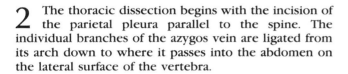

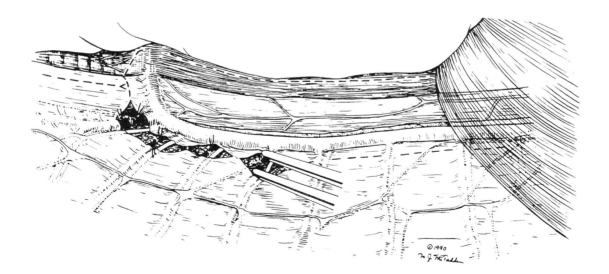

3   The posterior dissection is extended across to the left mediastinal pleura, along the intercostal arteries to the aorta and over the anterior surface of the aorta into the left side of the chest. This is done by elevating the intact azygos vein and its surrounding tissue, allowing the hemiazygos vein or veins to be seen as they cross over the spine underneath the aorta to join the azygos vein. These veins must be identified, ligated and divided. The aorta becomes visible when the hemiazygos veins are divided and serves as a guide for the extension of the posterior incision into the left side of the chest. Early division of the azygos vein at its entry into the superior vena cava should be avoided because the venous hypertension that ensues causes excessive bleeding during the mediastinal dissection.

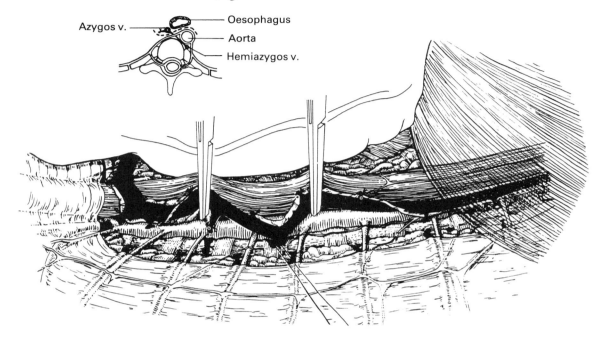

Azygos v. — Oesophagus — Aorta — Hemiazygos v.

3

4   At the caudal end of the posterior pleural incision, in the space behind the crura, the distal end of the azygos vein and the thoracic duct are identified, divided and ligated.

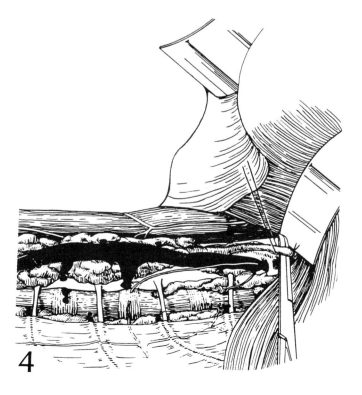

4

5 The anterior mediastinal dissection is developed by making an incision in the mediastinal pleura parallel to the posterior border of the right main stem bronchus and pericardium down to the diaphragm. The plane of dissection is carried across the midline through the left mediastinal pleura into the left pleural cavity, passing posterior to the left main stem bronchus and pericardium and anterior to the subcarinal lymph nodes. At this point the azygos vein is divided as it enters the superior vena cava.

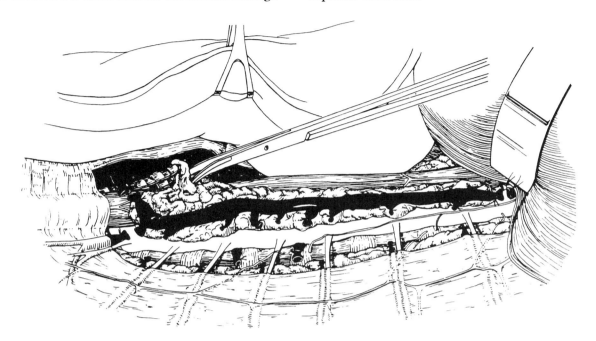

5

6 When the mediastinum has been dissected both anterior and posterior to the oesophagus, the oesophagus, along with its covering of perioesophageal areolar tissue, is surrounded by a Penrose drain, pulled into the right chest and freed completely by dissecting over the aorta and incising the left mediastinal pleura superiorly to the aortic arch and inferiorly to the left diaphragm. The block of tissue mobilized contains the oesophagus and adjacent subcarinal, paraoesophageal and parahiatal nodes.

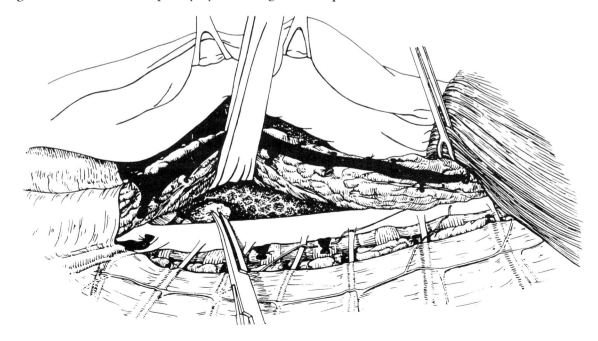

6

7 Care must be taken to avoid injury to the left recurrent nerve in the region of the aortic arch. Its common course is to pass directly to the trachea without redundancy and lie on the left lateral inferior cartilaginous wall of the trachea as it passes to the neck. Superior to the arch, the oesophagus is bluntly dissected into the neck, but is not divided. Inferiorly, a collar of diaphragmatic muscle is excised around the oesophageal hiatus. When the dissection is complete the thoracotomy incision is closed with the specimen remaining in the chest wrapped in a surgical sponge.

The patient is then moved to the recumbent position. The previously inserted double-lumen endotracheal tube, used for selected deflation of the right lung, is removed and a single-lumen tube is inserted. The anterior surfaces of the neck, chest and abdomen are prepared and draped and an upper midline abdominal incision made.

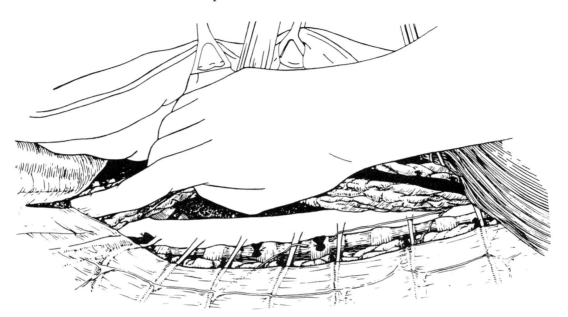

7

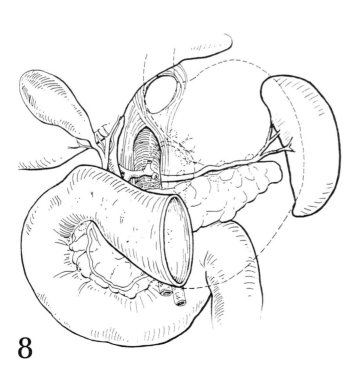

8

8 The abdominal portion of the procedure entails *en bloc* removal of all the posterior peritoneal periaortic areolar tissue down to the coeliac axis, the superior border of the common hepatic artery, and the surperior border of the neck and tail of the pancreas. It includes the splenic artery, the greater omentum, the proximal two-thirds of the stomach and lymph nodes around the left gastric artery and coeliac axis, superior to and underneath the common hepatic artery, medial to the portal triad, in the greater omentum and around the splenic artery. This extensive resection is performed so that all potentially involved peritumoural and regional lymph nodes, and the submucosal lymphatics of the stomach and oesophagus can be incorporated in the surgical specimen. The pancreas is not removed. The spleen and splenic artery with its associated nodes is taken with the specimen.

Curative *en bloc* dissection is abandoned if intraoperative staging reveals an unresectable primary tumour, cavitary spread of tumour, distant organ metastasis, extension of tumour through the serosa of the stomach, multiple gross lymph node metastases, or microscopic evidence of lymph node involvement at the margins of the *en bloc* resection (i.e. low paratracheal, portal triad or subpancreatic periaortic lymph nodes).

9 The abdominal dissection is started by freeing the greater omentum from its attachments to the transverse mesocolon and mobilization of the whole colon to the midline for its subsequent use as an oesophageal and gastric substitute. The gastrohepatic ligament is divided along the liver margin up to the oesophageal hiatus. The areolar tissue containing lymph nodes along the medial border of the portal triad and underneath and along the superior border of the common hepatic artery is swept toward the coeliac axis. Dissection of a collar of diaphragmatic muscle around the oesophageal hiatus, which was begun during the thoracic part of the operation, is continued down the right crus to the coeliac axis.

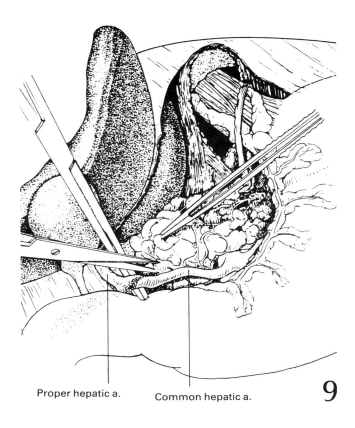

Proper hepatic a.   Common hepatic a.   **9**

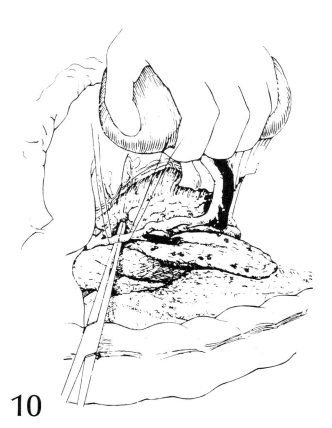

10

10 The spleen and tail of the pancreas are mobilized to the midline and the dissection of a collar of the diaphragmatic muscle that was started during the thoracic portion of the operation is continued down the margin of the left crus to the coeliac axis. The splenic artery and vein are dissected off the superior border of the pancreas. The vein is ligated near the body of the pancreas where it courses inferiorly away from the artery and prior to it joining the inferior mesenteric vein.

11 The splenic artery is further dissected off the pancreas until the coeliac axis is reached, where it is divided and ligated. This exposes the origin of the left gastric artery which is similarly divided and ligated.

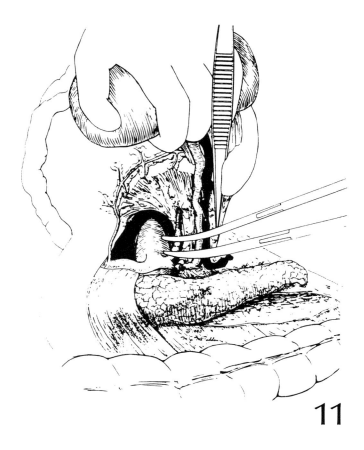

11

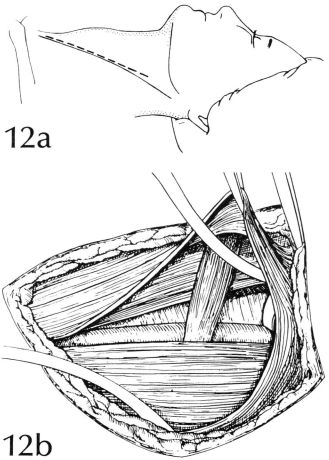

12a

12b

12a, b Exposure of the cervical oesophagus is obtained by making an incision in the left side of the neck along the anterior border of the sternocleidomastoid muscle from the suprasternal notch to the point just below the angle of the jaw. The platysma muscle is divided, exposing the muscles of the neck. The omohyoid muscle is divided at its tendon, and the sternothyroid and sternohyoid muscles at their sternoclavicular insertion. The contents of the carotid sheath are retracted laterally, exposing the cervical oesophagus.

13 Care must be taken to avoid injury to the left recurrent laryngeal nerve as it courses just anterior to the tracheo-oesophageal groove on the lateral aspect of the trachea and passes beneath the thyroid gland. The oesophagus is dissected circumferentially, mobilizing the entire cervical portion.

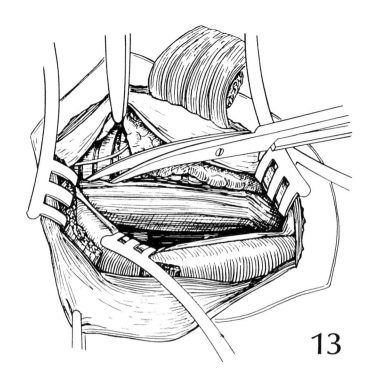

13

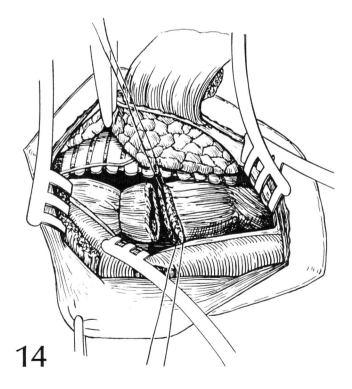

14

14 A ligature is tied distal to the point of proposed transection of the oesophagus and stay sutures are placed in the proximal oesophagus to prevent separation of the mucosa and muscle wall after division.

15 The specimen is removed from the posterior mediastinum through the diaphragmatic hiatus and the stomach is transected with a GIA stapling device, leaving the antrum and pylorus in place. A small pyloromyotomy is performed.

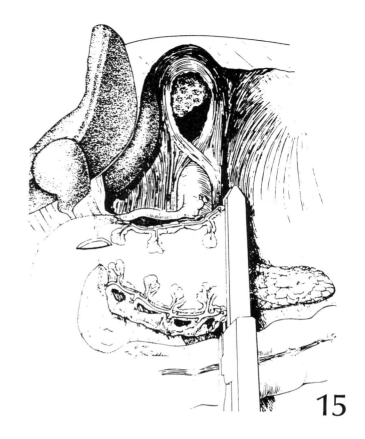

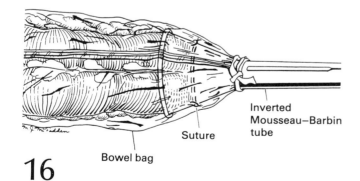

Inverted Mousseau–Barbin tube

Suture

Bowel bag

16 The colonic segment to be interposed is divided in the appropriate place with a GIA stapler. The proximal end of the colon graft is sutured to the inside of the funnel of a Mousseau–Barbin tube and wrapped in a bowel bag that has been trimmed to fit. This allows atraumatic passage of the interposed segment through the posterior mediastinum and out through the neck incision.

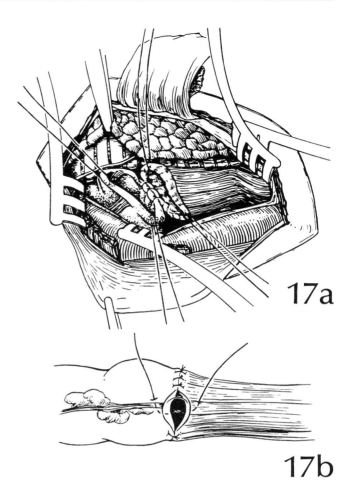

17a, b The bag and Mousseau–Barbin tube are removed. The staple closure on the colon is removed and an end-to-end anastomosis is performed to the oesophagus with interrupted 4/0 monofilament non-absorbable sutures. All sutures are tied within the lumen, except the last four or five which are placed in a modified Gambee fashion.

Left crus of oesophageal hiatus

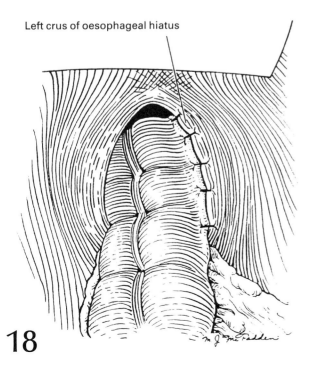

18 The colon is placed on a slight stretch from below to prevent redundancy in the chest and is anchored to the left crus of the diaphragm. The colon is not anchored circumferentially because this causes bowstringing and produces a functional obstruction.

19 The length of colon is measured so that no more than 10 cm extends below the oesophageal hiatus. The colon is transected and anastomosed to the remnant of the stomach. Continuity of the colon is then established by anastomosing the remaining colonic segments with a standard end-to-end closure. A feeding jejunostomy tube is placed, and the mesenteric defect in the colon is closed.

If the operation has lasted too long, or the patient is unstable, or the vascular supply to the colon segment is in doubt after the proximal marginal and middle colic artery and vein are ligated, the colon is not divided. The antral portion of the stomach is closed, an intramural jejunostomy tube is inserted, and a cervical oesophago-stomy is constructed. The transverse mesocolon is opened wide and the whole of the small bowel is brought up through the opening so that the transverse colon lies under the small bowel, low in the abdomen. The transverse colon is sutured to the abdominal wall in the right lower quadrant. This is to prevent it migrating into the left upper quadrant and adhering to the denuded posterior peritoneal surface. The patient is discharged on jejunostomy tube feedings to return in 90 days for re-establishment of gastrointestinal continuity with the previously delayed isoperistaltic descending colonic graft through a substernal route. The single-stage operation is preferred because postoperative adhesions and scarring of the transverse mesocolon can limit the length of the colonic transplant, but the reconstruction phase should not be undertaken unless everything is satisfactory.

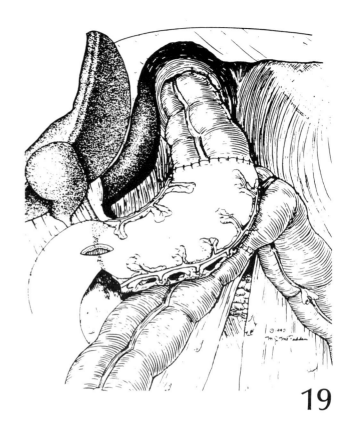

19

Postoperative care

Normally, fluid in the interstitium of the lung is cleared by its rich lymphatic network. After *en bloc* resection of the oesophagus the pulmonary lymphatics are inter-rupted, compromising the ability of the lung to clear interstitial fluid. This results in decreased compliance of the lung, reduced alveolar volume and increased resistance in airflow through the alveolar ducts, all of which adds to the work of breathing. As a result, ventilator support is usually required for 3–4 days until the excess fluid given has beeen mobilized and excreted. During this time the central venous pressure must be monitored and is a guide to fluid replacement. After 'third spacing' fluid has been replaced, colloid-containing fluids are preferable to minimize oedema and to maintain cardiovascular integrity. Blood is given as necessary to maintain the haematocrit at approximately 30% to ensure adequate oxygen carrying capacity.

Enteral feedings are commenced on the third day after surgery via the jejunostomy tube. This approach avoids parenteral nutrition and its inherent fluid load in nearly all patients. Oral feedings are started between the seventh and tenth day and, when reasonable, the jejunostomy feedings are continued only at night. On discharge from hospital a portable infusion pump is sent home with the patient to ensure adequate nutrition during the period of adaptation following colonic interposition.

Outcome

The authors have studied the survival of 69 consecutive patients with oesophageal cancer following *en bloc* or transhiatal oesophagectomy for carcinoma arising in the distal oesophagus and gastric cardia. Preoperative and intraoperative staging placed the patients in three distinct subgroups: (1) those with apparently limited disease and good physical fitness (*n* = 30) underwent *en bloc* resection; (2) those with apparently limited disease but poor physiological reserve (*n* = 16) underwent transhiatal resection, as did (3) those with evidence of more advanced disease (*n* = 23). The mean follow-up time of surviving patients was 26 months. Survival curves were calculated by the Kaplan–Meier method. Comparisons between groups were made using the log rank method.

Overall, survival was significantly better in the 30 patients who had *en bloc* resection (41%) than in the 39 patients who underwent transhiatal resections (14%) (*P* < 0.001, log rank). Using the WNM system of postoperative histological staging, 19 patients had early lesions (defined as intramural lesions associated with four or fewer involved nodes), 26 had intermediate lesions (defined as either transmural or associated with more than four involved lymph nodes), and 24 had late lesions (defined as both transmural and associated with more than four involved lymph nodes). Survival was significantly better in patients with early lesions following *en bloc* resection than in those having transhiatal resection (75% *versus* 20%, *P* < 0.01), and those with advanced lesions (27% *versus* 9%, *P* < 0.01). For intermediate llesions survival rates were similar (14% *versus* 20%), although the median survival following *en bloc* resection was longer (24 *versus* 8 months).

There are four possible explanations as to why transhiatal oesophagectomy failed to achieve the results obtained with *en bloc* oesophagectomy in favourably staged patients. First is the potential dissemination of tumour cells at the time of blunt dissection of the thoracic oesophagus. Secondly, an inadequate distal tumour margin may have been chosen in an effort to preserve a lengthy stomach with sufficient blood supply to perform cervical anastomosis. Thirdly, there may have been transfer of unrecognized perigastric metastatic nodes into the thorax with the gastric pull-up.

Finally, there is a chance that the blunt thoracic dissection can leave residual nodal disease in the mediastinum. *En bloc* oesophagectomy effectively eliminates all of these potential causes of recurrence.

On the basis of historical principles of surgical oncology, arguments derived from anatomical and histological observations, reports of other surgeons and the authors' personal experience, it is concluded that: (1) survival after surgical removal of a carcinoma arising in the distal oesophagus, cardia or proximal stomach is dependent upon the method of resection, i.e. transhiatal or *en bloc*; and (2) patients with early lesions have significantly better survival after *en bloc* resection.

Acknowledgements

The illustrations in this chapter have been reproduced with permission from Professor T. R. DeMeester, the copyright holder.

Further reading

Akiyama H, Tsurumaru M, Kawamura T, Ono Y. Principles of surgical treatment for carcinoma of the esophagus: analysis of lymph node involvement. *Ann Surg* 1981; 194: 438–46.

DeMeester TR, Zaninotto G, Johansson K-K. Selective therapeutic approach to cancer of the lower esophagus and cardia. *J Thorac Cardiovasc Surg* 1988; 95: 42–54.

Hagen JA, Peters JH, DeMeester TR. Superiority of extended *en bloc* esophagogastrectomy for carcinoma of the lower esophagus and cardia. *J Thorac Cardiovasc Surg* 1993; 106: 850–9.

Skinner DB. *En bloc* resection for neoplasms of the esophagus and cardia. *J Thorac Cardiovasc Surg* 1983; 85: 59–71.

Skinner DB, Dowlatshahi KD, DeMeester TR. Potentially curable cancer of the esophagus. *Cancer* 1982; 50: 2571–5.

Skinner DB, Ferguson MK, Soriano A, Little AG, Staszak VM. Selection of operation for esophageal cancer based on staging. *Ann Surg* 1986; 204: 391–401.

Sous HU, Borchard F. Cancer of the distal esophagus and cardia: incidence, tumorous infiltration and metastatic spread. *Ann Surg* 1986; 203: 188–95.

Wong J. Esophageal resection for cancer: the rationale of current practice. *Am J Surg* 1987; 153: 18–24.

Long oesophageal myotomy and excision of diverticula

André Duranceau MD
Professor of Surgery, Department of Surgery, University of Montréal, Division of Thoracic Surgery, Hôtel-Dieu de Montréal, Montréal, Québec, Canada

Principles and justification

Pulsion diverticula of the distal oesophagus are considered to be complications of abnormal intraoesophageal pressures. Cross et al.[1,2] supported the concept that spasm of the inferior sphincter accompanied by increased contraction pressures in the oesophageal body is responsible for both the symptoms and the appearance of the diverticulum. Allen and Claggett[3] and Benacci et al.[4] have reported significantly fewer leaks with secondary sepsis when a myotomy is combined with diverticulectomy than when a diverticulectomy alone is performed. When surgical treatment is indicated for distal oesophageal diverticula, the diverticulum should be excised if it is large enough and the underlying motor abnormality corrected. Following myotomy, a significant weakening of the gastro-oesophageal junction results, and an antireflux repair is added to the myotomy to prevent reflux damage to the oesophageal mucosa. A partial fundoplication is preferred, as a more complete wrap causes functional obstruction to an oesophagus made powerless by the myotomy.

Indications

Significant symptoms related to swallowing and to the presence of the diverticulum constitute the main indication for surgical treatment. Asymptomatic diverticula do not require operative treatment.

Preoperative

Assessment

Radiological assessment is important to identify the size and location of the diverticulum. Videoscopic radiology usually allows visualization of the accompanying motor dysfunction. Although optional, radionuclide transit studies using liquid and solid markers quantify oesophageal retention.

Oesophageal motility studies are essential to characterize the motor disorder accompanying the diverticulum and to determine the extent of dysfunction.

Endoscopy and 24-h pH monitoring are important for ruling out reflux disease and mucosal damage or other mucosal abnormality.

Patient preparation

The patient is put on a liquid diet for 24 h before the operation. If there is any possibility of significant oesophageal retention, lavage of the oesophageal cavity is performed in an awake state on the morning of the operation.

A cephalosporin and antibiotics active against anaerobes (such as metromidazole (Flagyl), 500 mg, or clindamycin, 600 mg) are administered before induction of anaesthesia. Subcutaneous heparin, 5000 units, is administered routinely 2 h before the operation and every 12 h thereafter until the patient is fully ambulatory and ready to leave hospital.

Operation

Incision

1 The oesophagus is approached through a left thoracic incision. The pleura is opened at the superior border of the eighth rib, and a small posterior segment of the rib is removed. Anaesthesia via a double-lumen endotracheal tube allows exclusion and retraction of the left lung during the operation.

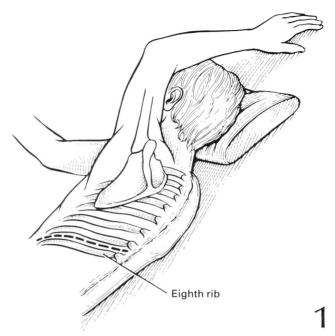

Eighth rib

1

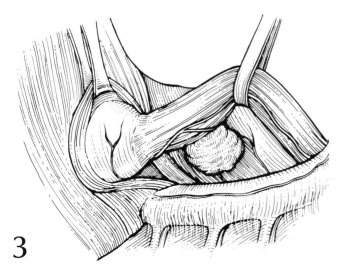

2

2 The mediastinum is opened 1 cm anterior to the aorta, from the aortic arch to the diaphragm. At the distal extent the pleura is incised as an inverted T in order to have free access to the hiatus. The inferior pulmonary ligament is divided up to the inferior pulmonary vein.

The oesophagus is mobilized proximally and at the level of the hiatus, below the diverticulum. Penrose drains are passed around it in order to facilitate traction and dissection.

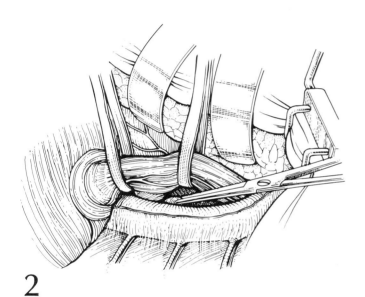

3

3 The oesophageal body is freed completely from its fascial and vascular attachments up to the inferior border of the aortic arch.

Progressive dissection of the diverticulum is then undertaken making sure that the right pleura is protected.

If the hiatus is small and without a hernia, free access to the peritoneal cavity is obtained through a peripheral diaphragmatic incision 2–3 cm from its insertion at the chest wall. This allows complete and easy dissection of the fundus, gastrosplenic vessels and hiatal structures. The phreno-oesophageal ligament and the peritoneum are opened, and the whole gastro-oesophageal junction is delivered into the chest through the hiatus. The gastro-oesophageal fat pad is removed.

4 When the oesophagus and proximal stomach have been fully mobilized, the diverticulum and the distal oesophagus are rotated towards the left chest. There is usually a layer of fibromuscular tissue investing the diverticulum. The mucosa of the diverticulum is freed progressively towards its neck, and the muscular defect surrounding the neck is thus clearly identified.

If the diverticulum is not directed towards the right chest, it may be necessary to include it in the planned myotomy and then suspend the diverticulum rather than remove it.

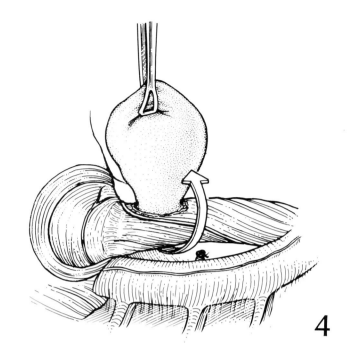

4

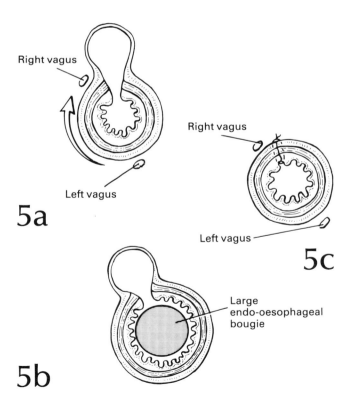

Right vagus

Left vagus

5a

Right vagus

Left vagus

5c

Large endo-oesophageal bougie

5b

5a–c On completion of the dissection, a large mercury bougie (no. 50) is placed into the oesophagus and stomach. This stent serves to distend the oesophageal lumen and prevent undue narrowing at the point of excision of the diverticulum.

With the bougie safely in place, resection of the diverticulum is now undertaken, using one of two methods.

6 The first technique is a manual one for resection of the diverticulum. Traction sutures are placed on the proximal and distal borders of the neck, and the diverticulum is resected opening a straight line of mucosa.

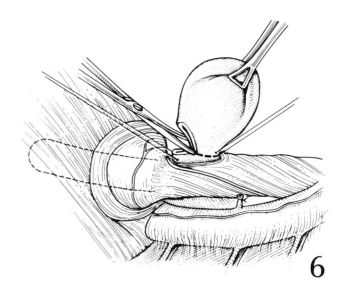

7 The oesophagotomy is closed longitudinally, as for any oesophageal anastomosis, with an interrupted single layer of inverting sutures, closing both ends with internal knots. The last three or four sutures are tied externally.

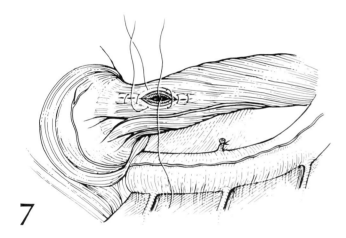

8 The second technique is to use a 5–6-cm stapler to close the neck of the diverticulum. This is again accomplished with a large bougie protecting the oesophageal lumen. A small cuff of mucosa is left distal to the stapling line, and a second row of sutures reapproximates the muscle over the staple line, anchoring it to the cut rim of the mucosa.

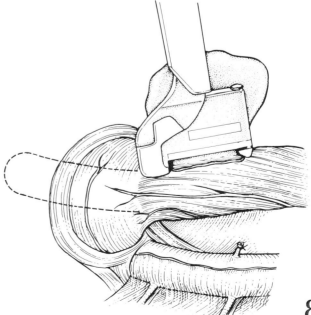

9 When the rotation traction is eased, the site of the diverticulectomy resumes its normal position facing the right chest. A long myotomy is performed on the left posterolateral oesophagus. The mercury bougie remains in place and serves as support for the mucosa. The use of magnifying spectacles helps in identifying the oesophageal structures and encourages stringent haemostasis. A no. 15 scalpel blade is used, and the longitudinal muscle is opened along the whole length of the planned myotomy. The myotomy is then completed through the circular muscle layer, making sure not to perforate the mucosa. The lower oesophageal sphincter area may be recognized as the muscle is usually thinner here.

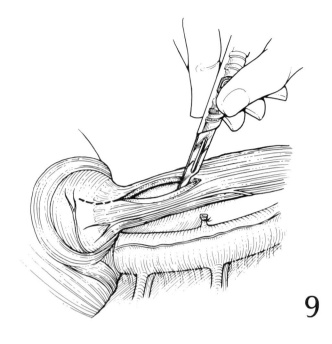

9

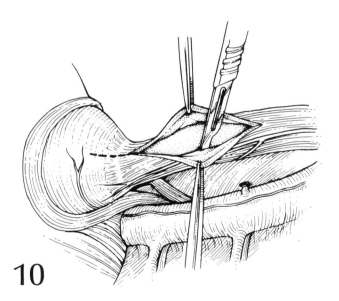

10

10 The myotomy is extended for 1 cm onto the gastric wall muscle and the gastric submucosa can then be seen as a richly vascularized layer.

11 Lateral dissection of the muscle from the mucosa is carried out with scissors. The assistant pulls the muscle outwards while the surgeon holds the mucosa against the bougie with a dissector swab. This exposes a cellular tissue plane between the layers which affords easy dissection. Approximately 50% of the oesophageal circumference is freed from the muscle. Once the myotomy is completed, haemostasis is obtained and the mucosa of the myotomized zone is checked to make sure that it has not been breached. The transverse sections show the points of dissection between layers and the placement of sutures to evert the dissected muscle and the position of the sutures in relation to the right and left vagi.

The bougie is removed, a nasogastric tube is placed in the oesophageal cavity and 50–100 ml air is introduced into the oesophagus while it is kept under saline. Any leak will be shown by bubbles of escaping air.

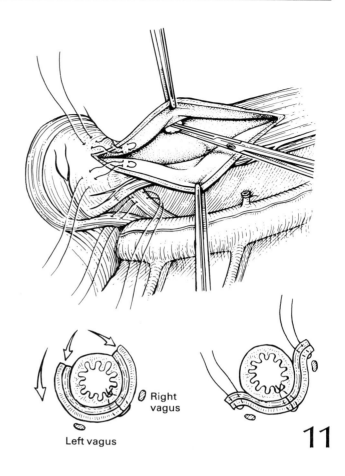

Right vagus

Left vagus

11

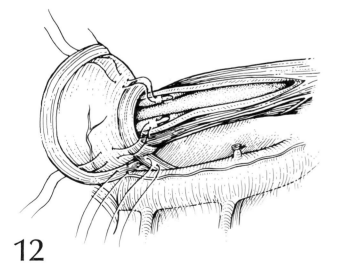

12

12 A two-thirds fundic wrap of the Belsey type is next carried out. Two 2/0 silk sutures anchor the fundoplication on each side of the myotomized zone and at two levels. The two layers of the muscle are transfixed from outside to inside in order to evert the muscle while anchoring the seromuscular layer of the fundus to the oesophageal wall. This is accomplished to prevent any closure of the myotomy at the gastro-oesophageal junction.

The first two sutures are completed at the level of the former insertion of the phreno-oesophageal ligament. The two sutures of the second layer are placed in a similar fashion, 2–3 cm more proximal, from the oesophagus to the fundus and then through the diaphragm in order to tie both sutures on the thoracic side of the hiatus.

13 With this partial fundoplication, the distal 4–5 cm of the myotomized oesophagus is reduced without any tension under the diaphragm. It affords good antireflux protection while allowing proper food transit at the gastro-oesophageal junction.

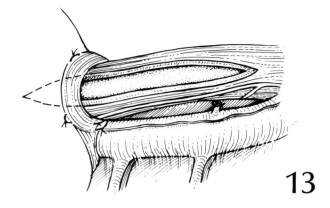

13

Postoperative care

The nasogastric tube is left in place until normal bowel activity has resumed. Once gastric drainage is discontinued, an oesophagram is obtained using water-soluble contrast medium. If the mucosal configuration is considered adequate, liquid barium is added to complete the immediate postoperative evaluation.

The chest tube is removed when normal pulmonary re-expansion is obtained with less than 100 ml of drainage over a 24-h period.

A liquid diet is resumed once the myotomy and diverticulectomy sites have been shown to be intact. The patient progresses to a semiliquid diet for the following 10 days. Normal alimentation is then resumed.

Complete functional reassessment is obtained 2 years after the operation and at regular intervals thereafter. It is particularly important to document emptying capacity and reflux damage over time in these patients.

References

1. Cross FS. Esophageal diverticula related neuromuscular problems. *Ann Otol* 1968; 77: 914–26.

2. Cross FS, Johnson GF, Gerein AN. Esophageal diverticula. *Arch Surg* 1961; 83: 525–33.

3. Allen TH, Claggett OT. Changing concepts in the surgical tratment of pulsion diverticula of the lower esophagus. *J Thorac Cardiovasc Surg* 1965; 50: 455–62.

4. Benacci JC, Deschamps C, Trastek V, Allen MS, Daly RC, Pairolero PC. Epiphrenic diverticulum: results of surgical treatment. *Ann Thorac Surg* 1993 (in press).

Illustrations by Peter Cox

Extramucosal enucleation of leiomyoma of the oesophagus

Guo Jun Huang MD, FRCS
Professor of Thoracic Surgery, Cancer Institute and Hospital, Chinese Academy of Medical Sciences, Beijing, People's Republic of China

Principles and justification

Leiomyoma is the most common of a relatively uncommon group of benign tumours of the oesophagus. It is usually slow growing with few symptoms. In some cases, however, after years of slow growth it will cause serious symptoms[1].

Surgical removal is preferred, except in elderly patients and those with a small tumour or who are a poor surgical risk. Extramucosal enucleation is the operation of choice, as it has a low risk of morbidity and mortality. In the author's experience extramucosal enucleation was successfully performed in 99 of 100 cases of oesophageal leiomyoma[2]. Oesophageal resec-tion and reconstruction was necessary in only very exceptional cases.

Large leimyomas situated at the gastro-oesophageal junction should be treated by antireflux repair following enucleation because of the extent of dissection required.

Preoperative

Unless mucosal abnormality or ulceration is obvious, preoperative endoscopic biopsy should be avoided because of the associated risk of inflammatory adher-ence of the tumour to the mucosa

The location, size and extent of the tumour and its relation to the surrounding structures should be assessed preoperatively using contrast oesophago-graphy, oesophagoscopy, computed tomography and/or magnetic resonance imaging. It is important to deter-mine the position of the tumour bulk in relation to the lumen of the oesophagus in order to decide the side of thoracotomy that will best expose the tumour, and which necessitates the least mobilization and dissection of the oesophagus for enucleation.

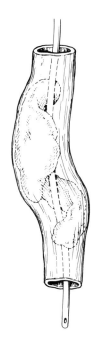

1 In about 20% of patients, the tumour is large and irregularly shaped – some look like root ginger encircling the oesophageal lumen. Extramucosal enucle-ation of such leiomyomas is much more difficult than that of smooth ovoid tumours and requires meticulous care to avoid rupturing the underlying mucosa.

Anaesthesia

As for other intrathoracic operations, endotracheal or endobronchial general anaesthesia is routinely used.

Operation

The patient is prepared as for any operation for oesophageal tumours (as described in the chapter on pp. 39–44). A nasogastric tube, preferably one with only one side hole close to its tip, is inserted before surgery to serve as a guide for the surgeon to define the extent of the oesophageal lumen and its relation to the tumour during enucleation. The tube may also be used to insufflate air into the oesophagus under water to ascertain mucosal integrity after enucleation.

Incision

2 A posterolateral thoracotomy incision is made along the fifth, sixth or seventh intercostal space or rib bed, depending on the location and extent of the tumour.

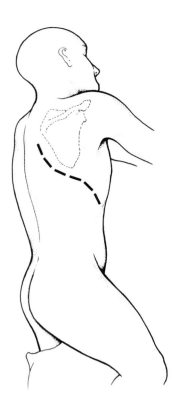

2

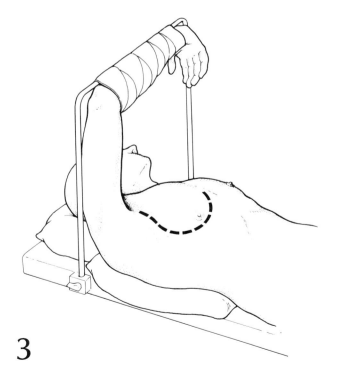

3

3 A right or left anterolateral thoracotomy through the third interspace is preferred for patients with a relatively small tumour situated above the aortic arch. This approach is much less traumatic and is quicker than the posterolateral thoracotomy.

In the author's series[2] the tumour was located in the upper third of the oesophagus in 15 patients, middle third in 71, and the lower third in 14. In no case was the tumour located above the upper border of the manubrium sterni. A right posterolateral thoracotomy was performed in 68 patients, a right anterolateral thoracotomy in 11, and a left posterolateral thoracotomy in 21.

Exposure and mobilization of the oesophagus

4 The pleural cavity is opened, and the lung is collapsed and retracted anteriorly and medially to expose the posterior mediastinum. In some patients it is desirable that the lung is completely collapsed: endo-bronchial anaesthesia should be chosen for these patients.

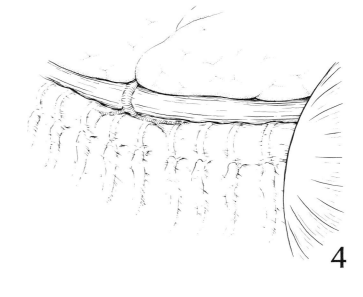

4

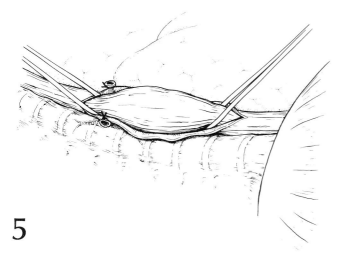

5

5 The mediastinal pleura is incised to expose the oesophagus at the site of the leiomyoma. When operating through the right chest, exposure may be improved by dividing the azygos vein. The tumour-bearing segment of the oesophagus is mobilized and traction tapes are passed around the oesophagus, one above and one below the tumour.

Extramucosal enucleation of leiomyoma

6 The size, shape, and extent of the tumour and its relationship to the oesophageal lumen are carefully assessed. (The last task is simplified by moving the indwelling nasogastric tube from one side of the lumen to the other.) The tumour is then lifted and its overlying muscle coat incised longitudinally. The muscle coat is then pushed aside to disclose the whitish, glistening, solid leiomyoma. Care is needed at this stage to ensure that the incision is made over the bulk of the tumour, and that the oesophageal lumen is not entered. While the surgeon is holding the tumour it tends to bulge out of the incised oesophageal wall so that excessive lifting should be avoided to ensure that the underlying mucosa does not rupture.

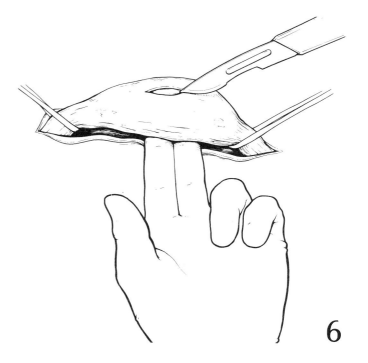

6

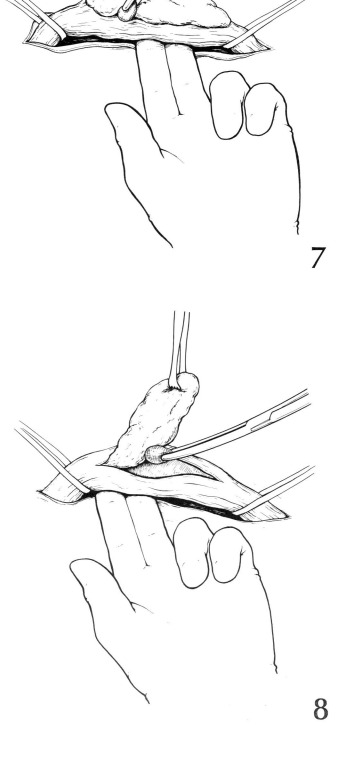

7, 8 The tumour is separated in all directions from the overlying muscle coat and the underlying submucosa and mucosa, mainly by blunt dissection using a 'gauze peanut' held in a curved clamp. Sharp dissection is used only to extend the muscle coat incision or if adhesions are encountered. Meticulous care is needed to keep the dissection plane close to the surface of the tumour at all times, even if it is irregular in shape and of the 'ginger root' variety. Greater care is required when dissecting the undersurface of the tumour, because it might contain pits and grooves with in-growths of submucosal or mucosal folds. Adhesions between the mucosa and the under surface of the tumour may be present at the site of previous endoscopic biopsy. These need to be freed carefully to avoid mucosal perforation.

7

8

Underwater inflation test for mucosal leakage

9 Following enucleation of the leiomyoma it is important to determine whether inadvertent damage to the mucosa has been caused. To carry out this check, the indwelling nasogastric tube should be withdrawn until its tip lies between the two traction tapes around the oesophagus. These tapes are now used as temporary air 'tourniquets' by passing each of them through a segment of tubing. The oesophageal lumen can thus be occluded above and below the enucleation site by gentle tightening.

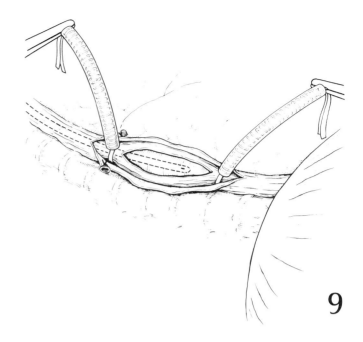

9

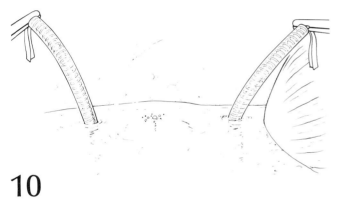

10

10 Saline is poured into the pleural cavity and the entire mobilized oesophagus is immersed. Injecting air through the nasogastric tube gently inflates the exposed mucosa and any leaks will be obvious at this point.

Repair of mucosal defects

During enucleation of leiomyoma the mucosa may be inadvertently perforated. In the author's series[2], perforation or rupture of the mucosa at enucleation occurred in seven patients. The causes were a very large and irregular tumour in two cases, multiple (six) tumours in one patient, high preoperative irradiation (7000 rad) in one patient, previous endoscopic biopsy in one patient, and operative accident in two.

11 Perforated mucosa should be sutured carefully with interrupted fine non-absorbable sutures, tying the knots inside the oesophageal lumen.

Extensively denuded mucosa should be excised and the defect carefully sutured to avoid ischaemic necrosis and fistula formation. The underwater insufflation test should be repeated after mucosal repair to ensure that the suture line is airtight.

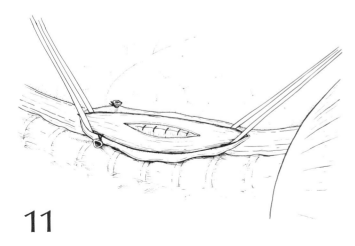

11

Repair of muscle coat defect

12 The defect in the muscle coat at the site of enucleation is repaired by suturing the two edges together. Any redundant muscle flaps may be sutured in an overlapping manner. In repairing the muscle coat attention should be paid to ensure that the mucosal suture line (if present) is well covered with muscle tissue, and that there is no gross dead space underneath the muscle coat.

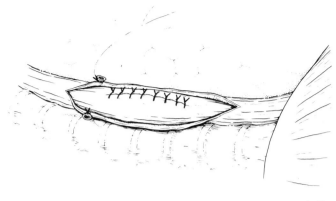

12

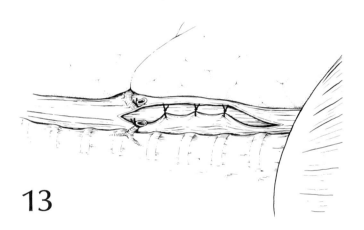

13

13 When feasible, a flap of pleura should be used to cover the oesophageal repair. A latissimus dorsi flap has been used to close a large defect left after excision of a giant leiomyoma[3].

Wound closure

14 Once satisfactory repair of the oesophagus has been achieved the traction tapes are removed and the mediastinal pleura is loosely approximated, leaving small gaps for drainage.

The lung is re-expanded and the pleural cavity irrigated with saline solution. A chest tube is inserted for closed drainage and the thoracotomy wound is closed in layers.

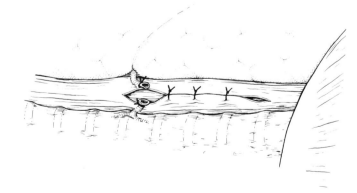

14

Postoperative care

This is one of the few procedures after which early oral intake is allowed. However, if the mucosa has been breached the same cautious approach should be used as with any major oesophageal surgery as described in the chapter on pp. 39–44.

Complications

In the author's experience postoperative complications are relatively few and included: one case of empyema without oesophageal leakage (which resolved on chest drainage); intrathoracic haemorrhage in two patients (who were successfully managed by conservative measures); and oesophageal leakage and empyema in one patient (in this patient the mucosa was perforated during enucleation and required repair). This last patient had a stormy postoperative course culminating on the 18th day in fatal haemorrhage from a perforation of the thoracic aorta. This was the only death in the author's series of 100 patients.

In summary, several measures are important in minimizing morbidity and mortality: avoiding endoscopic biopsy; avoiding mucosal perforation at enucleation; careful air insufflation to test for mucosal perforation after enucleation; and meticulous repair of any mucosal rupture.

If a postoperative oesophageal fistula occurs, prompt diagnosis, adequate closed chest drainage, and enteral or parenteral nutritional support are all important measures that may bring about a cure. Management of postoperative oesophageal fistula is discussed in the chapter on pp. 39–44.

Outcome

The results of extramucosal enucleation for leiomyoma of the oesophagus are generally good. In the author's experience of long-term follow-up in 65 patients, no tumour has recurred. All patients have returned to work and enjoy life. Only two have complained of mild dysphagia. No symptoms of reflux oesophagitis were observed in any of the patients. Barium swallow examination of 50 patients showed only a mild narrowing of the oesophageal lumen in three and a small diverticulum in one. All of these abnormalities occurred at the site of previous enucleation.

References

1. Peacock JA, Saleem SR, Becker SM. Sudden asphyxial death due to an oesophageal leiomyoma. *Am J Forensic Med Pathol* 1985; 6: 159–61.

2. Huang GJ, Zhang RG, Zhang DW, Wang LJ. Surgery for leiomyoma of the esophagus — experience in 100 patients. *Dis Esophagus* 1991; 4: 43–6.

3. Fujita H, Yoshimura Y, Yamana H *et al*. A latissimus dorsi muscle flap used for repair of the esophagus after enucleation of a giant leiomyoma: a case report. *Jpn J Surg* 1988; 18: 460–4.

Perforation of the oesophagus

Carlos A. Pellegrini MD, FACS
Professor and Chairman, Department of Surgery, University of Washington, Seattle, Washington, USA

Olivier Huber MD
Department of Surgery, University of California, San Francisco, California, USA

Principles and justification

Perforation of the oesophagus can be fatal unless diagnosed promptly and treated effectively[1-3]. The most common causes of perforation are passing instruments down the oesophagus, especially during forced dilatation of an oesophageal stricture[1-3], followed by external trauma due to stab or gunshot wounds. Other causes include the 'spontaneous' or emetogenic disruption of the oesophagus (Boerhaave syndrome – first described by Hermann Boerhaave (1668–1738) in the Baron of Wasenaar), perforation of an oesophageal cancer, sloughing of oesophageal wall after injection sclerotherapy of oesophageal varices and infectious processes in immunocompromised patients.

Most modern series report a mortality rate of 10–30%[1,4]. However, the risk of dying from an oesophageal perforation varies markedly with location and extent of the perforation, time elapsed before treatment, the general state of the patient and the presence of pre-existing oesophageal disease[5]. A key to understanding the pathophysiology of oesophageal perforation is the concept that it causes a rapidly evolving infection and rapid deterioration of the oesophageal wall at the site of the rupture. Thus, ideally an oesophageal perforation should be treated within 12 h of its occurrence – attempts at primary repair after the first 36–48 h are usually futile. The routine use of contrast radiography is recommended after pneumatic dilatation and whenever the circumstances related to oesophageal instrumentation cause any concern about the possibility of a perforation.

Preoperative

Clinical diagnosis

The most common symptom is pain which is first felt during, or immediately after, the completion of the instrumentation. Pain is constant, most often radiates to the back, and may be felt in the upper abdomen, the chest or the neck, depending on the site of the perforation. Most patients also complain of dysphagia, occasionally aphagia, and profuse salivation. High temperature is common within the first 4–6 h of perforation occurring. Perforations in the neck (and occasionally those in the chest) may lead to subcutaneous emphysema. Some patients develop hypotension, sweating and all the features of shock within a few hours of the event.

Radiological diagnosis

1, 2 Radiology is invaluable in the diagnosis of oesophageal perforation. The perforation may be suspected from plain films of the neck, chest or upper abdomen as free air may dissect adjacent tissues, creating subcutaneous emphysema, pneumomediastinum, pneumoperitoneum or even pneumothorax. A pleural effusion is also an indirect sign of oesophageal perforation. However, in the experience of the authors[1] and of others[6], these signs are present only in about 30% of cases.

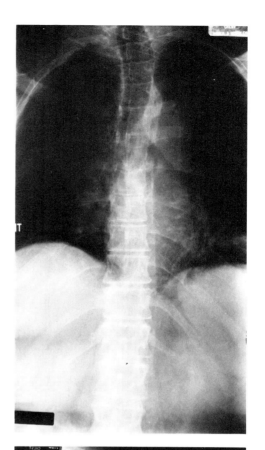

1

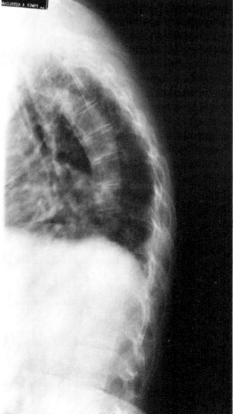

2

3 The most important radiological investigation in these patients is a contrast study of the oesophagus, which will reliably indicate an oesophageal perforation. More importantly, however, contrast studies will define the site and extent of the perforation, the amount of extravasation, the communication with the pleural or peritoneal cavity, and the presence of distal obstruction. Thus, a contrast study is not only important to diagnose oesophageal perforation, but it is essential in correct planning of surgery.

The authors prefer to use meglumine diatrizoate 66%, sodium diatrizoate 10% (Gastrografin) as contrast medium in the initial investigation. This water-soluble material is rapidly absorbed from the gastrointestinal tract and from the pleural or peritoneal cavity if extravasated and allows even small amounts of extravasation to be detected by a follow-up computed tomographic (CT) scan, which should be performed if the initial examination is negative.

Thin barium can also be used as contrast medium; however, barium makes the immediate use of CT scanning difficult and when extravasated is difficult to remove from the tissues, precluding the high-quality follow-up studies that are frequently needed. When using water-soluble materials every effort should be made to avoid aspiration.

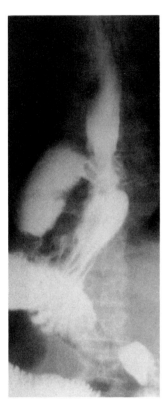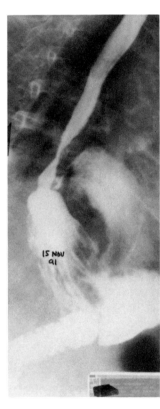

3

4 CT scanning may detect a small perforation that did not show up on the oesophagogram[7] and is indicated in patients in whom the swallow was negative but who are strongly suspected of having oesophageal perforation.

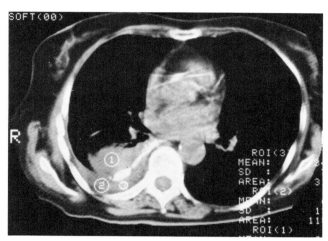

4

5 A CT scan will provide invaluable information on patients who present with delayed perforations. These are patients who survived the initial insult and who have developed an abscess that effectively contains the perforation and prevents further mediastinal or pleural soiling.

In order to plan adequate drainage, it is imperative to define the site, the extent, and the relation of the abscess to adjacent structures, and CT scanning is the test of choice.

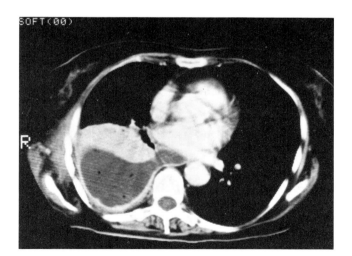

5

Endoscopic diagnosis

Endoscopic examination adds very little information to that gleaned from high-quality contrast radiography. However, in some patients endoscopy may help to identify and characterize the perforation. For example, a patient who has stab or gunshot wounds may also have a perforated oesophagus. As the patient is being anaesthetized to care for the other injuries oesophagoscopy immediately after induction of anaesthesia may help to identify an oesophageal perforation[1]. These patients are too unstable to undergo contrast oesophagography and the risk of oesophageal perforation is low to start with. Another example would be a patient undergoing dilatation of an oesophageal stricture and who is suspected of having had a perforation – insertion of the endoscope at the end of a difficult procedure may provide invaluable information at an early stage. It has been recommended that the endoscope should be passed through a perforated oesophagus to assess the damage inflicted to adjacent structures, but the authors believe the risks of this manoeuvre outweigh its potential benefit.

Initial management

The initial management of an oesophageal perforation involves several steps.

Aggressive resuscitation

These patients suffer rapid dehydration and overwhelming contamination if the perforation is large and in the chest.

Antibiotics

As soon as a perforation is suspected, the patient should be started on broad-spectrum antibiotics directed against oral flora to adequately cover aerobic Gram-positive and Gram-negative bacteria, as well as anaerobic micro-organisms.

Assessment of the injury

The surgeon should determine the following before deciding on the kind of treatment:

1. Whether the perforation is 'contained' (i.e., limited to the tissue immediately adjacent to the oesophagus) or 'free' (the most common type of perforation, with free extravasation of contents into the neck, the pleural cavity or the peritoneal cavity).
2. Time elapsed since the perforation occurred.
3. The location and extent of the perforation.
4. The presence of pre-existing oesophageal disease, most commonly an obstruction, usually distal to the perforated area.
5. The age and general health of the patient.

Indications for surgical intervention

The strategy for intervention should be chosen by following the steps described above.

Contained perforations

Contained perforations, which affect a small area of tissue adjacent to the oesophagus, may be treated without surgery, provided that: (1) the perforation is small[4,5]; (2) the contrast material flows immediately back into the oesophagus; (3) there is no underlying oesophageal disease distal to the perforation (i.e. stricture); and (4) the clinical manifestations are minimal (i.e. low-grade temperature, minimal pain, etc.).

One perforation that may be treated in this way is that which occurs a few weeks after injection sclerotherapy. The inflammatory reaction caused by the sclerosing agent plasters the perioesophageal tissues against the wall of the oesophagus, effectively blocking the perforation and decreasing the chance of mediastinal spread of infection. However, the underlying general state of the patient (cirrhosis) and the oesophagus (varices) would make any attempt at surgical intervention very difficult. When this strategy is followed, the patient should be given enteral or parenteral nutrition, as well as broad-spectrum antibiotics, for at least 7 days, or until there is no sign of infection. Most importantly, the oesophagus must be evaluated periodically with contrast radiography to monitor the progress. Any evidence of spread of infection or lack of adequate response to this treatment should elicit an immediate change of treatment, most probably surgical intervention.

Free perforations

Free perforations, which are much more common than contained perforations, should almost always be treated operatively, regardless of location or size.

Time elapsed since injury

The time elapsed since the perforation determines to some extent the intervention to be used. Patients who suffered their perforation 24–36 h previously should undergo an exploration of the area and if possible, the perforation should be closed with or without buttressing. Patients who present several days after perforation are likely to have perioesophageal abscess. In these cases closure of the perforation is no longer possible, and the use of interventional radiological techniques is recommended to drain the infected areas adequately.

Location and extent of perforation

Injuries to the oesophagus above the thoracic inlet should be treated by neck incision on the side of the extravasation, or on the left side (the oesophagus is easier to access from the left) if the injury is known to be in the neck but the exact location is not clear. Non-operative treatment of perforations in the neck has been advocated[8], on the basis that most heal by apposition of adjacent tissue (there is no 'real' space around the oesophagus in the neck). The authors believe that early closure of these injuries accelerates recovery and allows for treatment of associated injuries, which are common when external trauma is the cause of the perforation. If the perforation has occurred in a Zenker's diverticulum, resection of the diverticulum and a concomitant cricopharyngeal myotomy are recommended. Most other oesophageal perforations should be approached through a thoracotomy. High and mid-oesophageal lesions are best approached by thoracotomy through the right posterolateral fifth intercostal space. Most low lesions should be approached through the left posterolateral seventh intercostal space, even if the extravasation is in the abdomen.

Presence of underlying oesophageal disease

This plays a most important role in determining the kind of procedure to be performed. Because perforation occurs most commonly during dilatation of strictures, and because the mechanism of injury is such that the wall of the oesophagus is injured at or just above the stricture, therapy should be planned accordingly. If the stricture is fixed and fibrotic, the best treatment is to resect the stricture and perforated area, and immediately reconstruct the gastrointestinal tract[1,4–6]. If the perforation was caused by dilatation for achalasia, closure of the perforation and a Heller myotomy on the other side of the oesophagus is recommended. Whatever the choice, the important principle is *never* to close primarily a perforation above an oesophageal stricture.

General health of the patient

Unfortunately, a free perforation discovered early mandates an operation, regardless of the fitness of the patient. However, a poor general state of health may lead to a decision to treat non-operatively a perforation of the neck, or a small mediastinal perforation.

Preoperative preparation

The preoperative preparation involves adequate resuscitation (including tube thoracostomy if a pneumothorax is present), antibiotic administration and a thorough evaluation of the injury as described above

Anaesthesia

During induction of anaesthesia care must be taken to avoid causing tension pneumothorax, which is possible if vigorous mask ventilation is performed before intubation (because of the hole in the oesophagus). The anaesthetist must prevent aspiration of blood, secretions and any residual contrast medium from the oesophagography that may have accumulated in the oesophagus. It is unwise to insert a nasogastric tube blindly in these patients, as the tube is likely to exit through the perforation and cause further damage. Finally, a double-lumen endotracheal tube should be used, as independent ventilation of the lungs is required to be able to collapse the lung on the side of the operation.

Operations

UNOBSTRUCTED OESOPHAGUS

6 Most spontaneous and instrumental perforations occur in the distal oesophagus. The best way to approach these lesions is by thoracotomy through the left posterolateral seventh intercostal space. Once the chest has been entered and the lung adequately collapsed, the parietal pleura overlying the oesophagus should be opened at a site near the perforation. Occasionally the oesophageal lesion has also lacerated the pleura, and the site of perforation is obvious from the beginning. Taking care not to injure the contralateral mediastinal pleura, the oesophagus is dissected off its bed and surrounded with a tape above and below the perforation.

Adequate mobilization of the oesophagus may require extensive dissection, particularly if the perforation has occurred in the right side of the oesophagus. The area of injury must be clearly exposed, as well as the normal oesophagus above and below. If the perforation is not evident, the chest should be filled with saline while the anaesthetist blows air through the oesophageal lumen. Bubbles of air will appear at the site of perforation. At this stage a nasogastric tube should be carefully passed transorally and advanced into the stomach under direct vision to help during closure of the perforation.

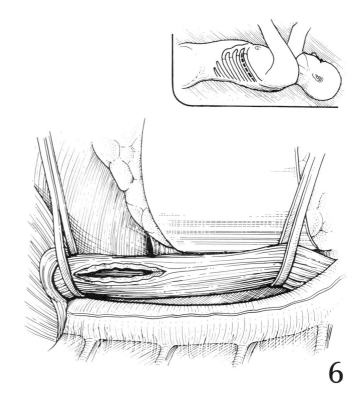

6

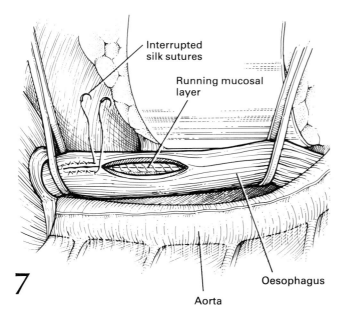

Interrupted
silk sutures

Running mucosal
layer

Oesophagus

Aorta

7

7 The edges of the perforation are trimmed with scissors in order to obtain 'clean' edges and to expose the mucosal rent entirely (the mucosal rent is often larger than the muscular defect). If the mucosa is healthy, it should be approximated using a running suture of 3/0 or 4/0 polyglyconate, and the muscular coat closed with interrupted sutures of non-absorbable material (3/0 silk or similar). If the perforation is several hours old and the tissues are oedematous, all the layers may have to be closed together. In this case, interrupted sutures of non-absorbable material of adequate size (2/0 or similar) are preferred, as thinner material tends to cut the inflamed tissues.

8   Whenever possible, the oesophageal closure should be buttressed by stripping a flap of pleura from the posterolateral chest wall, leaving it attached to the aorta and attaching it to the oesophagus with a few sutures. The pleura may be too oedematous to dissect because of the inflammatory reaction. If this is so, and if the stomach is accessible, the area may be buttressed using the stomach.

Finally, any fibrinous membrane is debrided and the lung re-expanded. The chest is drained with a thin (No. 22 or similar) straight tube placed with its tip in the apex of the pleural cavity and a larger (No. 36 or similar) right-angled tube left on the surface of the diaphragm with its tip near, but not touching, the area that has been repaired. The chest is then closed. Gastrostomy is not routinely performed, but it may be done percutaneously in high-risk cases.

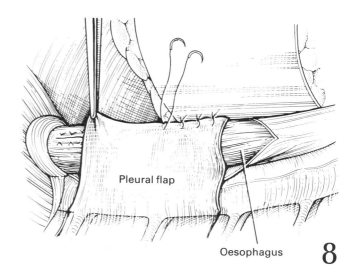

Pleural flap

Oesophagus   8

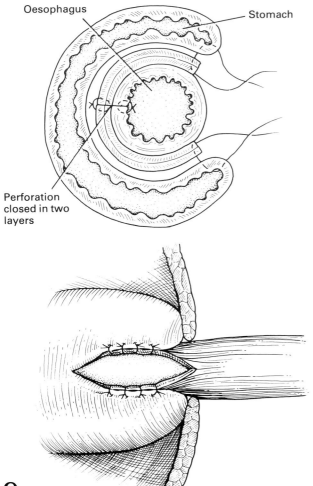

Oesophagus

Stomach

Perforation closed in two layers

9

OBSTRUCTED OESOPHAGUS

The two most common conditions are perforation occurring during pneumatic balloon dilatation of a patient with achalasia, and perforation occurring during instrumentation of a benign or malignant stricture.

Perforation from pneumatic dilatation

The approach and the initial procedure is similar to that described for the treatment of the unobstructed oesophagus. This perforation always affects the lower oesophagus and is approached from the left side.

9   Simply closing the perforation may result in early dehiscence (because of the concomitant obstruction) and leaves the patient with untreated achalasia. Thus, after closing the perforation in a manner similar to that described above, the opposite side of the oesophagus is exposed, exactly 180° from the perforated area, and a longitudinal myotomy performed[9]. After dividing the phreno-oesophageal ligament, the fundus of the stomach is brought up and a partial fundoplication over the area of the perforation made. The wrap is secured with interrupted sutures to each side of the myotomy. This not only buttresses the repair well, but also acts as an antireflux procedure and helps to keep the edges of the myotomy far apart, preventing it from healing.

Perforation above a fibrotic, benign or malignant stricture

Whenever possible resection of the oesophagus by the transhiatal approach and oesophagogastrostomy at the neck are recommended. This treats the perforation and underlying disease, and brings a graft of well-vascularized tissue into the posterior mediastinum which fills the space and helps treat the mediastinal infection. The patient is placed in the supine position, anaesthesia induced, and both lungs ventilated. A midline laparotomy is performed and, following a Kocher manoeuvre, the omentum is divided outside the gastroepiploic arcade, taking care to preserve this arcade.

10 The gastrohepatic ligament is divided, preserving the right gastric vessels. The gastro-oesophageal junction is then isolated, a tape passed around the distal oesophagus, and the short gastric vessels and the left gastric artery divided. The left diaphragmatic vessels are ligated and the diaphragm is opened anteriorly as far as needed to perform the mediastinal dissection.

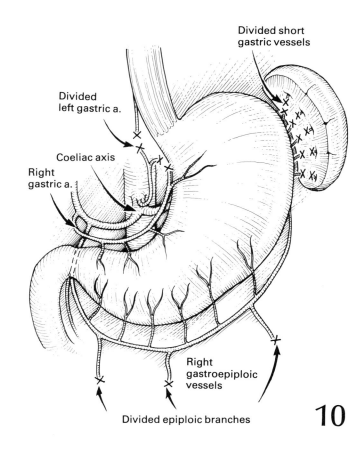

Divided short gastric vessels

Divided left gastric a.

Coeliac axis

Right gastric a.

Right gastroepiploic vessels

Divided epiploic branches

10

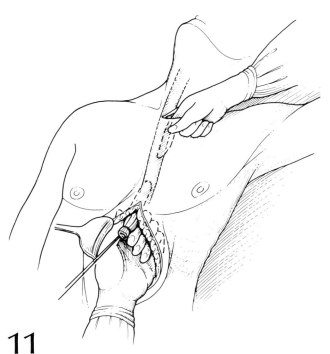

11

11 The lower oesophagus can usually be dissected under direct vision all the way to the inferior pulmonary vessels, and then bluntly to the thoracic inlet.

At this stage a pyloroplasty is performed and a 7-cm incision made in the left side of the neck following the anterior aspect of the sternocleidomastoid muscle. The muscles are separated laterally, and the lowest section of the cervical oesophagus is isolated and surrounded with tape.

12a, b The stomach is then divided, using a GIA instrument, starting 2–3 cm lateral to the gastro-oesophageal junction in the greater curvature, and continuing to the mid-portion of the lesser curvature.

A wide Penrose drain is sutured to the lower end of the divided oesophagus, and the oesophagus and top of the stomach removed by pulling from the neck to leave the Penrose drain in the posterior mediastinum. The inferior end of the drain is then attached to the fundus of the stomach to serve as a guide to direct the stomach to the neck, where a two-layer anastomosis is performed to the cervical oesophagus just above the thoracic inlet.

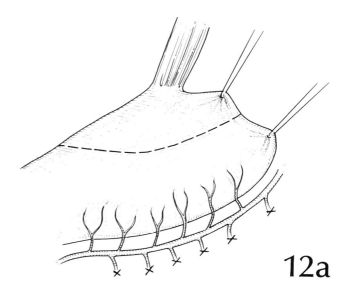

12a

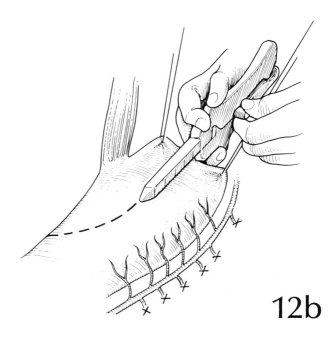

12b

PERFORATION DIAGNOSED SEVERAL DAYS AFTER OCCURRENCE

These patients are treated primarily by interventional radiological techniques[10], although some authors have used operative techniques[11]. The strategy is to drain the cavity adjacent to the perforation and the abscesses as adequately as possible.

13 This involves placing a transoral–transoesophageal tube through the perforation to aspirate the cavity. In addition, a percutaneous gastrostomy is performed and through it another tube is advanced retrogradely into the oesophagus. This tube may also be used to decompress the cavity. Finally, a thoracostomy tube may be placed to drain the abscess directly, but this may lead to a temporary oesophagocutaneous fistula.

Because the patient will not be able to eat for some time, a feeding jejunostomy catheter should be placed. This can be done laparoscopically to obviate the need for laparotomy.

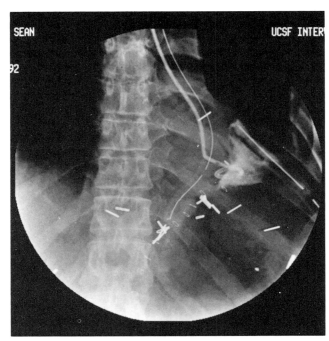

13

ALTERNATIVE APPROACH

In some patients it may not be possible to close the perforation because of a delay in diagnosis, because the patient is too sick for the thoracotomy, or because sepsis persists after interventional radiological management or dehiscence of a previous closure.

14 The treatment of choice in these cases is to divide the oesophagus at the neck, bringing out an end-oesophagostomy and closing the thoracic oesophagus as low as possible in the neck (just at the thoracic inlet), and to close the cardio-oesophageal junction with a stapling device via laparotomy or laparoscopy. This effectively isolates the perforated segment and stops mediastinal and pleural soiling.

Unfortunately, this procedure requires a second operation to re-establish continuity of the gastrointestinal tract. This is best accomplished 2–3 months later via a total oesophagectomy by the transhiatal approach and a gastro-oesophageal anastomosis at the neck.

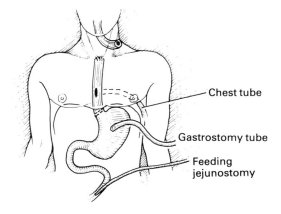

Chest tube

Gastrostomy tube

Feeding jejunostomy

14

Postoperative care

The patient is intubated for the first 12–24 h. Good ventilation and full lung expansion are essential to prevent atelectasis and pneumonia. Also if the endotracheal tube is removed at the end of the operation, not uncommonly emergency reintubation is necessary. Forceful mask ventilation before emergency reintubation increases oeosphageal pressure and may lead to dehiscence of the suture lines. These patients need intensive care during the first couple of days. The nasogastric tube must be carefully cared for, as it is important to drain the stomach continuously. To decrease gastric acid secretion H_2-receptor antagonists are administered. The apical chest tube is removed as soon as good lung expansion is achieved and there is no evidence of air leaks (usually 2 days after surgery).

Antibiotics are continued for 7–10 days, depending on the degree of contamination: in patients with preoperative positive blood cultures, antibiotics should be continued for 14 days. Total parenteral nutrition is administered for the first 8–10 days.

Approximately 8–9 days after surgery, a barium swallow examination should be made (water-soluble material should be used if there is any suspicion of dehiscence). If this shows no extravasation, the angled chest tube is removed and the patient is started immediately on a mechanically soft diet. Patients are discharged home as soon as they can eat and have no evidence of residual infection. If dehiscence is noted and it is contained and asymptomatic, they are kept on parenteral nutrition for an additional 10 days and the study is then repeated. If symptoms of abscess are present, treatment should be as if a delayed perforation is discovered.

Late diagnosed perforation

Management of the tubes is very important to the success of this procedure[10]. The tube placement should be inspected periodically (every 2–3 days or more frequently if there is evidence of infection) and cavity size measured by fistulography. The tubes are advanced back into the oesophageal lumen as soon as the cavity becomes smaller, to allow for more rapid closure of the perforation.

References

1. Flynn AE, Verrier ED, Way LW, Thomas AN, Pellegrini CA. Esophageal perforation. *Arch Surg* 1989; 124: 1211–15.

2. Jones WG 2nd, Ginsberg RJ. Esophageal perforation: a continuing challenge. *Ann Thorac Surg* 1992: 53; 534–43.

3. Skinner DB. *Instrumental Perforation and Mediastinitis*. Philadelphia: WB Saunders 1988: 783–98.

4. Attar S, Hankins JR, Suter CM, Coughlin TR, Sequeira A, McLaughlin JS. Esophageal perforation: a therapeutic challenge. *Ann Thorac Surg* 1990; 50: 45–51.

5. Tilanus HW, Bossuyt P, Schattenkerk ME, Obertop H. Treatment of oesophageal perforation: a multivariate analysis. *Br J Surg* 1991; 78: 582–5.

6. White RK, Morris DM. Diagnosis and management of esophageal perforations. *Am Surg* 1992; 58: 112–19.

7. Backer CL, LoCicero J 3rd, Hartz RS, Donaldson JS, Shields T. Computed tomography in patients with esophageal perforation. *Chest* 1990; 98: 1078–80.

8. Dolgin SR, Wykoff TW, Kumar NR, Maniglia AJ. Conservative medical management of traumatic pharyngoesophageal perforations. *Ann Otol Rhinol Laryngol* 1992; 101: 209–15.

9. Sauer L, Pellegrini CA, Way LW. The treatment of achalasia. A current perspective. *Arch Surg* 1989; 124: 929–32.

10. Maroney TP, Ring EJ, Gordon RL, Pellegrini CA. Role of interventional radiology in the management of major esophageal leaks. *Radiology* 1989; 170: 1055–7.

11. Gayet B, Breil P, Fekete F. Mechanical sutures in perforation of the thoracic esophagus as a safe procedure in patients seen late. *Surg Gynecol Obstet* 1991; 172: 125–8.

Anatomy of the hiatus and abdominal oesophagus

Hiram C. Polk Jr MD
Ben A. Reid Sr Professor and Chairman, Department of Surgery, University of Louisville School of Medicine, Louisville, Kentucky, USA

Mark A. Malias MD
Resident Surgeon, Department of Surgery, University of Louisville School of Medicine, Louisville, Kentucky, USA

G. G. Jamieson MS, FRACS, FACS
Dorothy Mortlock Professor of Surgery, University of Adelaide, Department of Surgery, Royal Adelaide Hospital, Adelaide, Australia

Anatomical relations of distal oesophagus and fundus of the stomach

In the lower thorax, the oesophagus first lies anteriorly and then anteriorly and to the left of the aorta. It then passes further to the left as it passes through the oesophageal hiatus to join the stomach. The segment of oesophagus that lies in the abdomen during repose is about 3 cm long. However, there is appreciable shortening of the oesophagus during swallowing, belching and vomiting. The abdominal oesophagus is more or less retroperitoneal with peritoneum covering its anterior and left side only. Posteriorly the oesophagus lies on the left hiatal pillar of the left (or right) crus of the diaphragm, which separates it from the aorta. The left lobe of the liver lies anterior to the abdominal oesophagus and to its right lies the caudate lobe. The physical presence of these structures means that the most direct access to the abdominal oesophagus is anterior and left.

As in all surgical procedures, exposure is the key to a successful operation. Much has been written about the length of the left triangular ligament. However, experience has shown that the thickness of the left morphological lobe of the liver is more often a limiting factor for adequate exposure of the oesophagus than the length of the left triangular ligament.

Visualization of the oesophagus can be improved by retracting the left lobe of the liver orad and to the right. If necessary, access can be improved further by dividing the left triangular ligament and folding the left lobe inferiorly on itself before retracting it to the right.

If the left lobe of the liver is too thick to fold up on itself, exposure may be difficult. It is worth noting that some surgeons do not think it is necessary to mobilize the left lobe of the liver at all in approaching the abdominal oesophagus.

1 The angle of entry of the oesophagus into the stomach, termed the angle of His, varies between 30° and 70° in healthly subjects, and in the cadaver averages about 20° (*see Table 1*).

The gastro-oesophageal junction is often, somewhat loosely, referred to as the cardia. The fundus of the stomach can be arbitrarily defined as the segment of stomach above an imaginary line drawn horizontally through the point of the angle of His. The height of the fundus above this point is 2–5 cm and averages about 3.6 cm in the cadaver.

The configuration of the fundus is usually round but occasionally it is short and conical, which makes manipulations such as a fundoplication difficult.

Table 1 Measurements made in fresh cadavers

	Mean (cm)
Length of triangular ligament	7.1
Thickness of sides of hiatus	
Left	0.3
Right	0.3
Distance apex hiatus to superior short gastric artery	8.8
Distance apex hiatus to superior left gastric artery	5.5
Height of fundus	3.6
Angle of His (cardiac notch) (°)	20.8
Distance between mucosal gastro-oesophageal junction and external gastro-oesophageal junction	1.6
Surface of bare area of stomach (cm^2)	18.1

Modified and reprinted from ref. 1 with permission of the publishers.

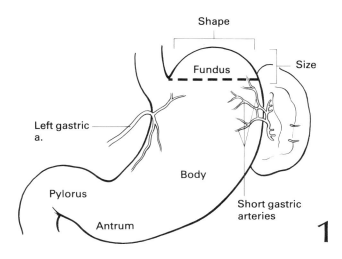

2 The fundus of the stomach is completely covered with peritoneum anteriorly, but posteriorly coverage is incomplete. The area above the upper reaches of the lesser omental sac is not covered by peritoneum and is known as the bare area of the stomach. This is most often a crescent-shaped area, with its greatest extent along the upper portion of the posterior lesser curvature and the right portion of the fundus. It then extends in an ever narrowing band towards the apex of the fundus. The extent of the bare area is 0–40 cm^2. A large bare area can be a limiting factor in mobilization of the fundus.

Posteriorly the fundus of the stomach lies directly on the diaphragm.

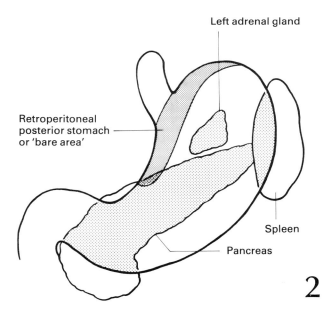

Musculature

3 As with the gastrointestinal tract in general, the oesophagus has an outer longitudinal layer and an inner circular layer of smooth muscle, the inner layer being the thicker of the two. Opinion is divided as to whether a morphological lower oesophageal sphincter exists. It is accepted that there is no thickening to correspond with the whole of the 2–3 cm of the manometrically measureable lower oesophageal sphincter. However, in the distal 1–2 cm of the oesophagus (and particularly on its left side) some thickening of the musculature has been described, which may represent the uppermost gastric sling fibres – oblique muscle fibres that sling around the gastro-oesophageal junction from the lesser curve.

The submucosa deep to the muscularis propria is composed of loose areolar tissue. Consequently the mucosa can be dissected away from the muscle easily. This laxity is useful in oesophagomyotomy for achalasia. Once a small incision has been made through the oesophageal muscle into the submucosa, a fine clamp can be inserted and gently opened and closed in order to separate the muscle from the mucosa. Division of the muscle overlying the jaws of the clamp is then simple.

Transection of the oesophagus at the level of the hiatus is followed by retraction of the proximal cut end into the posterior mediastinum as a result of contraction of the longitudinal layer which is fixed superiorly.

Contraction of the longitudinal muscle may also contribute to the development of sliding hiatus hernia.

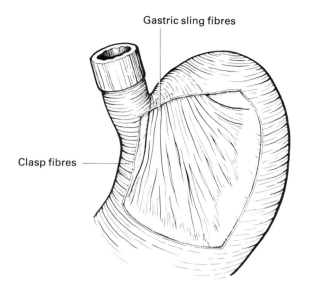

3

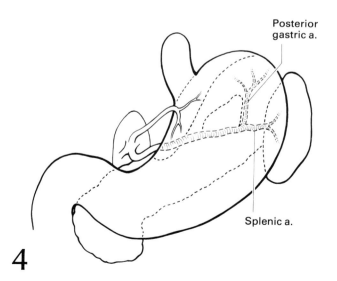

4

Blood supply

4 The anterior and right sides of the cardia of the stomach and the lower oesophagus (directly above it) are supplied by one or more ascending branches of the left gastric artery, and the posterior and left sides by branches of the posterior gastric or fundal branches of the splenic artery. The left inferior phrenic artery rarely has any role in the blood supply, despite its proximity to the area. The lower thoracic oesophagus may also receive one or more small direct branches from the aorta. The oesophagus has a rich intramural arterial anastomosis in its submucosal layer, which is continuous with a network in the submucosa of the stomach. This explains how, following a near-total gastrectomy, an upper gastric remnant retains its viability when its external blood supply has been completely divided.

Nerve supply

The distal oesophagus is autonomically innervated. Vagal inhibitory, non-cholinergic, non-adrenergic fibres are responsible for sphincteric relaxation associated with swallowing, belching, vomiting and at least some episodes of gastro-oesophageal reflux. There are also excitatory vagal cholinergic fibres responsible in part for basal sphincteric tone. The physiological role of the inhibitory sympathetic adrenergic innervation, which has been identified pharmacologically, remains to be defined. Vagal nerves innervating the distal oesophagus run a long downward course which is largely intramural after leaving the vagal trunks. This explains why skeletonization of up to 5 cm of the distal oesophagus, as practised in proximal gastric vagotomy, does not result in permanent dysfunction of the lower oesophageal sphincter.

Phreno-oesophageal ligament

This structure tends to be given greater prominence in surgical texts than in anatomy texts. It attaches the oesophagus anteriorly to the peritoneum and endo-abdominal fascia from the undersurface of the diaphragm. This fascia splits into two layers – a filmy layer that passes downwards to the gastro-oesophageal junction and a stronger superior layer that passes through the hiatus to blend with areolar tissue surrounding the oesophagus. When viewed from the thorax, the phreno-oesophageal ligament is the layer of tissue binding the oesophagus to the edges of the oesophageal hiatus. It is most easily demonstrated as a definite ligament or membrane from the abdomen. When the peritoneum in front of the hiatus is stretched by downward traction, the ligament can be seen to form a white line similar to that seen alongside the ascending and descending colon. Division of the peritoneum along the inferior aspect of the white line and the tissue immediately deep to it takes the surgeon into the mediastinum in front of the oesophagus.

Mobilization of the distal oesophagus

Mobilization of the distal oesophagus is achieved most simply by entering the lower mediastinum through the phreno-oesophageal ligament, allowing entry to the loose areolar tissue in front of the oesophagus. The normal oesophagus can then be encircled with the forefinger, passing from left to right behind the oesophagus. There is always fibroareolar tissue posteriorly, which must be broken through. The higher in the mediastinum the encirclement is undertaken, the weaker the posterior layer becomes. Mobilization posterior to the distal oesophagus should always be undertaken with great care, particularly when previous transmural peptic oesophagitis has resulted in perioesophageal inflammation and scarring. Under these circumstances it may be advisable to perform the mobilization using sharp dissection under direct vision, as the oesophageal wall (which is not robust) might otherwise be split by the mobilizing finger passing too anteriorly through the plane of least resistance.

When mobilized by blunt dissection, the encircling finger nearly always contains the anterior trunk of the vagus nerve and excludes the posterior trunk (which tends to lie between the pillar of the hiatus, posteriorly and to the right of the oesophagus). It is interesting that when the oesophagus is mobilized through a laparoscope, the posterior vagus nerve is often included with the oesophagus. This may be because the mobilization is undertaken from the right side of the oesophagus and is in a slightly deeper plane.

The amount of the oesophagus that can be mobilized upwards through the hiatus is limited by the dimensions of the oesophageal hiatus. If further mobilization is required, exposure can be improved either by dividing the right and left pillars of the hiatus or by dividing the hiatal opening vertically, anterior to the oesophagus, and extending forwards until the pericardium is reached. Care must be taken with such a median phrenicotomy, first because it is inadvisable to incise the pericardium and secondly because the anterior branch of the left inferior phrenic vein usually crosses in front of the oesophageal hiatus on its way to the inferior vena cava or left hepatic vein and thus must be ligated.

5 The distal mobilization of the oesophagus and upper stomach is limited at the cardia, or just below, by the left gastric trinity (the left gastric vein, the left gastric artery and the coeliac branch of the posterior vagal trunk). If mobilization distal to the cardia is required then the surgeon should commence to the right of the lesser curve about 3 cm below the gastro-oesophageal junction and cross obliquely below the cardia towards the angle of His. This should be done both anteriorly and posteriorly. Care must be taken not to damage the anterior vagal trunk in this dissection. The anterior vagal trunk, which is palpable as a thin cord when the region is stretched from below, is closely applied to the anterior surface of the oesophagus 5 cm above the cardia. As it passes inferiorly it crosses to the right of the oesophagus. At the level of the phreno-oesophageal ligament it is still close to the right side of the oesophagus; in the lesser omentum it is about 1 cm from the lesser curve. A similar mobilization to this is carried out during proximal gastric vagotomy and ensures that both vagal trunks are displaced to the right, away from the oesophagus.

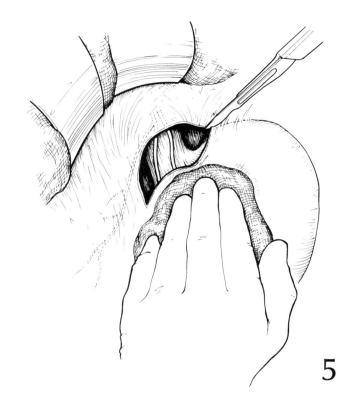

5

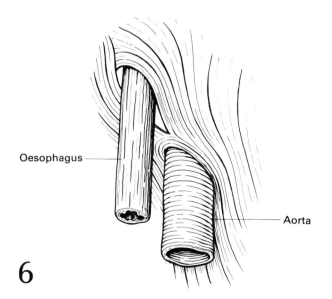

Oesophagus

Aorta

6

Oesophageal hiatus

6 The oesophageal hiatus is the opening in the diaphragm through which the oesophagus passes into the abdomen. The hiatus is at the level of T10 and lies to the left of the midline, with its anterior extent about 1 cm posterior to the central tendon of the diaphragm. The hiatus is formed from the left and right crura of the diaphragm. It is not only a somewhat longitudinal opening but also an oblique opening: its anterior and superior margins may lie more than 1 cm in front of its posterior and inferior margin. This obliquity adds to the difficulty of the radiologist when trying to define the level of the gastro-oesophageal junction relative to the hiatus. The tissue that forms the inferior margin of the oesophageal hiatus also forms the median arcuate ligament across the front of the aorta.

7 The crura of the diaphragm arise from the anterior surfaces and discs of L1–L3 as well as from the anterior longitudinal ligament of the spine. The right crus tends to reach slightly lower in its origin from the first three lumbar vertebrae, the left tending to arise from the first two lumbar vertebrae. Fibres arising from the right side of the lumbar vertebrae most commonly diverge and then reconverge to form the boundaries of the hiatus. Fibres on the right side of the hiatus are innervated by branches of the right phrenic nerve and those on its left side by branches of the left phrenic nerve.

The way in which the fibres of the crura cross each other is variable. The considerable debate over such variations probably has no surgical relevance. Two points, however, are relevant to antireflux surgery.

First, the tendinous tissue binding the right and left limbs of the hiatus together inferiorly, of which the median arcuate ligament is a part, is often poorly defined. Surgeons who use this structure to place anchoring sutures, in fact, use a variety of tissues lying in front of the aorta, including some of the neural tissue of the coeliac plexus. Nevertheless, these tissues hold sutures well.

Secondly, the limbs or pillars of the hiatus are musculotendinous structures, with their tendinous portions tending to lie posterior to the muscular portions. The tendinous portions are the most accessible portion of the pillars when operating from the chest, but for the surgeon operating from the abdomen they are the least accessible portions. From the abdomen the more tendinous portions are often best identified by palpation. When narrowing the hiatus, it is important to suture the tendinous portions: the hiatus is best narrowed behind and inferior to the oesophagus. This approach also maximizes the intra-abdominal length of the oesophagus. The hiatal pillars and the phreno-oesophageal ligament were previously thought to be important in maintaining gastro-oesophageal competence but at present their role is uncertain.

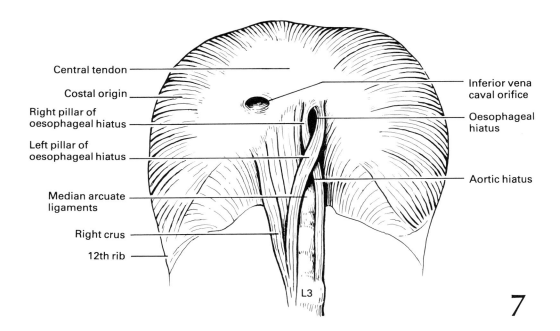

Acknowledgements

Table 1 and *Figure 1* are reproduced from reference 1 with permission from J. B. Lippincott Co., Philadelphia, USA.

Reference

1. Wald H, Polk HC Jr. Anatomical variations in hiatal and upper gastric areas and their relationship to difficulties experienced in operations for reflux esophagitis. *Ann Surg* 1983; 197: 389–92.

Further reading

Hollinshead WH. *Anatomy for Surgeons,* 2nd edn, vols 1, 2, and 3. New York: Harper and Row, 1971.

Jamieson GG, Martin CJ. Antireflux surgery. The anatomy of the distal oesophagus and associated structures. In: Jamieson GG, ed. *The Anatomy of General Surgical Operations.* Edinburgh: Churchill Livingstone, 1992: 59–62.

Williams PL, Warrick R, Dyson M, Bannister LH, eds. *Gray's Anatomy,* 37th edn. Edinburgh: Churchill Livingstone, 1989.

Myotomy for achalasia: thoracic approach

F. Henry Ellis Jr MD, PhD
Clinical Professor of Surgery, Harvard Medical School, and Chief Emeritus, Division of Cardiothoracic Surgery, New England Deaconess Hospital, Boston, Massachusetts, USA

History

The surgical treatment of oesophageal achalasia is a 20th century development, the most significant contribution being that of Heller who, in 1913, performed a double cardiomyotomy by the abdominal route on a 49-year-old woman who had experienced dysphagia for 30 years. This technique later underwent many modifications, the most important of which was restriction of the procedure to one myotomy. This has been further modified to include an antireflux procedure, an addition which, in the author's opinion, is unnecessary.

Principles and justification

Most physicians agree that patients whose general health does not permit an operative procedure should be treated by forceful dilatation. There is general agreement regarding circumstances that favour oesophagomyotomy to forceful dilatation including failure of dilatation, young children, advanced megaoesophagus, disclosure on oesophageal manometric studies of vigorous achalasia, and the coexistence of such associated disorders as hiatus hernia and an epiphrenic diverticulum which might require concomitant operative correction. The author believes that a transthoracic short oesophagomyotomy is the primary procedure of choice in the management of the symptomatic patient with oesophageal achalasia.

Preoperative

Diagnosis

A correct diagnosis is an essential part of the preoperative evaluation of the patient. In the early stages of disease before marked oesophageal dilatation has occurred, differentiation between oesophageal stricture and carcinoma of the cardia may be difficult. In such cases endoscopy constitutes an important part of the preoperative assessment. A definitive diagnosis, however, depends on oesophageal manometry which discloses the characteristic abnormalities of high resting pressures at the lower oesophageal sphincter with absence of or impaired deglutitory relaxation coupled with simultaneous (usually low-amplitude) non-peristaltic deglutitive contractions in the body of the oesophagus.

Preparation

Preoperative preparation of the patient is straight-forward. Few patients today seek medical attention so late in the course of the disease as to exhibit major weight loss and debilitation: over the past 20 years the author has not seen a patient with oesophageal achalasia who required preoperative hospitalization for restoration of normal nutrition. Some patients, however, may require preoperative respiratory therapy to relieve pulmonary complications secondary to regurgitation and aspiration. A clear liquid meal is prescribed the night before the operation and the oesophagus is completely lavaged and aspirated both the night before and the morning of the operation to minimize the danger of aspiration during the induction of anaesthesia.

Anaesthesia

The use of a double-lumen tube during transthoracic oesophagomyotomy permits deflation of the left lung, thus providing excellent exposure of the lower mediastinum for performance of the operative procedure. Inhalation agents such as isoflurane together with oxygen and intravenous fentanyl citrate coupled with a muscle relaxant such as vecuronium bromide are preferred.

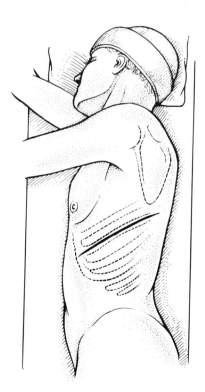

Operation

1 Incision through the bed of the non-resected left eighth rib provides direct access to the area of the lower oesophagus.

2 By incising the mediastinal pleura, the oesophagus is identified and encircled with a Penrose drain including the vagus nerves so as to prevent their subsequent injury. The oesophagus is then gently elevated using the encircling Penrose drain which results in the gastro-oesophageal junction being delivered for a short distance into the thorax without necessitating the division of any of the hiatal attachments. Incisions in the diaphragm and phreno-oesophageal membrane are thus avoided. A site is then selected on the left anterolateral surface of the oesophagus and proximal stomach for performance of the myotomy.

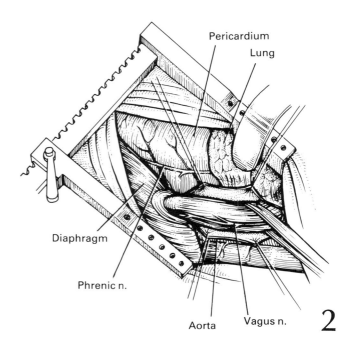

2

3 With the oesophagus under tension and compressed by the supporting fingers of the left hand, a longitudinal myotomy is performed and deepened through the encircling muscles of the lower end of the oesophagus down to the mucosa.

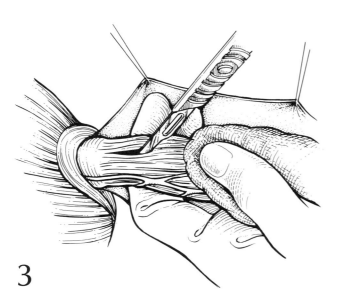

3

4 The incision is extended distally across the gastro-oesophageal junction just far enough to ensure complete division of the distal oesophageal musculature. External identification of the junction is difficult, but the greater vascularity of the gastric mucosa than the oesophageal mucosa can be identified by the presence of small veins traversing the upper portion of this organ and serves as a reasonably satisfactory landmark, identifying the stomach. The length of the gastric extension of the myotomy usually does not exceed a few millimetres and should be less than 1 cm.

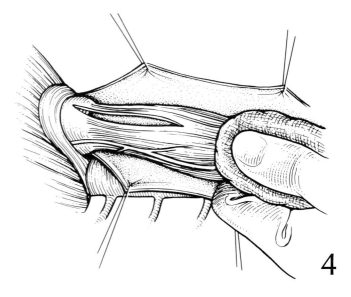

4

5 The incision is then extended proximally over the dilated thick-walled portion of the oesophagus. Proximal extension of the incision ensures total division of the circular muscle of the lower oesophageal sphincter. The length of the incision varies with the patient's build and the local anatomy, but usually extends for 6–8 cm.

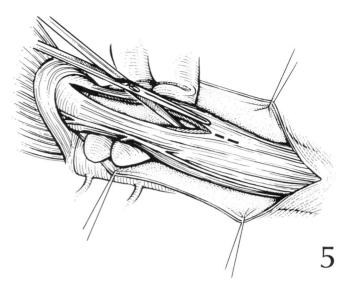

5

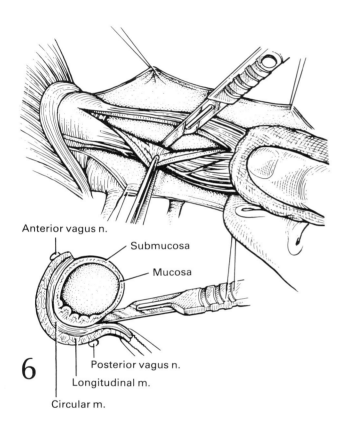

Anterior vagus n.

Submucosa

Mucosa

Posterior vagus n.

Longitudinal m.

Circular m.

6

6 In order to prevent healing of the myotomy, the muscle wall is then dissected laterally from the underlying mucosa so that approximately half of the circumference of the oesophageal mucosa is freed, permitting it to pout freely through the incision.

7 After completion of the incision, haemostasis is carefully obtained to prevent postoperative scarring and the oesophagus is returned to its position in the mediastinum, which restores the gastro-oesophageal junction to its normal intra-abdominal position. If the hiatal attachments are weak and the hiatus is patulous, two mattress sutures can be placed in the oesophageal muscular wall on either side of the myotomy, passed through the hiatus and brought out through the diaphragm where they are tied, thus ensuring maintenance of the gastro-oesophageal junction in an intra-abdominal position. The mediastinal pleura is then closed over the oesophagus with a running catgut suture and the thoracic incision is closed in layers with catheter drainage.

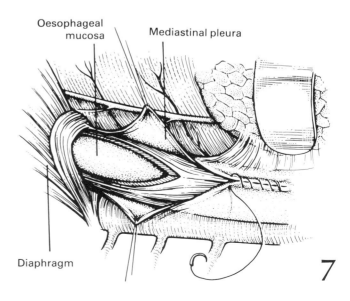

Oesophageal mucosa

Mediastinal pleura

Diaphragm

7

Postoperative care

Oral fluids may be permitted the night of surgery if the patient so desires and if mucosal integrity has not been violated. After institution of oral fluids, dietary restrictions are rapidly minimized so that the patient is able to resume a normal diet within 1–2 days. The intercostal drainage tube is removed on the day after operation and the patient is usually ready for discharge in 5–6 days.

Complications

Other than the usual postoperative complications that can occur after any surgical procedure, the postoperative period is not distinguished by any characteristic problems. If an opening has inadvertently been made in the mucosa and is not recognized, an oesophageal leak with development of an empyema is a potential complication that might require closed, or even open, pleural drainage. Incomplete mobilization of the muscle from the underlying mucosa may lead to healing of the myotomy with recurrent dysphagia. This is usually a delayed symptom occurring within weeks or months of the operative procedure. Inadequate myotomy that does not adequately reduce the lower oesophageal sphincter pressure can result in continued dysphagia and is a potential hazard of a limited myotomy if the gastro-oesophageal junction is not accurately identified. On the other hand, an over-zealous myotomy extending for more than a few centimetres onto the stomach predisposes to gastro-oesophageal reflux. Postoperative symptoms of regurgitation, heartburn and dysphagia herald this complication. The symptoms of heartburn may develop fairly rapidly, but an oesophageal stricture rarely develops early after surgery and may take months to develop. However, gastro-oesophageal reflux rarely occurs if the operative technique described above is employed.

Outcome

Between 1970 and 1992, 185 oesophagomyotomies have been performed by the author and colleagues on 183 patients with achalasia. The long-term results of 179 patients available for evaluation between 6 months and 20 years after operation showed an overall improvement rate of 89% with 93% of patients benefiting after a primary operation compared with a 70% success rate for patients undergoing reoperation. Clinically important gastro-oesophageal reflux developed in nine patients (5%).

Illustrations by Antoine Barnaud after Cedomir Vasić

Myotomy for achalasia: abdominal approach

Srdjan C. Rakić MD, PhD, FACS
Associate Professor of Surgery, Belgrade University School of Medicine, and Chief, Division of Oesophageal Surgery, Institute of Digestive Diseases, Belgrade, Yugoslavia*

History

Transabdominal oesophagomyotomy for achalasia was first described in 1914 by Heller, a German surgeon, and involved an extramucosal oesophagomyotomy on both the anterior and posterior walls of the gastro-oesophageal junction. Heller's operation was modified in 1918 by Groeneveldt of Holland who simplified the procedure to a single anterior myotomy. This modification was successfully popularized in continental Europe by Zaaijer in 1923 but its acceptance in the UK and North America took much longer. Numerous modifications of this method have been introduced but an extramucosal myotomy remains the basis of surgical treatment for achalasia.

*Present address: Department of Surgery, Leyenburg Hospital, Postbus 40551, The Hague 2504 LN, The Netherlands.

Principles and justification

The management of patients with achalasia is directed toward disrupting the lower oesophageal sphincter, thereby facilitating gravity-induced swallowing and relieving dysphagia. This goal can be achieved either by forceful dilatation or by surgical oesophagomyotomy. While a prospective randomized trial has reported superior results for oesophagomyotomy, dilatation gives a good to excellent result in 65% of patients[1]. Oesophagomyotomy can be approached transthoracically or transabdominally; there is no convincing evidence that either approach is superior to the other. The distal extent of the oesophagomyotomy is debatable, as is the value of the addition of a concomitant antireflux procedure. The transabdominal approach to the distal oesophagus with hiatal dissection and, especially, gastric extension of the myotomy, disrupts the antireflux mechanism. Reconstruction of the gastro-oesophageal junction is thus important for preventing gastro-oesophageal reflux and its complications[2]. The author's preference is to perform an anterior partial fundoplication after completion of the oesophagomyotomy, extending 1 cm on to the stomach. The limited gastric extent of the myotomy assures its completeness, while a partial wrap around the myotomized distal oesophagus provides satisfactory control of gastro-oesophageal reflux without causing obstruction.

Indications

Assuming the absence of general contraindications, the operation can be performed either as the initial treatment for achalasia or after dilatation fails. The transabdominal approach is preferable in patients with compromised cardiopulmonary function, those who have undergone previous thoracic surgery and those who require a concomitant abdominal procedure. This approach may not be satisfactory if more than 10 cm of the distal oesophagus has to be incised. When in doubt, the transthoracic route is recommended. This approach is also better for extremely obese patients with associated oesophageal disease (diverticulum), or when dense abdominal adhesions are expected.

A challenging group of patients are those with either previous unsuccessful oesophagomyotomy or a sigmoid-shaped megaoesophagus. After a failed myotomy, the preoperative diagnosis must be accurate and the reason for failure identified. A clear distinction should be made between unsuccessful myotomy and other postoperative complications, especially reflux or dysphagia resulting from an antireflux procedure. Transabdominal repeat myotomy can be performed when symptoms are due to either an inadequate or a healed initial myotomy. After multiple failures, oesophagectomy with visceral reconstruction is a more reliable option[3]. The treatment of megaoesophagus is even more controversial. The results of oesophagomyotomy in these patients are not as good as in those with mild dilatation of the oesophagus, but which patient will have a poor result from this procedure is clinically unpredictable. Oesophageal resection has been recently recommended as the primary treatment for patients with megaoesophagus[3]. In the author's opinion, initial treatment by standard myotomy is justified. If failure then occurs, oesophageal resection is the best option.

Preoperative

Assessment

The characteristic symptoms in achalasia are dysphagia and regurgitation. The diagnosis is often first made from a barium swallow examination.

Endoscopy should be performed to rule out neoplasm or other lesions obstructing the oesophagus.

Manometry confirms the diagnosis of achalasia. The manometric criteria for achalasia are: (1) absence of peristalsis in the body of the oesophagus; and (2) incomplete relaxation of the lower oesophageal sphincter with swallowing. Elevated lower oesophageal sphincter and oesophageal baseline pressures are frequently present but their demonstration is not essential for the diagnosis.

Preparation of patient

Preoperative hyperalimentation because of weight loss is rarely needed. Although complications due to recurrent aspiration are unusual nowadays, the pulmonary status should be routinely evaluated and preoperative respiratory therapy carried out in selected cases. Before the operation it is particularly important to evacuate the oesophageal contents completely to prevent aspiration during induction of anaesthesia. This may require a liquid diet for a day or two, and oesophageal lavage through a nasal tube both the night before and the morning of the operation. The tube is kept under suction to empty the dilated oesophagus completely; it is left in place during the operation.

Anaesthesia

General endotracheal anaesthesia is used.

Operation

Incision

1 An upper midline incision beginning over the base of the xiphoid process and extending below the umbilicus on the left side provides the best exposure of the lower oesophagus and upper stomach. A table mounted, self-retaining upper hand two-bladed retractor is positioned.

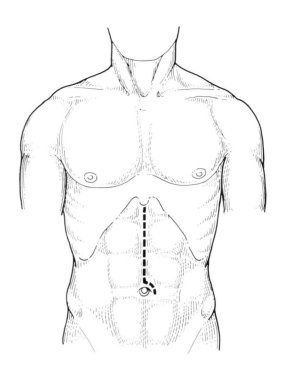

1

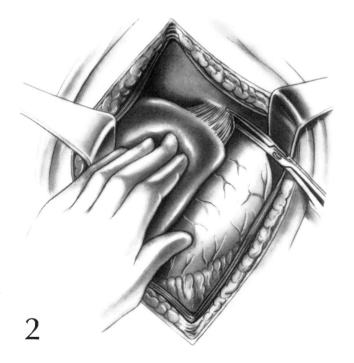

2

Mobilization of the left lobe of the liver

2 Mobilization of the left lobe of the liver is usually necessary for an adequate exposure. The left lobe is retracted by hand inferiorly to the right and the stretched left triangular ligament is divided with scissors or diathermy towards the midline (near the left hepatic vein). The mobilized left lobe is displaced downward and inward on itself and is retracted by a large S retractor which is placed over a saline-soaked pack. Bands extending between the stomach and the free edge of the spleen should be divided and a pack may be placed over the spleen.

Exposure of the gastro-oesophageal junction

3 While the first assistant maintains downward traction on the stomach using a gauze pad or a pair of Babcock forceps, the peritoneum over the gastro-oesophageal junction is incised and the underlying oesophagus exposed. Care must be taken to preserve the anterior vagus nerve, which should be mobilized from the oesophagus and retracted gently to the right with a tape.

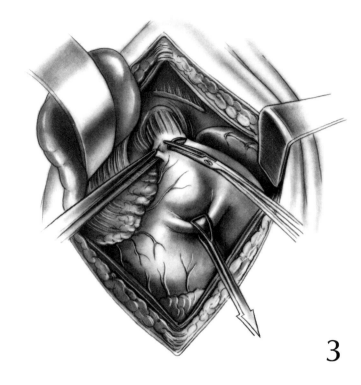

3

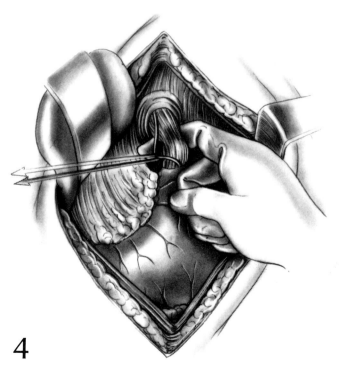

4

Mobilization of the oesophagus

4 Exposure of the anterior surface of the oesophagus is sufficient for a myotomy; however, mobilization of the whole oesophagus and downward traction provide better visibility of the oesophagus into the mediastinum, which is crucial for correct and safe performance of the myotomy. The oesophagus is mobilized by gently passing the right index finger around its distal end and it is encircled with a Penrose drain. Downward traction is applied while the phreno-oesophageal membrane is sectioned. A long, narrow, S retractor is inserted into the hiatus and the lower oesophagus is freed upwards from the adjacent structures using blunt and sharp dissection.

Myotomy

5 With the oesophagus under tension and gently elevated by the encircling Penrose drain, the incision is begun in the midline anteriorly and above the point of apparent constriction: the plane between the muscle and the mucosa is most easily identified at this level. The incision is deepened carefully through both the longitudinal and the circular muscles of the distal oesophagus down to the mucosa, which should remain intact.

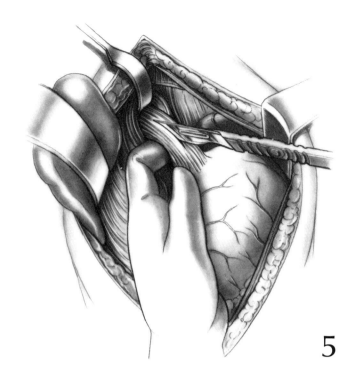

5

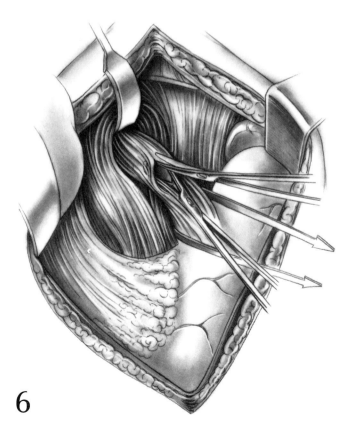

6

6 Once the oesophageal mucosa is exposed, further myotomy is carried out by following a cleavage plane between the overlying muscle layers and the mucosa. A right-angled clamp or a pair of blunt forceps is gently inserted into this plane and, by opening and closing the clamp, the muscle is separated from the mucosa. At the end of this manoeuvre, the tip of the semi-open clamp or forceps is gently elevated and the stretched muscle is cut with blunt-tipped scissors. Care should be taken not to cut the elevated muscle up to the very end of the clamp as tented mucosa may be perforated at this point. The sequence of division–elevation–cutting should be carried out at short intervals, not exceeding 1–1.5 cm in a single step. The oesophagus can be myotomized cranially in this manner for at least 10 cm, which is sufficient for achalasia. A metal clip is placed at the proximal corner of the myotomy to facilitate later radiographic evaluation.

7 After the myotomy is completed cranially, the incision is extended caudally. It is helpful to use a pair of right-angled forceps with the tips projecting caudally for this part of the myotomy. Ideally, the inferior boundary of the myotomy should be the stomach wall. A few small veins traversing the submucosa may help to identify the point when the stomach is reached but accurate identification of the gastro-oesophageal junction is usually difficult. The myotomy is therefore extended across the gastro-oesophageal junction for 0.5–1 cm over the anterior gastric wall. This limited incision on to the stomach assures an adequate caudal extent of the myotomy. Dense attachments make identification of the submucosal plane in the area of the gastro-oesophageal junction difficult. Care is taken to avoid mucosal perforation, which is most likely to occur at this point. Any opening in the mucosa made inadvertently must be closed with fine sutures.

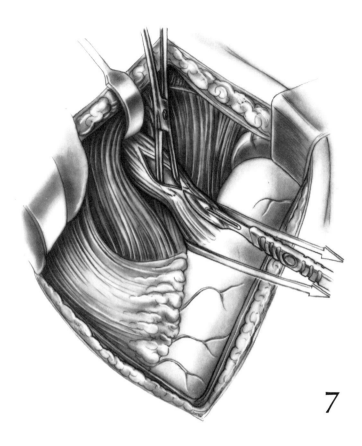

7

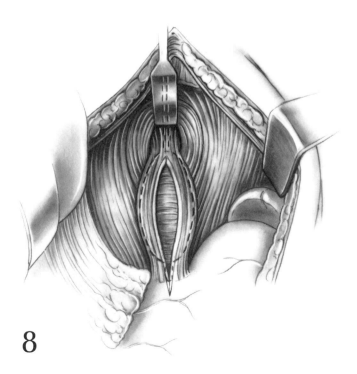

8

8 Care is taken to ensure that all muscular fibres are divided, at the same time avoiding perforation of the mucosa. It is helpful to insert a deflated oesophageal balloon dilator in the area of the myotomy with its distal end positioned across the gastro-oesophageal junction. The balloon dilator must be introduced carefully under manual and visual control in order to avoid the tip perforating the mucosa. The balloon is gently inflated, distending all constricting fibres, which are then divided.

9 The muscularis propria is dissected laterally and away from the oesophageal mucosa so that half of the mucosal circumference freely bulges through the myotomy. Haemostasis is secured using warm packs or fine ligatures. After the myotomy is completed, a metal clip is placed at the caudal margin of the myotomy. The balloon dilator is deflated and carefully replaced with a nasogastric tube. The anterior vagus nerve is released and returned to its normal position.

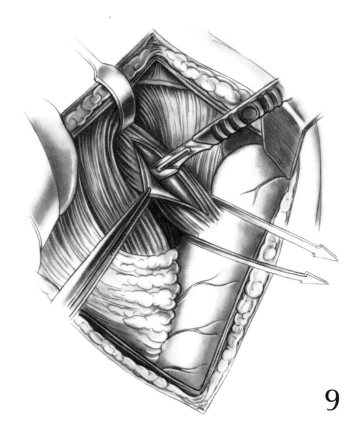

9

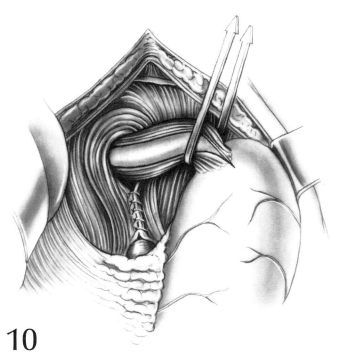

10

Approximation of crura

10 The crura of the diaphragm are reapproximated behind the oesophagus with interrupted 1/0 silk sutures placed 1 cm apart. After the sutures are tied, it should be possible easily to insert the index finger alongside the oesophagus through the hiatus.

Anterior partial fundoplication

11 To test whether mobilization of the gastric fundus is required, the fundus is rotated and its anterior surface laid over the myotomized oesophagus. Should any tension exist, division of the first few short gastric vessels is necessary. After the fundus is prepared for fundoplication, it is returned to its normal position. The serosa of the adjacent gastric fundus is now sutured to the left edge of the cut oesophageal muscle using 3/0 interrupted silk placed 1 cm apart or a 3/0 running polyethylene suture. The uppermost suture is placed first and includes the left diaphragmatic crus, fixing the fundoplication to the hiatus. The sutures must be seromuscular on the gastric side and include the full thickness of the cut muscle on the oesophageal side.

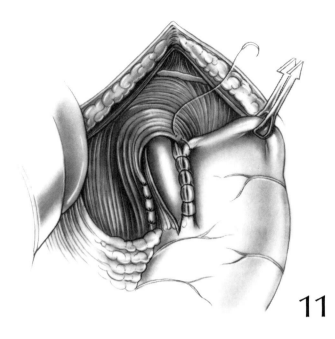

11

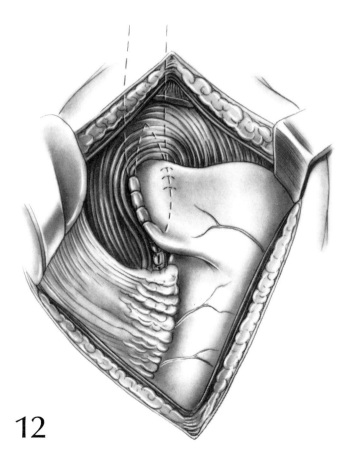

12

12 A flap of gastric fundus is placed anteriorly over the myotomy. The right edge of the gastric patch over the myotomy, which corresponds to the greater curvature of the stomach, is sutured to the right muscular border of the myotomy in the same manner as on the left side. The uppermost suture on this side should also be attached to the border of the hiatus. While suturing, care should be taken to avoid penetration into the oesophagus or the stomach, or damage to the vagi.

13 The total length of the gastric patch over the myotomy should be approximately 4 cm. A resulting partial anterior fundoplication of 180° does not add to the outflow resistance of the achalasic oesophagus and maintains the separation of muscular borders, thus preventing reunion of the myotomy. As it covers the exposed mucosa of the myotomized oesophagus, the anterior fundoplication also protects the suture line in case of inadvertent mucosal injury.

Wound closure

The wound is closed without drainage. The operation usually takes 60–70 min.

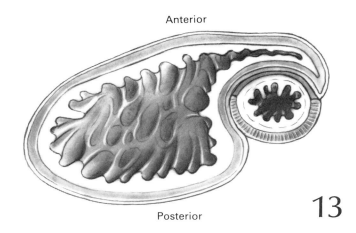

Anterior

Posterior

13

Postoperative care

The patient is ambulant on the evening of the operation. The nasogastric tube is removed on the morning after the operation, when sips of oral liquids are started. Diet is progressed to semisolid and then solid food by the third or fourth day after surgery. A barium swallow examination to demonstrate free passage of barium into the stomach is performed on the fifth day. The usual hospital stay is about 6–7 days.

If the oesophageal mucosa has been perforated and sutured the patient is kept on nasogastric suction for 3–4 days to prevent distension of the stomach and reflux during the healing period. Oral intake is suspended and fluids, antibiotics and gastric secretion blockers are administered intravenously. The suture line is tested for integrity by a water-soluble contrast study on the sixth day after operation. If no leaks are seen, oral liquids are started and the patient is gradually restored to solid food within a few days. A barium swallow examination is performed before discharge.

No significant morbidity has been recorded after this operation and potential complications are those that may follow any major abdominal surgical procedure. The single exception might be an unrecognized perforation of the oesophageal mucosa, which may lead to an oesophageal leak with development of an empyema or peritonitis. As the mucosal perforation, which is usually a pinpoint defect, is routinely covered by the fundic wrap, clinical evidence of perforation is exceptional.

Outcome

Good to excellent results have been reported following transabdominal Heller myotomy with a concomitant antireflux procedure in 85–95% of patients[1,4]. Failures are usually due to incomplete or healed myotomy and are more likely to occur in patients with previous unsuccessful myotomy or megaoesophagus. Severe gastro-oesophageal reflux and its complications are not likely after the procedure described here[1,4].

Between March 1970 and August 1991, 295 patients with oesophageal achalasia underwent a transabdominal myotomy with anterior fundoplication at the Institute of Digestive Diseases, Belgrade University Clinical Centre. There were 16 (5.4%) inadvertent injuries to the mucosa, all recognized during operation and managed by suture. Three inadvertent injuries to the spleen were managed by splenectomy. No significant postoperative morbidity was recorded. Excellent or good results were achieved in 89% of patients. Of the 24 unsatisfactory results, four patients (1.4%) had persistent symptoms due to inadequate or healed myotomy. Fourteen of the 52 patients with a preoperative oesophageal diameter larger than 6 cm and two of the seven patients who underwent repeat myotomy had a poor result. Four patients (1.4%) had severe gastro-oesophageal reflux. Three responded well to medical therapy, while one developed a stricture. The improvement rate was highest (94%) for those with a preoperative oesophageal diameter of less than 6 cm who underwent primary operation. It was, however, significantly lower for patients who underwent repeat myotomy (71%) or had an oesophageal diameter of more than 6 cm (73%).

References

1. Csendes A, Braghetto I, Henriques A, Cortes C. Late results of a prospective randomised study comparing forceful dilatation and oesophagomyotomy in patients with achalasia. *Gut* 1989; 30: 299–304.

2. Andreollo NA, Earlam RJ. Heller's myotomy for achalasia: is an added anti-reflux procedure necessary? *Br J Surg* 1987; 74: 765–9.

3. Orringer MB, Stirling MC. Esophageal resection for achalasia: indications and results. *Ann Thorac Surg* 1989; 47: 340–5.

4. Gerzić Z, Rakić S, Kneźević J *et al.* Achalasia of the esophagus: treatment controversies and evaluation of primary abdominal repair in 250 consecutive patients. *Arch Gastroenterohepatol* 1988; 7: 69–72.

Illustrations by Susan Darrington

Paraoesophageal hiatus hernia

Paul E. O'Brien MD, FRACS
Professor of Surgery, Monash University, Alfred Hospital, Melbourne, Victoria, Australia

Principles and justification

Paraoesophageal hiatus hernia is a true hernia of the abdominal cavity and, as such, may generate symptoms due to incarceration and to incomplete obstruction, and may be subject to the complications of obstruction and strangulation. Many paraoesophageal hernias are asymptomatic. When symptomatic, the common clinical patterns are of postprandial retrosternal or epigastric discomfort, dysphagia, vomiting following by dry retching, or melaena due to bleeding from contained erosions or ulceration.

The patient is generally middle aged or elderly. The aetiology is unclear. It is generally regarded as an acquired condition although persistence of the pericardiophrenic recess has been proposed. The lead point of the hernial contents is generally the ventral wall of the stomach on the greater curve at the region of the junction between antrum and body. As this point passes into the hernial sac, it draws with it the gastrocolic ligament and the transverse colon. It also generates an organoaxial rotation of the stomach about the fixed points of the left and right gastric pedicles. This can lead to partial or even complete occlusion of the stomach between the body and fundus above and more commonly at the level of the pylorus below. When well established the hernia may contain most of the stomach, a significant length of transverse colon and portions of the greater omentum. Inclusion of the spleen has been reported.

The principal points of controversy with regard to management are the place for surgical correction in the asymptomatic patient, the need for an antireflux procedure in combination with reduction and repair of the hernia, and the relative benefits of a transthoracic or transabdominal surgical approach.

Asymptomatic patients

Paraoesophageal hernia should be regarded as a true hernia, not different from inguinal or other abdominal hernias. Unless the patient is considered at high anaesthetic risk (ASA level 3 or greater), repair is indicated for the prevention of complications. The likelihood of complications is not well established. However, in one group of 21 patients who were not advised to have surgical correction of the hernia, there were six deaths due to complications[1].

Associated antireflux procedure

Gastro-oesophageal reflux is commonly present in this group of patients, presumably due to disturbance of the competence of the lower oesophageal sphincter in association with the anatomical abnormalities. When 24-h pH monitoring was conducted in a series of patients before elective repair of paraoesophageal hernias, abnormal findings were present in 11 of 18 patients[2]. Clearly, some patients should have an antireflux procedure in association with the hernia repair. The advocates of a selective policy imply that they can identify these patients. The author does not share their confidence, as the presence of the hernia itself may reduce the accuracy of pH testing, and therefore advocates an antireflux procedure in all patients with repair of the hernia.

Surgical approach

The abdominal approach is recommended. It provides the optimal approach for reduction of the hernial contents, good exposure of the defect for repair, and the capacity for treatment of any complications that have occurred to the incarcerated hernial content, or the performance of an antireflux procedure and/or the adequate fixation of the stomach within the abdomen at the completion of the repair.

Preoperative

The operation is subject to all the potential problems involved in making an upper abdominal incision in an elderly patient. Particular attention should be addressed to the preoperative respiratory status of the patient because of the expected reduction in vital capacity during the early postoperative phase. If the procedure is performed as an emergency or if there is suggestion of compromised viability of the hernial contents, appropriate perioperative antimicrobial prophylaxis should be given.

Operation

Incision and exposure

An upper abdominal midline incision is made as described in the chapter on pp. 70–78. A sternal raising retractor is an essential requirement for the optimal performance of this operation and should be placed at this stage. No other fixed retractors are needed. After a general laparotomy, the lateral segment of the left lobe of the liver is mobilized by division of the left triangular ligament and partial division of the left coronary ligaments. This liver segment is folded across the right side, covered by a moist pack and held with a Deaver retractor.

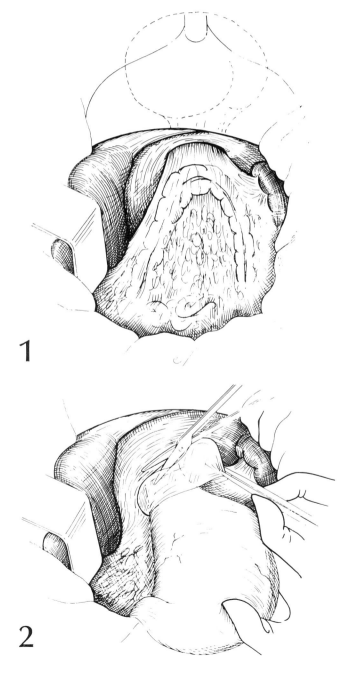

1 The hernial defect is now visualized. Typically, the tissues of the gastrocolic ligament or the transverse colon can be seen issuing from the site of the defect at this stage.

Reduction and excision of sac

2 The hernia is reduced by gentle and progresssive traction. In the elective procedure there is seldom any difficulty in this process. If obstruction has occurred, division of the diaphragm from the apex of the defect passing anteriorly should permit safe reduction of the content.

On completion of the reduction a large cavity lined by peritoneum remains. The author recommends complete removal of the peritoneal sac as this can be achieved easily in almost all patients by division of the peritoneum at the margin of the diaphragmatic defect. The margins of the sac are held by tissue forceps and, with blunt dissection (principally digital), the sac is drawn into the abdominal cavity and excised. Division of the peritoneum is continued down the lower oesophagus, which is then fully mobilized to provide a 4-cm segment about which a subsequent fundoplication will be performed.

Closure of hiatus

3 The defect in the diaphragm is commonly wide at the base and is more of an enlarged arc over the oesophagus than a hole anterior to the oesophagus. This can make closure of the defect by simple approximation somewhat difficult. The apex of the defect is grasped by a pair of tissue forceps drawn anteriorly to triangulate the arc as much as possible. The defect is then progressively closed by a series of interrupted non-absorbable sutures placed widely through the muscle of the diaphragm, e.g. 1 Ethibond. It is important to note that it is only the last of these sutures that carries the stress of the repair. Excessive tension in this last suture will cause it to fail and therefore a compromise between complete closure of the defect and excessive tension may need to be achieved. By this closure the oesophagus is pushed progressively posteriorly. It should be ensured that at least the index finger can pass easily alongside the oesophagus after completion of the closure.

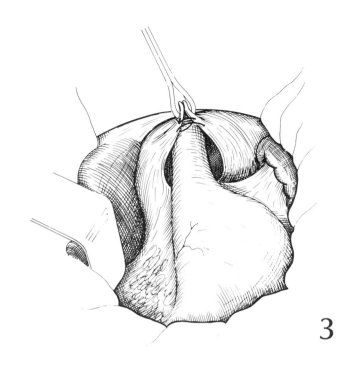

3

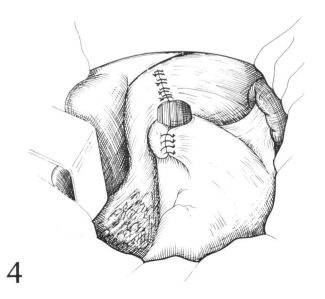

4

Fundoplication

4 The fundus must be freely mobile so that a complete wrap without tension can be achieved. This almost invariably requires division and ligation of the short gastric vessels. A wrap 4 cm in length is achieved by placing a series of non-absorbable sutures, e.g. 1 Ethibond. Each suture includes a full thickness of each aspect of the fundic wrap and a shallow bite of the anterior aspect of the lower oesophagus. This wrap should be performed with a 50-Fr bougie in place in the lower oesophagus.

Anterior gastropexy

5   If the diaphragmatic defect is a wide-based arc rather than a discrete defect, direct closure of the defect is often less than optimal. In this setting the author performs an anterior gastropexy to close the line of access of the lower stomach and other structures from the region of the hiatus. Using a series of interrupted non-absorbable sutures, the anterior surface of the fundus of the stomach is approximated to the diaphragm from the lesser curve on the right side to the greater curve well to the left of the hiatus.

A huge defect can also be treated by using a non-absorbable mesh, which is sutured to close the residual defect after partial closure.

Closure and completion

Routine closure of the anterior abdominal wall is performed with a continuous suture of 1 polydioxanone to achieve mass closure of the linea alba and a fine suture of 5/0 polydioxanone for subcuticular closure of the skin. No drain tubes are placed in the peritoneal cavity or in the wound, and a nasogastric tube is not left *in situ*.

Postoperative care

Adequate pain relief and chest physiotherapy are the most important aspects of early postoperative care. Sips of fluid are permitted early, but full oral fluid therapy is not commenced until evidence of good gastric emptying (lax abdomen and normal bowel sounds) is present.

Outcome

The long-term outcome is generally very satisfactory. The recurrence rate of the hernia is generally consi-

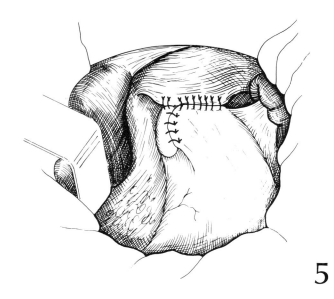

5

dered to be low, with some authors not recognizing any recurrence during the follow-up period[3]. However, Ellis *et al.*[4] noted a frequency of recurrence of 7% in 55 patients, indicating that secure closure is not always achieved.

References

1. Skinner DB, Belsey RH. Surgical management of esophageal reflux and hiatus hernia. *J Thorac Cardiovasc Surg* 1967; 53: 33–54.

2. Walther B, DeMeester TR, Lafontaine E, Courtney JV, Little AG, Skinner DB. Effects of para-esophageal hernia on sphincter function and its implications on surgical therapy. *Am J Surg* 1984; 147: 111–16.

3. Low DE, Hill LD. Paraesophageal hiatal hernia. In: Sabiston DC, Spencer FC, eds. *Surgery of the Chest*. 5th ed. Philadelphia: WB Saunders, 1990: 923–30.

4. Ellis FH Jr, Crozier RE, Shea JA. Paraesophageal hiatus hernia. *Arch Surg* 1986; 121: 416–20.

Oesophagogastrectomy for adenocarcinoma of the oesophagus and cardia

A. H. Hölscher MD
Assistant Professor of Surgery, Department of Surgery, Technical University of Munich, Munich, Germany

R. Bumm MD
Senior Resident in Surgery, Department of Surgery, Technical University of Munich, Munich, Germany

J. R. Siewert MD, FACS
Professor of Surgery, Chairman, Department of Surgery, Technical University of Munich, Munich, Germany

Classification

1 In this institution the term adenocarcinoma of the gastro-oesophageal junction is used to describe all tumours which have their centre within an area 5 cm orad or 5 cm aborad to the lower oesophageal sphincter (LOS). Oesophageal adenocarcinomas and subcardial gastric carcinomas are included in this category if they infiltrate the cardia, meaning the terminal oesophageal musculature. This therefore leads to the following classification for different types of adenocarcinomas at the gastro-oesophageal junction[1-3]:

1. Type I: adenocarcinoma in Barrett's oesophagus (centre of tumour 1–5 cm orad to the LOS).
2. Type II: carcinoma arising from the cardia proper (centre of tumour between 1 cm above and 2 cm below the LOS).
3. Type III: subcardial or fundal carcinoma of the stomach which infiltrates the lower oesophagus mostly within the submucosa (centre of tumour 2–5 cm below the LOS).

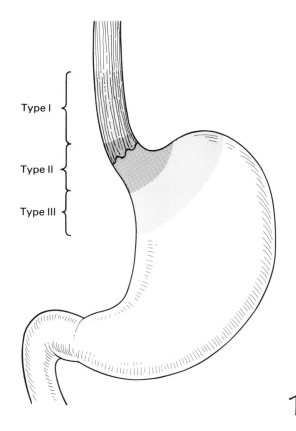

Type I

Type II

Type III

1

Principles and justification

2a–d
Four different procedures are available for the surgical treatment of these types of carcinomas, although the authors recommend only the first three.

The first is transmediastinal subtotal oesophagectomy and partial upper gastrectomy, which is appropriate for type I carcinomas (*Illustration 2a*).

The second is extended total gastrectomy with distal oesophageal resection via a transhiatal approach. This procedure can be used for type II tumours in the early stages (UICC stage 1 and 2) and type III tumours (*Illustration 2b,d*).

The third method of treatment is total oesophagogastrectomy (*Illustration 2c*). This is the authors' procedure of choice for advanced stages of type II (stage 3 and 4) tumours, especially if, by distal oesophageal resection (*Illustration 2b*), tumour-free resection margins cannot be achieved.

Although some authors advocate a proximal partial gastrectomy and distal oesophagectomy as a so-called regional cardia resection, the authors do not recommend such a resection because it seems insufficient from an oncological point of view. In addition, such a limited resection may be associated with troublesome alkaline reflux. It is used only rarely in a strictly palliative setting.

In this chapter the surgical technique for transmediastinal subtotal oesophageal resection and partial upper gastrectomy, as well as total oesophagogastrectomy, is described (*Illustration 2a,c*). Extended total gastrectomy is discussed on pp. 450–464.

Indications

Transmediastinal oesophagectomy is indicated when an adenocarcinoma of the distal oesophagus develops in a Barrett's oesophagus (type I cancer). These carcinomas metastasize mainly into the abdomen, so that a lower mediastinectomy seems to be sufficient. If the oesophageal hiatus is opened sufficiently, a proper radical resection of the tumour can be performed under direct vision. Regional lymphadenectomy in the upper abdomen is also performed (*see* chapter on pp. 142–153).

This operation is an important addition to the operative spectrum of oesophageal surgery[4]. However, it should not be seen as a simpler version of transthoracic oesophagectomy. Only surgeons with some experience in oesophageal surgery should perform this operation. With this prerequisite, the procedure has a low intraoperative risk. During the postoperative course, however, patients are exposed to similar complications as patients who have had a transthoracic oesophagectomy.

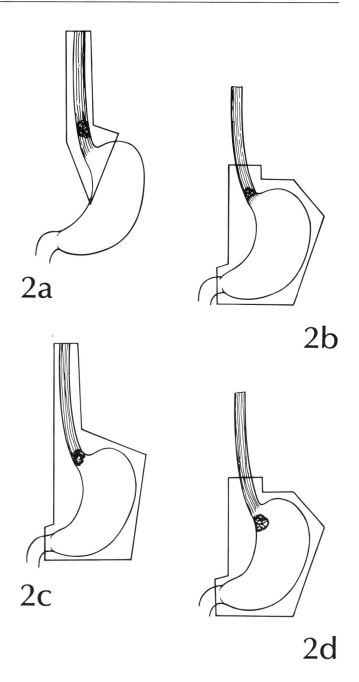

2a

2b

2c

2d

Preoperative

A careful preoperative diagnostic examination is necessary for surgery of adenocarcinoma of the gastro-oesophageal junction. The tumour is staged by endoscopy, endoscopic ultrasonography, barium swallow and computed tomographic scan. These investigations give quite exact information for TNM staging. If an advanced tumour of the gastro-oesophageal junction is present, neoadjuvant chemotherapy may be appropriate. It is also important in preoperative assessment to consider the risk factors which are present. These include an assessment of pulmonary, cardiac, renal and hepatic function. In most cases a reconstruction is performed by stomach interposition, but the colon should be prepared before operation by orthotopic bowel lavage and ideally, a colonoscopy so that an alternative is available should technical difficulties occur, as described on pp. 128–141.

Anaesthesia

The operation is performed under routine general anaesthesia. In contrast to a transthoracic oesophagectomy, a double-lumen endotracheal tube is not necessary.

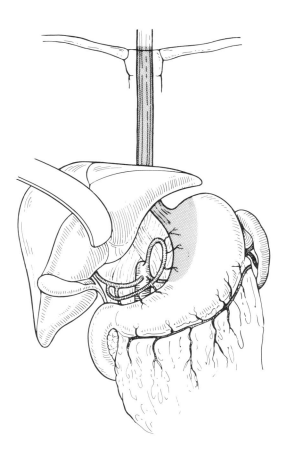

3

Operations

TRANSMEDIASTINAL OESOPHAGECTOMY AND PROXIMAL GASTRECTOMY

3 This procedure involves the subtotal removal of the oesophagus and proximal stomach by a transmediastinal route (without a thoracotomy), and is performed through an abdominal and cervical approach.

Position of patient

4 Transmediastinal oesophagectomy is performed with the patient lying supine. A bolster is used to bring the cardia region forwards to lessen the depth of dissection.

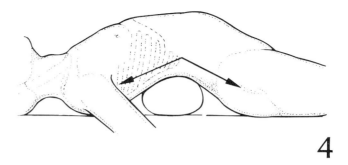

4

5 The neck is positioned as for thyroid gland surgery with the head turned to the right to expose the left part of the neck. Sterile draping is placed in such a way that two surgical teams (cervical and abdominal) can work simultaneously. The oesophagus is intubated with a large tube to facilitate palpation.

If the cervical dissection is performed endoscopically, the position of the video monitor on the right side of the neck of the patient has to be taken into account. In addition, enough space should be available for the movement of the mediastinoscope on the left side of the neck where the surgeon for the cervical approach is positioned.

A suprapancreatic lymphadenectomy is an important part of the operation for adenocarcinoma of the cardia[2, 5]. Therefore a wide abdominal approach is necessary. The authors perform the operation via a transverse upper abdominal incision with enlargement by an upper midline incision in the direction of the xiphoid process. This approach provides an excellent view of the whole upper abdominal cavity.

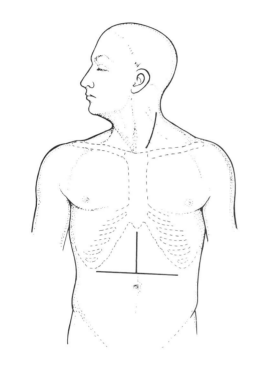

5

Preparation of the distal oesophagus

6 The first step in the operation is to divide the left triangular ligament of the liver and to hold the left lobe to the right side using a retractor. The oesophageal hiatus is next enlarged. It is crucial to enlarge the hiatus enough. This enlargement is performed in a ventral and slightly left lateral direction and should avoid opening the adjacent pericardium. This dissection of the anterior commissure of the diaphragm is nearly always sufficient. Very rarely an additional division of the left or right diaphragmatic crus is undertaken to improve exposure further. After dissection of the visceral peritoneum, the terminal oesophagus is bluntly dissected and a tape is passed around it. The lower mediastinum can now be palpated to decide the resectability of the tumour. If it is removable attention is turned to the stomach. The preparation of the stomach as an oesophageal substitute is described in the chapter on pp. 142–153.

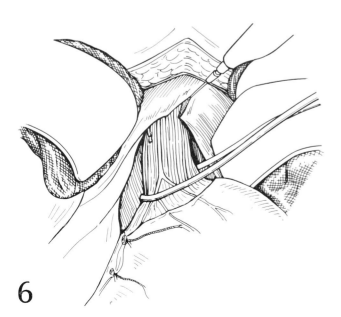

6

Preparation of the mediastinal oesophagus

7 After the stomach has been mobilized transmediastinal blunt dissection of the oesophagus is performed. Two or three fingers are moved close to the oesophageal wall and used to free the oesophagus using spreading and circular movements. A 42-Fr bougie is placed within the oesophagus to facilitate palpation. All pliable tissue can be dissected bluntly without danger, providing the dissection is kept close to the oesophageal wall. Direct aortic branches are very rare in the lower part of the mediastinum. The only structures which cannot be bluntly divided by the fingers are the vagal trunks. These are divided with scissors.

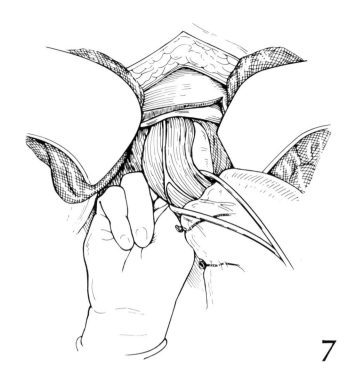

7

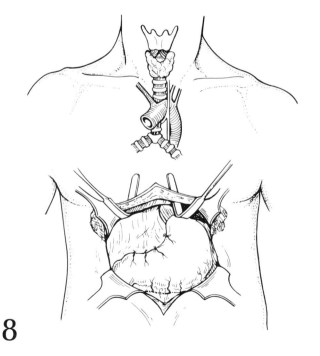

8

8 The oesophageal hiatus can be opened up using two very long hook retractors. This allows the whole posterior mediastinum up to the tracheal bifurcation to be inspected without difficulty. If bleeding occurs in this area, it can be controlled under direct vision. If bleeding is severe, it is not necessary to reposition the patient immediately and perform a thoracotomy because most of the bleeding points can be exposed and stopped through the abdominal approach.

The exposure afforded by this approach allows lymphadenectomy of the lower posterior mediastinum to be performed under direct vision. The ideal plane of dissection is the anterior wall of the aorta. The perioesophageal lymphatic tissue between the pericardium and the aorta, as well as between both diaphragmatic bundles, should be removed *en bloc* with the oesophagus. If the tumour is infiltrating the diaphragmatic bundles or the pericardium, these should be included in the resection.

Preparation of the proximal oesophagus

9 A second surgical team commences at the same time as the first operative team by opening the neck and exposing the cervical oesophagus. The approach is via a skin incision along the anterior edge of the left sternocleidomastoid muscle. The dissection of the cervical oesophagus is usually accomplished without difficulty. The recurrent laryngeal nerve is displayed and preserved. The left inferior thyroid artery is dissected, ligated and divided.

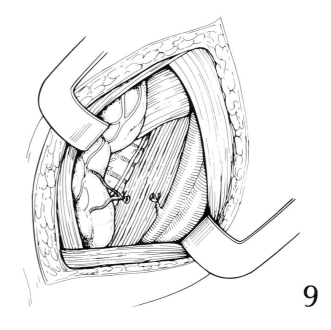

9

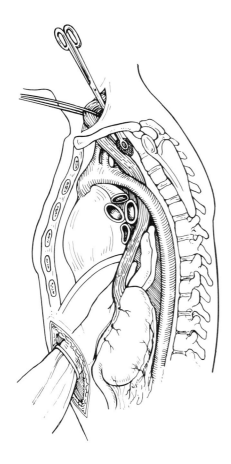

10

10 After circumferential mobilization a tape is placed around the cervical oesophagus. Further dissection of the oesophagus in the posterior mediastinum is performed bluntly using a sponge on a stick and goes as far as possible in the intrathoracic direction. The last step of the oesophageal dissection is performed by the first surgeon, who pushes his right hand from the oesophageal hiatus into the posterior mediastinum to meet his left hand or the sponge stick coming from the cervical approach. Often it is not possible to free the oesophagus completely by digital dissection, with there being a short section above the tracheal bifurcation which has to be dissected blind. It is very important to keep as close to the oesophageal wall as possible during dissection to prevent damage to the pars membranacea of the trachea and also the azygos vein.

11 Once mobilization of the oesophagus is complete, it is partially pulled up and out of the cervical incision and stapled closed. It is then divided proximal to the staple line. In this manner, a cervical oesophageal stump of sufficient length is preserved.

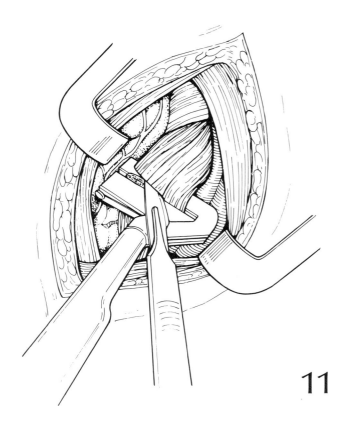

11

Endoscopic dissection of the cervical and intramediastinal oesophagus

The development of a novel mediastinoscope and suitable instruments has allowed the preparation of the mediastinal oesophagus under endoscopic view[6]. This is described in detail in the chapter on pp. 601–606. Endoscopic dissection of the oesophagus has advantages over conventional surgery for several reasons. First, it saves time because simultaneous work with the abdominal surgeon is possible. Secondly, initial experience suggests that damage to the recurrent laryngeal nerve is significantly less, and thirdly, postoperative pulmonary problems seem to be less frequent.

Transmediastinal pull-through and extirpation of the oesophagus

12 After conventional or endoscopic dissection of the oesophagus and division in the cervical part, the oesophagus can be pulled downwards by gripping it as high as possible to avoid tearing it.

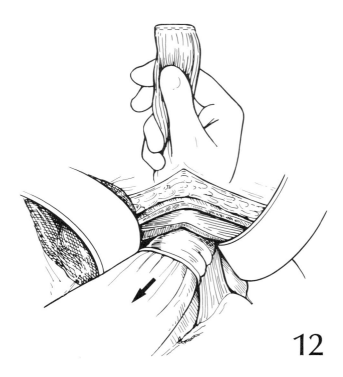

12

13 When the oesophagus has been removed the posterior mediastinum is tamponaded with a hot moist towel which is left *in situ* for 5–10 min. As the stomach has previously been prepared in a typical manner as described on pp. 142–153, the oesophagus, together with the stomach, can be placed in front of the abdominal cavity. The formation of the gastric tube or the preparation of the whole stomach as an oesophageal substitute is now performed using a stapler. Finally, the towel is removed from the posterior mediastinum and the oesophageal hiatus is again opened by two long hook retractors. Under vision, the posterior mediastinum is checked for bleeding points. In many cases the mediastinal pleura is inadvertently opened during the dissection on one or even both sides of the oesophagus. Closure of the pleura is not necessary, but the insertion of chest tubes is recommended. The oesophageal hiatus is narrowed around the gastric tube to avoid internal herniation and also to close the thoracic cavity off from the abdominal cavity. If the reconstruction is undertaken using the retrosternal route, the hiatus is closed completely.

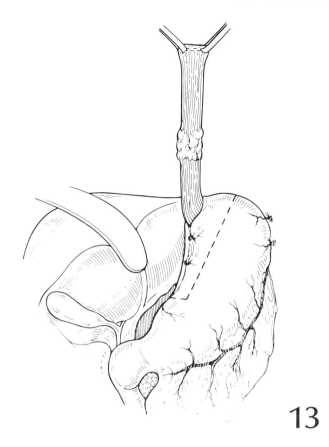

13

TOTAL OESOPHAGOGASTRECTOMY

Position of patient

The positioning and approach are the same as in transmediastinal oesophagectomy.

14 The shading in this illustration represents the extent of resection in total oesophagogastrectomy. After checking the oncological situation in the abdominal cavity with regard to distant metastases and making sure that the tumour is resectable, the procedure starts with the usual preparation of the stomach for gastrectomy as described on pp. 450–464.

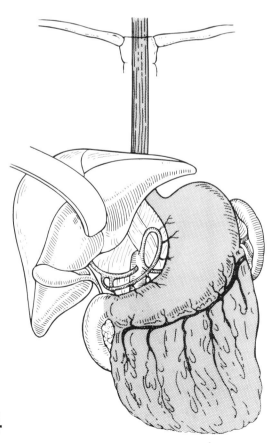

14

15 For this purpose the omentum is dissected from the transverse colon. The right gastro-omental (epiploic) artery and vein, as well as the left gastro-omental (epiploic) vessels are divided between ligatures.

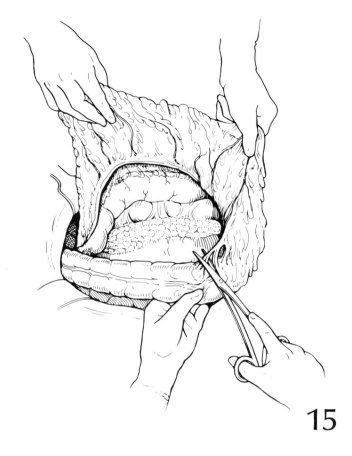

15

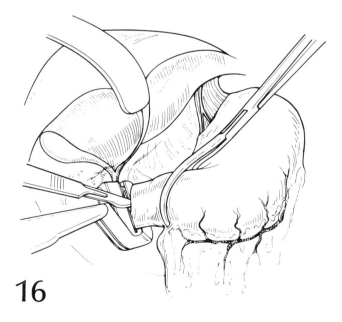

16

16 As the disease is at the cardia, the preparation of the duodenal stump is usually a relatively simple procedure. The duodenum should be closed 2 cm aborad to the pylorus using a TA-55 stapler; it is then divided. Further closure of the duodenal stump using seromuscular interrupted sutures is optional.

17 After the lesser omentum has been divided it is possible to elevate the stomach and to start preparing the tumour. Advanced tumours which initially seem difficult to remove can often be resected if dissection is performed as for a lymphadenectomy of compartment II of cancer of the body of the stomach, using the plane of the adventitia of the common hepatic artery[2].

The position of the common hepatic artery is usually easy to find if the gastroduodenal artery, which is exposed during dissection of the duodenal stump, is followed in a central direction. An incision in the adventitia of the common hepatic artery is continued from the right side towards the coeliac trunk. All tissue in front of the common hepatic artery is removed. Another important step is the dissection of the origin of the splenic artery. Once this has been achieved it is certain that the common hepatic artery has been completely freed and is safely preserved. The coronary (left gastric) vein is divided above the junction of the common hepatic artery and the splenic artery. The left gastric artery is easy to find and is ligated and divided near the coeliac trunk. If it is not possible to dissect free the common hepatic artery due to tumour infiltration, it may be sacrificed (so-called 'Appleby procedure') providing the arterial vascularization of the liver is guaranteed via the gastroduodenal artery or an accessory liver artery. In this way nearly all cardia carcinomas can be dissected from the aortic wall, even if it is necessary to resect some of the diaphragmatic crura to achieve a complete resection. In the authors' experience, carcinomas of the cardia infiltrate the arteries mentioned very infrequently.

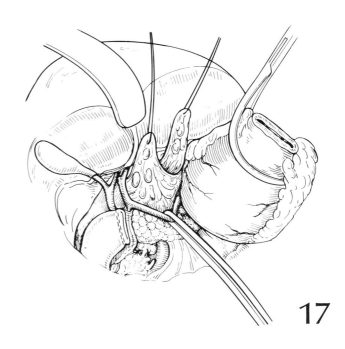

17

Extragastric extent of resection

Retroduodenal and para-aortic lymph nodes

The authors recommend that the lymph nodes of the so-called 'station 13', that is retroduodenal and retropancreatic lymph nodes, should be removed[2]. For this purpose, an extensive Kocher manoeuvre is performed. The duodenal stump is pulled via some retained seromuscular sutures in a medial and cranial direction to facilitate the lateral mobilization of the duodenum. Lymph nodes in this area are removed. Further mobilization of the cardia tumour is performed from the left side.

Pancreas-preserving splenectomy

In advanced cancer, tumour penetration is often found at the back wall of the fundus. If the tumour has not yet infiltrated the pancreas but has led to lymph node metastases at the splenic hilus and along the splenic artery, a so-called 'zone splenectomy' is also recommended. The authors try to avoid left pancreatectomy as

it leads to a high postoperative morbidity because of pancreatic fistulae.

Zone splenectomy refers to the meticulous dissection of the splenic artery from the coeliac trunk to the splenic hilus to remove the lymphatic tissue of this zone together with the spleen. The splenic artery is suture ligated half way between the coeliac trunk and the splenic hilus, whereas the splenic vein is suture ligated between the pancreatic tail and the spleen. After ligation and division of both vessels the splenectomy is performed *en bloc* with the cardia cancer.

Left pancreatic resection

If the tumour is infiltrating the tail or the corpus of the pancreas, a radical resection is only possible by adding a left side pancreatectomy. The authors find it helpful to tunnel under the pancreas above the mesenteric vein and to sever the organ at an early stage of the operation. Further on it is useful to ligate the splenic artery at the origin of the coeliac trunk and the splenic vein is ligated at its junction with the superior mesenteric vein. After severing these vessels, the left hemipancreas together with the spleen can be removed from the retroperitoneum *en bloc* together with the tumour.

Transmediastinal oesophagectomy

18 Transmediastinal oesophagectomy is performed by the method described above after widely opening the oesophageal hiatus. After completing this procedure, the whole of the stomach, together with the cardia and oesophagus, can be removed. A reconstruction is performed using a colon interposition (as described on pp. 128–141).

Postoperative care

Usual postoperative care involves artificial respiration for 24 h in the intensive care unit and afterwards a slow change to active respiration and extubation.

Intraoperative and postoperative complications which occur after transmediastinal oesophagectomy are shown in *Table 1*. Intraoperative complications are quite rare, with bleeding being seen only in exceptional cases. Damage to the trachea also represents a rare situation. During the early postoperative phase the development of pneumothorax often occurs. This is easily treated with a chest drain. Chylothorax resulting from damage to the thoracic duct is fortunately also quite rare. Recurrent laryngeal nerve palsy occurs more frequently. The reason for this may be related to the blunt digital dissection of the vagus nerve during the operation, resulting in intramediastinal damage to the nerves. The quite high rate of respiratory insufficiency in spite of avoiding a thoracotomy shows that transmediastinal oesophagectomy is not a lesser procedure than transthoracic oesophagectomy, and is associated with the same pathophysiological consequences.

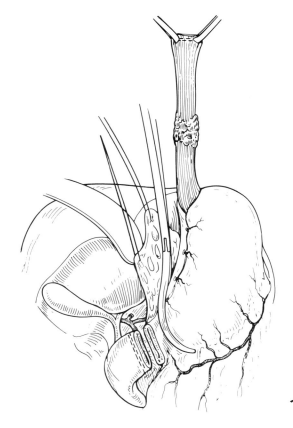

18

Outcome

In the authors' series of 106 patients with adenocarcinoma of the oesphagus treated by transmediastinal oesophagectomy, there was a 30-day mortality rate of 5.4% and a 3-month mortality rate of 10.8%[7]. In cases of advanced cancer of the cardia (type II), when total gastrectomy was added to the subtotal oesphagectomy the perioperative mortality rate was 14.2%[3]. In these cases neoadjuvant chemotherapy is recommended to try and downstage the tumour and so reduce the necessity for such radical procedures. In cases of adenocarcinoma in a Barrett's oesophagus treated by transmediastinal oesophagectomy a complete tumour resection (R_0) was achieved in nearly 80% of cases, although two-thirds of the patients had T3 or T4 tumours. Patients who had an R_0 resection had an estimated 5-year survival rate of 35%.

Table 1   Complications during and after transmediastinal oesophagectomy[5]

	Percentage
Intraoperative bleeding	0–8.6
Pneumothorax	13.2–51
Lesion of the trachea	0–2
Respiratory insufficiency	11.6–18
Chylothorax	0–3
Recurrent laryngeal nerve palsy	5–37

References

1. Siewert JR, Hölscher AH, Becker K, Gössner W. Cardiacarcinom. Versuch einer therapeutisch relevanten Klassifikation. *Chirurg* 1987; 58: 25–32.

2. Siewert JR (ed). *Chirurgie des Abdomens 2. Ösophagus, Magen und Duodenum*. München, Baltimore: Urban and Schwarzenberg, 1989.

3. Hölscher AH, Schüler M, Siewert JR. Surgical treatment of adenocarcinomas of the gastroesophageal junction. *Dis Esophagus* 1988; 1: 35–50.

4. Orringer MB. Transhiatal esophagectomy without thoracotomy for carcinoma of the thoracic esophagus. *Ann Surg* 1984; 200: 282–8.

5. Siewert JR, Hölscher AH, Horvath ÖP. Transmediastinale Ösophagektomie. *Langenbecks Arch Chir* 1986; 367: 203–13.

6. Bumm R, Hölscher AH, Feussner H, Tachibana M, Bartels H, Siewert JR. Endodissection of the thoracic esophagus: technique and clinical results in transhiatal esophagectomy. *Ann Surg* 1993; 218: 97–104.

7. Siewert JR, Hölscher AH, Bollschweiler E. Surgical therapy of cancer in Barrett's esophagus. *Diseases of the Esophagus* 1992; 5: 57–62.

Indications and preoperative assessment of patients for antireflux surgery

Glyn G. Jamieson FRACS, FACS
Dorothy Mortlock Professor of Surgery, University of Adelaide, Department of Surgery, Royal Adelaide Hospital, Adelaide, Australia

It may seem an unnecessary statement of the obvious to say that the single most important undertaking before carrying out antireflux surgery is to establish that the patient actually has gastro-oesophageal reflux disease. However, surgeons with an interest in this area continue to see patients with poor results following antireflux surgery who prove to have problems that such surgery could not have helped, e.g. achalasia or diffuse oesophageal spasm. The surgeon should therefore be guided by two important principles before carrying out antireflux surgery: (1) proof that abnormal reflux is occurring must be obtained; and (2) the fact that the reflux is causing the patient's symptoms and/or pathological damage to the oesophagus must be established.

The reflux of gastric contents into the oesophagus occurs in all of us for short periods after meals and so reflux alone should not be seen as an abnormal phenomenon. One very important means of assessing abnormality in reflux is also the simplest to ascertain, i.e. the patient's symptoms.

Symptoms

Abnormal reflux usually produces typical symptoms, for example retrosternal burning pain after meals or after bending over while gardening, etc., sometimes associated with the regurgitation of contents into the patient's mouth. The heartburn is typically relieved by antacids and worsened by certain dietary elements, e.g. spicy foods or alcohol. Up to 40% of people in Western communities experience such reflux symptoms at least once a month, and about 10% experience such symptoms at least once a day. However, in many of these people the symptoms are of a minor nuisance value only and the occasional ingestion of an antacid preparation provides adequate management of their problem. It is only when symptoms are spoiling the patient's enjoyment of life that consideration for surgery is given, and this usually presupposes that an adequate trial of drug therapy with H_2-receptor blockers and/or proton pump inhibitors has been undertaken.

Sometimes it is established that reflux is responsible for atypical symptoms and these can also lead to consideration for surgery. Examples are: (1) respiratory symptoms, particularly nocturnal regurgitation and aspiration; (2) dysphagia from stricture formation which sometimes develops in the absence of typical reflux symptoms; (3) chest pain of a sharper nature than typical heartburn; (4) recurrent anaemia, again sometimes in the absence of typical symptoms of reflux.

Objective assessment of reflux

Endoscopy

Strictly speaking, endoscopy assesses the effects of reflux rather than reflux itself. There is much observer variation for lesser degrees of reflux damage, such as erythema of the mucosa, so that it is only diffuse oesophagitis with erosions or ulceration that can be regarded as objective evidence of reflux disease.

Oesophageal stricturing and development of a columnar-lined lower oesophagus can also be determined endoscopically.

Biopsies to prove the endoscopic findings should be undertaken. It is a moot point whether it is useful to biopsy either erythema or a normal-appearing oesophagus. Biopsies should be taken of erythematous spots as these sometimes prove to be columnar mucosa or even erosions, somewhat to the surprise of the endoscopist.

Unless undertaken as part of a clinical trial, there is probably little benefit in performing a biopsy on a normal-appearing oesophagus because the pathological indicators of lesser degrees of reflux damage (increased basal cell layer and prominent rete pegs) are uncertain indicators of reflux disease.

Contrast studies

A barium meal is not a useful method for detecting abnormal reflux but is the best method of demonstrating a hiatus hernia objectively and also gives the surgeon a pictorial image of a stricture, if one is present. It is the author's practice always to obtain a barium meal before surgery.

Oesophageal manometry

In a patient with typical reflux symptoms, erosive oesophagitis on endoscopy, and particularly if the surgeon routinely performs either a partial or very loose total fundoplication, the usefulness of preoperative oesophageal manometry will be negligible. On the other hand, once symptoms are not typical, or there are other features which are in any way unusual, oesophageal manometry should be undertaken before surgery. It is the author's practice to obtain oesophageal manometry before operation in all patients as the operative approach is modified in the small percentage of patients who prove to have an adynamic oesophageal body, changing from a total fundoplication to a partial fundoplication.

At the same time short-term pH testing is carried out to establish that abnormal reflux is occurring.

pH monitoring

Twenty-four-hour pH monitoring should be undertaken whenever the patient's situation is atypical, and even in the typical situation if endoscopy is normal or equivocal and if reflux is not established on short-term testing with manometry. It is important to have a low tolerance for the performance of this investigation because it is not uncommon to see patients in whom (1) symptoms

are not matched by changes in oesophageal pH, or (2) changes in oesophageal pH are associated with atypical symptoms, e.g. coughing episodes. The usefulness of 24-h pH monitoring is shown in this latter situation because coughing episodes can cause reflux and it is therefore important to establish that a reflux episode occurs before coughing begins.

In situation (1), operation should not be considered; in situation (2), it may be. This is not to suggest that 24-h pH monitoring has a sensitivity of 100%. Sometimes it is necessary to repeat a 24-h study if the first has been normal; abnormality may be found on the second study. However, two normal studies and a normal endoscopy should be regarded as an absolute contraindication to carrying out antireflux surgery.

Histology

Pathological assessment of oesophageal mucosa is used to corroborate endoscopy findings, e.g. oesophagitis, ulceration, columnar mucosa, etc. Columnar mucosa should always be biopsied, particularly if it looks abnormal in any area. Lesser degrees of dysplasia can be associated with inflammation and can be ignored. However, high-grade dysplasia should never be treated by antireflux surgery. If high-grade dysplasia is proven to exist, which may mean multiple biopsies separated by several months, then the decision must rest between continued observation (if the patient is infirm) or resection (if the patient is fit for operation).

Is a columnar-lined oesophagus in the absence of severe symptoms an indication in its own right for antireflux surgery? As regression of columnar-lined oesophagus after surgery is uncommon, and as it is not known if the risk of cancer is lessened by antireflux surgery, the answer is probably no.

Summary

Antireflux surgery, including repeat antireflux surgery, is indicated when severe symptoms cannot be controlled by other means (or other means are too expensive) and when it has been proved that the symptoms in question are due to reflux.

The minimum acceptable assessment for antireflux surgery is typical severe symptoms and erosive/ulcerative oesophagitis seen on endoscopy. Whenever symptoms are not typical or endoscopic changes are less severe, then oesophageal manometry and 24-h pH monitoring should always be undertaken to prove that it is a reflux-related problem which is being dealt with.

Abdominal fundoplication

Christopher J. Martin FRACS
Professor of Surgery, University of Sydney, and Head of Surgical Division, Nepean Hospital, Penrith, New South Wales, Australia

History

The operation of abdominal fundoplication for gastro-oesophageal reflux disease was first described by Rudolf Nissen in 1956[1]. Although there have been various modifications of technique since then, the common feature that has persisted is plication of the gastric fundus around the distal oesophagus and cardia, so that the term Nissen fundoplication has come to be used interchangeably with distal oesophageal fundoplication. Perhaps the most important modification of the operation over the past 30 years is the fashioning of the fundoplication short and loose as described by Donahue and Bombeck in 1977[2]. This has resulted in reduction of the problematic postoperative sequelae of postprandial epigastric bloating, dysphagia and inability to belch and vomit.

Principles and justification

Heartburn and acid regurgitation are the common symptoms of gastro-oesophageal reflux disease. They are extremely prevalent in Western societies. For the majority of sufferers, for whom the symptoms are occasional, avoidance of known precipitants and an occasional dose of antacid are all that are required. When medical advice is sought for more persistent symptoms, it is worthwhile to establish the diagnosis by flexible fibreoptic upper gastrointestinal endoscopy before commencing a medical programme which might include a combination of weight reduction, postural advice and dietary modification, as well as the use of agents that neutralize gastric acid, reduce gastric acid secretion and enhance oesophageal and gastric clearance.

Indications

Surgical treatment should be considered only after a concerted effort with medical treatment has been tried and has failed. What constitutes a concerted effort and failure will obviously vary from patient to patient and will be affected by other factors, such as age and fitness of the patient, tolerance of symptoms, rapidity of recurrence after reduction or withdrawal of medication, compliance with treatment and attitude to the concept of long-term drug therapy.

Preoperative

Fibreoptic endoscopy should always be performed before operation. The possibility that changes have occurred justifies repeating the procedure if the interval since diagnostic endoscopy is considerable. The preoperative endoscopy should specifically define the severity and extent of peptic oesophagitis, the presence and size of an associated hiatus hernia, and the presence and histological type of a segment of Barrett's oesophagus including the presence of dysplasia. A radiological contrast study of the oesophagus and gastro-oesophageal junction before surgery might demonstrate an associated hiatus hernia. More importantly from a planning point of view, it might demonstrate the presence of oesophageal stenosis, or definite or equivocal oesophageal shortening in conjunction with an irreducible hiatus hernia. In these cases consideration will need to be given to a thoracic rather than an abdominal approach.

Oesophageal manometry and oesophageal pH monitoring, although not mandatory, are recommended. Traditionally, oesophageal manometry has been performed in reflux disease to assess lower oesophageal sphincter tone and position. These measurements, however, are of limited use to the surgeon. Much more important is the recognition of the occasional patient with an unsuspected motility disorder of the oesophageal body, such as scleroderma or perhaps even achalasia, which will result in a change in clinical strategy. Lower oesophageal pH monitoring clearly defines the severity of oesophageal acidification. This is imperative in patients without ulcerative oesophagitis. This assessment is more sensitive and specific than other diagnostic criteria such as mucosal friability or erythema at endoscopy or abnormal morphometric scores of distal oesophageal mucosal biopsies, which have been used previously to establish the diagnosis of gastro-oesophageal reflux disease in the absence of ulcerative oesophagitis.

Counselling is also an important step in the preoperative preparation. As medical therapy can occasionally be as effective as surgical therapy, the patient should be aware that surgical control of reflux symptoms in the long term is not guaranteed and that there might be significant side effects of surgery, such as dysphagia (which is usually transient), early postprandial satiety and increased flatus production (which is universal). Other possible sequelae, which are now believed to be partly dependent on technique but which should be discussed, include difficulty with belching and vomiting, postprandial epigastric distension and borborygmus.

Operation

Incision

An upper midline incision from the xiphisternum to at least the umbilicus is required for good exposure. The incision can be extended below the umbilicus if necessary, as described in the chapter on pp. 70–78.

General exposure

Exposure can be optimized by: (1) displacing the mobile organs inferiorly by tilting the head of the operating table upwards; and (2) elevating the costal margins away from the operating table, as well as retracting them laterally and superiorly, using a retractor fixed to the operating table as described in the chapter on pp. 70–78.

Local exposure

1 Access to the gastro-oesophageal junction can be improved further by: (1) decompression of the stomach with a nasogastric tube; (2) retraction of the stomach inferiorly by the assistant using the nasogastric tube to achieve atraumatic purchase on the stomach (which also tends to reduce any hiatus hernia); (3) division of small peritoneal bands to the visceral surface of the spleen to prevent an inadvertent capsular tear; and (4) gentle retraction of the liver to the right after dividing the left triangular ligament and folding the left lobe inferiorly. This step is not regarded as necessary by some surgeons.

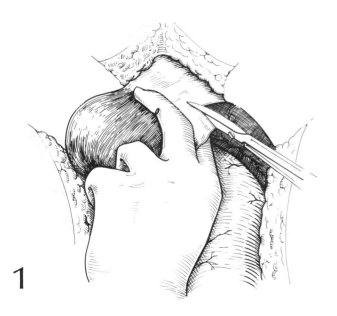

1

Initial mobilization of fundus

2 A small window is made in the peritoneum of the gastrosplenic ligament adjacent to the stomach at the level of the middle of the anterior border of the spleen. Individual leashes of vessels in this layer are ligated and divided progressively up as far as the angle of His, with division of the intervening peritoneum. Metal clips can be used to ligate the splenic ends of these cords as they are unlikely to become dislodged. This mobilization of the fundus allows progressively greater retraction of the stomach anteriorly, inferiorly and to the right.

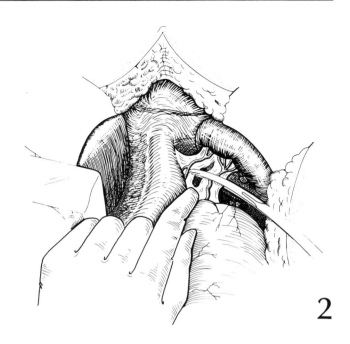

2

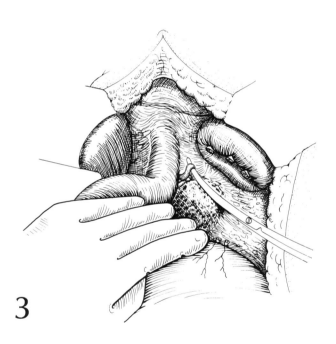

3

Further mobilization of fundus

3 The initial mobilization exposes further leashes of vessels entering the fundus from the bare area. These are progressively divided until the posterior branches of the left gastric artery on the lesser curve are reached. At the same time avascular adhesions that tend to obliterate the upper reaches of the lesser sac are divided.

Initial mobilization of distal oesophagus

4 The relatively avascular plane surrounding the oesophagus must be developed. This is best entered by dividing the peritoneal reflection of the phreno-oesophageal ligament to the left of the oesophagus and cauterizing and dividing small vessels to the left of the oesophagus.

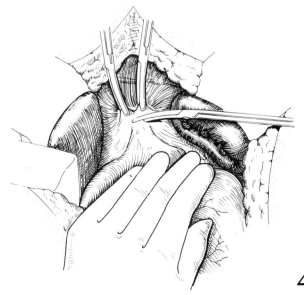

4

Identification and preservation of anterior and posterior vagal trunks

5 At this stage the anterior vagal trunk is visible and palpable as a cord just to the right and anterior to the oesophagus. This is best gently retracted with a fine rubber sling. The posterior vagal trunk is visible between the crura posterior to the plane of dissection.

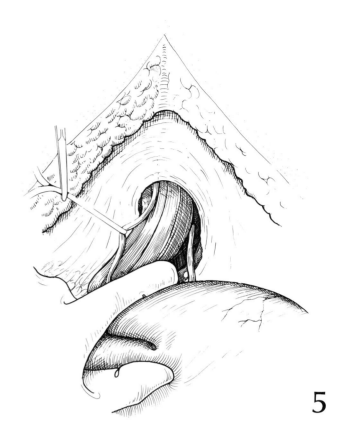

5

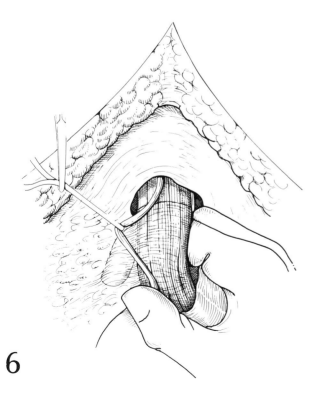

6

Encircling the oesophagus

6 The oesophagus is encircled from the left by passing the index finger behind it and the thumb between the anterior vagal trunk and the oesophageal wall to make a small window in the residual tissue anchoring the right side of the distal oesophagus. A narrow Penrose drain, passed through the window and around the oesophagus, thereafter acts as the principal oesophageal retractor.

Completion of distal oesophageal mobilization

7 With the oesophagus and anterior vagal trunk gently retracted to the left and right, respectively, the residual tissue anchoring the right side of the oesophagus can be mobilized, cauterized and divided under direct vision. At completion three fingers should be able to pass behind the oesophagus and through the window to the left of the anterior vagal trunk without tension. Any tension requires further mobilization in whichever is the appropriate direction.

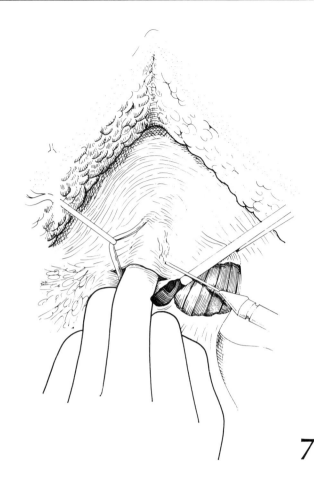

7

Crural plication

8 With the oesophagus retracted to the right, the margins of the hiatus are identified by a combination of sharp and blunt dissection and loosely plicated with one to three 0 polypropylene (Prolene) sutures, anterior to the posterior vagal trunk.

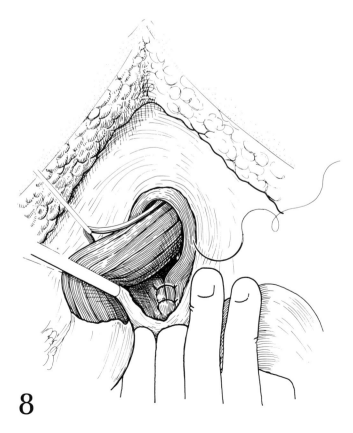

8

Testing the adequacy of fundal mobilization before fundoplication

9 The fundus is pushed behind the oesophagus into the window between the anterior vagal trunk and the oesophagus with the tips of the operator's right fingers. The ties on the short gastric vessels should appear at the leading edge. The leading edge is grasped with a pair of Babcock's forceps and approximated to the portion of anterior fundic wall to which it will be plicated, also grasped with Babcock's forceps. Tissue tension on the greater curve means that further mobilization is required.

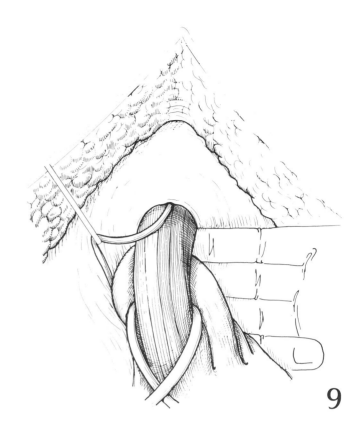

9

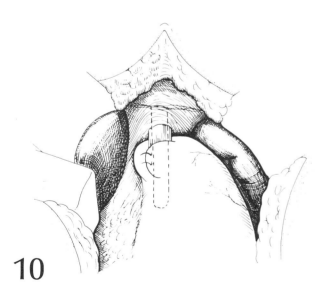

10

Fixing the fundoplication

10 The anaesthetist passes a 52–56-Fr Hurst mercury bougie orogastrically, which acts as a stent for the fundoplication. The fundoplication is secured with two or three 2/0 Prolene sutures. The oesophageal wall does not need to be incorporated in these sutures, as is commonly practised, as the fundoplication sits on the left gastric leash of vessels and cannot slip inferiorly. A single suture between the left wall of the oesophagus and the fundus prevents eversion of this aspect of the fundoplication.

Buttressing the fundoplication

11 The bougie is removed and the fundoplication may be overlaid by a 4 × 1 cm polytetrafluoroethylene (Teflon) felt patch secured at each corner by a 2/0 Prolene suture.

Wound closure

Haemostasis and the position of the nasogastric tube are checked and the abdomen is closed without drainage.

Postoperative care

Intravenous fluids and free nasogastric drainage are continued until peristaltic activity returns. The consistency of the food is progressively increased. The patient is warned first about the need to chew all foods carefully in order to avoid dysphagia, and second about the need to take small, frequent meals in the early postoperative period in the event of early satiety.

Complications

With careful attention to surgical technique, specific early complications of the operation should be extremely rare. These complications include oesophageal or fundic perforation (secondary to damage or ischaemia caused intraoperatively) and splenic haemorrhage.

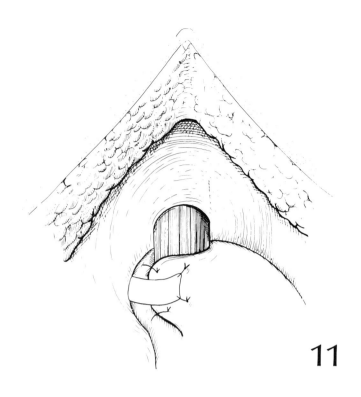

11

References

1. Nissen R. Eine einfache Operation zur Beeinflussung der Reflux-oesophagitis. *Schweiz Med Wochenschr* 1956; 86: 590–2.

2. Donahue PE, Bombeck CT. The modified Nissen fundoplication – reflux prevention without gas bloat. *Chir Gastroenterol (Surg Gastroenterol)* 1977; 11: 15–27.

Illustrations by Paul Richardson

Antireflux surgery by the thoracic approach

Clement A. Hiebert MD, FACS
Chairman Emeritus, Department of Surgery, Maine Medical Center, Portland, Maine, USA

History

Ideas get fixed in names. For much of this century surgeons treated a hiatus hernia as a muscle to be repaired, a rim to be snugged or an organ to be tethered. In 1951 Allison[1] put an end to this preoccupation with bulging stomach and showed that the symptoms of an ordinary sliding hernia derive from gastro-oesophageal reflux rather than the supposedly throttled stomach implicit in the name of the condition. Although Allison's thesis proved to be correct his repair failed the test of the follow-up clinic; it remained for Belsey and Nissen, more or less simultaneously, to develop useful and more durable operations to curb reflux. Nissen's fundoplication was a serendipitous discovery. Belsey's Mark IV operation[2], on the other hand, was the culmination of operative trials and years of observations in the endoscopy suite and follow-up clinic of Frenchay Hospital. Both operations may be performed through the chest; the Belsey operation *must* be done via that route.

The thoracic approach has a number of advantages: (1) mobilization of the oesophagus permits reduction and repair without tension; (2) when panmural oesophagitis has shortened the gullet other corrective measures are possible, e.g. Collis/Belsey (Pearson procedure), resection and interposition, or Thal patch; (3) better access to the cardia is afforded, especially in obese patients and in individuals who have undergone previous operations at the gastro-oesophageal junction.

Operation

BELSEY MARK IV PROCEDURE

The operation is performed by double-lumen tracheal intubation with collapse of the left lung.

Technique

1 With the patient in the full right lateral position a left seventh or eighth interspace is used. The higher level is chosen in obese patients where the diaphragm may be high. Postoperative intercostal pain is markedly reduced by spreading the retractor blades to a (measured) interval of less than 5 cm.

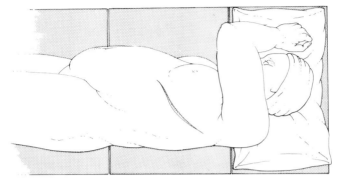

1

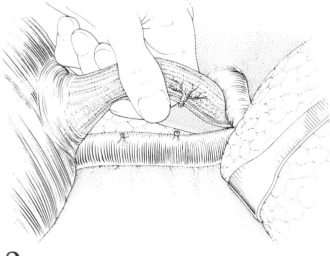

2

2 The mediastinal pleura is incised medial to the aorta from the diaphragm to the inferior pulmonary vein, thereby gaining entrance to the areolar tissue plane surrounding the (uninflamed) oesophagus. The inferior pulmonary ligament is divided and its vessel is secured. An oesophageal artery arising from the aorta is ligated and divided. The left forefinger encircles the oesophagus and both vagus nerves, the left nerve being palpable on the medial side of the oesophagus and the right nerve coming into view with elevation of the oesophagus.

3 Caudal dissection is begun with division of the pleural reflection between the muscular hiatal rim and the end of the original longitudinal mediastinal incision. The dissection is carried posteriorly to expose the two halves of the right crus of the diaphragm. Note that the muscle of both diaphragm and oesophagus is fragile.

A rubber drain is passed around the oesophagus and vagi for exposure and protection. Upon opening the endothoracic fascia at the anteromedial aspect of the hiatus the retroperitoneal fat will bulge and the inexperienced operator may mistake it for a tab of omentum. However, the peritoneum lies deep to the fat. Once the peritoneum has truly been entered it is incised laterally close to the rim until the first short gastric vessel is seen and then to the right until a thickened band of tissue is encountered. There is a variably sized vessel here that Belsey believes to be a communication between an ascending branch of the left gastric artery and the inferior phrenic artery. Division of this pedicle opens the lesser sac and exposes the caudate lobe of the liver. Circumferential clearing of the attachments of the cardia to the diaphragm is now complete.

Non-absorbable 0 sutures are passed through the two halves of the right crus of the diaphragm and the ends are set aside for later approximation. The object is both to narrow the hiatus and to provide a buttress against which the intra-abdominal oesophageal segment may press when the abdominal pressure increases. Three sutures ordinarily suffice; the tissue bites must be broad. The upper one is placed last and, for the time being, encompasses only the medial half of the crus[3].

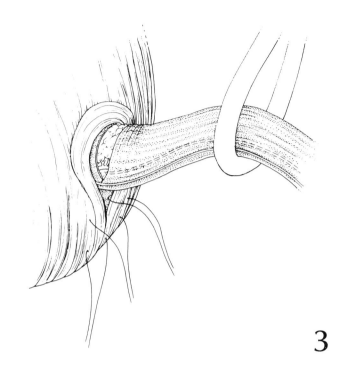

3

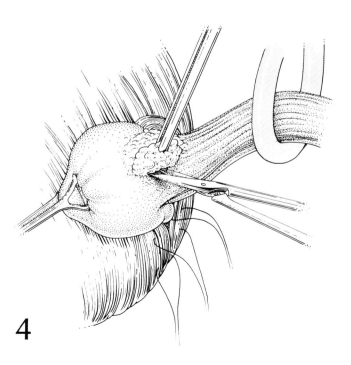

4

4 Removal of the fat pad overlying the anterior aspect of the gastro-oesophageal junction provides raw surfaces to encourage union. Numerous fine vessels here are a nuisance. As the fat pad is released from left to right the left vagus will be mobilized at its lower end and will fall posteriorly. These manoeuvres are facilitated by traction on the stomach with a non-crushing clamp.

Because the lower oesophagus is soon to be angulated by the operation the anaesthetist passes a no. 18 nasogastric tube and the surgeon manually ensures its passage into the stomach.

5 The fundoplication of the Belsey procedure is begun by placing a row of 3/0 silk or linen sutures mattressed between the stomach and adjacent oesophagus to initiate a crescentic fold, approximately 1.5 cm in width, as measured in the axis of the oesophagus. These three sutures span the interval between the two vagi. Care should be taken to avoid snaring them.

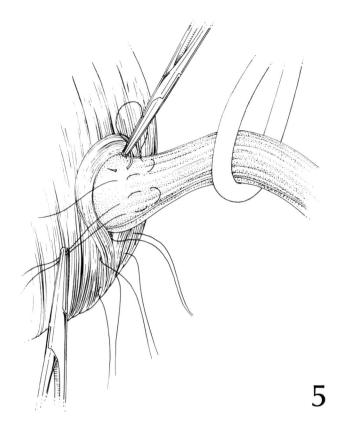

5

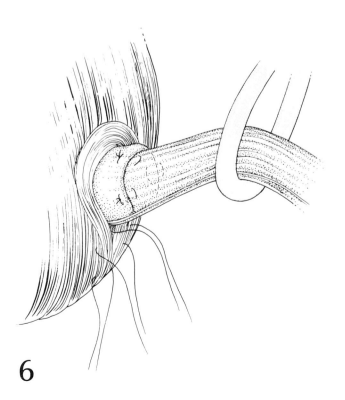

6

6 The first row of the fundoplicating sutures are knotted. The integrity of the repair depends on them not being tied so tightly as to produce necrosis and is better done by *viewing* the tissue than by feeling the tautness of the suture. Necrosis can also result from misjudging the depth of the variably thick oesophageal or gastric wall. Superficial bites may result in recurrence, and sutures that penetrate the lumen invite a fistula.

7 The second line of three sutures is placed 1.5–2 cm from the junction created by the first row and they are then passed through the diaphragm from below upwards. Lateral and medial sutures are placed first to approximate the proclaimed ideal of 240° plication as closely as possible. The vagal nerves mark the lateral extremities of the fundoplication.

Location of the sutures and the depth of their placement are critical. The length of oesophagus that can be durably anchored beneath the diaphragm is debatable; too skimpy a reduction invites reflux, too much reduction results in tension and recurrence.

A spoon retractor aids in passing the second row of sutures so that needle points emerge at the junction of the central tendon and the edge of the muscular ring without impinging on unseen abdominal viscera. Precision here can also avert the nuisance of bleeding that follows hapless stabbing of the undersurface of the diaphram.

The reconstructed cardia is now tucked into the abdomen by pushing on the cardia and tugging on the sutures. Each suture end is gently eased through the diaphragm independently of the other member of the pair so that sawing of the fragile oesophageal muscle is avoided. The fundoplication should lie below the diaphragm *without tension*. If in doubt the lines are slackened and the oesophagus is further mobilized in the region between the inferior pulmonary vein and the aortic arch. If tension still remains the operator must decide whether a lengthening procedure, as introduced by Collis and refined by Pearson, ought to be performed.

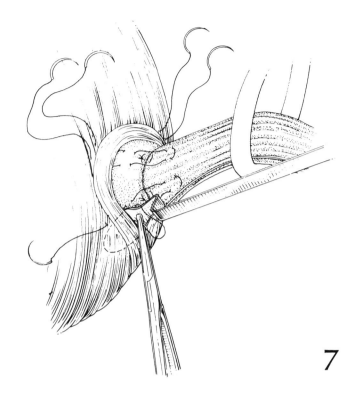

7

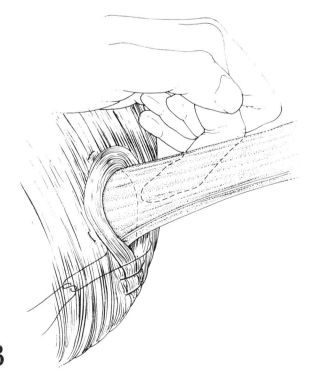

8

8 When the longitudinal aspect of the repair is deemed to be satisfactory the surgeon must ascertain that the hiatal opening is of optimal size. Beginning at the back, the two sutures uniting the halves of the right crus are knotted (again this is done by viewing rather than feeling).

The uppermost suture is completed by passing it through the oesophageal muscle beside the more posterior vagus nerve and thence through the lateral half of the right crus, this being done to discourage early herniation through the otherwise unprotected posterior hiatus. After placing the first throw of the final knot an index finger is passed to the distal interphalangeal joint behind and medial to the oesophagus. It should feel loose. If it does not the uppermost transhiatal stitch should be slackened, cut out and/or replaced.

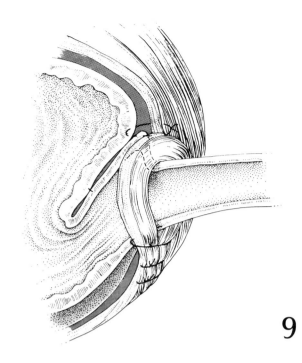

9 The 3–4-cm length of intra-abdominal oesophagus is now embraced by a 240° crescent of stomach. This seromuscular fundic fold serves, arguably, as a sphincter, probably discourages dilatation of the terminal oesophagus, and certainly gives the tethering lines a more reliable purchase than if they were passed through naked oesophageal muscle.

Postoperative care

The goal is to avoid unnecessary stress on the repair though retching, vomiting, or abdominal distension.

An analgesic is selected that has no emetogenic effect on the particular patient. A convenient way to ensure this is to use the same narcotic as was used in the premedication for endoscopy. Meperidine 25–50 mg every 2 h is usually sufficient. An antiemetic (e.g. prochlorperazine 10 mg intramuscularly) is administered every 6 h for the first 24 h.

The nasogastric tube is placed on low suction and irrigated with normal saline every 2 h. The tube is kept in place until flatus is passed and peristalsis is active. Diet is slowly advanced from clear liquids to a mechanically soft diet by the sixth or seventh postoperative day, at which point the patient usually may go home. The first oral fluids consist of tea, broth, water, gelatin dessert and flat ginger ale.

Patients are encouraged to avoid lifting anything or anyone weighing more than 18–20 kg for at least 6 months. The mechanically soft diet is advanced to full fare at 6 weeks, providing that the patient understands that chewing well and eating slowly are part of the long-term formula for success.

In addition to clinical follow-up at 3 months, 6 months, and yearly intervals, a barium study is done before discharge and repeated at 1 year. Additional radiological, endoscopic and oesophageal function studies are done as circumstances require.

Outcome

The purpose of the treatment is to eliminate gastro-oesophageal reflux while preserving the other functions of the oesophagus such as unimpeded passage of masticated food, the venting of gastric gas, and a capacity for vomiting when necessary. To assess the success of treatment those points should be addressed and the presence or absence of wound pain or numbness should be established.

Our experience of 282 patients followed for up to 20 years has shown that heartburn was either absent or occurred less than once a week in 80% of the group and about the same percentage had effortless agreeable swallowing. Ability to belch was recorded in 86% but half of the entire number felt they were excessively gassy. Of the total, 56% had had occasion to vomit and could do so, 16% had tried but were unable to and 28% had never tried.

Wound numbness or pain had been a problem in 3%; most of these problems occurred in the first years of the study. With institution of a policy of spreading the ribs no more than 5 cm, comfortable incisions became the rule.

Overall, 84% of patients were pleased with their result and 'would go through with it again' knowing what they do now.

References

1. Allison P. Reflux esophagitis, sliding hiatal hernia and anatomy of repair. *Surg Gynecol Obstet* 1951; 92: 419–31.

2. Skinner DB, Belsey R. *Management of Esophageal Disease*. Philadelphia: WB Saunders, 1988: 576–99.

3. Hiebert CA. Surgical management of esophageal reflux and hiatal hernia. *Ann Thorac Surg* 1991; 159–60.

Operations for uncomplicated gastro-oesophageal reflux: miscellaneous procedures

P. G. Devitt FRACS, FRCS
Senior Lecturer in Surgery, Department of Surgery, Royal Adelaide Hospital, Adelaide, Australia

Glyn G. Jamieson FRACS, FACS
Dorothy Mortlock Professor of Surgery, University of Adelaide, Department of Surgery, Royal Adelaide Hospital, Adelaide, Australia

Principles and justification

As with all operations designed to cure reflux, the important features are to bring the lower oesophagus into the abdomen and for it to enter the stomach at an acute angle. Protecting the lower oesophageal sphincter against the effects of proximal gastric distension may also be important. The best accepted surgical procedures for achieving these aims are the Nissen fundoplication and the Belsey (Mark IV) operations. Other procedures which probably achieve similar aims, but which have not been as widely accepted, are described below.

Operations

OESOPHAGEAL EXTENSION

1 This procedure was introduced for 'complicated' reflux when oesophageal shortening meant that the gastro-oesophageal junction could not be placed below the diaphragm. The principle is that the oesophagus is 'lengthened' by converting part of the proximal stomach into a tube, which is then sometimes referred to as the neo-oesophagus. Some surgeons have advocated the use of this procedure in uncomplicated reflux disease. Although it is possible to perform the operation by the abdominal route, as described here, a thoracic approach gives better access for the placing of staplers. To perform an extension alone, it is not necessary to mobilize the oesophagus, only to dissect the angle of His between the lower end of the oesophagus and the greater curve of the stomach. The peritoneum over this angle is divided and a finger can gently dissect bluntly down behind the stomach for 6–7 cm to open a plane for placement of the posterior jaw of an automatic stapling device.

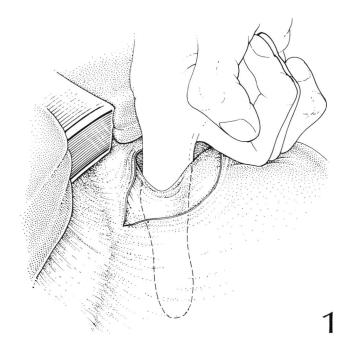

1

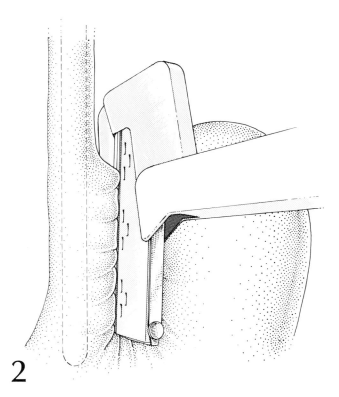

2

2 A large (>50-Fr) bougie is introduced through the mouth and passed across the gastro-oesophageal junction. The bougie is held against the lesser curve, the stapling device is inserted, and the stomach is clamped close to the bougie. The stapler should be applied so that a 3–5-cm length of neo-oesophagus is fashioned.

A potential drawback of this technique is that when the staples have been crimped there is a hole through the anterior and posterior walls of the stomach at the limit of the line of staples where the guidepin of the instrument has pierced the organ. These holes are small and may not cause problems but it may be prudent to close them with interrupted absorbable sutures. To do so, it is necessary to enter the lesser sac through the gastrocolic omentum to provide access for the hole in the posterior wall of the stomach to be repaired. It is obvious that this procedure differs little from some of the gastroplasty techniques used in the surgical treatment of obesity.

OESOPHAGEAL EXTENSION AND FUNDOPLICATION

As with oesophageal extension alone, this technique was introduced for use in situations where disease had led to shortening of the oesophagus. It is now being undertaken more widely for uncomplicated reflux. The lower end of the oesophagus is approached through a left thoracotomy. The oesophagus is mobilized up to the aortic arch and the fundus of the stomach is mobilized through the oesophageal hiatus. Several short gastric vessels need to be divided.

3 When the diaphragmatic hiatus has been cleared and the crura identified, interrupted non-absorbable sutures are placed through the medial and lateral crura in readiness to narrow the hiatus. These sutures are left loose and can be tied after the fundoplication has been fashioned and placed below the diaphragm (shown for the abdominal approach).

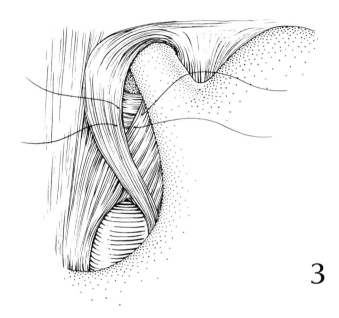

3

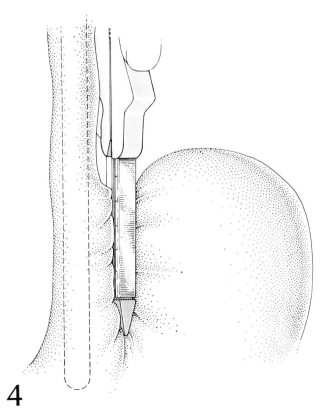

4

4 A large (>50-Fr) bougie is passed by mouth and held against the lesser curve of the stomach. If it is planned to cut the gastroplasty, a four-layered stapling device with cutter is introduced and placed parallel and close to the bougie, clamping at least 5 cm of stomach.

5 The staples are crimped and the tissue is divided. If there is any bleeding the cut edges may be oversewn with 3/0 polydioxanone. Otherwise, inversion of the suture line is not necessary. The apex of the divided stomach is now the new gastro-oesophageal junction and a 3-cm fundoplication can be fashioned around the new oesophagus (with the bougie still in place).

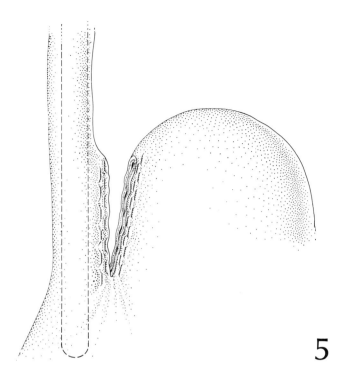

5

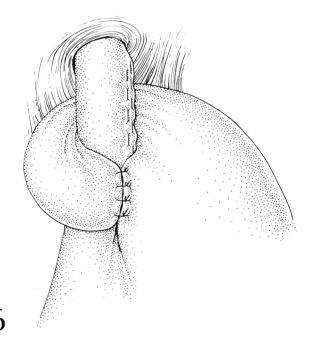

6

6 This 360° wrap around the neo-oesophagus (the Collis–Nissen operation) is reduced below the diaphragm and the crural sutures are tied. The hiatus should be narrowed so that one finger can be comfortably introduced alongside the oesophagus. The chest is closed in the usual manner with a single apical drain.

An uncut version of this operation is gaining in popularity. In this procedure the stapler is fired without cutting the stomach. The fundus lateral to (to the left of) the suture line is then wrapped around the neo-oesophagus.

ANATOMICAL REPAIR

7 This operation is designed to restore normal anatomical relationships in the region of the gastro-oesophageal junction, albeit usually exaggerating the angle of His. Although the operation was first described using a left thoracic approach, the procedure may be satisfactorily performed by the abdominal approach. This repair may be suitable for a para-oesophageal hernia, but was initially designed for gastro-oesophageal reflux. Essentially, the operation consists of reduction of the hiatus hernia and anchorage of the stomach to its normal anatomical neighbours by narrowing the hiatus (sutures inserted behind the oesophagus) and repairing the phreno-oesophageal ligament. This is done by suturing the ligament to the diaphragm. Sutures are also placed to restore the acute angle of His. Anatomical repairs have lost popularity because of a high rate of recurrent reflux when the patients are followed for a long period of time.

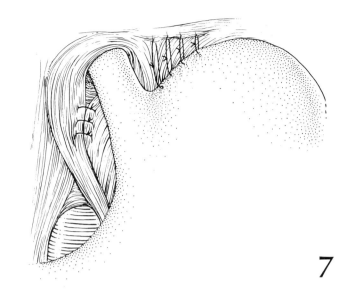

7

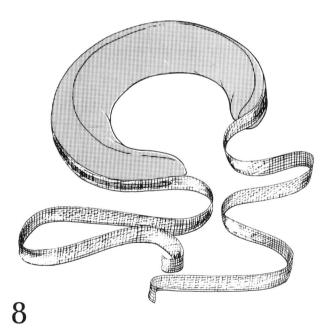

8

CIRCUMFERENTIAL PROSTHESIS (ANGELCHIK)

8 The insertion of a prosthetic collar around the lower end of the oesophagus to reduce reflux is a procedure that is technically easier to perform than many of the standard antireflux operations. The advocates of the Angelchik collar argue that it is as efficacious as conventional antireflux surgery in the prevention of reflux.

The device described by Angelchik consists of a collar-shaped tube, tapered at each end. Once in position, the ends of the collar are approximated and tied with two Dacron-reinforced ties which have been banded to the collar.

9 The lower end of the oesophagus is approached through an upper midline incision, with suitable retraction of the costal margin and left lobe of the liver. The peritoneum over the gastro-oesophageal junction is divided and the lower 2 cm of oesophagus is dissected free. One of the ties of the collar is run behind the oesophagus and the collar is slid into position. The collar is tied in front of the oesophagus. The diameter of the collar is sufficient to allow a loose fit between it and the oesophagus. Apart from problems with occasional migration, the major problem with the prosthesis is postoperative dysphagia, which is troublesome enough to require removal of the collar in about 10% of patients.

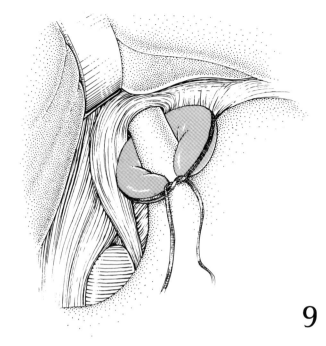

9

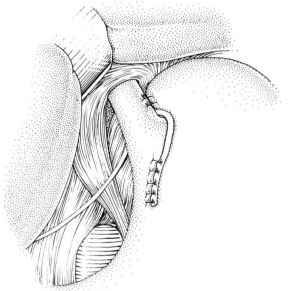

10

LIGAMENTUM TERES FIXATION

10 This procedure is used mainly in Spain, although it has also been used for laparoscopic antireflux surgery elsewhere. The gastro-oesophageal junction is approached through an upper midline incision. The overlying peritoneum is divided and a finger tunnelled around the oesophagus. The ligamentum teres is identified in the free edge of the falciform ligament and divided where it reaches the anterior abdominal wall. It is dissected free, back to its point of entry into the liver. The ligamentum teres is then slung around the gastro-oesophageal junction and sutured to the lesser curve of the stomach. The procedure is usually accompanied by stitching the greater curvature of the stomach to the left wall of the oesophagus in order to exaggerate the acute angle of His.

SUPPLEMENTAL PROXIMAL GASTRIC VAGOTOMY

The reasons advanced for incorporating this procedure with an antireflux operation include: (1) facilitation of a posterior gastropexy: opening up the lesser curve of the stomach allows more precise insertion of sutures into the median arcuate ligament and the preaortic fascia; (2) treatment of the frequent coexistence of peptic ulcer and reflux disease; and (3) reduction of the acid production of the stomach to lessen the acidity of any refluxate, i.e. a 'belt and braces' approach to the reflux problem.

11 Proximal gastric vagotomy may be combined with posterior gastropexy or fundoplication. The vagotomy is performed first. Once the nerves of Latarjet have been identified, the leaves of the lesser omentum are divided and the dissection is taken down to within 5 cm of the pylorus. The posterior gastropexy is then performed.

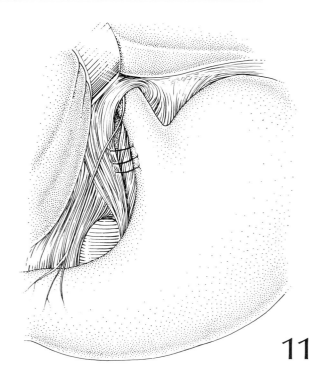

11

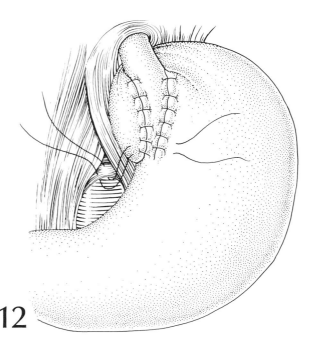

12

12 Alternatively, the proximal gastric vagotomy may be followed by a partial fundoplication and anchorage of the gastro-oesophageal junction to the median arcuate ligament.

13 Another option is to perform a proximal gastric vagotomy and total fundoplication. With the extensive dissection of the lesser curve and gastro-oesophageal junction, there is a small risk of lesser curve necrosis. Whether this risk is greater than the low risk associated with proximal gastric vagotomy alone is an open question.

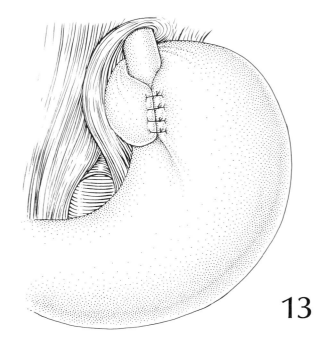

13

POSTERIOR GASTROPEXY

14 The object of this procedure is to anchor the gastro-oesophageal junction posteriorly to the median arcuate ligament. The junction is approached through an upper midline incision. The overlying peritoneum is divided and the oesophagus mobilized. A tape is passed round the oesophagus, which is retracted to the left so that the median arcuate ligament can be defined. A finger is placed behind the preaortic fascia and the median arcuate ligament. Provided the finger is kept in the midline, a plane of cleavage becomes apparent.

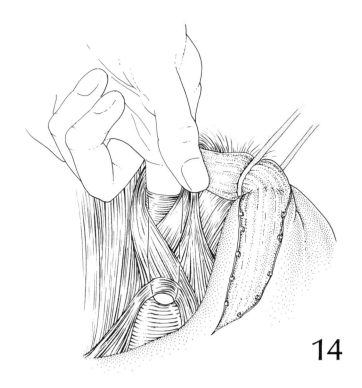

14

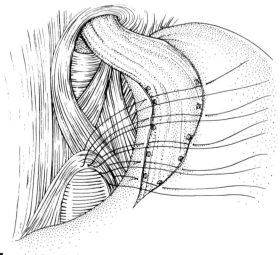

15

15 If necessary, several interrupted sutures are placed through the hiatus to narrow it. Interrupted sutures are also placed through the phreno-oesophageal bundles, the median arcuate ligament and the preaortic fascia.

16 Tightening these sutures will result in the anterior part of the fundus of the stomach being wrapped around the gastro-oesophageal junction and anchored posteriorly.

Postoperative care

Postoperative care and complications are discussed in the chapter on pp. 39–44.

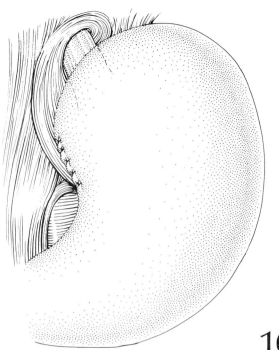

16

Reoperative antireflux surgery

Glyn G. Jamieson FRACS, FACS
Dorothy Mortlock Professor of Surgery, University of Adelaide, Department of Surgery, Royal Adelaide Hospital, Adelaide, Australia

The long-term results of modern antireflux surgery are excellent. A failure rate of 10–20% over a long period of time, however, has been recorded with all operations currently undertaken. The majority of these failures occur in the first 2 years after operation. The commonest cause is recurrence of the original problem, i.e. recurrent reflux. In a smaller proportion of patients, there may be new problems such as dysphagia or chronic abdominal pain.

The requirement of reoperative surgery therefore falls into two categories. First is the management of patients with recurrent reflux. The decision for further surgery is here based on exactly the same criteria as for primary antireflux surgery, i.e. either intractable oesophagitis or complications from the reflux as described in the chapter on pp. 292–293. In this group of patients the aim of surgery is the same as in primary reflux disease, but the technique for achieving that aim may have to be modified. Second, there is the much smaller group of patients in whom the reason for further surgery is related to a complication of the surgery itself. This may be:

1. Dysphagia – the repair may have been made too tight, the oesophagus may be adynamic above a total wrap, or the hiatus may have been narrowed excessively by sutures.
2. Bloating after meals. It is very uncommon for this symptom to be so severe that it is necessary to undo a previous wrap.
3. Chronic postprandial pain syndrome. This occurs infrequently, but is sometimes a difficult problem.

On occasions a gastric ulcer is found in the region of the fundoplication, or a paraoesophageal hernia associated with the fundic wrap. Often no cause for the pain is found. In this situation the surgeon should only reoperate when a gastroenterological colleague, and possibly a psychiatrist, are in agreement that the patient's pain is apparently related to the previous surgery. When no overt cause for pain is found at operation, the surgeon has little alternative but to take the wrap down and substitute some other procedure, e.g. a partial fundoplication. Even with this cautious approach it should be stressed to the patient that the likelihood of a successful outcome is low.

Principles and justification

Early in the author's career it made good sense to operate via a previously unoperated approach. Thus, if the patient had previously undergone operation via an abdominal approach, the operation was carried out using the thoracic approach, or vice versa. Increasingly, the author has used the abdominal approach even when the previous surgery has been from the abdomen. This approach causes considerably less morbidity than a thoracic approach and also provides better access to the often dense adhesions associated with recurrent problems in this area. This approach will therefore be described here.

Operation

Incision

An upper midline incision is used. The findings in the region of the oesophageal hiatus are quite unpredictable. Sometimes it is almost as if no previous surgery has actually been carried out. At the other end of the spectrum are patients who have had some form of associated surgery, e.g. proximal gastric vagotomy, antiobesity surgery, or myotomy. In these patients the lesser curve is densely adherent to the liver, and there are other fibrous adhesions in the region. Whatever the circumstances, it is best first to define the upper limit of the dissection by seeking the oesophagus. A nasogastric tube should be passed to aid in this identification.

1 If adhesions are particularly dense in the region, the oesophagus is best approached by incising the diaphragm above and anterior to the hiatus and entering the thorax immediately proximal to the hiatus. It is then usually a relatively simple matter to mobilize the oesophagus and place a sling around it.

It is also important to mobilize the whole of the oesophagus distal to this point, the gastro-oesophageal junction and the upper stomach. This is done anteriorly by dividing adhesions from the stomach to the liver and diaphragm, using sharp dissection. Posteriorly, the lesser sac is entered and the stomach is dissected free from the pancreas and retroperitoneal tissues.

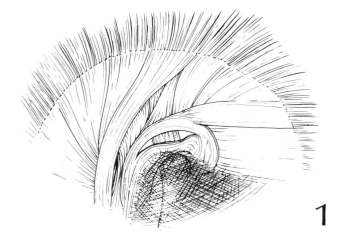

1

2 It is only when the gastro-oesophageal junction and the proximal stomach are completely free that any assessment can be made of the cause of the failure. Even then it is not always easy to be certain of the exact nature of the problem. Perhaps most commonly the fundoplication is around the stomach, rather than the oesophagus, either because it was constructed in that way in the first place, or because the oesophagus has pulled the stomach up through the fundoplication.

If possible, the fundoplication should be taken down in its entirety. This is a tedious process and can prove difficult to achieve without perforating the stomach. Any perforation should be closed immediately.

If the fundoplication has come undone, or was originally incomplete, it is permissible to leave it and construct a new fundoplication proximal to or around the old fundoplication.

It is usually necessary to divide all of the short gastric vessels in order to have enough stomach to carry out a new fundoplication. The author uses a double-wrap technique to make sure that the fundoplication will not come undone at a later date. Three sutures of 3/0 Prolene are inserted to create a 2-cm-long wrap, with a 50–60 French bougie in position. The sutures incorporate layers of stomach, oesophageal wall and stomach. Once this wrap has been constructed, two further sutures are placed in such a way as to bury the previous suture line. It is better not to anchor the wrap in any way within the abdominal cavity, as this provides the potential for the oesophagus to pull stomach up through the wrap.

If the dissection has been difficult, it is often unclear at the end of the procedure whether or not the vagus nerves have been divided. It was the author's previous practice to add a pyloroplasty if it was thought that the vagi had been divided, particularly if preoperative gastric emptying was demonstrated to be delayed.

Because it was found that patients having a pyloroplasty after previous antireflux surgery seemed to have more problems than patients not having a pyloroplasty, the technique of using a pyloroplasty primarily in this situation has now been abandoned.

If, after the whole area has been mobilized, the gastro-oesophageal junction is at or above the level of the hiatus, some form of oesophageal extension gastroplasty is added before carrying out the fundoplication as described in the chapter on pp. 307–315.

If the reoperation is a third operation in the area, then unless there is a clear reason why a further fundoplication should be attempted, the author progresses straight to a Roux-en-Y antrectomy as described in the chapter on pp. 335–344.

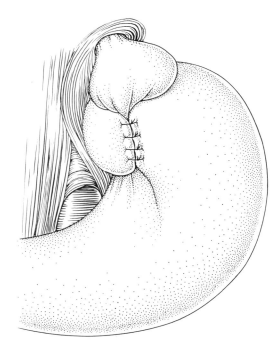

2

Outcome

Since 1978 the author has operated on 45 patients for recurrent reflux and ten patients for dysphagia following previous antireflux surgery. The author had undertaken the original surgery in 14 of the patients. Previous surgery consisted of a total fundoplication in 25, a Belsey mark IV operation in seven, a proximal gastric vagotomy and fundoplication in eight, and in 15 patients the type of previous repair was unknown. Eleven patients had undergone two or more previous procedures. In 20 patients the previous fundoplication had probably come undone, in 11 the fundoplication appeared to be around the stomach, indicating either slippage or pull-through, and in 14 patients it was difficult to be certain whether the repair had partially come undone, had undergone partial pull-through, or was not working for unknown reasons. Three of the cases of dysphagia were due to an Angelchik prosthesis, an over-tight fundoplication and a too-narrow closure of the hiatus; the remaining seven had a fundoplication performed distal to an atonic oesophagus, five patients having had a long myotomy for 'spasm', one patient a short myotomy for achalasia and one patient a

'scleroderma' oesophagus. The reoperations carried out were total fundoplication in 24 (four with a proximal gastric vagotomy and six with a pyloroplasty), oesophageal extension gastroplasty in four, antrectomy and Roux-en-Y in four, repair of paraoesophageal hernia in three and one each of total gastrectomy, division of hiatus and removal of an Angelchik prosthesis.

There were two postoperative deaths, both from cardiac causes, at day 2 and day 6 after operation. Median follow-up in the patients was 38 months (range 6–170 months). The results were rated by the patient and an independent observer as good to excellent in 83% of cases. Sixteen patients had either a drainage procedure or a gastric resection, and seven patients experienced dumping symptoms. Eight of the 11 patients having a third or further operation achieved a good result.

Thus, reoperative surgery can produce results that are in many ways comparable with primary antireflux operations, particularly when the operation does not interfere with pyloric function.

Intrathoracic fundoplication

James W. Maher MD
Section of Gastrointestinal Surgery, Department of Surgery, University of Iowa Hospitals and Clinics and
College of Medicine, Iowa City, Iowa, USA

History

The Nissen fundoplication provides extremely effective protection against gastro-oesophageal reflux and has become the benchmark antireflux procedure. Part of the appeal of fundoplication lies in the large number of ways in which it may be modified to accommodate the needs of individual patients. Most patients with gastro-oesophageal reflux and oesophagitis may be treated by transabdominal fundoplication. Intrathoracic (supradiaphragmatic) fundoplication may be defined as a variant of fundoplication in which the operation is performed via a left thoracotomy and the wrap is deliberately left partially in the chest. It was first described by Krupp and Rosetti[1] and has proved extremely useful in the therapy of patients with acquired oesophageal shortening. Their overall results were excellent, but there were two episodes of gastric fistula in the early postoperative period that resulted in death. No details of these complications were provided. They reported four deaths from peritonitis in patients who had undergone transabdominal fundoplication,

underscoring the point that none of the antireflux procedures are without complications. Many surgeons have regarded supradiaphragmatic fundoplication as the procedure of choice in the occasional patient with marked oesophageal shortening.

Nicholson and Nohl-Oser in their review of 141 patients in which the wrap was deliberately left in the supradiaphragmatic position reported that excellent long-term results were achieved, with no complications that were attributable to the presence of the wrap in the chest[2].

Despite the usefulness of this approach, two reports have documented an unusual number of life-threatening complications in relatively small numbers of patients with intrathoracic wraps[3,4]. These reports led the author and colleagues to a critical review of the records of all patients in whom fundoplications had been left above the diaphragm, paying special attention to both complications and long-term results[5]. The results of that review are included in this chapter.

Principles and justification

Indications

The assumption that most patients with oesophagitis should undergo transabdominal fundoplication is the starting point. Transthoracic fundoplication is reserved for patients in whom shortening of the oesophagus may place tension on the completed repair. This includes patients who have had a previous antireflux procedure, patients with radiographic evidence of acquired oesophageal shortening from long-standing reflux, and patients with a longitudinal oesophageal stricture that is not easily dilated in the preoperative period. When used in these situations, the surgeon may mobilize the scarred oesophagus extensively. In many cases this will allow the wrap to be replaced into the abdomen without tension. However, if scarring from a previous antireflux procedure or transmural oesophagitis has led to acquired oesophageal shortening, this precludes restoration of the wrap to an intra-abdominal position without tension. Attempts at intra-abdominal reduction in this situation may ultimately lead to dehiscence or intussusception of the wrap down on to the body of the stomach because of the tension on the oesophagus. This situation results in recurrent severe reflux. Another approach is to lengthen the oesophagus by the Collis technique so that the wrap can lie in the abdomen. The author's preference in this situation has been to leave some of the wrap in the chest, securing it circumferentially to the diaphragm.

Preoperative

A thorough preoperative assessment of all patients felt to be candidates for fundoplication should detect most patients who should undergo transthoracic fundoplication. The preoperative assessment of patients undergoing antireflux procedures is described in the chapter on pp. 39–44. Here we will focus on the special needs of those requiring transthoracic fundoplication. Attention should be given to any history of previous antireflux surgery. Previous transabdominal antireflux procedures frequently produce rather marked scarring of the distal oesophagus. Additionally, a repeat transabdominal procedure may be fraught with hazard if adhesions between the liver and stomach are severe. A transthoracic approach to this situation allows the surgeon to side-step the 'footprints' of the previous operator, which in turn allows a more precise anatomical dissection of the fundus and construction of a better wrap. A history of Raynaud's phenomenon should be sought since this may be the first indication of oesophageal scleroderma. If the presence of scleroderma is confirmed, surgery should be avoided if at all possible because fundoplication may make these patients worse. This is understandable if it is remembered that fundoplication works by creating a pressure gradient that prevents reflux of gastro-oesophageal contents. However, this pressure barrier may also create an antegrade barrier to passage of solid food if the oesophagus is aperistaltic, as it is in scleroderma.

Barium swallow

All patients should undergo a barium swallow examination before surgery. Attention must be paid to the presence of a hiatus hernia, reflux, stricture (annular or longitudinal), oesophageal shortening and the quality of peristalsis visible on fluoroscopy. If the hernia is of the sliding type, whether or not it is reducible and whether there is any tortuosity of the distal oesophagus should be noted. An irreducible hiatus hernia should alert the surgeon to the possibility that he or she might be dealing with a shortened oesophagus that should be approached transthoracically. However, the author has noted that if the distal oesophagus is somewhat tortuous, the fundoplication may usually be performed transabdominally even in the presence of an irreducible hiatus hernia. There are no hard and fast rules that make identification of a short oesophagus completely reliable. It just looks short on barium studies and has the appearance of drawing the stomach up into the chest. An annular stricture, by itself, is not an indication for a transthoracic approach. Such strictures can be dilated before operation and treated with a simple transabdominal fundoplication. However, longitudinal strictures (also referred to as transmural strictures) should be approached through the chest, especially if the stricture is difficult to dilate before surgery. These strictures are commonly associated with oesophageal shortening because of involvement of the longitudinal muscle by the transmural scarring. Additionally, if the stricture cannot be dilated before surgery the patient may be treated by combining a Thal fundic patch with fundoplication through the chest.

Upper gastrointestinal endoscopy

Most patients will have undergone endoscopy with establishment of the diagnosis of oesophagitis before surgical referral but it is sometimes wise to repeat this study.

If the patient has an oesophageal stricture, even a long-standing one, the surgeon must be sure that the possibility of malignancy has been excluded by both brushings and biopsy. This is especially important if the patient has a history of Barrett's metaplasia. Ideally, all strictures should be dilated in the preoperative period because this establishes that the stricture can indeed be dilated. Many strictures that are difficult to dilate intraoperatively can be easily dilated at endoscopy with Savary or balloon dilators. There is the additional advantage of having a conscious patient who can respond to pain, thus minimizing the risk of perforation. If the stricture cannot be dilated a transthoracic approach should be elected.

Oesophageal manometry

Ideally, manometry should be undertaken on all patients undergoing surgery for oesophageal reflux to establish the presence of normal peristalsis. Manometry is especially important in patients with dysphagia because the incidence of motility disorders in these patients is higher.

Preparation of patient

A healthy oesophageal lumen is sterile. Swallowing produces a transient contamination of the lumen, but the flora are rapidly cleared by peristalsis. Oesophageal obstruction leads to an accumulation of both bacteria and saliva that gradually produces a colonic-type flora. This is aggravated by H_2 antagonists which inhibit acid production, leading to an increase in bacterial colony counts. Gastric colony counts of the order of 10^6 are common in patients on H_2 blockers. The following steps may be taken to try to reduce the incidence of infectious complications:

1. If the oesophagus has not been dilated, the patient should receive only clear liquids for 24 h before operation.
2. To reduce the risk of aspiration the oesophagus should be emptied with a nasogastric tube before induction of anaesthesia.
3. The oesophagus is lavaged with kanamycin, 1 g, in saline after induction of anaesthesia.
4. Cephazolin, 1 g, is given on transfer to the operating theatre and every 8 h for three doses.
5. If there is any possibility of oesophageal resection, the colon should be prepared mechanically and with antibiotics.

Anaesthesia

One lung ventilation is particularly helpful in achieving adequate exposure but can be somewhat tricky unless the anaesthetist has substantial experience with the technique.

Operation

After induction of anaesthesia a nasogastric tube is passed into the stomach and the patient is placed in a standard left thoracotomy position. The operation is performed transpleurally through the bed of the resected sixth or seventh rib.

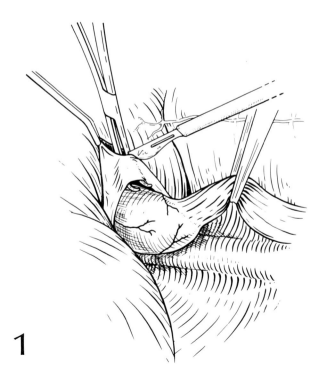

1 After dividing the inferior pulmonary ligament to just below the left inferior pulmonary vein the oesophagus is mobilized bluntly and encircled with a Penrose drain. The diaphragm is incised radially from the oesophageal hiatus. Care is taken to preserve the branches of the phrenic nerve. The hiatal incision provides access to the left upper quadrant and prevents constriction of the wrap at the diaphragm if the wrap cannot be reduced. The vasa brevia are ligated to allow the fundus to flop into the chest.

2 The anaesthetist passes a 42-Fr bougie perorally alongside the nasogastric tube. The fundoplication is performed over this bougie on the left lateral border of the oesophagus with non-absorbable sutures (2/0 braided Dacron). (The author prefers not to use monofilament because of its stiffness.) No oesophageal bites are included at this point because they would leave the fundoplication with a permanent 120° twist compared with its position when performed intra-abdominally. This poses no problems if the repair is reducible; however, should scarring or acquired shortening necessitate leaving the wrap in a supra-diaphragmatic position, this twist could create a functional obstruction at the diaphragmatic closure.

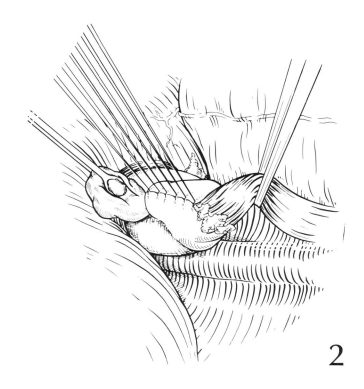

2

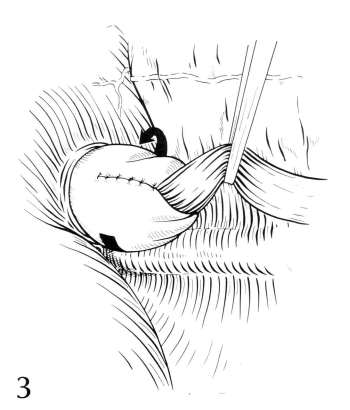

3

3 The fundoplication is now rotated clockwise so that the suture line is on the right-hand border of the oesophagus.

4 The wrap is secured to the oesophagus with interrupted sutures of 2/0 silk.

An attempt is then made to reduce the wrap to an intra-abdominal position. Mobilization of the oesophagus to the aortic arch may facilitate this. It is not necessary to worry about compromising the blood supply of the oesophagus: longitudinal collaterals are more than adequate to compensate for the loss of direct aortic branches.

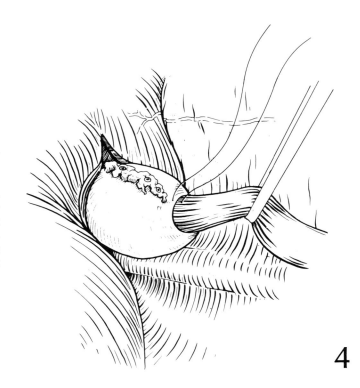

4

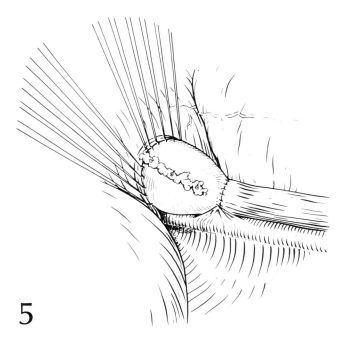

5

5 If the wrap cannot be reduced intra-abdominally without tension, it is sutured circumferentially to the hiatus with 2/0 braided Dacron sutures after reducing as much fundus as possible. Care must be taken not to create a 'waist' in the stomach by closing the hiatus too tightly. This mistake may result in functional obstruction of the supradiaphragmatic stomach.

Diaphragmatic closure is an irremediable weakness of all transthoracic procedures on abdominal organs. This is easily understood when one considers that the diaphragm contracts 900 times per hour. It is therefore imperative that the surgeon exercises special care during this portion of the operation so that the risk of diaphragmatic hernia is minimized. The chest is closed in standard fashion. Two chest tubes are used. A 28-Fr tube is placed anteriorly in the apex of the left chest to ensure full pulmonary re-expansion. A 32-Fr angle tube is placed posteriorly in the costodiaphragmatic sulcus near the wrap.

Postoperative care

Nasogastric decompression is maintained for 3–5 days to allow return of normal peristalsis. Most of these patients cannot vomit. An ileus can therefore create a closed loop obstruction and a life-threatening situation. When effective peristalsis has resumed, the nasogastric tube is removed. All patients are started on intravenous metoclopramide, 10 mg four times daily, which has been found empirically to reduce gas bloat symptoms. When oral intake can be tolerated they may be switched to oral metoclopramide, which is continued for 6 weeks.

The anterior chest tube is removed on the first day after operation if the lung is fully expanded. The posterior tube is not removed until the patient is tolerating oral intake.

Any signs suggestive of a leak (tachycardia, fever, leucocytosis, etc.) should prompt the surgeon to obtain a water-soluble contrast study of the oesophagus and stomach. This is a very rare complication unless the gastric lumen has been violated during surgery.

Outcome

Forty-four patients (25 men, 19 women) of mean age 56 (range 27–74) years underwent supradiaphragmatic fundoplications between 1970 and 1982. Follow-up was obtained by chart review, clinic visits and telephone interviews with the patients, referring physicians, or next of kin if the patient had died.

The indications for surgery in this group of patients represented a wide spectrum of the complications of advanced oesophagitis. Many had multiple indications. Twenty-one patients had strictures which could not be dilated before surgery, but which were dilatable in the operating room. The author maintains that patients with strictures that are difficult to dilate before surgery should undergo a transthoracic approach to allow performance of a combined Thal patch–Nissen fundoplication if there is a longitudinal transmural oesophageal stricture because the results of dilatation and antireflux procedure alone in this group are poor. Eight of the patients with stricture had had previous antireflux procedures. These included nine fundoplications that had either slipped or disrupted, presumably because of acquired oesophageal shortening. Two individuals had undergone previous fundoplications that were intact but had apparently been wrapped too tightly. Symptoms in this group included severe dysphagia. Radiographic and manometric findings simulated achalasia. Four patients had obvious acquired shortening of the oesophagus on barium swallow examination, despite the absence of previous oesophageal surgery.

Three of the 44 (7%) patients were lost to follow-up at periods ranging from 3 weeks to 9 months. Mean follow-up was 42 (range 4–98) months. There were two hospital deaths (5%). One patient died from anoxic brain damage several days after a respiratory arrest sustained in the recovery room. The other had undergone a fundoplication with vagotomy and drainage 3 years previously and this had failed to control his symptoms. Extensive adhesions encountered during the operation made dissection difficult and apparently led to devascularization of the proximal stomach. An oesophagogastrectomy was performed at the same procedure but the patient developed an oesophago-cutaneous fistula with uncontrolled sepsis and died. This death therefore represents a technical error, not a fundamental defect in the operation itself.

There was one late postoperative death which illustrates the danger of intestinal obstruction in patients with a fundoplication, as the patient developed a perforation of the stomach before nasogastric aspiration was instituted. This case clearly documents the urgency of establishing nasogastric decompression in patients with suspected intestinal obstruction following fundoplication.

Two patients were considered to have had poor results (5%). In one patient this was associated with scleroderma of the oesophagus and subsequent colon replacement alleviated her problem. The other patient developed a severe gas bloat syndrome after surgery and was subsequently shown to have developed herniation of most of the stomach into the chest. This was repaired with a satisfactory result.

There were two other incidences of diaphragmatic hernia in the early postoperative period. This is a troublesome problem which it was originally thought would be eliminated by meticulous attention to the details of diaphragmatic closure. This has reduced the incidence of the problem, but not eliminated it. It appears that suture closure of a muscular organ which contracts cannot be successfully accomplished all of the time. It is nevertheless worth noting that these patients have subsequently had the hernia repaired and ultimately achieved a satisfactory result.

Gastric ulceration was seen in two patients but the ulcers were not noted to be in or near the wrap in either of these cases.

Good to excellent results were achieved in 82% of patients (68% excellent, 14% good). This represents 88% of patients not lost to follow-up. Sixteen patients have now been followed for longer than 5 years and there have been no late complications in this group.

The results of 68 combined Thal patch–Nissen fundoplication procedures, in which the wraps remain in an intrathoracic position, have also been reviewed and similar results found.

Complications

A review of the recent literature warning of the dangers of supradiaphragmatic fundoplication reveals three general categories of complication: (1) diaphragmatic hernia; (2) gastric ulceration; and (3) gastric fistula.

Meticulous attention to the details of diaphragmatic closure with heavy non-absorbable suture is the best method for reducing the potentially hazardous complication of diaphragmatic hernia.

Gastric ulceration is a more serious problem[3,4] and has been reported to occur in from 3% to 10% of patients undergoing transabdominal fundoplication[6]. The high incidence reported in intrathoracic fundoplication appears to be due to technical differences in the operations that various surgeons choose to term 'intrathoracic' or 'supradiaphragmatic' fundoplication. It is possible that an inadequately patulous hiatus might lead to constriction of the supradiaphragmatic stomach. The author routinely requires that the hiatus be fist-sized to allow for any subsequent contraction of the hiatal ring from scarring.

Fistula formation is another serious complication but this also has been reported after transabdominal wraps. The nasogastric tube may be left in place until normal gastric emptying and peristalsis has resumed as it is felt that this avoids distension of the fundoplication with the possibility of leakage.

Since the previous published reports, the author has performed an additional 20 intrathoracic fundoplications. Good control of reflux has been obtained in all patients. One individual developed a diaphragmatic hernia 6 months after the initial surgery; it required operative repair.

Conclusions

Supradiaphragmatic fundoplication offers effective protection against complicated gastro-oesophageal reflux, with an acceptable morbidity and low mortality. It should be emphasized that these results were not achieved in cases of primary oesophagitis, but in the small percentage of patients who presented as either failures of previous operative procedures or with severe transmural oesophagitis with oesophageal shortening.

The alternative to a supradiaphragmatic fundoplication in an individual with acquired shortening is a Collis gastroplasty combined with a fundoplication and good results have been reported with this approach. In previously operated patients, any alterations in blood supply to the fundus might render the neo-oesophageal suture line ischaemic. Thus, it does not seem prudent to add a possible complicating factor to a proven operation unless there is a demonstrable benefit.

Fundoplication represents the most effective procedure available for the therapy of reflux oesophagitis. In the patient with a shortened oesophagus, whether from transmural oesophagitis or previous surgery, supradiaphragmatic placement of the fundoplication results in uniform control of gastro-oesophageal reflux with an acceptable morbidity and low mortality.

References

1. Krupp S, Rosetti M. Surgical treatment of hiatal hernias by fundoplication and gastropexy (Nissen repair). *Ann Surg* 1966; 164: 927–34.

2. Nicholson DAS, Nohl-Oser HC. Hiatus hernia: a comparison between two methods of fundoplication by evaluation of the long-term results. *J Thorac Cardiovasc Surg* 1976; 72: 938–43.

3. Mansour KA, Burton HG, Miller JI, Hatcher CR. Complication of intrathoracic Nissen fundoplication. *Ann Thorac Surg* 1981; 32: 173–8.

4. Richardson JD, Larson GM, Polk HC. Intra-thoracic fundoplication for shortened eosphagus: treacherous solution to a challenging problem. *Am J Surg* 1982; 143: 29–35.

5. Maher JW, Hocking MP, Woodward ER. Supra-diaphragmatic fundoplications: long-term follow-up and analysis of complications. *Am J Surg* 1984; 147: 181–6.

6. Bremner CG. Gastric ulceration after a fundoplication operation for gastro-oesophageal reflux. *Surg Gynecol Obstet* 1979; 148: 62–4.

Combined Collis–Nissen operation

Victor F. Trastek MD, FACS
Consultant, Section of General Thoracic Surgery, Mayo Clinic and Mayo Foundation and Associate Professor of Surgery, Mayo Medical School, Rochester, Minnesota, USA

W. Spencer Payne MD
Emeritus Consultant, Section of General Thoracic Surgery, Mayo Clinic and Mayo Foundation and Emeritus Professor of Surgery, Mayo Medical School, Rochester, Minnesota, USA

Principles and justification

The sensitivity of oesophageal mucosa to certain digestive secretions has been implicated in almost all the complications of gastro-oesophageal reflux. Gastro-oesophageal incompetence permits free reflux of the gastroduodenal contents to the oesophagus. The recognized oesophageal consequences of this reflux are directly related to the effects of the secretions on the oesophagus and to the tissue's response to chemical injury. These consequences are: desquamation; erosion; ulceration; inflammation; pain; bleeding; motility disturbances; oesophageal shortening; stricture formation and Barrett's disease (columnar epithelial lining of the lower oesophagus). Complications vary from patient to patient, and the pathological processes are often reversed by eliminating the contact between the corrosive secretions and the oesophagus.

Surgical control of the complications of gastro-oesophageal reflux depends upon restoring gastro-oesophageal competence. Many different surgical approaches have been used to accomplish competence, but the authors currently advocate a combined Collis–Nissen operation. This technique is a modification of Nissen's 360° fundoplication and Collis's technique for lengthening the oesophagus, to provide a tension-free wrap.

The uncut Collis–Nissen gastroplasty, which uses a stapling device applied to the stomach, allows a 3-cm neo-oesophagus to be developed and a 360° Nissen fundoplication to be made around it. This restores gastro-oesophageal competence and provides excellent protection from oesophageal reflux. By minimizing the length of the uncut Collis manoeuvre (3 cm) and the fundoplication (2 cm) a reasonably low rate of dysphagia is possible without sacrificing control of reflux.

Preoperative

Placement of a double-lumen endotracheal tube following induction of anaesthesia collapses the lung and gives a quiet operative field. The patient is placed in the right lateral decubitus position and stabilized with appropriate bolsters.

Operation

Incision

1 A left thoracotomy is performed, and the pleural space is entered through the periosteal bed of the non-resected eighth rib. Following a posterolateral thoracotomy, the chest cavity and lung should be thoroughly explored.

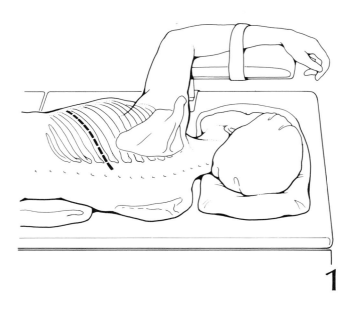

1

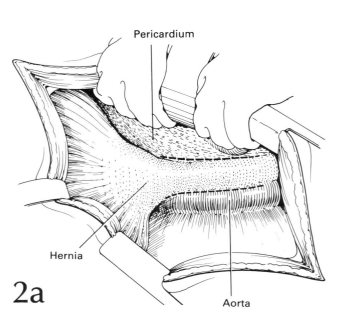

2a

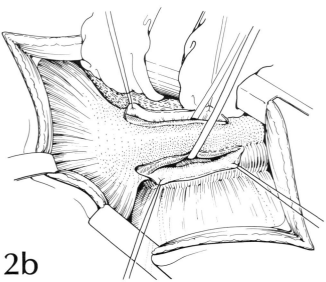

2b

Exposure

2a–c The inferior pulmonary vein is divided and the lung collapsed, retracted cephalad, and packed away out of the operative field. The oesophagus, gastro-oesophageal junction, stomach, and hernia sac (if present) should be freed from the mediastinum extending from the inferior pulmonary vein to the hiatus. The mediastinal pleura along the pericardium is divided and dissected down through the associated plane to the parietal pleura of the opposite chest cavity. A second incision is made parallel to the aorta through the mediastinal pleura and carried down, freeing the hernia sac and oesophagus from the parietal pleura down to the hiatus. The intrathoracic protrusion of proximal stomach and gastro-oesophageal junction is usually apparent. The oesophagus (including the vagal nerves) is then surrounded with a Penrose drain.

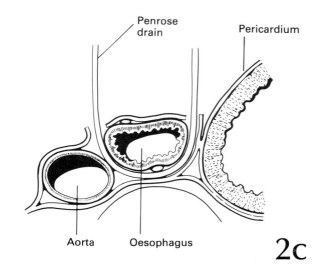

2c

Dissection of oesophageal hiatus

3a–d The posterior or right crus is identified during the exposure of the hiatus, the lesser sac is entered and the liver edge identified. Anteriorly, the phreno-oesophageal ligament should be freed from the anterior or left crus using cautery to increase the portion of sac available for division. The sac is then entered and the phreno-oesophageal ligament and sac are resected medially by placing the fingers of the left hand astride the attachments between the gastro-oesophageal junction and the crura of the diaphragm, dividing the hepatic branches of the vagus nerve and joining up with the posterior division of the sac made previously. The anterior sac is then divided laterally, stopping at the level of the short gastric vessels. This completely frees the sac circumferentially from all hiatal attachments except the short gastric vessels.

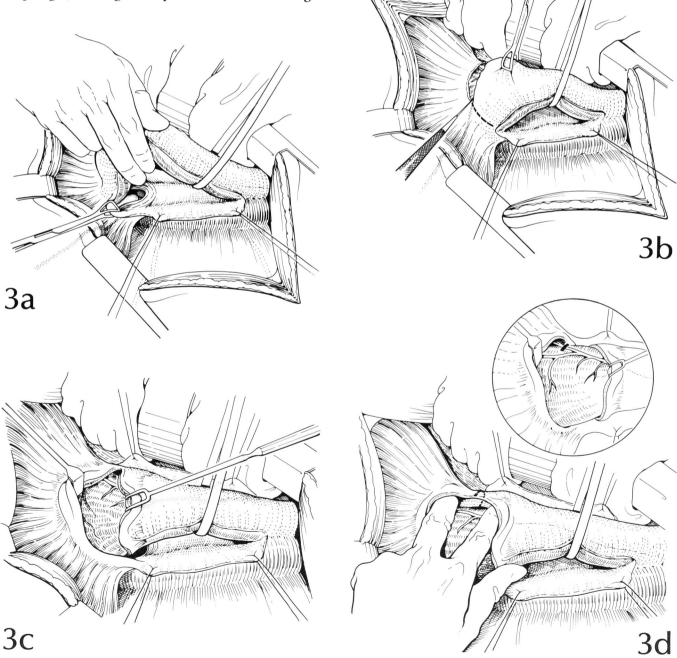

3a

3b

3c

3d

Division of short gastric vessels

4 A small Richardson retractor is placed in the caudad position and a lung clamp on the stomach in the cephalad direction just below the gastro-oesophageal junction and the short gastric vessels are exposed, ligated with 2/0 silk and divided. If the hernia is large, this task is relatively easy as the short gastric vessels are elongated. However, if the hernia sac is very small, this portion of the operation may need to be completed through a separate radial incision in the diaphragm. The short gastric vessels are divided until the right gastroepiploic arcade is visible. This completes the exposure and mobilization of the oesophagus, gastro-oesophageal junction and fundus, from the inferior pulmonary vein to mid-stomach on the greater curve side.

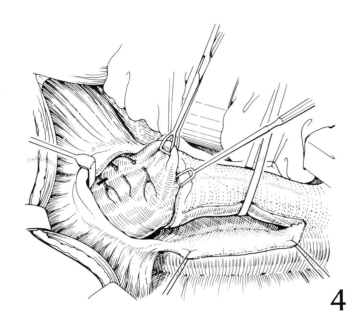

Placement of crural sutures for closure of hiatus

5 The stomach and gastro-oesophageal junction are reduced to ensure that they will easily go below the hiatus. The need for a lengthening procedure is rare, except in the case of reoperations. At this stage the hiatal crural sutures should be placed and tagged, because they will allow the hiatus to be closed as the last step of the procedure. Figure-of-eight sutures of 1 polypropylene (Prolene) are placed through the right and left crura, taking up the right crus to the insertion of the pericardium but using only half of the left crus. This allows space for the oesophagus and gastro-oesophageal junction when the sutures are tied. Care must be taken not to drive the sutures within the pericardium and that they do not become twisted during placement.

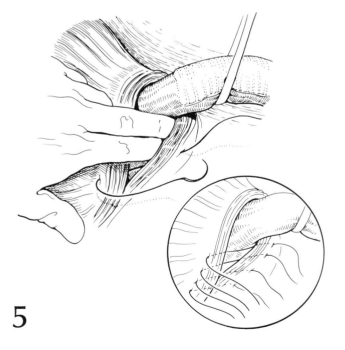

Removal of gastro-oesophageal fat pad

6 The gastro-oesophageal fat pad is divided in the midline and removed, moving cephalad from the stomach to the gastro-oesophageal junction and oesophagus. Both vagal trunks should be carefully preserved. The trunks may be visualized and palpated, but at no time should they be put in jeopardy. The remaining fatty tissue, including the vagus nerves, is allowed to retract and will be included within the wrap. Meticulous cauterization or ligation of multiple gastric nutrient vessels is required to avoid formation of a haematoma. This manoeuvre clears a portion of the gastric serosa and gastro-oesophageal junction for the later steps of the operation and exposes sound tissue in which to place the fundoplication sutures.

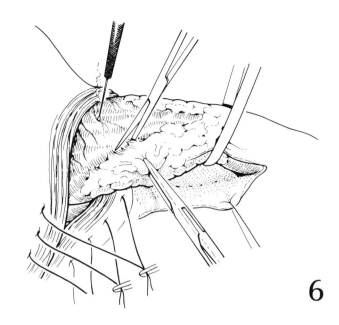

6

Uncut Collis gastroplasty

7a, b A 50-Fr Maloney dilator is passed by mouth through the gastro-oesophageal junction into the stomach, for use as a mandrel about which an uncut tubular extension of the oesophagus will be fashioned from the lesser curvature of the stomach. This is accurately and simply achieved by applying a TA 30 stapler to the stomach at the angle of His, parallel to the lesser curvature of the stomach and the indwelling dilator. Because the alignment pin is not used in this application, special care should be taken to ensure that the staples and crimping anvil are accurately aligned.

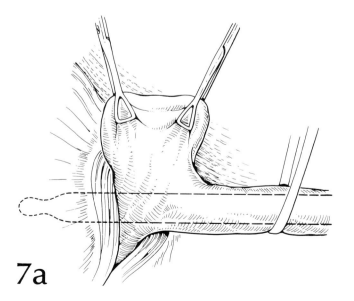

7a

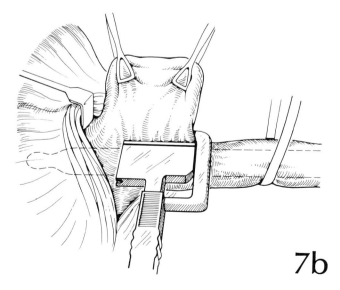

7b

Nissen fundoplication

8a, b After the staples have been placed and the stapling device removed, the previously mobilized fundus is imbricated 360° around the 30-mm uncut Collis gastroplasty tube or neo-oesophagus, following the technique developed by Nissen. The wrap is fashioned loosely with the dilator in place and is maintained with one row of interrupted seromuscular 2/0 silk sutures, which initially approximate the fundus to the Collis gastroplasty tube over a 2-cm length. A second, outer, row of 3/0 silk is used to reinforce these sutures, going from stomach to stomach. The vagi are located within the fundal wrap in their normal position. At each step of the procedure injury to these nerves must be avoided – accidental vagotomy is the most common cause of 'gas bloat' syndrome in the postoperative period. It is noteworthy that the fundoplication, as described, avoids placing sutures near the vagal trunks: the anchoring sutures for the plication are all on the stomach, not the oesophagus. The purpose of the uncut staple line is to establish a frenula that will prevent the neo-oesophagus telescoping out of the fundoplication and to reduce tension.

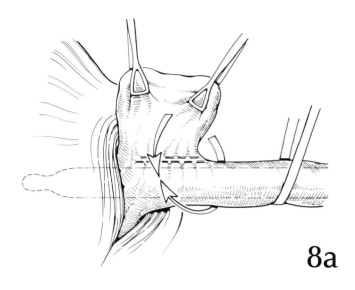

8a

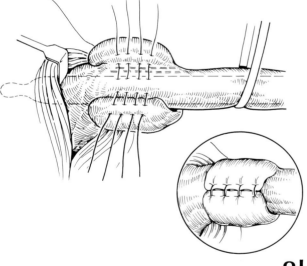

8b

Reduction of wrap and closure of hiatus

9a–c Once the fundoplication is complete, the reconstructed area is reduced below the diaphragm and is held in place with three interrupted horizontal mattress sutures of 2/0 Prolene (Johnsrud sutures). These sutures catch the oesophagus just above the gastro-oesophageal junction, passing through the stomach and underneath the crus and diaphragm. These sutures cover 270°, beginning medially at the level of the last posterior crural suture at the insertion of the pericardium. The second suture should be positioned half-way between the first and third sutures. The final suture should be placed at the last suture of the left or anterior crus. The wrap is then reduced with the dilator in place, and the anchoring Johnsrud sutures tied and divided. The crural sutures are then tied and divided, working from the aorta to the pericardium, ensuring that there is one finger's breadth posteriorly between the oesophagus and the crus with each suture tied. If the last suture is too tight, one throw (or an entire suture) should be removed to allow adequate space posteriorly. This ensures a hiatus large enough to prevent dysphagia. At this stage the dilator is removed and a nasogastric tube passed into the stomach. Haemostasis is secured, a chest tube placed, and the incision closed in the usual manner.

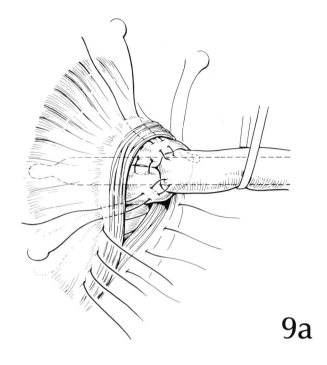

9a

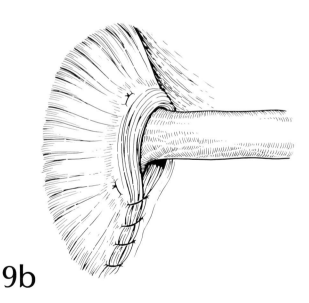

9b

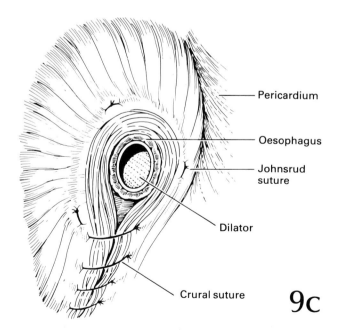

Pericardium

Oesophagus

Johnsrud suture

Dilator

Crural suture

9c

Postoperative care

The morning after the day of the operation the oesophagus is studied fluoroscopically following ingestion of a water-soluble contrast medium (Gastrografin). If no leakage from the oesophageal or gastric suture site is evident, the nasogastric tubes may be removed. Oral feeding may begin safely on the next day and will progress from a liquid to a general diet during the next 2–3 days. Chest tubes are removed once drainage has reduced to less than 150 ml. Total hospitalization time is approximately 7 days.

Complications

Minor leakage from any site evident on radiographic examination is usually asymptomatic, localized and confined. If leakage is observed, chest and nasogastric tube suction should be continued, parenteral central nutrition started and broad-spectrum antibiotics administered for 7–10 days. After this period, repeat radiographic examination almost invariably shows that the leaks have sealed completely. Oral feeding may be resumed safely after tapering off parenteral feeding and removing all the drainage tubes.

Acknowledgements

All the illustrations used in this chapter have been redrawn from originals supplied by the Mayo Foundation, for which copyright is held by the Mayo Foundation.

Illustrations by Antoine Barnaud

Roux-en-Y diversion and fundoplication for gastro-oesophageal reflux

François Fekete MD
Professor of Surgery and Chief, Department of Digestive Surgery, University Paris VII, Hôpital Beaujon, Clichy, Paris, France

Yves Panis MD
Department of Digestive Surgery, University Paris VII, Hôpital Beaujon, Clichy, Paris, France

History

In 1949 Wangensteen and Levin noticed that a distal gastrectomy resulted in improvement in patients suffering from peptic stenotic oesophagitis. Others[1-3] have also promoted the use of an antrectomy with Roux-en-Y diversion to treat peptic stenosis. Duodeno-gastric reflux when associated with peptic acid reflux plays an important role in the development of severe oesophagitis[4] and perhaps also of Barrett's metaplasia, and it is for this reason that duodenal diversion is advocated in complicated cases.

Principles and justification

The goal of duodenal diversion is indirectly to cure gastro-oesophageal reflux. Duodenal diversion involves truncal vagotomy and antrectomy to reduce peptic acid activity and a Roux-en-Y gastrojejunal anastomosis to prevent duodenogastric reflux. An antireflux procedure can also be added to the procedure.

Indications

A recurrence after a previous hiatal repair is usually treated by a new antireflux procedure, although one randomized study suggested that duodenal diversion gives better results than the Nissen procedure, even in cases of uncomplicated oesophagitis. However, the authors believe that in patients who have undergone several hiatal repairs, duodenal diversion is preferable to a further fundoplication and the results in terms of cure of gastro-oesophageal reflux are better. Also, in the authors' experience the quality of the results of duodenal diversion in the treatment of acquired short oesophagus encourages its use in this condition. The regression of Barrett's oesophagus following duodenal diversion and an antireflux procedure is still a matter for discussion. The prevalence of increased alkaline exposure in patients with complicated columnar-lined oesophagus is a further indication for performing a duodenal diversion.

A stricture alone is not used as an indication for duodenal diversion, the procedure being reserved for those patients with long or high dilatable stenoses. The authors believe that duodenal diversion is especially useful for the treatment of severe oesophagitis following Heller's myotomy. It is also indicated for the treatment of reflux following gastro-oesophageal resection, with or without colonic interposition. In these circumstances duodenal diversion avoids a total gastrectomy or coloplasty[5].

Preoperative

The usual investigations and preoperative assessment described in the chapter on pp. 39–44 are undertaken.

Operations

NORMAL TECHNIQUE

1 The usual technique includes truncal vagotomy, antrectomy, and Roux-en-Y gastrojejunal anastomosis; an antireflux procedure is added when possible.

The abdominal approach as described in the chapter on pp. 70–78 is used.

Vagotomy

A bilateral truncal vagotomy is performed using a transhiatal approach. This includes division of the left triangular ligament of the liver with coagulation of the small vessels running with it which allows the left liver lobe to be retracted if it hinders exploration, and division of the lesser omentum. Some small nerves and vessels require coagulation. A hepatic branch of the left gastric artery may run in the lesser omentum. When it is small, it may be coagulated; when it is larger, it should be occluded before division to make sure there is no change in liver colour. If so, the artery should be preserved.

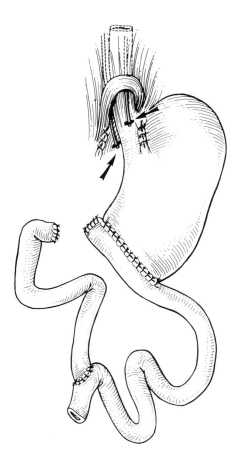

1

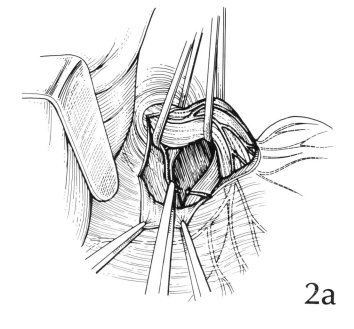

2a

2a, b The peritoneal incision is continued in front of the hiatus and oesophagus and the gastrophrenic ligament is divided. The diaphragmatic crura are then cleared, the oesophageal dissection is completed and the vagus nerves located. Both the oesophagus and the vagus nerves are then held in a sling and freed into the mediastinum for about 6 cm. The single trunk of the posterior vagus and the single or multiple trunks of the anterior vagus are divided. Pieces of the nerves are excised and sent for histological examination.

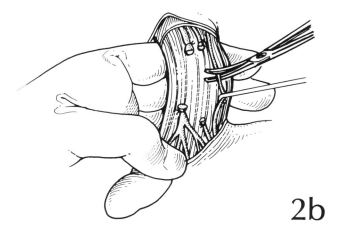

2b

Antireflux procedure

3a, b This is performed when possible to increase the patient's comfort by preventing reflux of food and other material.

The assistant pulls the oesophagus forwards and the surgeon puts one or two non-absorbable sutures in the diaphragmatic crura posterior to the oesophagus (*Illustration 3a*). The authors perform a 180–270° fundic wrap, which they believe is as efficient as a Nissen procedure but less troublesome. The gastric fundus is driven behind the oesophagus by means of a pair of special forceps. There is no need to divide short gastric vessels. The valve is fastened by four sutures to the right diaphragmatic crura, then on the anterolateral right and left surfaces of the oesophagus with non-absorbable thread; the upper suture includes the hiatal margin. The vagus nerves are divided (*Illustration 3b*).

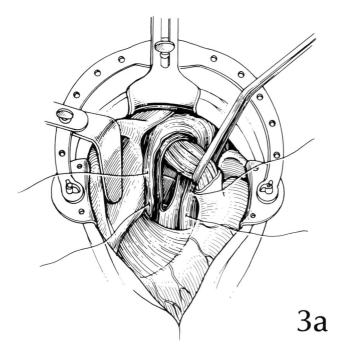

3a

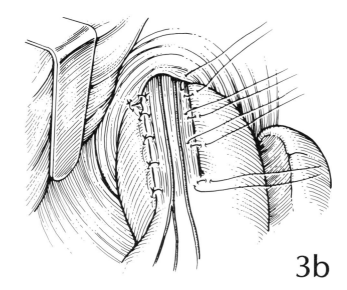

3b

Antrectomy

A Kocher procedure is performed. The gastrocolic ligament is severed, maintaining the gastroepiploic vessels along the stomach in the unlikely event of a reoperation being required.

On the right, the division of the gastrocolic ligament proceeds to the duodenum. On the left, the division stops at the point where the vertical and horizontal parts of the stomach meet.

Vessels to the pylorus are divided, as is the first part of the duodenum, taking away the duodenal bulb. This section is performed either by hand suture or by stapling. Regardless of the method, the stapled suture line is buried by a running suture.

4 Gastric resection is limited: the line of resection goes from the lesser curvature (at the meeting point of the horizontal and vertical parts of the stomach) to the greater curvature, which it cuts perpendicularly (interrupted line B). The muscular layer is cut and submucosal vessels are tied with absorbable sutures.

If too large a gastric resection is carried out (e.g. interrupted line A) this is often followed by gastric stasis and other undesirable gastric sequelae.

Roux-en-Y gastrojejunal transmesocolic anastomosis

An opening is made in an avascular area of the mesocolon, the posterior edge of which is fastened to the posterior face of the stomach 2 cm above the line of gastric resection.

A loop of jejunum supplied by the second jejunal arcade is prepared and divided with a TA stapler on the distal part. The stapled suture is buried by a running 4/0 suture. The jejunal loop is brought behind the colon. The gastrojejunal anastomosis is an end-to-side one. The authors first perform a posterior running seromuscular suture with absorbable thread, following which the gastric mucosa is divided. The antroduodenal resection is completed and an anterior seromuscular running suture is inserted. The anterior margin of the hole in the mesocolon is sutured to the stomach 2 cm above the anastomosis.

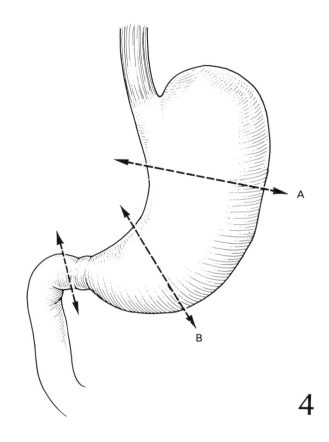

4

Jejunojejunal terminolateral anastomosis

The proximal end of the divided jejunum is anastomosed to the ascending loop. The authors measure 70 cm on the antimesenteric border from the superior point of the vertical part of the Y loop. The anastomosis is performed with two running sutures of absorbable thread. The hole in the mesentery is closed. Both gastrojejunal and jejunojejunal anastomosis can be constructed with staplers, rather than by hand.

OTHER TECHNIQUES

The operation described above was carried out in 70% of the authors' patients. However, reflux sometimes results from previously performed operations and then different strategies may have to be adopted. These will now be considered.

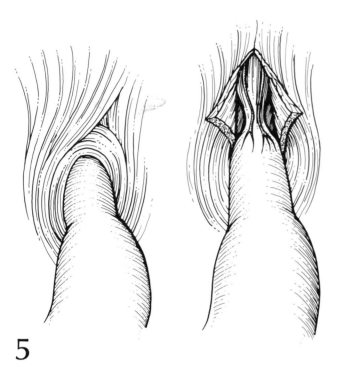

5

Problems related to vagotomy

Possible previous inadequate vagotomy

The authors believe that total truncal vagotomy is important to prevent the development of an anastomotic ulcer. When a previous vagotomy and pyloroplasty or vagotomy and gastrectomy has been performed, it is essential to make sure that the vagotomy is total, either by a study of gastric acid secretion preoperatively or, preferably, by peroperative assessment. The authors frequently find residual trunks at operation.

Hiatal opening easily reached but vagotomy difficult

5 This occurs in cases where there is extensive perioesophagitis, especially in cases with oesophageal shortening. The hiatal approach is performed as above, but access to the oesophagus is made easier by enlarging the hiatus by section of its anterior margin and extending onto the centre of the diaphragm for about 5 cm. The pericardium has to be progressively pushed back from the diaphragm using closed scissors or a swab on a stick. It is usually necessary to suture a phrenic vein which runs on the diaphragm anterior to the oesophagus. This approach usually provides sufficient exposure of the oesophagus to perform an adequate vagotomy.

Hiatal opening difficult or dangerous to reach

It is sometimes very difficult to expose the hiatal region after multiple previous operations. Over-enthusiastic dissection under these circumstances can result in an oesophageal perforation and this may even lead to the necessity for a gastro-oesophageal resection. This risk is particularly high during reoperation for peptic oesophagitis following a Heller's myotomy. The absence of muscle makes the oesophageal mucosa especially vulnerable.

A classic vagotomy cannot therefore be undertaken. However, vagotomy remains a necessity to reduce acidity and avoid gastrojejunal anastomotic ulceration. A two-thirds gastrectomy is not a good solution, as it does not protect the oesophagus against peptic reflux, it does not prevent anastomotic ulceration, and it produces its own digestive sequelae. The simple solution to this problem is to perform a transthoracic vagotomy. This is undertaken through a short left thoracotomy in the seventh interspace. Both vagi are found as trunks at this level, and they are easily identified and resected.

More recently vagotomy has been performed by a thoracoscopic approach.

6 Another solution is to carry out a transdiaphragmatic vagotomy[6]. It is performed by the abdominal approach. A diaphragmatic incision is made 2–3 cm above the hiatus in a transverse line for 5 cm in the aponeurotic part of the diaphragm. The pericardium is pushed away, as is the left pleura, and the oesophagus is sought, mobilized and encircled by a tape. The two vagus nerves are then resected, and the diaphragmatic opening is closed with non-absorbable material. If the pericardium is opened it does not need to be sutured. A pleural opening is treated by placing an underwater seal drain into the chest.

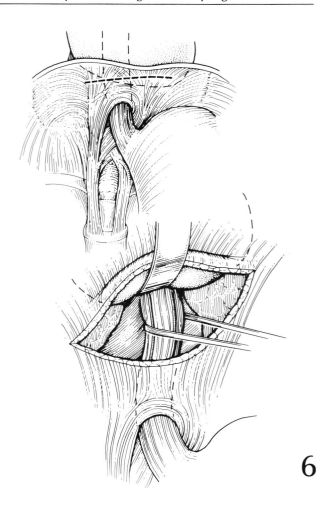

6

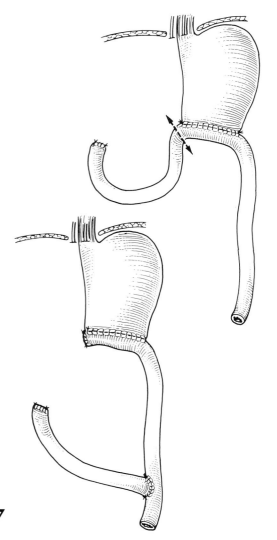

7

Duodenal diversion after partial gastrectomy

After a previous partial distal gastrectomy, bile and pancreatic reflux can be poorly tolerated by gastric or oesophageal mucosa.

If it has not been performed previously, a truncal vagotomy is performed by a hiatal approach.

If a gastroduodenal anastomosis has been performed previously then, after a Kocher procedure, the duodenum is divided immediately downstream from the anastomosis and a gastrojejunal Roux-en-Y anastomosis is performed.

7 If a gastrectomy with a gastrojejunal anastomosis has been performed previously, it is sufficient to divide the afferent loop at the level at which it joins the stomach, using a stapler to close the distal end. A jejunojejunal anastomosis is then constructed between the afferent and efferent loops, 70 cm below the gastrojejunal anastomosis.

Duodenal diversion after previous partial gastro-oesophagectomy

8a–d After gastro-oesophageal resection a peptic (or mixed) reflux may occur, particularly if a pyloroplasty has been performed. In these cases, the duodenum is divided using a stapler and a gastrojejunal Roux-en-Y anastomosis is performed. The authors also like to perform an antrectomy to suppress acid secretion (*Illustration 8a, b*).

Two dangers are to be avoided: (1) damage to the right gastroepiploic pedicle, which is the only blood supply to the stomach (for this reason the greater curvature must be freed close to the stomach wall, *Illustration 8c*); and (2) damage to the colonic pedicle if a previous colonic interposition has been performed; in such cases, the colonic pedicle usually lies in the retrogastric position (*Illustration 8d*).

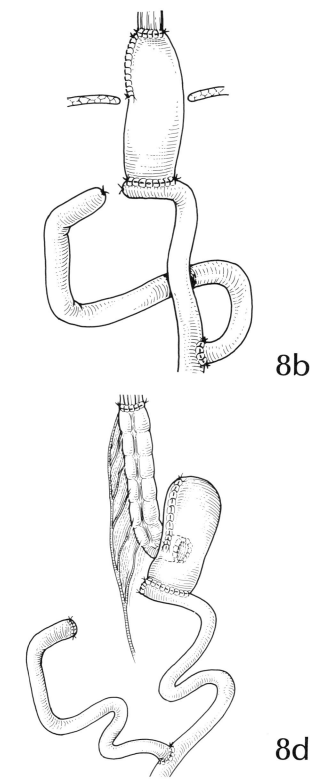

8b

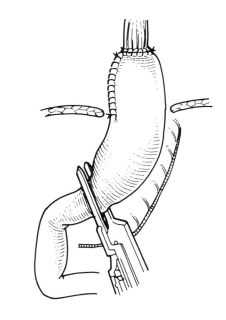

8a

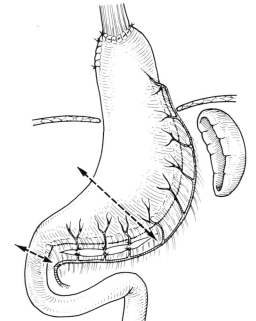

8c

8d

Duodenal diversion after total gastrectomy

9 Duodenal reflux may be intolerable after previous total gastrectomy with oesophagojejunal omega anastomosis, with or without an accompanying jejuno-jejunal anastomosis.

If a jejunojejunal anastomosis is present, the two joined loops are separated using a stapler. The afferent loop is divided with a stapler to close the distal end. The proximal loop is implanted in the efferent loop 70 cm distal to the oesophagojejunal anastomosis.

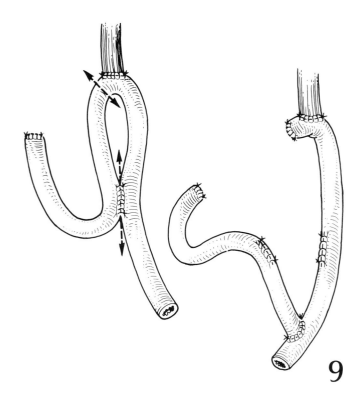

9

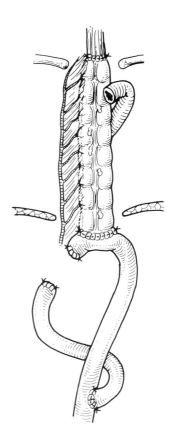

10

Duodenal diversion after total gastro-oesophagectomy and colonic interposition replacement

10 If a total gastrectomy combined with total oesophagectomy has been performed with digestive continuity restored by a colonic interposition anastomosed with the duodenum or the first jejunal loop, duodenal reflux may lead to colitis or tracheal regurgitation and aspiration pneumonia. Duodenal diversion is then performed with stapled closure of the coloduodenal or colojejunal anastomosis, and the construction of an end-to-side Roux-en-Y colojejunal anastomosis.

Postoperative care

Routine nasogastric suction, intravenous parenteral nutrition and antibiotics are used.

Outcome

Between 1979 and 1989 150 patients with severe peptic oesophagitis (including oesophageal stenosis, columnar-lined oesophagus and postoperative oesophagitis) underwent surgery, 83 of whom had a duodenal diversion.

Complications

Two patients developed duodenal fistulae which healed after drainage and total parenteral nutrition. One patient developed acute pancreatitis and one patient developed acalculous cholecystitis. Two patients died from pulmonary embolism in spite of systemic antiembolic treatment. Delay in gastric (or gastrojejunal) emptying occurred in five patients and required total parenteral nutrition for up to 20 days. The authors have not observed this complication since the size of the distal gastrectomy was reduced. Perhaps sparing of the proximal stomach retains the gastric pacemaker.

Heartburn disappeared completely in all patients in the immediate postoperative period. In 25 patients with a stricture, dysphagia was cured without postoperative bougienage in 18. One to three dilatations were required for six patients, while one patient with a tight stricture requires regular bougienage.

Endoscopy showed that peptic oesophagitis disappeared after 3 months except in four patients, all of whom had had a gastrectomy without vagotomy. In these cases, ulceration persisted in the distal oesophagus.

Among the 31 patients who had a preoperative columnar-lined oesophagus, six showed partial regression (20%) and in one patient the columnar-lined oesophagus progressively disappeared. No carcinoma or dysplasia was observed during follow-up (158 patient years).

Twenty patients complained of minor difficulties during the first postoperative year, with postprandial discomfort and disordered gastric emptying in 14, including eight bezoars, moderate dumping in four and postprandial diarrhoea in two.

Severe digestive discomfort and a persistent dumping syndrome were observed in only two patients, both of whom had had a two-thirds gastrectomy. Stomal ulcer occurred in four of nine patients receiving a two-thirds gastric resection without vagotomy following a Heller's procedure. The authors believe that stomal ulcer is prevented by truncal vagotomy. If vagotomy cannot safely be performed through a transhiatal approach, a transthoracic or transdiaphragmatic retropericardial approach should be used.

The result in terms of lasting cure of symptoms of gastro-oesophageal reflux is a major advantage of the procedure when compared with procedures such as repeat fundoplication and Collis gastroplasty.

Most patients have a relatively normal digestive function 1 year after duodenal diversion. Troublesome digestive symptoms have a tendency to decrease with the passage of time and in the authors' series persisted in only six patients.

References

1. Holt CJ, Large AM. Surgical management of reflux esophagitis. *Ann Surg* 1961; 153: 555–62.

2. Payne WS, Thompson GB, Trastek VF, Piehler JM, Pairolero PC. Gastric secretion suppression and duodenal diversion: the Roux-en-Y principle in the management of complex reflux problems. In: DeMeester TR, Matthews HR, eds. *Benign Esophageal Disease in International Trends in General Thoracic Surgery*. St Louis: Mosby, 1987: 162–71.

3. Spencer J. Roux-en-Y diversion for complicated reflux disease. In: Jamieson GGJ, ed. *Surgery of the Esophagus*. Edinburgh: Churchill Livingstone, 1988: 337–40.

4. DeMeester TR, Attwood SEA, Smyrk TC, Therkildsen DH, Hinder RA. Surgical therapy in Barrett's esophagus. *Ann Surg* 1990; 212: 528–42.

5. Perniceni T, Gayet B, Fekete F. Total duodenal diversion in the treatment of complicated peptic esophagitis. *Br J Surg* 1988; 75: 1108–11.

6. Narbona B. Transphrenic access to the lower mediastinum. *Dig Surg* 1987; 4: 204–6.

Illustrations by Gillian Lee Illustrations

Resection of oesophageal strictures

Robert O. Mitchell MD
Resident Surgeon, Department of Surgery, University of Louisville School of Medicine, Louisville, Kentucky, USA

William G. Cheadle MD
Assistant Professor of Surgery, Department of Surgery, University of Louisville School of Medicine, Louisville, Kentucky, USA

Hiram C. Polk Jr MD
Senior Professor and Chairman, Department of Surgery, University of Louisville School of Medicine, Louisville, Kentucky, USA

History

Symptomatic gastro-oesophageal reflux can usually be managed non-operatively but, when stricture occurs, most informed physicians agree that an antireflux procedure is necessary. Nissen fundoplication has become the preferred operation for complicated reflux disease, and most strictures will resolve after control of reflux and two or three oesophageal dilatations. For those patients who have persistent stricture that is fibrotic, shortened, or does not respond to operative control of reflux, resection is indicated. Merendino and Dillard[1] proposed the use of a jejunal segment for interposition between the oesophagus and stomach because of its isoperistaltic nature, relative resistance to acid injury, and lack of reflux into the proximal oesophageal segment[2,3]. Their study of both animals and humans demonstrated the jejunal segment to be the conduit of choice, and we have had long-term successful experience with its use[4].

Principles and justification

The procedure may be performed regardless of whether the original antireflux procedure was carried out through the abdomen or the chest. There are few contraindications; other conduits such as the stomach or colon are usually more appropriate when the entire length of the oesophagus is to be resected. The operation is performed to remove the stricture and to cure subsequent gastro-oesophageal reflux disease with its attendant symptoms of recurrent dysphagia, heartburn and regurgitation.

Preoperative

All patients must have had an upper gastrointestinal series and an upper endoscopy with thorough biopsies of the stricture to exclude malignancy. A general medical evaluation is indicated, since the operation usually requires opening both the abdomen and left chest.

Anaesthesia

A general anaesthetic is essential with endotracheal intubation. A double lumen Carlin's endotracheal tube is usually not necessary because the thoracic portion of the procedure is performed in the inferior aspect of the left chest and the lungs are typically normal. Since the abdominal portion of the procedure is done with the patient in the supine position and the patient is then repositioned for the left thoracotomy, good preoperative communication with the anaesthetist is imperative.

Operation

Selection of jejunal segment

1 The abdomen is entered by an upper midline incision and a general exploration is carried out. The selection of the appropriate jejunal segment is at least as important as its surgical preparation. Generally, the fourth or fifth jejunal trunk is the largest. The arcades given off this trunk can be examined by backlighting or with intraoperative Doppler ultrasonography, but this does not replace careful palpation and observation by the experienced surgeon.

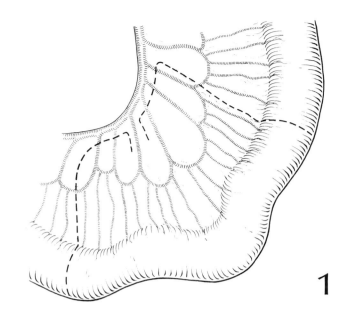

1

Preparation of jejunal segment

2a, b The marginal arcade should be able to support a 20-cm jejunal segment, and at least 12 cm is required for effective function. By opening the peritoneal covering of the mesentery in a series of darts, the mesentery itself will stretch and the proximal end, which is to be used for the oesopha-

gojejunal anastomosis, literally unkinks to facilitate end-to-end anastomosis. The proximal end of the jejunal segment should be marked with a long suture (see arrows) so that later there is no confusion as to which end is proximal.

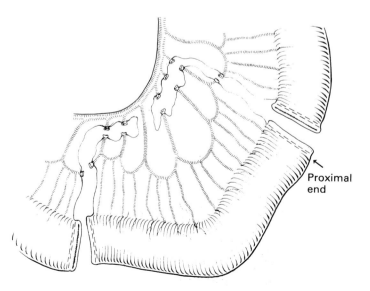

Proximal end

2a

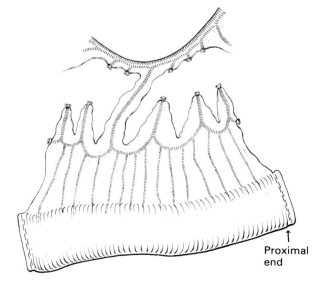

Proximal end

2b

Resection of gastro-oesophageal junction, pyloroplasty and gastrostomy tube

3 The upper stomach is transected and often stapled with the GIA instrument near the gastro-oesophageal junction. A truncal vagotomy is also performed. A Heineke–Mikulicz pyloroplasty is performed to facilitate gastric emptying after vagal disruption and is essential after gastro-oesophageal transection. Before abdominal closure a Witzel gastrostomy is fashioned with a no. 18 straight catheter. This alleviates the discomfort of prolonged nasogastric decompression and may even permit feeding in the postoperative period if an anastomotic leak or obstruction occurs.

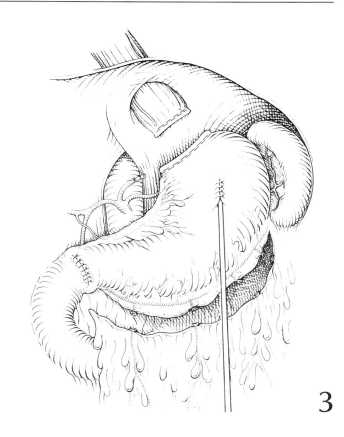

3

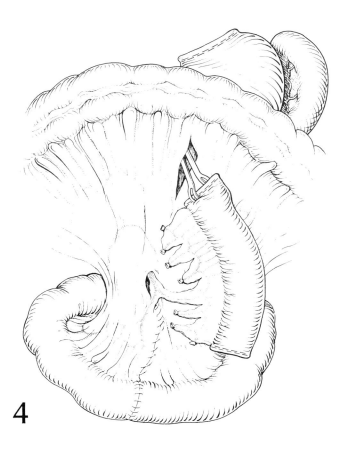

4

Passage of jejunal segment through oesophageal hiatus

4 The jejunal segment is passed through the transverse mesocolon in a retrocolic fashion and passes behind the stomach, special care being taken not to twist the blood supply of the segment and to protect the venous return. Compromise of venous outflow is responsible for immediate early failure in this operation[5]. The oesophagus is dissected free of its attachments up into the mediastinum until the oesophageal mucosa is encountered. The proximal portion of the segment is then pushed into the hiatus in an isoperistaltic position.

Jejunogastric anastomosis

5   The distal jejunum is sutured to the fundus of the stomach with an inner layer of running 3/0 chromic catgut and an outer layer of interrupted 3/0 silk. The anastomosis should be separated from the transected gastro-oesophageal junction by 4–5 cm to take advantage of the mobility of the fundus and to protect the blood supply of both suture lines. The jejunal segment is again checked for viability and gently pushed further into the chest with a tacking suture at the hiatus. Haemostasis is achieved and the abdomen is then closed with a running suture of 0 polypropylene.

Thoracotomy and oesophagectomy

The patient is repositioned and a standard left posterolateral thoracotomy incision is made. The chest is entered through the fifth or sixth interspace, depending on the expected level of anastomosis. Resection of a rib will not add to the morbidity and often improves exposure. The oesophagus is then resected above the level of stenosis and the jejunal segment is gently pulled further into the chest with care not to rotate the segment. Often there is surrounding inflammation with direct adherence of the oesophagus to the periaortic pleura.

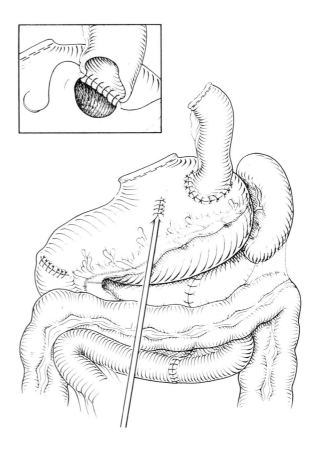

5

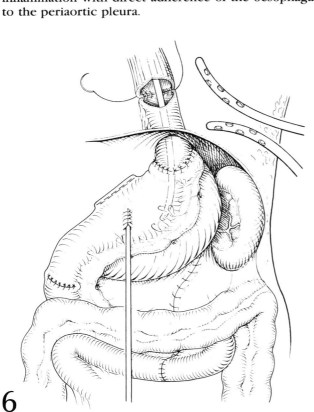

6

Oesophagojejunostomy

6   The oesophagus is sutured end-to-end to the jejunal segment with an inner layer of running 3/0 chromic catgut and an outer layer of interrupted 3/0 silk. A right-angled thoracostomy tube is placed along the diaphragm and a second thoracostomy tube is usually placed to the apex. The tubes should have the ends clipped so that they extend into the chest cavity but do not come in contact with the graft. A nasogastric tube is placed through the entire jejunal segment and into the stomach if possible. The nasogastric tube serves as a stent to prevent kinking of the jejunal graft.

Postoperative care

Systemic antibiotics should be used during the operation and adequate intravenous fluids and nutrition should be maintained postoperatively. The superior thoracostomy tube can usually be removed 48 h after the operation. At 7 days a Gastrografin swallow should be performed to check for anastomotic leakage, followed by barium confirmation if no leak is seen on the Gastrografin study. The lower chest tube should not be removed until anastomotic leaks are excluded radiographically. The gastrostomy tube is then clamped for 24 h and clear liquids are started the following day.

Outcome

In a personal series of 41 patients excellent results have been achieved in 37. These include complete resolution of symptoms due to gastro-oesophageal reflux including dysphagia due to stricture. There has been one death in the series and only two patients required reoperation. Two other patients have had long-term digestive functional complaints that preclude labelling their results as entirely satisfactory, and the second operation was successful in one of the two other reoperative cases.

Once the clinical situation is severe enough, jejunal interposition is clearly the operation of choice. First recurrences are generally treated by dismantling the failed antireflux procedure with a new, proper fundoplication which also includes crural repair. We believe the weight of evidence now supports jejunal interposition when two or more previous operations have failed.

References

1. Merendino KA, Dillard DH. The concept of sphincter substitution by an interposed jejunal segment for anatomic and physiologic abnormalities at the oesophago-gastric junction. *Ann Surg* 1955; 142: 486–509.

2. Dillard DH, Merendino KA. New studies in the dog supporting the concept of equal resistance of various levels of the intestinal tract to acid-peptic digestion. *Surg Gynecol Obstet* 1956; 103: 289–302.

3. Skinner HH, Merendino KA. An experimental evaluation of an interposed jejunal segment between the oesophagus and the stomach combined with upper gastrectomy in the prevention of esophagitis and jejunitis. *Ann Surg* 1955; 141: 201–7.

4. Polk HC Jr. Jejunal interposition for reflux esophagitis and esophageal stricture unresponsive to valvuloplasty. *World J Surg* 1980; 4: 731–6.

5. Brain RHF. The place for jejunal transplantation in the treatment of simple strictures of the oesophagus. *Ann R Coll Surg Engl* 1967; 40: 100–18.

Operations for complicated gastro-oesophageal reflux: miscellaneous procedures

Glyn G. Jamieson FRACS, FACS
Dorothy Mortlock Professor of Surgery, University of Adelaide, Department of Surgery, Royal Adelaide Hospital, Adelaide, Australia

Operations

FUNDIC PATCH

For those surgeons familiar with the Dor patch technique following myotomy for achalasia (as described on pp. 267–275), this procedure is similar. It is only used when the oesophagus is shortened and cannot be dilated.

Technique

Through a midline incision, the hiatus is exposed and the oesophagus and upper stomach are dissected free. Although it is sometimes possible to use the anterior wall of the stomach without dividing any short gastric vessels, because of the shortening of the oesophagus it is better to mobilize the stomach as far as the anterior border of the spleen.

1 A tapered bougie such as a 52-Fr Maloney is passed with the tip through the oesophageal stricture. A longitudinal incision is made through the stricture extending into the healthy oesophagus above and the stomach (or healthy oesophagus) below. The bougie is then advanced into the stomach.

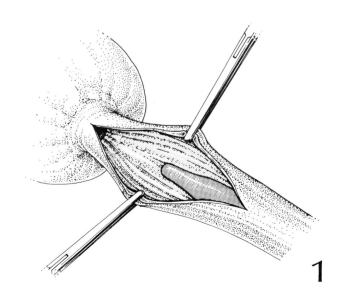

1

2 In order to produce an acid-resistant lining, a split skin graft is now taken and sutured to the stomach in the region to be used as the patch. The needles are left on the sutures, which are then used to sew the fundus and skin graft first to the left wall of the opened oesophagus and then to the right wall.

The remaining fundus is brought round the patch as a complete 3-cm long fundoplication. This fundoplication will lie above the level of the hiatus. It is important to make sure the hiatus is widely open, so that there is no constriction of the stomach as it lies in the mediastinum. Because of the greatly widened hiatus that is required, it is a good idea to close the remaining gap between the stomach and the hiatus to prevent further herniation of the stomach or large intestine.

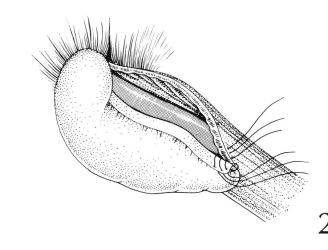

2

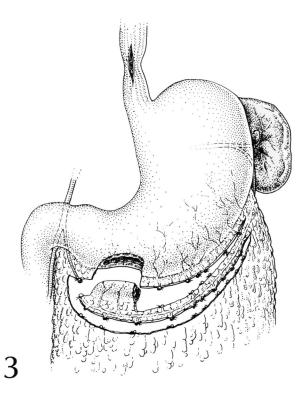

3

ANTRAL PATCH

This procedure should only be used if a stricture that cannot be dilated is present. It utilizes the same principle as the fundic patch, but is a more precise method of plastic repair of the oesophagus. Furthermore, it uses mucosa that is acid resistant.

Technique

3 A patch of antrum is developed, supplied by the gastro-omental arch from the left gastro-omental (epiploic) artery. It is best to mobilize the gastro-omental arcade before constructing the antral patch, as sometimes the arcade is deficient in its mid-portion and this technique should not then be used.

T. Hugh, the originator of this technique, recommends using a pH probe and a pentagastrin infusion to stimulate acid secretion, to be certain that the patch being developed is devoid of acid-secreting cells. The patch is developed about 8 cm proximal to the pylorus. If the patch is developed closer to the pylorus, it is less necessary to use the pentagastrin test.

4 A full-thickness patch, approximately 5 cm × 2 cm, is constructed and brought behind the stomach to the posterior mediastinum. Care must be taken to make sure that the pedicle is not twisted in its ascent. The oesophagus is mobilized well into the mediastinum, incised vertically through the stenosis, and the scar tissue sent for frozen section to ensure that a carcinoma is not present. A large bougie is passed and the patch is sewn into the oesophageal defect, using a one-layer technique and the surgeon's preferred method of suturing.

A fundoplication is now constructed around the lower oesophagus. If this cannot be brought into the abdomen, it is left in the chest with several tacking sutures attaching it to the edges of the wide diaphragmatic hiatus.

The construction should be tested for leakage before closure.

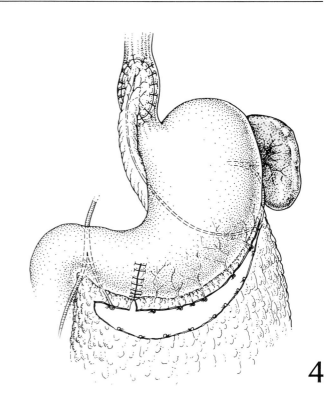

4

SCHATZKI'S RING

This is a mucosal ring at the squamocolumnar junction, always associated with a small hiatus hernia, gastro-oesophageal reflux, or both. It is usually associated with intermittent episodes of aphagia. There is no agreement as to the best method of management. If dilatation fails to relieve the aphagic episodes (and it often does), the alternatives are (1) intraoperative forceful dilatation and an antireflux procedure, or (2) excision of the ring (sleeve resection) and an antireflux procedure. The former can be achieved by passing a 60-Fr bougie through the mouth or by carrying out a small high gastrotomy and using a forefinger to 'fracture' the ring. The technique for sleeve resection is described below.

Technique of sleeve resection

5 The lower oesophagus is mobilized as for a standard fundoplication. A vertical incision is made into the oesophagus, commencing at the anatomical gastro-oesophageal junction and extending up to the ring, which is usually about 3 cm proximal to the anatomical gastro-oesophageal junction. The mucosa, including the ring, is separated from the oesophageal muscle for the full circumference of the oesophagus. It is then a simple matter to excise the ring and its mucosa with scissors.

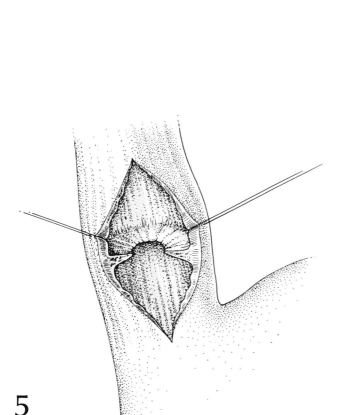

5

6 The defect produced in the mucosa should be no more than 5–7 mm, and it is closed with an absorbable suture such as Maxon or polydioxanone (PDS).

The oesophagus is similarly closed. A total fundoplication is then constructed, long enough to cover the oesphageal suture line.

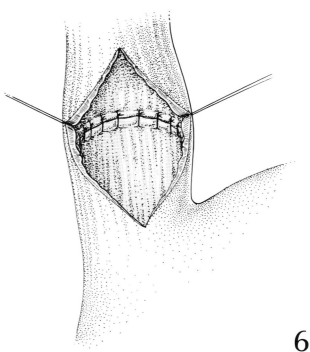

6

Illustrations by Gillian Oliver

Surgical anatomy of the vagus nerves

Haile T. Debas MD
M. Galante Distinguished Professor of Surgery and Dean of the School of Medicine, University of California, San Francisco, California, USA

From the perspective of operative surgery of the upper gastrointestinal tract, the important aspects of vagal anatomy are relationships and distribution in the cervical and upper mediastinal regions and at and below the diaphragmatic hiatus. Central vagal anatomy, therefore, will not be dealt with in any detail. The importance of the cervical anatomy of the vagus relates to the need to protect the vagus and its laryngeal branches during surgery on the upper oesophagus. A thorough knowledge of vagal anatomy at the hiatus is essential for the performance of various types of vagotomy.

Besides meticulous anatomical dissection, the combination of anterograde and retrograde staining with horseradish peroxidase and immunocytochemistry has resulted in the definition, in great detail, of the central projections of the vagi as well as the type of neurones contained within them. This degree of detail will not be provided in this chapter, but the interested reader is referred to some excellent papers in the field[1,2].

Central vagus complex

The fibres of the vagus nerves that control secretion and motility of the gastrointestinal tract originate in the medulla oblongata from neurones of the dorsomotor nucleus of the vagus (DMNV), as well as the nucleus ambiguus (NA) and the nucleus tractus solitarius (NTS). Of the 60 000 fibres that constitute the abdominal vagi in humans, visceral efferents comprise approximately only 3%. Most secretory neurones arise from the DMNV, while most of the gastric motor efferents originate in the NA. Primary visceral sensory information is relayed to the DMNV via the tractus solitarius. General somatic afferent fibres of the vagus arise from the superior ganglion. The larger inferior ganglion (nodose ganglion) is the source of both general and special visceral afferent fibres. The vagus nerves issue from the cranium through the jugular foramen and the superior and inferior ganglia are outside the skull.

Functional anatomy of the vagus has been defined using central stimulation with electrical impulses or by hypoglycaemia. Electrical stimulation of the DMNV in cats leads to vigorous, prolonged gastric acid secretion. Hypoglycaemia stimulates the DMNV indirectly by acting on the lateral hypothalamus.

Cervical anatomy of vagus

1 After issuing from the skull via the jugular foramen, the right and left vagi enter the carotid sheath where they come to lie between and deep to the carotid artery and jugular vein.

The first surgically important branch of the vagus in the neck is the superior laryngeal nerve, which divides into the internal and external laryngeal nerves. The internal laryngeal nerve pierces the thyrohyoid membrane and is sensory to the larynx above the vocal cords. The external laryngeal nerve runs deep and parallel to the superior thyroid artery and is motor to the cricothyroid muscle (the tuning fork of the larynx) and the inferior constrictor.

Within the carotid sheath the vagus gives off cardiac branches, but the next surgically important branch of the cervical vagus is the right recurrent laryngeal nerve, which comes off the right vagus as the latter crosses the subclavian artery. The right recurrent nerve hooks around the vessel, and passes behind the common carotid to reach the groove between the trachea and the oesophagus. It runs up the tracheo-oesophageal groove, along the medial surface of the right lobe of the thyroid, and enters the larynx behind the right cricothyroid joint. The left recurrent laryngeal nerve comes off the left vagus behind the aortic arch, loops anteriorly around the vessel to go up the neck where it also travels in the tracheo-oesophageal groove. The recurrent laryngeal nerves are motor to all the intrinsic muscles of the larynx and are sensory to the larynx below the vocal cords.

Potential damage to the external laryngeal nerve occurs at the time of division of the superior thyroid artery during thyroidectomy. Damage to the recurrent laryngeal nerves can occur during cervical oesophagectomy, the excision of a pharyngo-oesophageal diverticulum or during gastro-oesophageal anastomosis in the neck following transhiatal oesophagectomy. In the last two procedures, neuropraxia of the left recurrent laryngeal nerve may result from pressure caused by retractors.

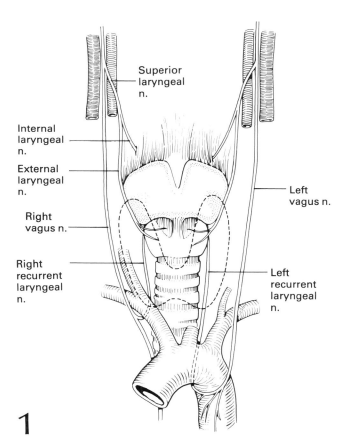

Superior laryngeal n.

Internal laryngeal n.

External laryngeal n.

Right vagus n.

Right recurrent laryngeal n.

Left vagus n.

Left recurrent laryngeal n.

1

Vagal anatomy within thorax

2   The vagus enters the thorax by crossing the first part of the subclavian artery on the right, and by passing anterior to the subclavian on the left. The superior cervical branches are given off in the neck within the carotid sheath and also enter the chest anterior to the subclavian artery. Within the chest, each vagus forms a network of nerves that surround the oesophagus. Although several small branches are given off to the tracheobronchial tree and lungs, pericardium, aorta and diaphragm, there are no major branches that the surgeon has to attempt to preserve during oesophagectomy.

Over the distal oesophagus, single anterior and posterior nerve trunks emerge from the neural reticulum around the oesophagus. Anatomists are in agreement that the left vagus forms the major portion of the anterior vagus but receives branches from the right vagus, and that the right vagus is mainly formed from the posterior vagus but receives branches from the left vagus[3, 4]. The right thoracic vagus lies mainly posterior to the oesophagus and usually to its left side. The two trunks are linked by several long and short communicating strands.

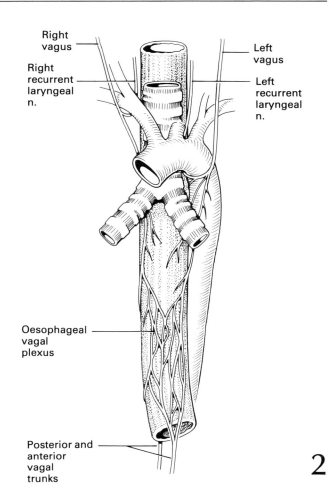

3   The vagal anatomy at the diaphragmatic hiatus is particularly important for the surgeon. The posterior vagus forms a single trunk 3–4 cm above the diphragm and remains a single trunk at the hiatus in 92% of cases, while the anterior vagus is a single trunk at the hiatus in only 66% of cases.

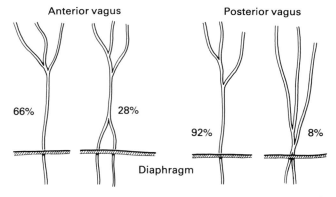

Abdominal vagus

A knowledge of the major divisions of the abdominal vagus is essential in the performance of vagotomy (see above). The anterior vagus trunk is usually found closely applied to the anterior surface of the abdominal oesophagus. The posterior vagus, on the other hand, is separated from the oesophagus by areolar tissue and may lie at any location from behind the oesophagus medially to the right crus of the diaphragm laterally. In about one-third of cases the posterior vagus runs along the right crus of the diaphragm at some distance from the oesophagus.

Divisions of anterior vagus

4 The anterior vagus has three main divisions: hepatic gastric, and antral. In addition, it often gives off a communicating branch to the coeliac axis[4].

Hepatic branches

These are the first branches of the anterior vagus below the diaphragm and travel in the layers of the lesser omentum from the vagus towards the liver. These branches are multiple. When there is only one anterior vagal trunk in the abdomen, it gives two or more hepatic branches. When there are two or more anterior vagal trunks, usually each gives at least one hepatic branch.

On reaching the liver, the hepatic branches give off nerves to that organ before passing downward on the hepatic artery, forming a plexus from which branches are given off to the gallbladder, bile duct and pancreas. Besides these branches, a pyloric branch is given off that travels along the right gastric artery, and a deeper branch that travels along the gastroduodenal artery and subsequently along the right gastroepiploic artery to supply a small portion of the greater curvature of the stomach.

Gastric branches

A variable number of gastric branches comes off the anterior vagal trunk after it gives off the hepatic branches. The gastric branches arise as between five and ten thin twigs or as one to four main divisions which then subdivide to supply the anterior portion of the proximal stomach including the fundus[4]. At the lesser curvature these branches run in close relationship to the vessels of the stomach. The gastric branches penetrate the gastric wall at the lesser curvature and then travel between the serosa and muscle for a distance of 1–2 cm before penetrating to the submucosal and mucosal layers. Thus, these nerves can be effectively divided by anterior seromyotomy of the stomach.

The gastric branches innervate the parietal cell mass and the smooth muscle cells of the body and fundus. In highly selective vagotomy these branches are divided, leaving intact the hepatic branches and the innervation to the antropyloric region. When the gastric branches are divided basal acid secretion is reduced by about 70–80% and maximal acid output by about 50%. In addition to the division of the secretory fibres, motor nerve fibres that mediate receptive relaxation of the stomach during deglutition are also interrupted.

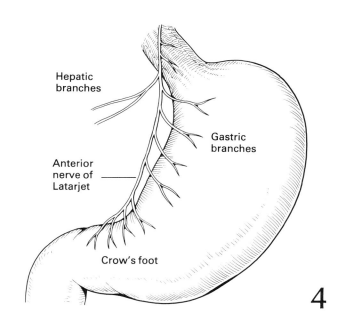

Hepatic branches

Gastric branches

Anterior nerve of Latarjet

Crow's foot

4

In some patients, one or more gastric branches may come off the anterior vagal trunk very high in the hiatus and travel in the peritoneal fold at the angle of His. It becomes necessary, therefore, that this peritoneal fold is completely divided towards the fundus to ensure completeness of highly selective vagotomy.

Anterior long nerve of antrum: anterior nerve of Latarjet

After giving off the hepatic and gastric branches, the anterior vagus continues distally towards the antrum about 1–2 cm from the lesser curvature. This nerve is often referred to as the anterior nerve of Latarjet, in honour of the French surgeon[5] who described it in 1921. It is also sometimes referred to as the greater anterior nerve of Mitchell. The anterior nerve of Latarjet passes onto the anterior wall of the stomach near the incisura. Over the antrum it fans out into branches akin to the digits of a crow's foot[6]. The most superior digit of the crow's foot is usually 7 cm from the pylorus.

The anterior nerve of Latarjet and its posterior counterpart supply the antropyloric mechanism which is responsible for antral 'milling' and pyloric sphincter functions. When performing proximal gastric vagotomy these nerves must be carefully preserved to avoid the need for pyloroplasty.

Divisions of posterior vagus

5 The divisions of the posterior vagus are analogous to those of the anterior vagus except that, instead of hepatic branches, the posterior vagus gives off coeliac branches. The divisions of the posterior vagus are, therefore, coeliac branches, gastric branches and the posterior long nerve to the antrum or the posterior nerve of Latarjet.

Coeliac branches

Coeliac branches originate from the posterior vagus below the diaphragm, although sometimes they may arise at the level of the diaphragm or even above. These branches join the left gastric artery 2–4 cm from the origin of the vessel and go to the coeliac axis. The exact distribution from there on has not been fully worked out but branches supply the pancreas, the small intestine and the right colon to the mid-transverse colon. As mentioned above, the coeliac branches of the posterior vagus not infrequently receive a communicating branch from the anterior vagus. They may also give fibres that join the hepatic plexus from the anterior vagus by coursing along the hepatic artery.

Gastric branches

On average, six gastric branches originate from the posterior vagus distal to the origin of the coeliac branches. They go to the posterior wall of the proximal stomach and are distributed in the stomach in a manner analogous to the gastric branches from the anterior vagus.

Posterior long nerve to antrum: posterior nerve of Latarjet

After giving off the coeliac and gastric branches, the posterior vagus courses towards the antrum as the posterior nerve of Latarjet. It is located within 1.5–2 cm of the lesser curvature of the stomach. Its distribution on the posterior surface of the antrum is similar to that of the anterior nerve of Latarjet on the anterior surface of the antrum. It, too, branches, giving the semblance of a crow's foot.

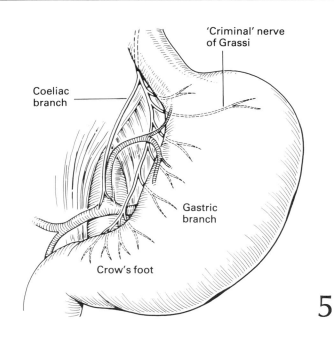

5

Anatomical points with special surgical significance

Distal oesophageal plexus

The gross anatomical distribution of the vagus has been described. What gross anatomy fails to show is that there is important vagal supply to the proximal stomach that is distributed over the distal 6–8 cm on the oesophagus. For most of this distance the oesophagus is usually abdominal. However, the proximal 2–3 cm may be at the hiatus or even above the diaphragm in many; the vagal trunks form 3–5 cm above the diaphragm. Hence the oesophageal fibres that supply the stomach derive either from high branches from the vagal trunks or from a residual neural plexus over the distal oesophagus. It is essential that the distal 7–8 cm of the oesophagus is skeletonized to achieve complete vagotomy of the parietal cell mass as described in the chapter on pp. 373–381. Hallenbeck *et al.* have quantified the difference that skeletonization of the distal 6–7 cm makes, and have shown significant reductions in acid response to hypoglycaemia and in the rate of ulcer recurrence when this is done[7].

Crow's foot of nerves of Latarjet

The distribution of the nerves of Latarjet resembles the digits of a crow's foot, the most proximal digit being about 7 cm from the pyloroduodenal junction. Amdrup and Jensen, who have defined the proximal limit of the antrum by intragastric pH probe, have indicated that the mucosal junction between the antrum and the body may be 3–4 cm higher up than the crow's foot[8]. On the basis of this, many surgeons have used as their starting point for proximal gastric vagotomy a point 3–4 cm proximal to the crow's foot, which would, therefore, be 10–11 cm from the pylorus. While the distal end of dissection may not be an important cause of incomplete vagotomy, the author believes the dissection should start at the crow's foot, or even one digit distal[9].

Angle of His

Vagal fibres that supply the fundus may be distributed within areolar tissue in the peritoneal fold to the left of the oesophagus at the angle of His. A special point should be made during the performance of proximal gastric vagotomy to ensure complete division of the tissue to the left of the oesophagus towards the most proximal short gastric artery.

'Criminal' nerve of Grassi

Grassi has called attention to an errant branch of the right vagus that crosses transversely behind the cardia to supply a portion of the fundus or proximal stomach. If this nerve is not cut, a portion of the stomach will remain innervated and test positive on pH probing during pentagastrin stimulation[10].

Gastroepiploic vagal innervation

A recurrent division of the hepatic vagal branches is distributed along the gastroduodenal and right gastro-epiploic arteries to the greater curvature of the stomach. Standard proximal gastric vagotomy leaves these vagal fibres intact, and some have suggested that this defect of the operation may add to ulcer recurrence. As a result, the so-called operation of 'extended proximal gastric vagotomy' has been suggested, in which division of these fibres at the junctions of the two gastroepiploic vessels at the greater curvature is added to the standard procedure of proximal gastric vagotomy[11]. However, Braghetto et al. have studied prospectively the effect of division of gastroepiploic nerves and could show no significant difference in postoperative gastric acid secretion beyond that achieved by standard proximal gastric vagotomy[9].

References

1. Fox EA, Powley TL. Longitudinal columnar organization within the dorsal motor nucleus represents separate branches of the abdominal vagus. *Brain Res* 1985; 341: 269–82.

2. Yamamoto T, Satomi H, Ise H, Takahashi K. Evidence of the dual innervation of the cat stomach by the vagal dorsal motor and medial solitary nuclei as demonstrated by the horseradish peroxidase method. *Brain Res* 1977; 122: 125–31.

3. Jackson RG. Anatomy of the vagus nerves in the region of the lower esophagus and the stomach. *Anat Rec* 1949; 103: 1–18.

4. Ruckley CV. A study of the variations of the abdominal vagi. *Br J Surg* 1964; 51: 569–73.

5. Latarjet CR. *C R Seanc Hebd Soc Biol* 1921; 84: 985.

6. Goligher JC. A technique for highly selective (parietal cell or proximal gastric) vagotomy for duodenal ulcer. *Br J Surg* 1974; 61: 337–45.

7. Hallenbeck GA, Gleysteen JJ, Aldrete JS, Slaughter RL. Proximal gastric vagotomy: effects of two operative techniques on clinical and gastric secretory results. *Ann Surg* 1976; 184: 435–42.

8. Amdrup E, Jensen HE. Selective vagotomy of the parietal cell mass preserving innervation of the undrained antrum. A preliminary report of results in patients with duodenal ulcer. *Gastroenterology* 1970; 59: 522–7.

9. Braghetto I, Lazo M, Leiva V et al. A prospective study of intraoperative histologic antrum and corpus boundary in patients undergoing highly selective vagotomy for duodenal ulcer. *Surg Gynecol Obstet* 1987; 164: 213–18.

10. Grassi G. A new test for complete nerve section during vagotomy. *Br J Surg* 1971; 58: 187–9.

11. Donohue PE, Bombeck CT, Yoshida Y, Nyhus LM. Endoscopic Congo red test during proximal gastric vagotomy. *Am J Surg* 1987; 153: 249–55.

Illustrations by Gillian Oliver

Total abdominal vagotomy and drainage

Haile T. Debas MD
M. Galante Distinguished Professor of Surgery and Dean of the School of Medicine, University of California, San Francisco, California, USA

History

Vagotomy has emerged as the cornerstone of surgical therapy in peptic ulcer. Total abdominal or truncal vagotomy not only denervates the acid-secreting part of the stomach but also the antropyloric mechanism that controls gastric emptying. Hence, truncal vagotomy causes significant impairment of gastric emptying. It must, therefore, be combined with a drainage procedure (pyloroplasty or gastroenterostomy) to obviate the problem of gastric stasis. Although truncal vagotomy and drainage can be performed transthoracically, the procedure is more easily accomplished through the abdominal route.

In the early 1940s Dragstedt popularized truncal vagotomy for the treatment of duodenal ulcer disease[1]. Initially, his operations were performed transthoracically and were not accompanied by a gastric drainage procedure. It soon became clear that two-thirds of the patients developed postoperative gastric stasis, and one-half of these patients eventually required a gastric drainage operation. In 1951 Dragstedt advised that a drainage procedure in the form of either a pyloroplasty or a gastrojejunostomy be added[2]. For nearly two decades truncal vagotomy and drainage enjoyed popularity as the operation of choice for peptic ulcer disease. Although the ulcer recurrence rate was acceptable at 6–10%, significant side effects, particularly the dumping syndrome and postvagotomy diarrhoea, led to a search for more selective operations. Now, in most parts of the world, proximal gastric or highly selective vagotomy has replaced vagotomy and pyloroplasty as the elective operation of choice for duodenal ulcer. Despite this, truncal vagotomy still remains an important operation in the armamentarium of the peptic ulcer surgeon.

Principles and justification

Indications

Truncal vagotomy and drainage is now used with decreasing frequency in the elective treatment of uncomplicated duodenal ulcer. Truncal vagotomy and pyloroplasty continues to be the procedure of choice, however, in the emergency treatment of patients with bleeding duodenal ulcers. Truncal vagotomy and drainage may also be the operation of choice in very old or very frail patients, particularly in the presence of gastric outlet obstruction. For most patients requiring an elective operation for duodenal ulcer, proximal gastric vagotomy is the procedure of choice. In the USA, many surgeons still favour truncal vagotomy and antrectomy with Billroth I anastomosis as the elective operation, mainly because of the very low rate of ulcer recurrence. Truncal vagotomy and pyloroplasty is sometimes employed in the treatment of frail patients with gastric ulcer. In this situation, the ulcer should be excised and submitted for frozen section. Life-threatening, uncontrollable bleeding from stress ulceration in critically ill patients is seldom seen nowadays. This is primarily because of aggressive control of gastric pH in postoperative patients and in those in intensive care units. Vagotomy and pyloroplasty combined with gastrotomy and suture control of the major bleeding sites may occasionally be useful in selected patients with uncontrollable bleeding from stress ulcers.

Operations

Position of patient

The patient is placed supine on the operating table with a least one arm secured to an armboard for venous access. A 15–20° reverse Trendelenburg position aids in displacing the intestine downwards away from the upper abdomen.

Incision

The abdomen is prepared and draped. The author routinely uses Steridrapes. A midline incision is employed extending from the umbilicus up to the left side of the xiphoid process and for 2–3 cm onto the sternum. It may often also be necessary to extend the incision below the umbilicus.

Exploration

Once the abdomen is opened, exploration is used to rule out unsuspected pathology. The supracolic compartment is first inspected, palpating the oesophageal hiatus, both the left and the right lobes of the liver, the gallbladder and spleen. With the stomach retracted inferiorly, the body of the pancreas may be palpated through the lesser omentum. The stomach is palpated. The first portion of the duodenum is examined for scarring and ulceration. A gentle rubbing of the external surface of the duodenum with a damp sponge may result in the development of stippled erythema on the serosal surface characteristic of the presence of an active ulcer within the duodenum. It should be noted that an active ulcer will not always be present at the time of operation. Often, however, the first portion of the duodenum will be foreshortened, scarred and deformed as a result of repeated ulceration and healing.

The head of the pancreas is now palpated within the C loop of the duodenum. If there is some reason to suspect the presence of a gastrinoma, the duodenum should be mobilized thoroughly by a Kocher manoeuvre to palpate the head of the pancreas. The gastrocolic omentum should be divided to expose the entire length of the pancreas for careful examination and palpation. Intraoperative ultrasonographic examination of the pancreas, the liver and the upper retroperitoneum may even be necessary. The transverse colon is then delivered out of the abdomen and retracted superiorly to enable examination of the contents of the infracolic compartment and the pelvis.

Exposure

1 A decision must be made as to whether it is necessary to divide the left triangular ligament to aid in the retraction of the liver to expose the hiatus. This manoeuvre is seldom necessary if the modified technique described below (where the oesophagus is not mobilized) is used. The author prefers to use either the 'Iron Intern' or Bookwalter retractor. Both of these provide excellent elevation of the sternum and retraction of the liver using well padded body wall retractor and a modified Deaver retractor, respectively. If the Iron Intern is used a Balfour retractor is necessary to retract the wound edges. With the Bookwalter retractor, however, body wall retracting elements can be attached to the oblong ring of the instrument to retract the wound edges. An excellent exposure of the hiatus is thus obtained.

The surgeon can improve visibility further by wearing a head-mounted light and, extremely occasionally, by removing the xiphoid process.

Two techniques of vagotomy will be described. The first (the traditional one) mobilizes and encircles the oesophagus as a necessary step to identification of the vagus trunks. In so doing, however, a degree of disruption of the hiatus is caused. The second technique of vagotomy requires neither oesophageal mobilization nor extensive dissection[3].

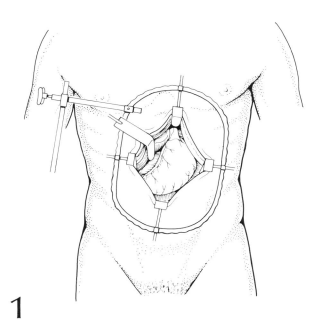

1

TRADITIONAL TECHNIQUE OF TRUNCAL VAGOTOMY

2 With the stomach retracted downward, the region of the oesophagus is palpated. The nasogastric tube within the oesophagus greatly simplifies the identification of this organ. The peritoneal reflection over the abdominal oesophagus is divided transversely about 0.5 cm from the diaphragm. The incision is extended to the right towards the liver by dividing the uppermost part of the lesser omentum. Bleeding is controlled with electrocautery. Similarly, the incision is extended to the left towards the spleen.

It is seldom necessary to pack away the spleen. Should this be necessary, however, the left hand is passed between the diaphragm and the superior surface of the spleen. The spleen is gently retracted downward, and a moist laparotomy sponge is packed above and to the right of the spleen, displacing the organ inferiorly and to the left away from the oesophagus.

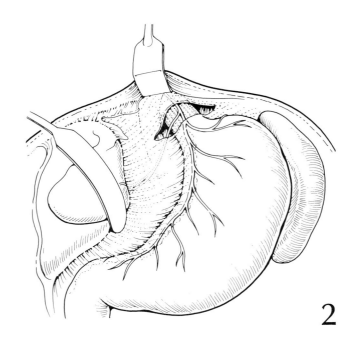

2

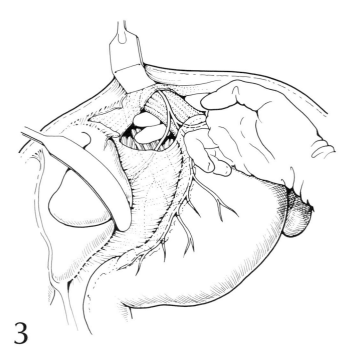

3

3 Next the oesophagus is mobilized bluntly. Two fingers are passed beneath the oesophagus on the left side. The aorta is readily palpable behind the oesophagus, and finger dissection proceeds to the right in the areolar tissue between the oesophagus and abdominal aorta. The posterior vagal trunk is often encountered at this stage. If so, it is mobilized with the oesophagus. As the dissecting finger passes to the right of the oesophagus, firm connective tissue, composed of portions of the phreno-oesophageal and the uppermost extension of the hepatogastric ligaments, is encountered. This has to be divided with curved scissors or with a cautery, often by the assistant, who is on the left side. Once this is done, the index finger can be passed clear around the oesophagus. The dissection behind the oesophagus is easily widened so that both the index and middle finger can be passed from the left side of the oesophagus to the right.

Using a long dissecting forceps, a 19 mm Penrose drain can now be passed to the fingers, grasped, and pulled around the oesophagus. A Kelly haemostat is used to clamp the two ends of the Penrose drain together. The drain can now be used to retract the oesophagus to the left, so that the area between the oesophagus to the left and the right crus of the diaphragm and caudate lobe of the liver can be dissected.

Anterior vagotomy

4 Anterior vagotomy is performed first. The trunk(s) of the anterior vagus is identified by palpation over the anterior surface of the oesophagus. The vagal trunk is raised off the oesophagus using the tips of a pair of right-angled forceps, or a nerve hook, and dissected up and down using the forceps so that about 2.5 cm of it is cleared. The nerve is doubly clamped with the right-angled forceps and divided. Another pair of forceps is applied about 1.25 cm below the distal forceps and the nerve segment between these clamps is excised and submitted for histological identification.

The author prefers to ligate the ends of the vagus with 2/0 silk sutures rather than apply haemoclips to them. A search for additional vagal fibres is made by palpation over the anterior surface of the oesophagus. In about 40% of patients, one or more additional trunks will be found and these must be divided between haemoclips or ligatures. A final inspection of the anterior surface of the oesophagus is made for small nerve fibres that need to be divided.

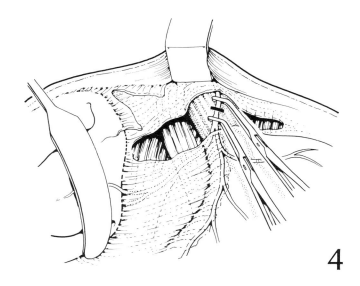

Posterior vagotomy

5 Posterior vagotomy begins by retracting the oesophagus to the left and exposing the interval between the oesophagus and the right crus of the diaphragm. The posterior vagus may have been identified earlier during oesophageal mobilization. If not, the surgeon uses palpation and direct visualization to identify the nerve. Most commonly, the nerve travels obliquely behind and to the right of the oesophagus to lie in the interval between the oesophagus itself and the right crus of the diaphragm. The nerve may lie, however, entirely behind the oesophagus, on the right crus at some distance from the oesophagus, or somewhere in between.

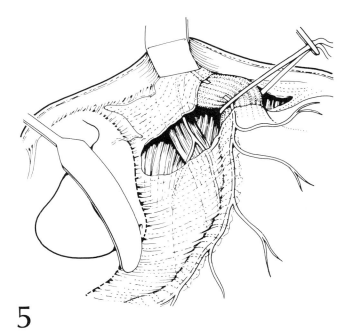

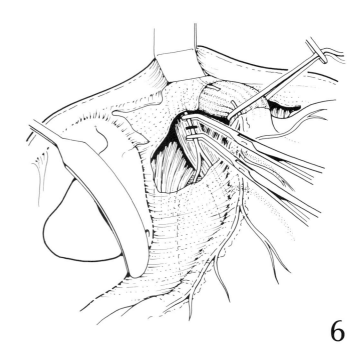

6 Once palpated, it is dissected under direct vision using a pair of right-angled forceps. It is handled in much the same way as the anterior vagus. A segment of it is also excised and sent for histological identification. The posterior vagus is usually larger than the anterior vagus and is found as a single nerve trunk in 95% of patients. Nevertheless, it is always wise to look for extra nerve fibres after the major trunk is divided. It is important to look for connecting branches from the anterior vagus above its division to either the posterior vagus below the point at which it is divided or the coeliac branch. If found, all communicating nerves must be divided. It should be noted that in most patients with ulcer recurrence after a previous incomplete truncal vagotomy, it is the posterior vagal trunk that is found intact.

Following completion of the vagotomy, the operative area is inspected for bleeding. If a laparotomy sponge had been used to displace the spleen, it is now removed carefully and the spleen is inspected for inadvertent damage. Next, a drainage procedure is performed.

Drainage procedure

The choice between pyloroplasty and gastroenterostomy as the drainage procedure depends on the status of the duodenal bulb. In most cases, a Heineke–Mikulicz pyloroplasty can be performed safely. If an inflammatory mass is associated with a severely distorted duodenal bulb, a gastrojejunostomy is a safer drainage procedure. Other types of drainage procedures that may be considered in the appropriate situations are the Finney and the Jaboulet pyloroplasties. The techniques for these types of pyloroplasty and for gastroenterostomy are described fully on pp. 394–402 and pp. 403–413.

Once the drainage procedure has been completed, the sponge from the subhepatic space is removed, as is the sponge at the hiatus. The operative sites are examined for haemostasis and the upper abdomen is irrigated with saline. The abdomen is closed without drains.

MODIFIED TECHNIQUES OF VAGOTOMY

The author prefers a simplified technique of vagotomy that does not require full mobilization of the oesophagus or extensive dissection at the hiatus. Following the traditional technique of truncal vagotomy, described above, a small percentage of patients develop a hiatus hernia and/or gastro-oesophageal reflux, presumably because of anatomic disruption caused by the operation.

The modified technique not only avoids extensive dissection but greatly simplifies the identification and sectioning of the vagal trunks.

Exposure is obtained as described above. It is seldom necessary to divide the left triangular ligament of the liver to perform this operation. The peritoneum over the abdominal oesophagus is incised transversely.

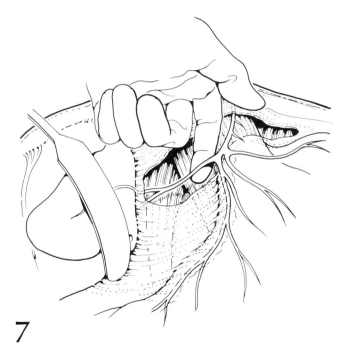

7

Anterior truncal vagotomy

7 The incision is carried to the right onto the lesser omentum short of the hepatic vagal branches within the lesser omentum. The hepatic branches, constant in their presence and location, are easily seen in most patients because the lesser omentum is not fatty at this level. Even when not clearly visible, the surgeon can place the left index finger above the incised edge of the lesser omentum. Gentle caudad retraction brings the hepatic branches taut. This manoeuvre brings the anterior vagal trunk into prominence and enables the surgeon to see or readily palpate it with the middle finger over the anterior surface of the oesophagus. The nerve trunk is then dissected with right-angled forceps for a distance of several centimetres. Two pairs of right-angled forceps are applied to the trunk and the nerve is divided between the forceps.

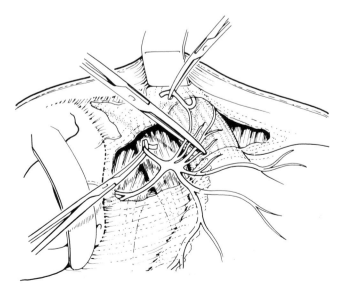

8

8 After division, the cut ends of the nerve are placed under traction sequentially to bring into prominence any other trunks of the anterior vagus and any branches originating at a point higher than the cut end of the trunk. A 2–3-cm section of the anterior trunk is sent for pathological identification.

Posterior truncal vagotomy

9 Exposure for the posterior truncal vagotomy is obtained by retraction of the oesophagus to the left and undertaking a minor degree of dissection between it and the right crus of the diaphragm. The key to identifying the posterior vagal trunk is its coeliac branch, which is constant in its course along the left gastric artery. If the index finger is placed on the aorta behind the oesophagus, and is then moved caudad along the anterior surface of the aorta, further distal progress of the index finger will be stopped by the left gastric artery as it comes off the coeliac axis. Gentle traction on the left gastric artery and the coeliac branch of the vagus with it will bring into prominence the posterior vagus, making it easily palpable. The posterior trunk is divided between right-angled forceps. Cephalad and caudad retraction of the proximal and distal cut ends of the vagus, respectively, will identify any additional branches or trunks that may need to be severed. A 2–3-cm piece of the trunk is removed and submitted for histological identification. The cut ends of the vagus are ligated with 2/0 silk sutures to prevent bleeding from any accompanying vessels. Secondary branches, if present, are divided between haemoclips.

The anterior and posterior surfaces of the oesophagus are then examined thoroughly for any uncut nerve twigs. Haemostasis is assured before pyloroplasty and closure.

Closure

The abdomen is closed, without drain, using continuous 0 Maxon sutures approximating the linea alba; several reinforcing, interrupted 0 Maxon sutures are also used. No subcutaneous sutures are necessary unless the patient is obese. Skin edges are approximated either with metal clips or with interrupted sutures of 3/0 silk.

Postoperative care

The postoperative management after abdominal vagotomy is described in the chapter on pp. 39–44.

Complications

Patients undergoing truncal vagotomy and drainage may develop the early complications that might occur in any patient undergoing an upper abdominal operation. Only specific complications and their management are discussed here.

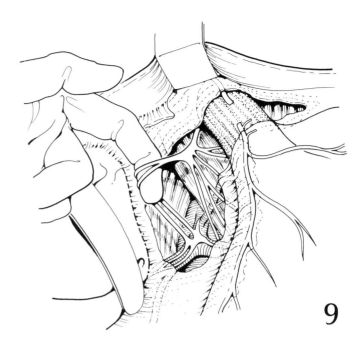

9

Oesophageal injury

A tear in the oesophagus may occur either as a result of the mobilization or dissection of nerve closely applied to the wall. When the injury is recognized, it is treated with direct suturing. The closure is reinforced further by pulling up some of the fundus and suturing it with 3/0 silk to the oesophagus or even performing a formal Nissen fundoplication. If an oesophageal injury has occurred, the perioesophageal area should be drained with a closed drainage system. A more serious problem arises when the oesophageal perforation is unrecognized at the time of operation. The patient will usually develop early signs and symptoms of sepsis and leucocytosis. Occasionally, these symptoms are delayed and appear only when the patient starts to take oral fluids. If other more common causes of sepsis are excluded, the patient should have a diatrizoate (Hypaque) swallow to locate any leak. If there is a leak, the patient is placed on triple antibiotics and taken back to the operating room. The goals of surgery are to repair the perforation, to reinforce it with a fundic wrap and to drain the area.

Splenic injury

Splenic injury is not uncommon. It is usually caused by medial retraction of the stomach, particularly when adhesions to the splenic capsule are present. The complication is more common in patients who have had a previous operation. It can be prevented by examination of the spleen for adhesions, early division of these adhesions and minimizing medial retraction of the stomach. Every effort should be made to conserve the spleen. If bleeding persists, however, the spleen should be removed.

Gastric outlet obstruction

This complication occurs as a result of suture line haematoma, technical problems with the pyloroplasty closure (inadvertent suturing of posterior wall to anterior wall; too much tissue inverted), oedema, or a minor suture line leak. The problem will resolve in most patients in 7–10 days. If not, a Hypaque swallow is required. If the obstruction has not resolved in 2 weeks, a careful endoscopic examination is necessary. In the meantime the patient is given total parenteral nutrition. If the obstruction is due to technical problems, the pyloroplasty should be revised as soon as possible. If the pyloroplasty is involved in an inflammatory mass, a retrocolic loop gastroenterostomy may be a safer procedure.

Postoperative pancreatitis

Fortunately this serious complication is uncommon after truncal vagotomy and drainage. The serum amylase concentration is often elevated, and no mechanical obstruction at the pyloroplasty is identifiable. The treatment is expectant, with the patient placed on total parenteral nutrition.

Postoperative jaundice

When postoperative obstruction jaundice occurs in a patient who has undergone suture control of a bleeding duodenal ulcer and vagotomy, the possibility of injury to the common bile duct should be seriously entertained. The diagnosis may be confirmed with ultrasonography, HIDA radionuclide scanning and/or transhepatic cholangiography. If obstruction of the common bile duct is identified, an operative approach will be required. The issue is the timing. It may be best to wait 3–4 weeks to allow for the bile duct to dilate. Also at that time, endoscopic retrograde cholangiography may be possible. It is unlikely, however, that the problem can be corrected endoscopically. Operative management will include cholecystectomy and Roux-en-Y choledochojejunostomy.

Leaking pyloroplasty

This is also an uncommon complication. The patient will either develop an acute abdomen or a subhepatic collection. In the former situation, an emergency operation will be required. In the latter, percutaneous drainage of the subhepatic collection may be possible.

The size of the leak can then be assessed by diatrizoate swallow and/or sinography. Further management depends on the findings. The patient should receive total parenteral nutrition, H_2-receptor antagonists to decrease gastric secretion and perhaps even the long-acting analogue of somatostatin. Eventually, however, surgical correction may be required.

The following late complications may also be encountered.

Recurrent ulcer disease

The incidence of recurrent ulcer after vagotomy and drainage for duodenal ulcer is 6–10%[4]. The causes of ulcer recurrence include:

1. Inadequate operation, usually because of incomplete vagotomy and occasionally because of inadequate drainage procedure. In about 70% of patients with incomplete vagotomy and ulcer recurrence, an intact posterior vagus is found at reoperation.
2. Zollinger–Ellison syndrome, a condition present in only 2% of patients with recurrent ulcer.
3. Excessive ingestion of ulcerogenic drugs, such as non-steroidal anti-inflammatory drugs.

If the recurrent ulcer is in the stomach, malignancy should always be excluded by endoscopy and biopsy.

The surgeon should have a well-formulated strategy for the diagnosis and treatment of recurrent ulcer. The diagnosis is usually suggested by recurrence of dyspeptic symptoms or by the development of complications: bleeding (overt or occult), perforation, or obstruction. The diagnosis is best established by endoscopy, although contrast studies of the upper gastrointestinal tract may also be useful. Having established the presence of recurrent ulcer, the next task is to establish the cause. The most important consideration is the possibility of incomplete vagotomy. This is best assessed by gastric secretory studies of acid. The basal acid output should be 2 mmol/h or lower. A basal acid output of 5 mmol/h or more is almost always indicative of incomplete vagotomy. The more direct way of testing completeness of vagotomy, however, is to stimulate the vagal centres in the brain either by insulin hypoglycaemia or by modified sham feeding (patient chews and spits without swallowing). The insulin test has been almost completely abandoned because of the risk of severe hypoglycaemia. Acid response to insulin hypoglycaemia or to sham feeding is evidence of incomplete vagotomy.

Zollinger–Ellison syndrome is ruled out by measuring plasma gastrin levels. It must be remembered, however, that vagotomy itself causes hypergastrinaemia. Hence, if a modestly elevated serum gastrin level is discovered, e.g. twice or three times normal, a provocative test with secretin should be performed. The intravenous administration of secretin, 2 units/kg, will cause a paradoxical increase of plasma gastrin (up to 100 pg/ml over basal) in Zollinger–Ellison syndrome, but will either have no effect or reduce plasma gastrin level in postvagotomy hypergastrinaemia. If a positive secretin test is obtained, a search for a gastrinoma should be initiated.

If the evidence suggests incomplete vagotomy, a decision must be made whether to treat the patient medically or to operate. Medical treatment requires a lifelong commitment to taking expensive medications. Except in the elderly, therefore, operative management will be necessary. The surgical options are to complete the vagotomy or to complete the vagotomy and perform antrectomy in addition. If at operation an intact vagal trunk, usually the posterior one, is found, completion vagotomy may suffice. If, on the other hand, the completion vagotomy is less than completely satisfactory, antrectomy with Billroth I anastomosis should be performed. If the primary operation included gastrojejunostomy, it is better to revise this and perform either a pyloroplasty or an antrectomy.

Dumping syndrome

This complication is seen in 10–15% of patients after vagotomy and pyloroplasty[5]. The symptoms may be mild and easily controllable with dietary measures. Occasionally, however, the symptoms can be quite severe. Two aspects of the syndrome are recognized. The early form, occurring within 30–60 min of eating, is manifested as abdominal pain, weakness, tachycardia with palpitation, and sometimes flushing and diarrhoea. The late dumping syndrome occurs 2 h or more after eating, and the symptoms are those of hypoglycaemia including lightheadedness, tachycardia, sweating and variable neuropsychiatric manifestations including seizure disorder or even coma. Early dumping syndrome is due to rapid entry of hyperosmolar chyme into the duodenum, leading to fluid shifts from the circulation into the gut lumen and to the release of a number of vasoactive substances from the gut, such as kinins, neurotensin and substance P. Late dumping syndrome is due to hyperinsulinism. The syndrome appears to be more common in slender women.

Most patients can be managed conservatively. Conservative measures include eating small dry meals, avoiding carbohydrates, lying down for 20–30 min after eating and drinking fluids about 30 min after eating. Severe symptoms can be effectively managed with the somatostatin analogue, octreotide; however, the drug has to be given by subcutaneous injection two or three times/day and long-term compliance of patients is poor. Surgical techniques to correct dumping include:
1. Pylorus reconstruction, a simple procedure that is 50–60% effective long-term.
2. Revision of gastroenterostomy with, or preferably without, pyloroplasty.
3. Antrectomy and Roux-en-Y gastrojejunostomy.
4. Insertion of a 10-cm antiperistaltic jejunal segment between the stomach and the duodenum.

The last procedure is seldom performed, because it tends to produce more problems than it solves.

The most important point to be made, therefore, is that it is easier to prevent than to treat dumping syndrome. In rare cases, dumping syndrome is a worse affliction for the patient than the primary peptic ulcer disease for which the operation was performed. Substituting proximal gastric vagotomy for truncal vagotomy as the primary elective operation for duodenal ulcer will prevent the development of this difficult side effect in almost all patients.

Postvagotomy diarrhoea

Diarrhoea develops in 10–20% of patients after truncal vagotomy and drainage[6]. The diarrhoea is usually mild, but in about 2% of patients it can be disabling. Typically, the diarrhoea is episodic and is associated with great urgency and the passage of much flatus with liquid stools. The exact pathophysiology of this complication is still unknown, and conservative measures to treat it are unsatisfactory. Interposition of a reversed segment of jejunum has been used to treat patients with the most severe postvagotomy diarrhoea. The results have been mixed and the operation is indicated only on very rare occasions.

Gallstone formation

An increased incidence of gallstone formation after truncal vagotomy has been reported on many occasions; the increase, however, is not significant[7]. Truncal vagotomy denervates the gallbladder and may also decrease the release of cholecystokinin from the duodenum. Both of these changes favour stasis in the gallbladder and stone formation.

References

1. Dragstedt LR, Owens FM Jr. Supradiaphragmatic section of the vagus nerves in the treatment of duodenal ulcer. *Proc Soc Exp Biol Med* 1943; 152–4.

2. Dragstedt LR, Woodward ER. Appraisal of vagotomy for peptic ulcer after 7 years. *JAMA* 1951; 145: 795–800.

3. Roberts JP, Debas HT. A simplified technique for rapid truncal vagotomy. *Surg Gynecol Obstet* 1989; 168: 539–41.

4. Stabile BE, Passaro E Jr. Recurrent peptic ulcer. *Gastroenterology* 1976; 70: 124–35.

5. Goligher JC, Pulvertaft CN, DeDombal FT, Conyers JH, Duthie HL, Feather DB *et al.* Five-to-eight-year results of Leeds/York controlled trial of elective surgery for duodenal ulcer. *BMJ* 1968; 2: 781–7.

6. Johnston D, Goligher JC. Selective, highly selective or truncal vagotomy? In 1976 – a clinical appraisal. *Surg Clin North Am* 1976; 56: 1313–34.

7. Thompson JC, Wiener I. Evaluation of surgical treatment of duodenal ulcer: short and long-term effects. *Clin Gastroenterol* 1984; 13: 569–600.

Total (selective) gastric vagotomy

Haile T. Debas MD

M. Galante Distinguished Professor of Surgery and Dean of the School of Medicine, University of California, San Francisco, California, USA

History

Selective gastric vagotomy was introduced in 1947 by Jackson[1]. Modifications of the procedure were suggested by Moore and Franksson[2, 3]. None of these surgeons combined selective gastric vagotomy with a drainage procedure. As a result, the operation was abandoned until Griffith and Harkins demonstrated the need for a drainage procedure, first in animals in 1955, and then in man in 1960[4, 5]. Subsequently, the operation was popularized by several surgeons in the treatment of duodenal ulcer. The main benefit claimed for selective gastric vagotomy over truncal vagotomy was a marked decrease in the incidence of episodic postvagotomy diarrhoea. The most significant, prospective, double-blind, randomized clinical trial comparing selective and truncal vagotomy was published by Kennedy *et al.* in 1973[6]. They showed that patients undergoing selective vagotomy had less postvagotomy diarrhoea, less ulcer recurrence, and superior Visick clinical status. Based on this study and that of Harkins *et al.*[7], the author believes that selective gastric vagotomy is superior to truncal vagotomy in the treatment of duodenal ulcer. The operation takes slightly longer to perform, however, and few surgeons have learnt to do it well. For this reason, it has not attained the same popularity as truncal vagotomy.

Principles and justification

Selective gastric vagotomy is designed to accomplish the following three goals: (1) total vagotomy of the stomach, (2) preservation of the hepatic division of the anterior vagus, hence preservation of the innervation of the liver, biliary tree and duodenum, and (3) preservation of the coeliac division of the posterior vagus, and hence preservation of the vagal innervation of the pancreas, the entire small intestine and the right colon to the midpoint of the transverse colon.

Because total gastric vagotomy is achieved, a drainage procedure is always needed with selective gastric vagotomy.

Indications

The indications for selective gastric vagotomy are identical to those for truncal vagotomy, the major ones being duodenal and prepyloric ulcer. Unless it is combined with antrectomy it requires a drainage procedure, either pyloroplasty or gastrojejunostomy. Because of the infrequency of elective surgery for peptic ulcer disease, the surgeon is wise to perform the procedure with which he/she is most comfortable. On the other hand, the surgeon who is experienced in selective gastric vagotomy is well advised to perform it, because the clinical results are superior to those of truncal vagotomy.

Operation

Incision

A supraumbilical midline incision provides a satisfactory approach.

Exposure

Exposure is obtained in a manner identical to that for truncal vagotomy, as described on page 361. The oesophagus is mobilized and encircled with a Penrose drain. The operation is performed in four steps:

1. Anterior selective gastric vagotomy with the preservation of the hepatic division.
2. Posterior selective gastric vagotomy with the preservation of the coeliac division.
3. 'Skeletonization' of the distal 6–8 cm of the oesophagus.
4. Performance of pyloroplasty.

Anterior selective gastric vagotomy

The hepatic division of the anterior vagus is easily seen if the assistant firmly retracts the stomach downward and to the left. The hepatic division will be seen as several whitish strands of nerve coursing towards the liver in the upper portion of the lesser omentum overlying the caudate lobe of the liver.

1 The peritoneal reflection over the abdominal vagus is incised transversely close to the diaphragm using scissors or electrocautery. This incision is carried onto the lesser omentum but short of the hepatic branches. An opening is made in the lesser omentum distal to the hepatic division. A vessel loop is passed around the hepatic division and the isolated lesser omentum. Gentle traction on the vessel loop will bring the anterior vagal trunk into prominence over the anterior surface of the oesophagus. The nerve trunk is bluntly dissected off the oesophagus using a pair of right-angled forceps, and a vessel loop is passed around it for retraction.

2 With the two vessel loops gently retracted to the right, everything contained within the lesser omentum along a line drawn between the two vessel loop retractors and the lesser curvature of the stomach is divided. Within the divided tissue is included the anterior nerve of Latarjet and all anterior gastric branches. This procedure completes anterior selective gastric vagotomy while preserving the anterior vagal trunk and its hepatic division.

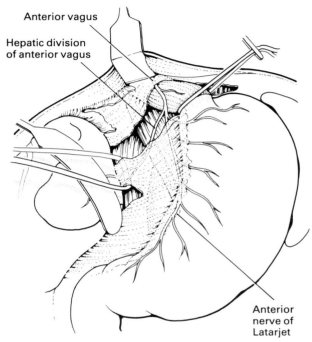

Anterior vagus

Hepatic division of anterior vagus

Anterior nerve of Latarjet

1

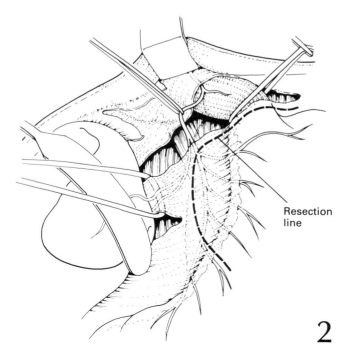

Resection line

2

Posterior selective gastric vagotomy

With the lesser omentum having been divided, an excellent approach is obtained to the region of the coeliac axis.

3 The abdominal aorta is palpated with a finger behind the oesophagus. As the finger is drawn distally over the anterior surface of the aorta, the left gastric artery is reached. Further gentle traction on the left gastric artery brings taut the coeliac division of the posterior vagus bringing the posterior vagus into prominence. The posterior vagus is dissected with a pair of right-angled forceps and encircled with a vessel loop for retraction. With the right vagus retracted to the right and the stomach firmly retracted to the left and downward, the coeliac division is easily felt as a piano string in close proximity to the left gastric artery over its proximal 3–4-cm course. The relationship, as well as the terminal branches of the left gastric artery beyond the coeliac division of the vagus, is noted.

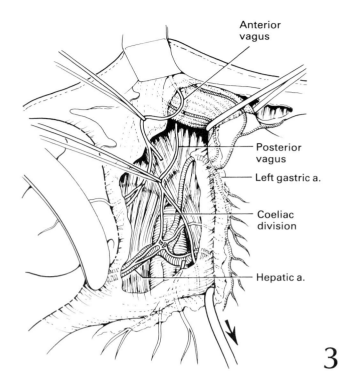

3

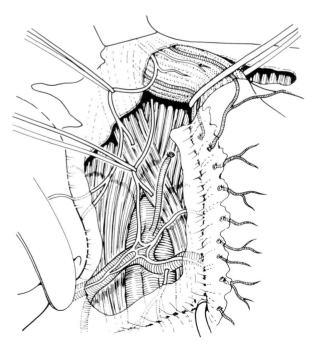

4

4 It is now possible to divide all the tissue between the posterior vagal trunk and the course of the coeliac division on the right and the stomach on the left. Thus, the posterior nerve of Latarjet, all the gastric vagal branches and the terminal branches of the left gastric artery are divided.

Skeletonization of the distal oesophagus

5 Analogous to the procedure in proximal gastric vagotomy, nerve fibres over the distal 6–8 cm of the oesophagus are carefully divided both on the anterior and posterior surface of the oesophagus. The dissection should also extend to the left of the gastro-oesophageal junction, so that the areolar tissue and peritoneal fold in this location are divided. Unless this step of the procedure is carefully performed, vagal fibres to the stomach coming off the anterior trunk above the diaphragm or from the distal oesophageal plexus and nerve branches at the angle of His will not be divided. The result is incomplete gastric vagotomy.

At this point the operative field should be inspected, ascertaining the preservation of the anterior vagus and its hepatic division, the posterior vagus and its coeliac division, and the adequacy of distal oesophageal skeletonization and haemostasis.

Performance of pyloroplasty

A Heineke–Mikulicz pyloroplasty (some prefer a Finney pyloroplasty) is performed as described in the chapter on pp. 394–402. The abdomen is irrigated with saline and closed without drainage.

Postoperative care

This is identical to that described for other types of vagotomy, as described on pp. 39–44.

Complications

Early complications are those of any vagotomy, and include inadvertent damage to the oesophagus and

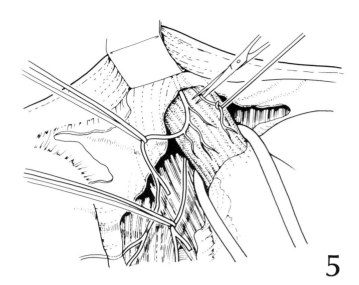

5

bleeding either from splenic injury or from uncontrolled vessels. Late complications are the same as those described for truncal vagotomy on pp. 369–372. The long-term complications of selective gastric vagotomy have been compared with those of truncal vagotomy in prospective randomized trials by Kronborg et al.[8]; the results of the trial by Kennedy et al. are summarized in *Table 1*. The reduction in the incidence of diarrhoea is significant. While the differences in the incidence of a positive Hollander (insulin) test and recurrent ulcer did not achieve significance, the data suggest that better denervation can be achieved with selective than with truncal vagotomy.

References

1. Jackson RG. Anatomic study of the vagus nerves and technic of transabdominal selective gastric vagus resection. *Univ Hosp Bull, Ann Arbor* 1947; 13: 31–5.

2. Moore FD. Follow-up of vagotomy in duodenal ulcer. *Gastroenterology* 1948; 11: 442–52.

3. Franksson C. Selective abdominal vagotomy. *Acta Chir Scand* 1948; 96: 409–12.

4. Griffith CA, Harkins HN. Partial gastric vagotomy: an experimental study. *Gastroenterology* 1957; 32: 96–102.

5. Griffith CA. Gastric vagotomy vs. total abdominal vagotomy. *Arch Surg* 1960; 81: 781–8.

6. Kennedy T, Connell AM, Love AHG, MacRae KD, Spencer EFA. Selective or truncal vagotomy? Five-year results of a double blind, randomized, controlled trial. *Br J Surg* 1973; 60: 944–8.

7. Harkins HN, Stavney LS, Griffith CA, Savage LE, Kaj T, Nyhus LM. Selective gastric vagotomy. *Ann Surg* 1963; 158: 448–60.

8. Kronborg O, Malmstrom J, Christiansen PM. A comparison between the results of truncal and selective vagotomy in patients with duodenal ulcer. *Scand J Gastroenterol* 1970; 5: 519–24.

Table 1 Comparison of the results of selective and truncal vagotomies. Reproduced with permission from Kennedy et al.[6]

	Truncal vagotomy and pyloroplasty	Selective vagotomy and pyloroplasty
Number of patients	50	50
Follow-up (years)	5	5
Positive Hollander test (%)	18	4
Recurrent ulcer (%)	7	0
Dumping (%)	11	26
Diarrhoea (%)	27	8
Clinical grading:		
Perfect (%)	63 } 87	55 } 96
Good (%)	24	41
Fair (%)	4	0
Poor (%)	9	4

Proximal gastric vagotomy

Haile T. Debas MD

M. Galante Distinguished Professor of Surgery and Dean of the School of Medicine, University of California, San Francisco, California, USA

Principles and justification

Proximal gastric vagotomy (PGV) selectively denervates the acid-producing part of the stomach (the body and fundus). The operation preserves the vagal innervation of the antrum and pylorus, making a gastric drainage procedure unnecessary. The operation is sometimes also referred to as highly selective vagotomy (HSV) or parietal cell vagotomy (PCV). Strictly speaking, the latter appellation should only by used when the operation is performed while the effect on parietal cell function is monitored either with an intragastric pH electrode or Congo red spray. PGV reduces both acid and pepsin secretion. Basal acid secretion is reduced by 80%, while maximal acid response to pentagastrin or to a meal is reduced by 50–60%. The rate of ulcer recurrence has varied from 2% to 22% among different surgeons, presumably because of variations in operative technique[1]. Although several potential sites of incomplete vagotomy are possible, the most important determinant of ulcer recurrence appears to be the thoroughness with which the distal 6–8 cm of the oesophagus is 'skeletonized' of vagal fibres. Hallenbeck *et al.* compared the results of PGV in which only the distal 1–2 cm was skeletonized with that in which the distal 5–7 cm of the oesophagus was denervated[2]. The former operation was associated with a 15.4% incidence of proven recurrent ulceration and a 10.2% incidence of suspected recurrence. By comparison, when 5–7.5 cm of the distal oesophagus was skeletonized, only one of 14 patients developed a recurrent ulcer.

PGV requires meticulous operative technique, not only to accomplish complete vagotomy but also to preserve the innervation of the antropyloric mechanism, critically important in promoting normal gastric emptying postoperatively.

Indications

Worldwide, PGV is the choice for elective operation in duodenal ulcer disease. It is a safe operation with a rate of operative mortality of less than 0.3%[3]. It is also associated with the lowest incidence of such undesirable side effects as dumping and diarrhoea[4]. However, the incidence of ulcer recurrence after PGV (10–15%) is significantly higher than after vagotomy and antrectomy. Despite this, recurrent ulcer after PGV appears to be more responsive to H_2-receptor antagonists than does primary duodenal ulcer. In addition, should surgical management become necessary for ulcer recurrence, antrectomy with or without truncal vagotomy appears to be highly efficacious[5].

Prospective randomized clinical trials have established that patients with perforated duodenal ulcer should undergo PGV in addition to closure of the perforation[6]. Routine application of PGV in perforated duodenal ulcer is indicated unless the perforation has existed for longer than 24 h, is associated with significant peritoneal contamination, or the patient is unstable with severe cardiopulmonary, renal or other serious illness.

The application of PGV in the management of emergency or urgent complications of duodenal ulcer has not been unanimously accepted. When an emergency operation is performed to control bleeding, suture control of the bleeding ulcer can be accomplished via a duodenotomy that does not violate the pylorus[7]. The operation can then be completed with the performance of PGV providing the patient is stable, otherwise healthy and not old or frail. This approach is particularly appealing in women who are believed to be more susceptible than men to the development of dumping and other undesirable side effects following truncal vagotomy and pyloroplasty or vagotomy and antrectomy. The use of PGV and balloon dilatation of the pylorus in the surgical management of an ulcer that has caused gastric outlet obstruction appears unjustified. When this procedure was utilized in the past, acute pyloric perforation or postoperative obstruction occurred. Most surgeons in the USA prefer to treat duodenal ulcer with pyloric obstruction by vagotomy and antrectomy. The experience with PGV and pyloroplasty in this setting is insufficient to recommend the approach.

Some have advocated the use of PGV combined with ulcer excision in the treatment of benign gastric ulcer. Collected series from the literature show a rate of ulcer recurrence of 3–23% after follow-up of 2–12 years[8]. However, most surgeons prefer to treat gastric ulcer by antrectomy because it removes all the susceptible mucosa and results in a rate of ulcer recurrence of only 2%. At present, therefore, the prime indications for PGV are elective operation for duodenal ulcer, in perforated duodenal ulcer, and in good risk patients, particularly women, with bleeding from a duodenal ulcer.

Preoperative

Patients requiring PGV have the routine preoperative management of any patient of comparable age. Cardiopulmonary and renal evaluation is routine in patients over 40 years of age. Perioperative antibiotic use is probably unnecessary because the gastrointestinal tract is not entered and, even if it were, the stomach and duodenum in these patients are sterile because of the hypersecretion of acid. In practice, however, patients are given a second generation cephalosporin on arrival in the operating theatre and three more doses postoperatively, so that they receive antibiotic coverage for 24 h.

Immunoreactive plasma gastrin levels are measured routinely before surgery to rule out Zollinger–Ellison syndrome. The yield is small but the test is simple and relatively inexpensive. Although only one in 1000 patients with duodenal ulcer disease will have a gastrinoma, the incidence in those patients with severe enough disease to require an operation is unknown.

It is also advisable to discontinue H_2-receptor antagonists at least 24 h before operation and omeprazole 5–7 days preoperatively to restore acidity in the gastroduodenal lumen and to reverse any bacterial colonization that might have occurred over a long course of medical treatment. Again, this consideration is probably less important in PGV where the gastrointestinal tract is not entered than in vagotomy and drainage or gastric resection procedures.

Operation

General endotracheal anaesthesia is used. The patient is placed supine on the operating table and a nasogastric tube is inserted as soon as anaesthesia is induced. The abdomen is prepared and draped exposing the lower chest for 5–7 cm above the xiphisternal junction and the abdomen midway between the umbilicus and pubic symphysis. Tilting the operating table 15–20° in the reverse Trendelenburg position will allow the intestines to be displaced away from the upper abdomen. A midline incision is employed. Depending on the habitus of the patient, the incision may need to extend around the umbilicus. The upper limit of the incision should extend along the xiphoid process for 2–3 cm onto the sternum. Once the abdomen is entered, complete exploration is performed to rule out other unexpected pathology. The first portion of the duodenum is inspected for ulcer disease and the pyloric vein of Mayo, usually present, is identified. The first portion of the duodenum is often shortened, scarred and distorted. Sometimes the presence of an active ulcer is suggested by a characteristic stippling that develops when the serosal surface of the duodenum is gently rubbed with gauze.

Exposure

1 The left triangular ligament of the liver is divided, taking care not to injure the inferior phrenic vein at the extreme right extent of the ligament. Once this ligament is divided, retractors can be used to expose the hiatus. The author prefers to use the Bookwalter retractor. Alternatively, the double-arm 'Iron Intern' may be used. One arm of the latter retractor is used to pull up the sternum, while a Deaver-type retractor is applied to the other arm to pull upwards and to the right the left lobe of the liver which frequently can be folded under the right lobe, protected with a moist laparotomy sponge and retracted.

With this retractor a self-retaining Balfour retractor needs to be used to keep the wound edges open. The advantage of the Bookwalter retractor, however, is that all the necessary blades to retract the sternum, the liver and the body wall can be attached to and optimally positioned on the oval ring of the instrument. If the above retractors are not available, the sternum can be retracted upwards using a Richardson retractor attached to a rope which can be tied to the rigid anaesthetic frame as originally suggested by Goligher. An excellent exposure is usually achieved with these retractors. A headlight significantly improves visibility.

It is now possible to retract the stomach downwards and to the left out of the abdomen and to examine the distribution of the anterior vagus nerve. Except in rare circumstances it is possible to visualize the hepatic branches within the lesser omentum near the gastro-oesophageal junction, and the anterior nerve of Latarjet as it courses along the lesser curvature 1.5–2 cm from the stomach. Distally, the nerve of Latarjet will cross the anterior surface of the stomach to divide into its terminal branches. Goligher has coined the term 'the crow's foot' to describe the appearance of the terminal branching of the anterior nerve of Latarjet.

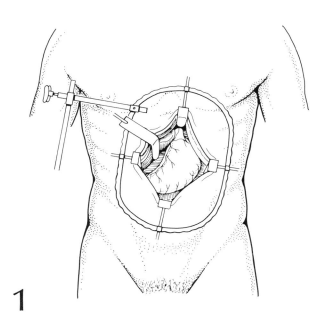

1

Mobilization of oesophagus and vagal trunks

With the stomach retracted inferiorly, the oesophagus and the nasogastric tube within it are palpated. The peritoneal reflection over the abdominal oesophagus is incised and the incision carried to the right towards the hepatic branches in the lesser omentum. The oesophagus is then bluntly dissected with the finger.

2 As the finger is passed behind the oesophagus, the posterior vagus nerve is often palpable. The oesophagus should be dissected leaving behind the posterior vagus nerve. Once the oesophagus is dissected circumferentially, a 0.75-inch Penrose drain is passed around it for retraction. Next, the anterior vagal trunk(s) is identified. This is best done by retracting the hepatic branches inferiorly with the right index finger while palpating with the middle finger over the anterior surface of the oesophagus. This manoeuvre brings the anterior vagal trunk(s) taut.

Using right-angled forceps, the anterior vagal trunk is dissected off the oesophagus and encircled with rubber vessel loops (or silk thread) for retraction to the right. The posterior vagus nerve is next identified. The oesophagus is retracted to the left and the areolar tissue between the oesophagus and the right diaphragmatic crus is dissected. The simplest way of locating the posterior vagal trunk is by retracting downwards its constant branch, the coeliac division. The coeliac division of the posterior vagus courses along the left gastric artery. The aorta below the diaphragm can be palpated with the right index finger. If the index finger is now drawn downwards over the anterior surface of the aorta, further downward progression of the finger will be stopped by the left gastric artery as it originates from the coeliac axis. Application of further traction on the left gastric artery, and hence on the coeliac division, will bring taut the posterior vagus wherever it is, thereby making it readily palpable. It is dissected and encircled with a vascular loop or silk ligature in a manner analogous to the anterior vagus nerve. The identification and dissection of the anterior and posterior vagal trunks at this stage is not always necessary, but this manoeuvre simplifies the subsequent steps of the operation. Having identified and gently retracted the anterior and posterior vagal trunks, the surgeon is now ready to start the vagotomy. Retraction of the stomach downwards and to the left, manually or with Babcock's clamps, is an essential manoeuvre.

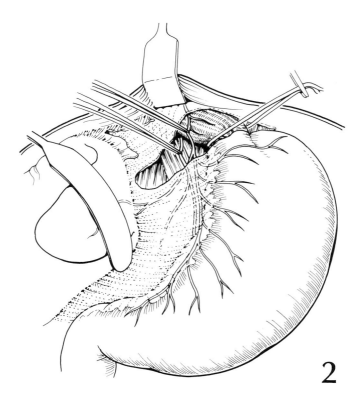

2

Anterior vagotomy of the proximal stomach

PGV is started by identifying the distal limit of dissection. Frequently the crow's foot of the anterior vagus can be seen. If so, anterior vagotomy is started by taking the uppermost digit of the crow's foot. If the anatomy is not obvious, a point on the lesser curvature 7 cm from the pylorus (the pyloric vein of Mayo) is selected by ruler measurement and marked with a 3/0 suture on the antrum. Dissection will start here and proceed proximally.

Goligher has pointed out that there are three tissue layers at the lesser curvature where the lesser omentum inserts onto the stomach: an anterior layer in which vessels and the gastric branches of the anterior vagus are found; a middle areolar layer containing some vessels; and the posterior leaf of the omentum containing the gastric branches from the posterior vagus and vessels[9]. Taking these three layers individually greatly simplifies the operation.

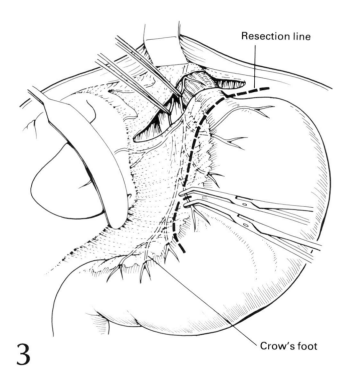

Resection line

Crow's foot

3

3 Starting at the selected distal point of dissection, a curved haemostat is passed under the vessels of the anterior layer. The vessels are clamped, divided and tied with 4/0 silk sutures very close to the gastric wall. The process is repeated serially up the lesser curvature, dividing the neurovascular structures in the anterior leaf, until the gastro-oesophageal junction is reached. Only small bites must be taken. Haemoclips should be avoided because they come off, causing annoying bleeding. Electrocautery must be avoided because the nerve branches being cut may transmit the current to the nerves of Latarjet.

The previously dissected anterior vagal trunk must be retracted and visualized. In the same manner, the middle layer is dissected and divided. It is easier at this point to proceed with division of the gastric branches from the posterior nerve of Latarjet and to leave the oesophageal dissection until later.

Posterior vagotomy of the proximal stomach

4 When PGV was first undertaken the author used to identify the posterior nerve of Latarjet by dividing the gastrocolic omentum to enter the lesser sac and by retracting the stomach superiorly. Now no attempt is made to identify the posterior nerve of Latarjet as an initial step, and the lesser curvature is dissected close to the stomach to divide the neurovascular structures in the posterior leaf of the lesser omentum. It is important to hug the lesser curvature but to take care to avoid including the wall of the stomach in the ligatures.

The first step in this posterior dissection is to enter the lesser sac with a curved haemostat at the distal point of dissection. Once a few vessels are divided, the anterior surface of the pancreas is clearly seen behind the stomach. Again, the devascularization–denervation procedure is carried up the lesser curve of the stomach towards the gastro-oesophageal junction. Near the cardia and behind it, the so-called 'criminal' nerve of Grassi may be seen coming off the posterior vagus nerve and coursing behind the stomach to the left. It must be divided.

At this stage it is often possible to visualize the posterior nerve of Latarjet on the posterior surface of the cut edge of the lesser omentum usually 1–1.5 cm from the edge.

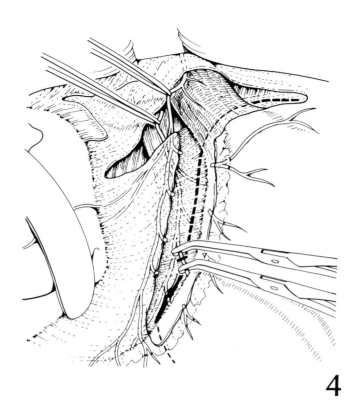

4

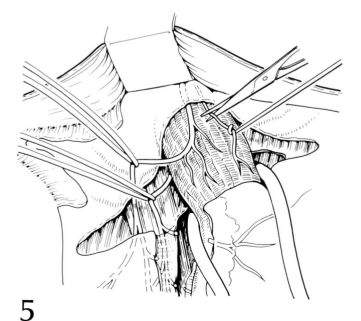

5

Oesophageal 'skeletonization'

5 The next task is to vagally denervate the distal 6–8 cm of the oesophagus, first anteriorly and then posteriorly. The anterior vagal trunk is gently retracted to the right and all neurovascular structures on the anterior surface of the oesophagus are divided. It is necessary to carry out this dissection carefully and meticulously. Some vagal fibres will be found embedded in the oesophageal muscle. These must be divided without injuring the oesophagus. The dissection must also extend beyond the oesophagus at the angle of His and all fibrous and areolar tissue in this location must be divided.

Next, the posterior surface of the distal oesophagus is skeletonized. The oesophagus is retracted to the left, and the posterior vagus to the right. The assistant can rotate the oesophagus with his fingers to expose the posterior surface to the surgeon. Again, meticulous division of all neural fibres over the distal 6–8 cm of the oesophagus is necessary. When this is done vagotomy is complete.

Inspection of completed vagotomy

6 It is now necessary to trace the anterior and posterior vagus nerves distally, following the nerves of Latarjet to the pylorus and ensuring that both these nerves are intact. The posterior surface of the oesophagus must be inspected and any undivided nerve fibres sought behind the cardia. Haemostasis must be adequate. The Penrose drain around the oesophagus and the vessel loops around the vagal trunks are removed.

At this point the surgeon has the option of imbricating the lesser curvature with 3/0 silk sutures that bury the dissected surface. Those who perform lesser curve imbrication cite two potential advantages; first, the procedure may minimize nerve regeneration, and secondly, it may help to prevent gastric perforation if lesser curve devascularization has occurred. It must be stated, however, that lesser curve necrosis is an extremely rare complication and probably occurs because the stomach wall is incorporated in a ligature.

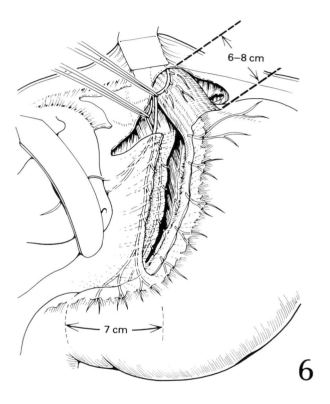

Potential pitfalls

7 The potential pitfalls in PGV are (1) inadequate margins of dissection resulting from a failure to denervate the distal 6–8 cm of the oesophagus or because of an inappropriate distal limit of denervation; and (2) secondary sites of incomplete vatogotomy, such as the angle of His fibres, the 'criminal' nerve of Grassi, or gastroepiploic nerves.

Of these, by far the most important is failure to skeletonize the distal 6–8 cm of the oesophagus. The study by Hallenbeck *et al.* showing the importance of this has already been cited[2]. Similar experience was reported by Liedberg and Oscarson[10]. These authors reported ulcer recurrence in four of 20 patients, and an 83% positive Hollander test when they performed PGV with limited denervation of the distal oesophagus. After modifying their procedure to include denervation of the distal 6–8 cm of the oesophagus, none of 60 patients developed ulcer recurrence and only 31% had a positive Hollander test.

The distal limit of denervation has not been found to be as critical as the proximal. For example, Johnston *et al.*, using anatomical landmarks, left only 6.5 cm of distal antrum innervated. By contrast, Amdrup *et al.*, employing either a pH electrode or Congo red spray to determine the antral–fundic junction, left an average of 9 cm of antrum innervated[9]. Despite these differences, both procedures were equally effective in inhibiting basal and maximal acid secretion. This type of comparison, however, gives little idea of long-term results with respect to ulcer recurrence. It has come to light, for instance, that ulcer recurrence in patients operated upon by the Copenhagen group was about 38% in a 25-year follow-up[11].

The results of incomplete vagotomy because of failure to divide the 'criminal' nerve, the nerves at the angle of His, or the gastroepiploic branches at the greater curve have not been quantified. However, on theoretical grounds the minor degree of incomplete vagotomy so caused may, with the passage of time, cause problems. Hypergastrinaemia develops after PGV. Any parietal mucosa left innervated will be chronically stimulated by the elevated levels of gastrin, not only to secrete acid but also to undergo hyperplasia. Because of these concerns, Braghetto *et al.* have proposed that the

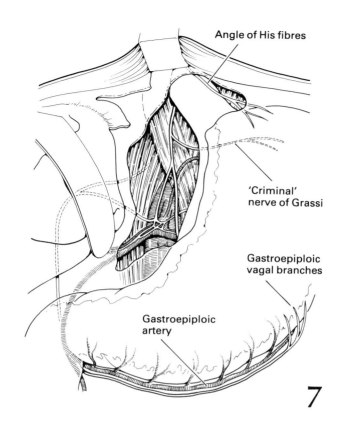

gastroepiploic fibres should be cut by dissection at the greater curvature at the junction of the left and right gastroepiploic arteries[12]. This procedure has been referred to as extended PGV.

Postoperative care

The nasogastric tube placed at the time of operation is kept on continuous low suction for 24 h and then removed. By the second or third postoperative day the patient may be started on clear fluids. Some surgeons prefer to wait until gastrointestinal motility returns as evidenced by the passage of flatus. If the patient tolerates clear fluid, the diet can be advanced quickly to a regular diet. The patient is typically discharged from the hospital any time between the fourth and sixth postoperative day. Because patients lose gastric accommodation after PGV, they are advised to eat smaller meals 4–6 times a day for 4–8 weeks. The author prefers to place the patient back on H_2-receptor antagonists for 2–3 weeks postoperatively, but this practice is based on preference and not on any documented evidence of advantage.

References

1. Jaffe BM. Parietal cell vagotomy: surgical technique, gastric acid secretion, and recurrence. *Surgery* 1977; 82: 284–6.

2. Hallenbeck GA, Gleysteen JJ, Aldrete JS, Slaughter RL. Proximal gastric vagotomy: effects of two operative techniques on clinical and gastric secretory results. *Ann Surg* 1976; 184: 435–42.

3. Johnston D. Operative mortality and postoperative morbidity of highly selective vagotomy. *BMJ* 1975; 4: 545–7.

4. Johnston D, Goligher JC. Selective, highly selective or truncal vagotomy? In 1976 – a clinical appraisal. *Surg Clin North Am* 1976; 56: 1313–34.

5. Herrington JL Jr, Bluett MK. The surgical management of recurrent ulceration. *Contemp Surg* 1986; 28: 15–24.

6. Boey J, Branick FJ, Alagaratnam TT *et al*. Proximal gastric vagotomy: the preferred operation for perforations in acute duodenal ulcer. *Ann Surg* 1988; 208: 169–74.

7. Johnston D, Lyndon PJ, Smith RB, Humphrey CS. Highly selective vagotomy without a drainage procedure in the treatment of haemorrhage, perforation and pyloric stenosis due to peptic ulcer. *Br J Surg* 1973; 60: 790–7.

8. Heberer G, Teichmann RK. Recurrence after proximal gastric vagotomy for gastric, pyloric and prepyloric ulcers. *World J Surg* 1987; 11: 283–8.

9. Goligher JC. A technique for highly selective (parietal cell or proximal gastric) vagotomy for duodenal ulcer. *Br J Surg* 1974; 61: 337–45.

10. Liedberg G, Oscarson J. Selective proximal vagotomy – short time follow-up of 80 patients. *Scand J Gastroenterol Suppl* 1973; 20: 12.

11. Hoffman J, Jensen H-E, Christiansen J, Olesen A, Loud FB, Hauch O. Prospective controlled vagotomy trial for duodenal ulcer. Results after 11–15 years. *Ann Surg* 1989; 209: 40–5.

12. Braghetto I, Csendes A, Lazo M *et al*. A prospective randomized study comparing highly selective vagotomy and extended highly selective vagotomy in patients with duodenal ulcer. *Am J Surg* 1988; 155: 443–6.

Illustrations by Gillian Oliver

Complications of ulcer surgery: prevention and reoperative management

Haile T. Debas MD
M. Galante Distinguished Professor of Surgery and Dean of the School of Medicine, University of California, San Francisco, California, USA

Sam H. Carvajal MD
Research Fellow, Department of Surgery, University of California, San Francisco, California, USA

Principles and justification

Reoperative gastric surgery is technically challenging and is fraught with pitfalls. The dissection may be difficult because of dense adhesions to surrounding structures including the spleen, the transverse colon, pancreas, and structures of the porta hepatis. With appropriate preoperative management and an effective operative plan, the risks of reoperative ulcer surgery can be minimized.

Indications for reoperative ulcer surgery include bleeding, obstruction, anastomotic dehiscence, recurrent ulcer disease, dumping syndrome, intractable diarrhoea, afferent loop syndrome and alkaline reflux gastritis. Accurate diagnosis of the complication must be established. Understanding the pathophysiology of the complication is also essential to choosing the appropriate corrective operation.

Indications for reoperative ulcer surgery may be divided into early and late. Early indications are for septic complications, bleeding and obstruction. The two most common late indications are recurrent ulcer disease and alkaline reflux gastritis.

The undesirable sequelae of ulcer surgery can lead to profound metabolic abnormalities, extracellular fluid depletion and nutritional deficit. This is particularly true in patients with gastric outlet obstruction. Without adequate correction of these abnormalities preoperatively, successful resolution of the complication by surgery may be difficult.

Technical manoeuvres in abdominal re-exploration

1 Whatever the specific indication for gastric reoperation, the same precautions apply both in entering the abdomen and in the dissection of the stomach. The small intestine and the transverse colon may be adherent to the undersurface of the incision. To avoid injury to these structures during entry, the incision is best extended beyond the scar so that the abdomen may be opened at a site free of adhesions. Alternatively, if the original incision was vertical, the abdomen can be safely entered in the upper portion of the scar over the liver.

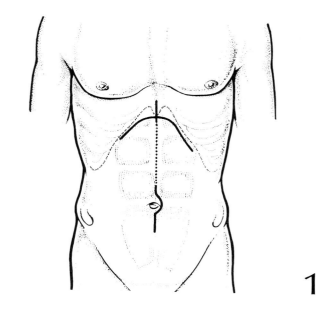

1

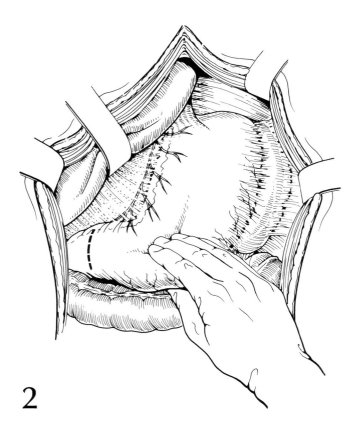

2

2 The spleen is at highest risk of injury in reoperative gastric surgery because of the formation of capsular adhesions. Traction on these adhesions readily tears the spleen. This can be avoided by two manoeuvres: first, by exposing the spleen and dividing all evident adhesions between the stomach and the spleen; and secondly, by avoiding medial retraction of the stomach. The stomach is more safely retracted laterally and inferiorly.

The stomach and the duodenum, if present, are often densely adherent to the undersurface of the liver. These structures are best dissected by separating the adhesions to the liver very close to the liver capsule. A combination of scissors, knife and electrocautery dissection is often necessary. Occasionally the adhesions are so dense that the stomach is not readily identified, in which case a previously inserted nasogastric tube may be felt by palpation. Alternatively, air may be insufflated into the stomach.

Careful dissection is also necessary in identifying previous suture lines such as pyloroplasty or gastrojejunal stomas. The gallbladder may be used as a guide to dissecting the first portion of the duodenum. Gastrojejunal stomas are readily identified when antecolic. When retrocolic, however, the transverse colon should be dissected and lifted upwards to identify the stoma which should be below the mesocolon.

Operations

EARLY COMPLICATIONS

The early complications are often the result of technical problems and typically require emergency surgery. It is important to recognize the complications early and to treat them promptly to minimize morbidity and mortality.

Septic complications

The incidence of septic complications after gastric surgery is reported to be 2–3%. Most septic complications following gastric surgery are due to technical failure which may include suture line leak, anastomotic dehiscence, unrecognized oesophageal perforation during vagotomy, and partial or complete gastric necrosis. In addition, conditions not directly related to the technical procedure may cause peritonitis. Important among these are pancreatitis and acalculous cholecystitis. Peritonitis following laparotomy can be difficult to diagnose clinically. The usual symptoms of abdominal pain and signs of rebound tenderness, ileus and fever are often explained away as normal postoperative events. As soon as peritonitis is diagnosed, the patient should be placed on intravenous triple antibiotics for coverage of Gram-positive, Gram-negative and anaerobic bacteria. The development of significant leucocytosis, hypotension, respiratory distress, tachycardia, persistent abdominal pain, or prolonged ileus should prompt investigation. This may include imaging studies by ultrasonography and/or computed tomography which will provide diagnosis of cholecystitis, pancreatitis or abscess formation if present. Upper gastrointestinal views with a water-soluble contrast medium may be obtained if a leak is suspected. If a leak is strongly suspected but not observed with a water-soluble contrast medium, barium may then be used as it may be a more sensitive indicator of small leaks.

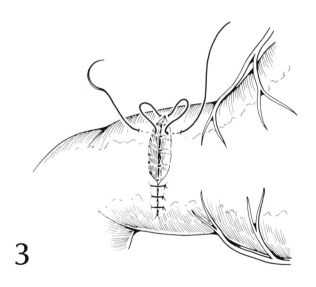

3

Prevention

3 Since most of these complications are caused by technical error, prevention becomes important. After gastric surgery, suture line dehiscence is rare. The most common sites are at the corners which may have been difficult to visualize or construct. Surgeons have referred to these sites as 'corners of grief'. A corner leak is best prevented by a special suture technique designed to invert the corner completely. A Lembert stitch is started on one side of the suture line about 5 mm from the corner. The tissue adjacent to the corner is then incorporated and, finally, the second half of the Lembert suture is placed. When the suture is tied, the corner is safely tucked in.

The duodenal stump may provide a serious challenge to the surgeon. Duodenal stump blow-out is a serious complication that usually occurs between the 7th and 12th postoperative days. The experienced surgeon prevents this tragedy in two ways. The most important principle in ulcer surgery is to examine the duodenal bulb very carefully before an operation is selected. When the duodenum is severely scarred or involved in an inflammatory mass, any direct attack on the duodenum should be avoided. Patients with this problem should be treated by vagotomy and gastroenterostomy. Secondly, if after duodenal transection the surgeon finds that closure of the duodenal stump will be difficult, he would be prudent to accept a controlled duodenal fistula.

4 The duodenum is closed with a 2/0 silk purse-string suture around a 20-Fr or 24-Fr Foley catheter. This is further reinforced with omentum. When this manoeuvre becomes necessary, additional procedures are required for safety including: (1) adequate drainage of the subhepatic space with Penrose drains or preferably with a closed, soft drainage system; (2) provision of a tube gastrostomy, if possible; and (3) a feeding jejunostomy. The Foley catheter is left in place for 3 or more weeks and is removed only when the Penrose drainage is minimal and the patient appears to be clinically out of trouble.

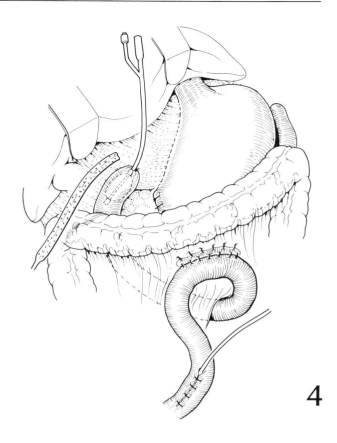

4

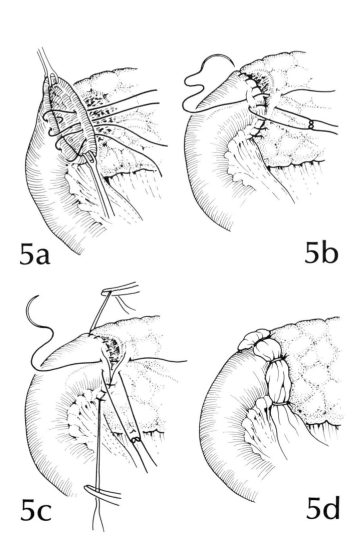

5a

5b

5c

5d

5a–d Several other techniques are available to close a difficult duodenal stump. One of these is the Nissen technique suitable for a posterior ulcer that has penetrated into the head of the pancreas. The duodenal stump is closed with a continuous inner layer of absorbable suture. The discrepancy between the anterior wall and the deficient posterior duodenal wall is dealt with by suturing the anterior wall of the duodenum to the pancreatic capsule at the inferior edge of the ulcer penetration.

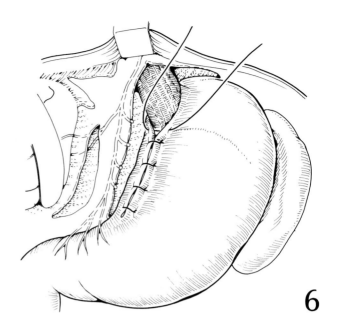

6

6 A rare cause of septic complication after proximal gastric vagotomy is lesser curve necrosis. This complication occurs not because of devascularization of the stomach, but rather as a result of the incorporation of the gastric wall in a ligature. This complication may be prevented by more careful ligation of vessels and by enfolding the lesser curvature with several inverting Lembert 3/0 silk sutures. This enfolding manoeuvre has the additional theoretical advantage of preventing nerve regeneration.

Operative management

Subphrenic abscess
Nearly all subphrenic abscesses are now drained percutaneously with ultrasound or computed tomographic guidance. Some, however, are not accessible to percutaneous drainage and must be drained operatively. One approach in which the abscess is drained through the bed of the 12th rib is discussed here. This procedure is suitable only for posterior subphrenic abscesses.

7 Depending on the location of the abscess, the patient is placed with the right or left side upwards. The 12th rib is palpated and an incision is made along its length.

7

8   The rib is exposed and resected subperiosteally. A syringe with a 20-gauge needle is used to aspirate for the abscess. Once the abscess is located, a transverse incision is made across the rib bed at the level of the first lumbar vertebra.

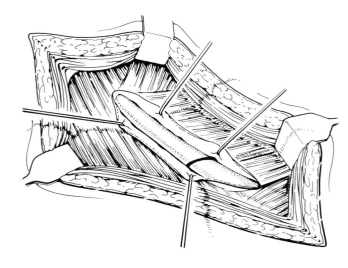

8

9   This incision should not be along the bed of the rib because of the danger of entering the pleural cavity. The erector spinae muscle must be retracted upwards and posteriorly. The incision should be large enough to accommodate the surgeon's hand. Once the abscess is entered, loculations are gently broken manually and, if on the right, the space between the liver and the kidney is readily explored.

The space is now irrigated thoroughly with saline using a no. 16 Robinson red rubber catheter. At least two large soft drains (Penrose or closed drainage system) are inserted into the abscess cavity. The wound is then closed around these and the drains are secured to the skin.

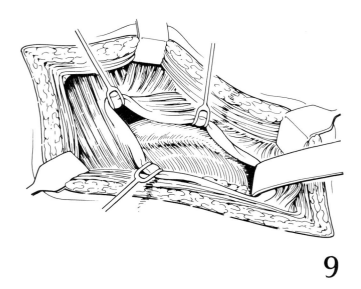

9

Suture line dehiscence

This is a rare complication after ulcer surgery. Infrequently, the lesser curve suture line, pyloroplasty, or even gastroduodenal or gastrojejunal anastomosis may fail. The patient develops peritonitis and systemic signs of sepsis. Plain films of the abdomen may show more free air than expected. Diagnosis is established by upper gastrointestinal study using water-soluble contrast medium.

Unless the leak is small and can be controlled with percutaneous and intraluminal catheters, the patient will require re-exploration. The dehisced area should be closed with suture, reinforced with omental patch, and drained adequately. Sometimes, however, the suture line will have to be taken down and reconstructed, or even resected.

Duodenal stump blow-out

Prevention of this disastrous complication has been discussed above. Percutaneous catheter control of the leak may be possible depending on whether the process is localized. Otherwise, operative intervention will be necessary to provide a controlled duodenal fistula with catheter drainage (see above) and feeding jejunostomy.

Unrecognized oesophageal perforation

10 This, too is a rare complication of vagotomy. Oesophageal perforation, if it occurs, is usually evident during the operation. However, small perforations may be missed or go unsuspected. The clinical picture is that of any perforated viscus, and will require contrast studies to establish the diagnosis. Almost always, an emergency operation will be needed.

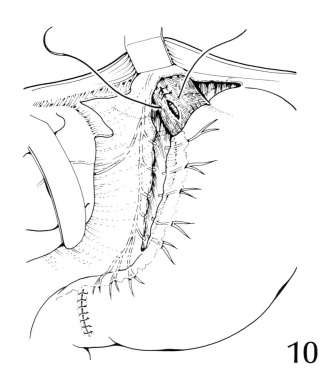

10

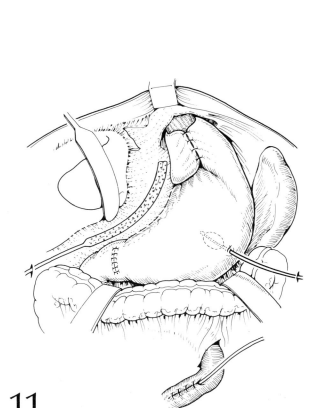

11

11 The goals of the operation are to close the perforation and protect the closure with some sort of gastric wrap. The authors prefer to use a Nissen fundoplication to completely surround the repair. Again, gastrostomy, drainage, and feeding jejunostomy are important adjuncts to treatment.

Bleeding

Postoperative bleeding can occur into the peritoneal cavity or into the gastrointestinal tract. Intraperitoneal bleeding may result from splenic injury or stem from previously divided and ligated vessels. Upper gastrointestinal bleeding following ulcer surgery, particularly if the indication for operation has been bleeding, is likely to be from the ulcer bed. However, bleeding into the lumen can occur as a result of bleeding from suture lines.

Intraperitoneal haemorrhage will become evident with the development of hypovolaemia and falling haematocrit when no bleeding is evident in the nasogastric suction. While a computed tomographic scan may help to diagnose a splenic tear, expeditious re-exploration is the best course of action. Haemorrhage can then be controlled appropriately.

Significant gastrointestinal bleeding, particularly after an operation for a bleeding ulcer, requires early exploration. The goal is to identify the site of bleeding and to control it. If this represents early rebleeding from the ulcer bed, a more extensive ulcer operation may be necessary. If the primary operation was truncal vagotomy, pyloroplasty and suture control of bleeding, further attempt at suture control, including ligation and division of the gastroduodenal artery outside the duodenum, may be attempted. Alternatively, antrectomy with excision of the ulcer may be necessary.

Gastric outlet obstruction

Obstruction becomes evident only 7–10 days after operation when nasogastric suction remains high and contains no bile and/or the patient fails to tolerate clamping of the tube. Gastric outlet obstruction may be due to technical error, oedema, suture line haematoma, a localized leak or obstruction of the efferent loop after Billroth II anastomosis. The problem could also be caused by postoperative pancreatitis. The main decision to be made is when to reoperate. If the obstruction persists beyond 3 weeks, endoscopic examination should be performed. If the obstruction appears to be secondary to oedema or haematoma at the anastomosis, further conservative management may be indicated. The patient should be on total parenteral nutrition. Obstruction that persists beyond 4–6 weeks requires reoperation. At reoperation, if the anastomosis was gastrojejunal, it is revised. However, if the anastomosis was gastroduodenal, it may be revised or a gastrojejunostomy may be constructed. The decision depends, to a large extent, on the operative findings.

LATE INDICATIONS

The most important late indications for reoperation in ulcer disease are recurrent ulcer and alkaline reflux gastritis. Rarely, attempts are made to correct surgically severe dumping syndrome and disabling postvagotomy diarrhoea. Exceedingly rare complications that may require reoperation are retrograde jejunogastric intussusception and afferent limb syndrome.

Recurrent ulcer[1, 2]

Ulcer recurrence rates vary with the type of the primary operation (Table 1). The causes of recurrent ulcer may be classified as follows:

1. Incomplete operation:
   (a) incomplete vagotomy;
   (b) inadequate resection: e.g. retained antrum syndrome.

Table 1   Ulcer recurrence rates

Proximal gastric vagotomy	10–15%
Truncal vagotomy and drainage	8–10%
Truncal vagotomy and antrectomy	0.5%
Subtotal gastrectomy	5–6%

2. Inappropriate operation: e.g. proximal gastric vagotomy for pyloric/prepyloric ulcer.
3. Zollinger–Ellison syndrome (gastrinoma).
4. Drugs, e.g. non-steroidal anti-inflammatory drugs.

Most patients with recurrent ulcer will suffer from a return of their symptoms. A significant number of patients, however, may have no typical symptoms and recurrence is diagnosed by endoscopy or because of complications (bleeding, perforation, obstruction, gastrojejunocolic fistula). The cornerstone to the investigation of patients with recurrent ulcer is endoscopy. When the recurrence is in the stomach, biopsy and brushings are needed to rule out malignancy. Once a recurrent ulcer is diagnosed, the cause must be investigated. All patients with recurrent ulcer should have their fasting plasma gastrin determined. A gastrinoma should be suspected if hypergastrinaemia is either very marked (more than five times normal) or has occurred in a patient with previous antrectomy. Patients with an intact antrum and previous vagotomy will have mild hypergastrinaemia. The best way to establish the diagnosis of gastrinoma is, therefore, by the secretin stimulation test (2 units/kg intravenously). A rise in plasma gastrin of more than 100 pg/ml with secretin is diagnostic of gastrinoma. Another rare cause of hypergastrinaemia is the retained antrum syndrome after Billroth II gastrectomy. Such a patient will have a negative secretin test. The retained antrum may be demonstrated by technetium scan.

The most common cause of ulcer recurrence, however, is incomplete vagotomy. Completeness of vagotomy is best assessed by the modified sham feeding test which is much safer and more physiological than the insulin test used in the past.

Patients with recurrent ulcer are successfully treated with either H_2-receptor antagonists or omeprazole. Because of the high incidence (>90%) of *Helicobacter pylori* infection, a course of appropriate antibiotic therapy is also indicated. The indications for reoperation are similar to those for the primary ulcer operation, i.e. failure of medical therapy, bleeding, perforation, and obstruction. When a stomal ulcer develops after Billroth II gastrectomy, it could erode into the adjacent transverse colon causing a gastrojejunocolic fistula. This complication causes severe diarrhoea and weight loss.

The primary ulcer operation performed determines the nature of the procedure for the recurrence. The choices of operation for recurrence are summarized below.

Recurrence after proximal gastric vagotomy (PGV)

12 The operation of choice is antrectomy with or without truncal vagotomy depending on the ease with which the latter procedure can be performed. In performing antrectomy after PGV, the single most important consideration is not to damage the spleen. At PGV the left gastric artery is ligated.

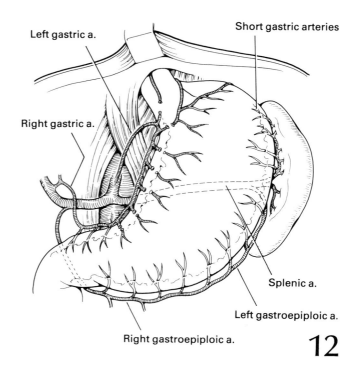

12

13 During subsequent antrectomy, both the right gastric and the right gastroepiploic arteries are ligated, leaving only branches from the splenic artery to supply the stomach. This sole blood supply might be removed during splenectomy. Hence, injury to and removal of the spleen must be avoided. If splenectomy is necessary, the splenic artery must be ligated at the splenic hilum so that the left gastroepiploic artery and as many of the short gastric arteries as possible are preserved. If the stomach becomes ischaemic after splenectomy, total gastrectomy with a 50-cm Roux-en-Y oesophagojejunostomy will be needed.

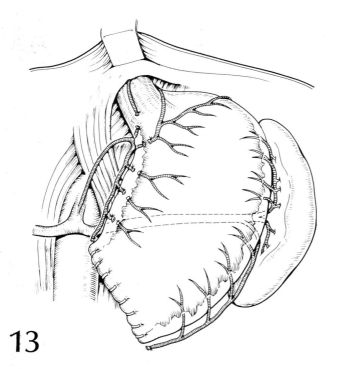

13

Recurrence after vagotomy and drainage

If incompleteness of vagotomy has been established, the hiatus should be explored to complete the vagotomy. In over 70% of patients an intact posterior vagus trunk will be found. If this is the case, completion vagotomy may suffice. In most patients, however, particularly in those with bleeding or with a gastric recurrence, antrectomy with gastroduodenostomy should be added.

14 If dense adhesions make dissection at the hiatus difficult, truncal vagotomy may be performed transdiaphragmatically from the abdomen (Dragstedt vagotomy). Alternatively, truncal vagotomy may be performed transthoracically.

Recurrence after vagotomy and antrectomy

Recurrence after this procedure is less than 0.5%, hence a gastrinoma or retained antrum syndrome must be excluded. If these are excluded, the operation of choice is to complete the vagotomy. If an intact vagal trunk is found and divided, this may suffice. Otherwise a repeat vagotomy and further gastric resection will be necessary.

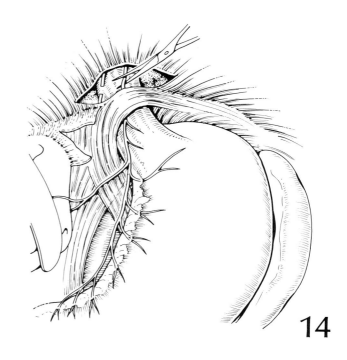

14

Alkaline reflux gastritis[3]

Excessive reflux of bile and other enteric contents into the stomach after procedures that have resected, destroyed, or bypassed the pylorus may result in a syndrome of continuous, burning epigastric pain unrelieved by antacids. Other accompanying manifestations are bilious vomiting, weight loss, and hypochromic, microcytic anaemia. Frequently, patients with this syndrome are achlorhydric or hypochlorhydric. Endoscopy may show friable mucosa with erythema and oedema. Biopsy may show gastritis but is often not striking. Reflux of bile may be sometimes documented with scintigraphy using technetium dimethylimimoacetic acid. The syndrome is more common after Billroth II gastrectomy than after Billroth I. Since most postgastrectomy patients have bile reflux, the true incidence of the syndrome is unknown but is estimated to be 2–5%. Despite enthusiastic early reports of successful surgical intervention, late results are not as encouraging; hence, patient selection is important. Patients must have severe symptoms, weight loss, achlorhydria or severe hypochlorhydria, and evidence of reddened, friable, and oedematous gastric mucosa on endoscopy. If scintigraphy is performed, the extent of reflux must be at least ten times that of control asymptomatic patients.

Operative management

After previous vagotomy and gastrojejunostomy
Simple take-down of the gastrojejunostomy without pyloroplasty is the best initial treatment.

After previous vagotomy and pyloroplasty
Pyloric reconstruction (see below in section on 'Dumping syndrome') may be a good initial operative management.

After previous gastrectomy (Billroth I or Billroth II)
The operative treatment of choice is the conversion of the anastomosis to a 45-cm Roux-en-Y gastrojejunostomy. The operative techniques in construction of a Roux-en-Y gastrojejunostomy after either Billroth I or II gastrectomy are described in detail in the chapter on pp. 335–344. Because the Roux syndrome (stasis in the Roux-en-Y limb) is an important complication, the temptation to create a Roux limb longer than 45 cm must be avoided. Some surgeons have recommended performing a 90–95% gastrectomy before the construction of the Roux-en-Y to remove a flaccid, atonic stomach that might impede gastric emptying. There is little evidence to recommend this approach.

Dumping syndrome[4]

Rapid emptying of chyme after operations that destroy, remove, or bypass the pylorus results in a constellation of symptoms that include epigastric fullness, pain, vasomotor symptoms, and urgent diarrhoea. This postgastrectomy syndrome is known as the 'early' dumping syndrome. Some patients experience signs and symptoms of severe hypoglycaemia 2–3 h after eating. This 'late' dumping syndrome is associated with postprandial hyperinsulinaemia. Following gastrectomy about two-thirds of patients experience some symptoms of dumping. Symptoms persist beyond 2 years in only 20% of patients. In most of these patients, simple dietary manipulation (low carbohydrate diet, no liquids with a meal, lying down for 30 min postprandially) will control the symptoms. Hence, it is the rare patient that may

require operative intervention. Since operations for the dumping syndrome have a low success rate they should be considered as a last resort, except in the patient with pyloroplasty where simple pyloric reconstruction may be successful.

Various surgical approaches have been tried including conversion from Billroth II to Billroth I or vice versa, creation of a Roux-en-Y limb, pyloric reconstruction, and the insertion of a reversed jejunal segment. In this section the last two procedures will be discussed.

It must be emphasized, however, that dumping is far better prevented than treated. Indeed, if proximal gastric vagotomy is selected as the primary ulcer operation, dumping can be completely prevented.

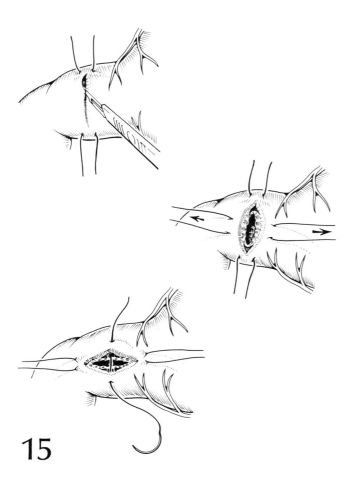

15

Pyloric reconstruction[5]

15 The abdomen is opened through the previous incision as described before. The stomach is identified and the pylorus mobilized by dissecting along the undersurface of the liver. Once the pyloroplasty is identified, stay sutures are placed at each end. The pyloroplasty is opened with a knife along the old incision. A finger is then inserted into the lumen and the posterior ridge of the pyloric sphincter is palpated. The finger is then moved laterally on each side feeling the residual pyloric sphincter. A stay suture of 3/0 silk is placed on each side where the pyloric muscle attenuates. The stay sutures that marked the corners of the initial pyloroplasty are removed. The pyloric muscle from each end is approximated with one or two 3/0 silk sutures. The gastroduodenal opening is then closed longitudinally with interrupted Lembert 3/0 silk sutures. An omental patch is sewn onto the closure for reinforcement. The abdomen is then closed in the usual fashion.

Antiperistaltic jejunal interposition loop[6]

The success of this operation in reversing dumping has been mixed. The procedure involves the interposition of a 10-cm reversed segment of jejunum between the stomach and the jejunum after take-down of the initial anastomosis. The major problem with this operation is knowing the optimum length of the jejunal segment. Even with a 10-cm reversed jejunal segment, patients have developed obstruction. Hence, extreme care must be used in performing this operation.

Postvagotomy diarrhoea

Nearly all patients experience some diarrhoea following truncal vagotomy. However, only 3–6% will experience continuing symptoms 1 year or more after vagotomy. Less than 1% of postvagotomy patients, however, will experience disabling diarrhoea. Diarrhoea can be completely prevented if proximal gastric vagotomy is used instead of truncal vagotomy. The incidence of diarrhoea is also significantly lower after selective gastric vagotomy than after truncal vagotomy.

Surgical correction in postvagotomy diarrhoea is a procedure of last resort. A 10-cm reversed segment of jejunum is interposed in the small intestine 50–90 cm beyond the ligament of Treitz. Again, the possibility of obstruction exists[1–6].

References

1. Mulholland MW, Debas HT. Chronic duodenal and gastric ulcer. *Surg Clin North Am* 1987; 67: 489–507.

2. Stabile BE, Passaro EJ. Recurrent peptic ulcer. *Gastroenterology* 1976; 70: 124–35.

3. Ritchie WP. Alkaline reflux gastritis. Late results of a controlled trial of diagnosis and treatment. *Ann Surg* 1986; 203: 537–44.

4. Herrington JL. Remedial operations for postgastrectomy syndromes. *Curr Probl Surg* 1970; Apr: 1–63.

5. Cheadle WG, Baker PR, Cuschieri A. Pyloric reconstruction for severe vasomotor dumping after vagotomy and pyloroplasty. *Ann Surg* 1985; 202: 568–72.

6. Poth EJ. Use of gastrointestinal reversal in surgical procedures. *Am J Surg* 1969; 118: 893–9.

Pyloroplasty

Sean J. Mulvihill MD
Attending Surgeon, The Medical Center at the University of California, and Associate Professor of Surgery, Department of Surgery, University of California, San Francisco, California, USA

History

Pyloroplasty is used to promote gastric emptying following vagotomy or to relieve obstruction of the gastric outlet, usually due to peptic ulcer disease. Three main types of pyloroplasty have been described and are now known by the eponyms Heineke–Mikulicz, Finney and Jaboulay. Of these, the first is the most commonly used. Weinberg[1] contributed significantly to the popularity of the Heineke–Mikulicz pyloroplasty by demonstrating the safety and improved gastric emptying of a modified one-layer closure.

Principles and justification

In addition to inhibiting acid secretion, truncal vagotomy interferes with regulated motility of the antrum and pylorus and, consequently, gastric emptying. Dragstedt recognized early in his clinical experience with truncal vagotomy that an emptying procedure was required to prevent gastric retention. The surgeon has four main options in aiding gastric emptying following vagotomy: antrectomy, gastrojejunostomy, pyloroplasty and pyloromyotomy. The decision as to which procedure to undertake depends on the main indication for operation (i.e. bleeding, perforation, obstruction, or intractability), the degree of duodenal inflammation, the type of ulcer being treated, the overall condition of the patient and the training of the surgeon.

Of the three types of pyloroplasty, the Heineke–Mikulicz variation is simplest and satisfactory in most settings. Occasionally, chronic inflammation from duodenal ulceration produces retraction of the pylorus toward the liver hilum. In this situation, the Finney pyloroplasty may be preferred. There appear to be few long-term functional differences between the Heineke–Mikulicz and Finney variations[2]. It should be recognized that in the presence of severe inflammatory changes at the pylorus, gastrojejunostomy is a safer alternative emptying procedure.

Pyloromyotomy is mainly used for the management of infants with hypertrophic pyloric stenosis. Occasionally it is used to promote emptying following oesophagogastrectomy. It is not recommended in the presence of pyloric inflammation such as in peptic ulcer disease.

Partial pylorectomy was initially used to excise anterior duodenal ulcers in an attempt to reduce recurrence rates; this was unsuccessful. Recently, partial pylorectomy has found a small role in conjunction with proximal gastric or truncal vagotomy in the management of duodenal ulcer complicated by pyloric stenosis[3].

Preoperative

Assessment and preparation

Upper gastrointestinal tract endoscopy is the most important diagnostic tool in patients with symptoms suggestive of peptic ulcer disease and should be performed before surgery. Specific information to be gained from endoscopy includes the nature of the peptic disease (duodenal, gastric, or prepyloric ulcers, or gastritis), the presence or absence of pyloric or postbulbar stenosis and, in the case of gastric ulcer, the benign or malignant nature of biopsied specimens. In the emergency setting of haemorrhage, endoscopy is valuable in excluding varices or diffuse gastritis. Endoscopy is unnecessary and potentially dangerous in patients with perforation.

Barium contrast studies are complementary to endoscopy and are particularly valuable when symptoms of gastric outlet obstruction are present, when malignancy is suspected, or in reoperative gastric surgery.

Prophylactic intravenous antibiotics (usually a first-generation cephalosporin) are indicated in operations for bleeding, perforation, or gastric ulcers, but are unnecessary in the elective setting for intractable duodenal ulcer. In patients with gastric outlet obstruction, bezoars should be removed by endoscopy or nasogastric tube lavage before operation. A final gastric lavage with 100–200 ml 1% neomycin sulphate solution may reduce the rate of postoperative wound infection.

Prophylaxis against deep vein thrombosis with sequential compression stockings or low-dose subcutaneous heparin is begun immediately after operation. Bladder and nasogastric catheters are placed following induction of anaesthesia.

Anaesthesia

In all but rare instances the operation is performed under general anaesthesia with adequate muscle relaxation.

Operations

HEINEKE–MIKULICZ PYLOROPLASTY

Position of patient

The patient is positioned supine 5–10° in the reverse Trendelenburg position. The right arm is tucked and padded. The left arm is secured to an armboard for venous access.

Incision

Exposure is best gained through an upper midline incision from the xiphoid process to near the umbilicus. A self-retaining retractor frees the assistant. Two blades are used on the abdominal wall, one retracts the liver cephalad, and a fourth retracts the hepatic flexure of the colon caudad. All blades must be well padded.

1 Stay sutures are placed in the pylorus on either side of the mid-axis. A longitudinal gastroduodenal incision is made, extending for 5–6 cm, centred on the pylorus, or in the case of gastric outlet obstruction, on the narrowest portion of the pyloroduodenal channel. Bleeding vessels in the incision are lightly electrocoagulated. The stay sutures are used to distract the edges of the incision, allowing inspection of the duodenal bulb.

In emergency operations for haemorrhage, haemostasis is rapidly achieved by digital pressure on the bleeding gastroduodenal artery in the posterior ulcer. Blood and clots are then aspirated from the stomach and duodenum, so that accurate oversewing of the bleeding artery can be undertaken in a dry field.

2 Oversewing of an actively bleeding posterior ulcer is accomplished with three interrupted sutures of 2/0 silk. Two figure-of-eight sutures are placed deeply in the cephalad and caudad extents of the ulcer bed with the intention of occluding feeding branches of the gastroduodenal artery proximal and distal to the bleeding point. A third U-stitch is placed at the bleeding site to occlude any transverse pancreatic branch[4]. Failure to control this small branch is an occasional cause of recurrent haemorrhage. The surgeon should be conscious of the location of the common bile duct 1.0–1.5 cm to the right of the gastroduodenal artery.

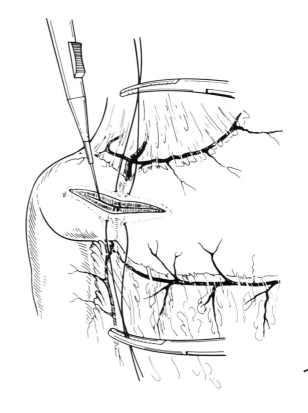

1

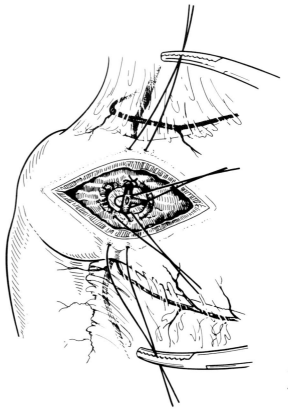

2

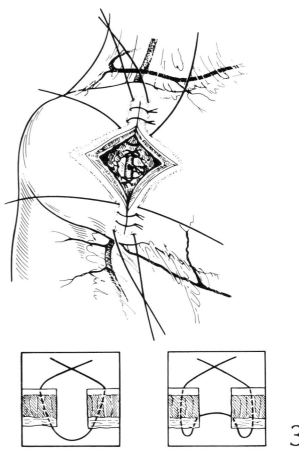

3 The pyloroplasty incision is closed transversely by distracting the stay sutures in cephalad and caudad directions. Interrupted 3/0 monofilament synthetic absorbable sutures of polyglycolate are placed at 4–5-mm intervals. Simple sutures may be alternated with Gambee sutures to ensure accurate approximation of all layers of the gastric and duodenal walls. The closure is begun at each end, working towards the middle.

Alternatively, a two-layer closure may be used, with an inner running, full-thickness 3/0 polyglycolate suture reinforced with outer, interrupted 3/0 silk Lembert sutures. Special care must be taken to avoid obstruction of the pyloric lumen from excessive infolding of tissue.

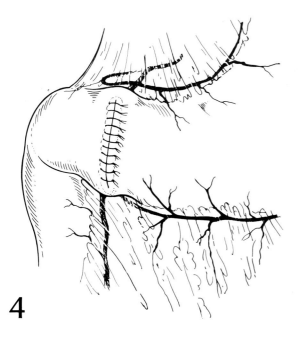

4 The completed pyloroplasty is widely patent. Omentum may be sutured over the closure if desired. A nasogastric tube is positioned along the greater curvature of the stomach before abdominal closure.

FINNEY PYLOROPLASTY

The abdominal incision and exposure for a Finney pyloroplasty are similar to those noted above.

5 Mobilization of the second part of the duodenum (Kocher manoeuvre) is required to relieve tension on the pyloroplasty closure. As the assistant provides traction on the second part of the duodenum towards the left, the surgeon divides the lateral peritoneal reflection with scissors or electrocautery. The duodenum is then swept anteriorly and to the left, exposing the vena cava posteriorly. Care must be taken to avoid injury to the bile duct superiorly and the hepatic flexure of the colon inferiorly.

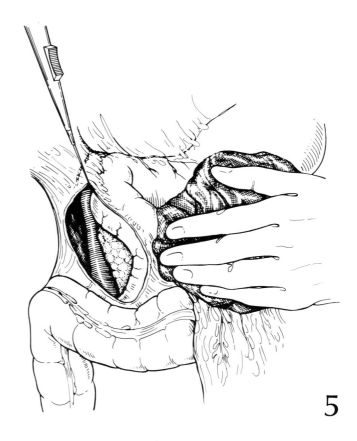

5

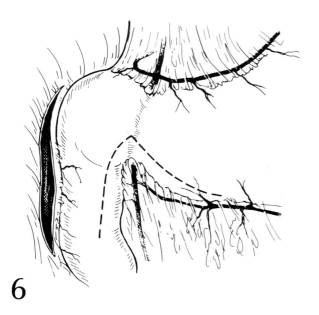

6

6 The gastroduodenal incision is made as an inverted U, close to the gastric greater curvature and medial duodenal wall. Placement of the incision closer to the gastric lesser curvature or lateral duodenal wall results in excessive tension on the anterior gastroduodenal closure. The incision extends for 10 cm, evenly divided between stomach and duodenum, and centred on the pylorus.

7 Three stay sutures are placed, one at each end of the incision and one at the apex of the inverted U.

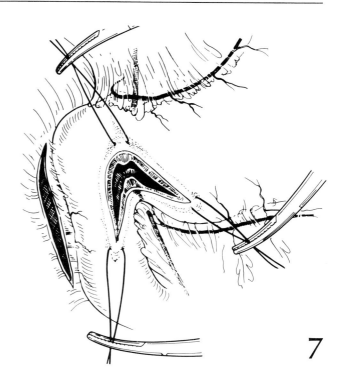

7

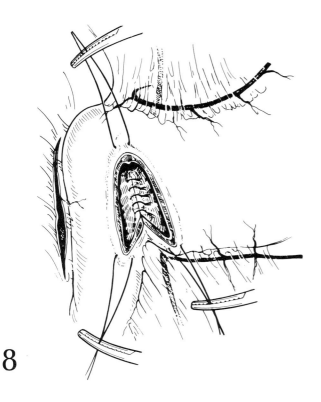

8

8 Closure is achieved with interrupted full-thickness simple sutures of 3/0 polyglycolate, beginning posteriorly between the stomach and duodenum. As the posterior layer progresses, the two stay sutures at the ends of the gastroduodenal incision are brought together.

9 Closure is continued anteriorly and superiorly towards the third suture at the apex of the inverted U. Inversion of the mucosa is achieved by taking larger bites of serosa and smaller bites of mucosa. Gambee-type sutures may be used to aid this inversion and to provide accurate approximation of tissue layers.

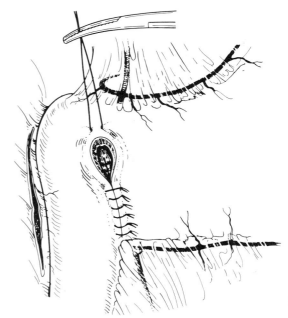

9

JABOULAY GASTRODUODENOSTOMY

Adequate mobilization of the duodenum with a wide Kocher manoeuvre is mandatory. If a tension-free anastomosis between the stomach and duodenum in non-inflamed tissue cannot be achieved, the surgeon should consider gastrojejunostomy as a safer alternative.

10a–c
A posterior layer of interrupted 3/0 silk sutures using seromuscular bites is placed over a distance of 6–7 cm. The end sutures are distracted as stays, the others may be cut. Longitudinal incisions are made in the stomach and duodenum. Small bleeding vessels are lightly coagulated. Closure of the anastomosis is in two layers. For the inner layer, full thickness bites of 3/0 polyglycolate are taken between the stomach and duodenum. Two strands are used, running in opposite directions, carried around each corner and tied to each other anteriorly. This is reinforced with anterior seromuscular 3/0 silk Lembert sutures.

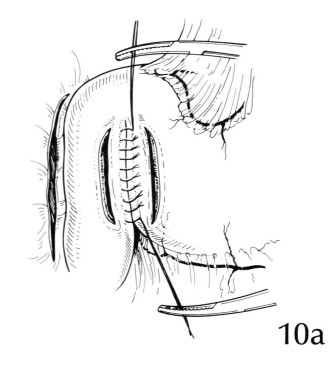

10a

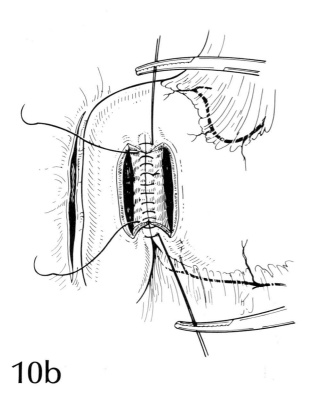

10b

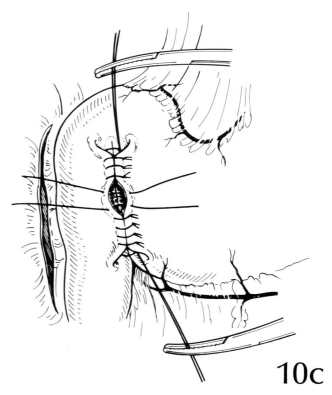

10c

PARTIAL PYLORECTOMY

11a–c The excision is planned to encompass the anterior half of the scarred pylorus. Stay sutures are placed at the cephalad and caudad aspects of the pyloric ring. Transverse incisions are made with cautery through the gastric and duodenal walls just proximal and distal to the pylorus. The anterior half of the pyloric ring is then excised. A gastroduodenal anastomosis with interrupted sutures of 3/0 polyglycolate is performed. Simple sutures may be interspersed with Gambee-type sutures to ensure accurate reapproximation of all layers. Occasionally, a discrepancy exists between the gastric and duodenal openings. Larger bites on the gastric side generally solve the problem. A Kocher manoeuvre may be necessary to relieve tension on the anastomosis.

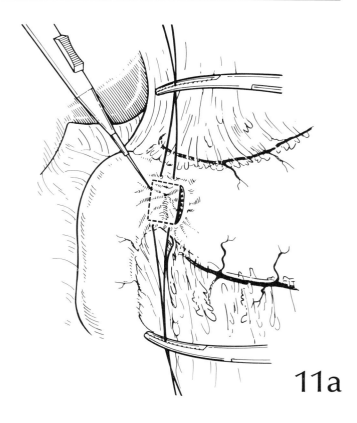

11a

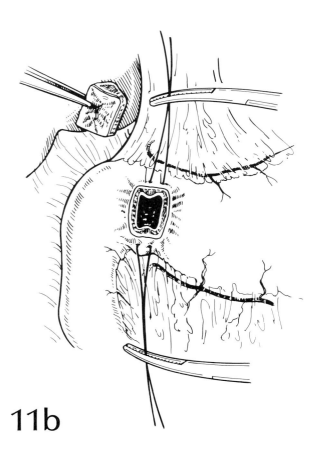

11b

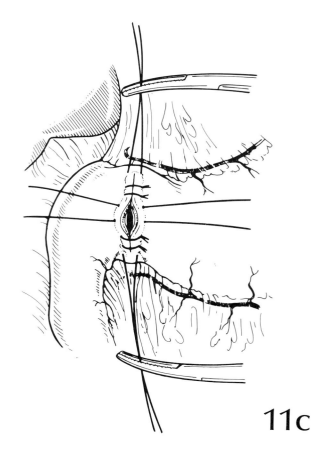

11c

PYLOROMYOTOMY

12 A longitudinal incision is made from the distal stomach to the first part of the duodenum across the pylorus, without opening the mucosa. A gentle spreading motion with a clamp opens the incision and facilitates identification of residual muscle fibres. Special care must be taken at the duodenal end of the incision to avoid inadvertent mucosal injury. As the muscle fibres are divided, the mucosa is encouraged to bulge outwards. This dissection is difficult in the setting of pyloric inflammation or scarring.

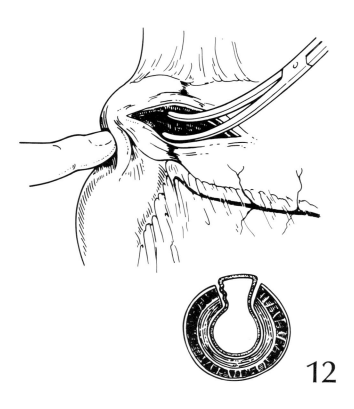

12

Postoperative care

Nasogastric tube decompression is usually used for 2–3 days after operation, although its benefits are debated. Intravenous fluids are required until satisfactory oral intake of liquids is present (usually the fourth day after operation). Analgesia is provided by patient-controlled intravenous injections of morphine via a dedicated infusion device.

Outcome

Suture line leakage is rare, unless the surgeon has unwisely attempted pyloroplasty in the face of marked acute pyloric inflammation. A gastrojejunostomy is the better option in this case. Delayed gastric emptying is uncommon following pyloroplasty and usually relates to oedema from excessive tissue infolding, as in a two-layer Heineke−Mikulicz closure, or to haematoma at the suture line in a one-layer closure. Generally, emptying improves with time. Significant symptoms of dumping or diarrhoea occur in about 15% of patients undergoing truncal vagotomy and pyloroplasty. In 1% the symptoms may be severe enough to consider remedial surgery such as pyloroplasty reversal[5].

References

1. Weinberg JA. Vagotomy and pyloroplasty in the treatment of duodenal ulcer. *Am J Surg* 1963; 105: 347−51.

2. Thompson BW, Read RC. Long-term randomized prospective comparison of Finney and Heineke−Mikulicz pyloroplasty in patients having vagotomy and peptic ulceration. *Am J Surg* 1975; 129: 78−81.

3. Donahue PE, Yoshida J, Richter HM, Liu K, Bombeck CT, Nyhus LM. Proximal gastric vagotomy with drainage for obstructing duodenal ulcer. *Surgery* 1988; 104: 757−64.

4. Berne CJ, Rosoff L. Peptic ulcer perforation of the gastroduodenal artery complex: clinical features and operative control. *Ann Surg* 1969; 169: 141−4.

5. Cheadle WG, Baker PR, Cuschieri A. Pyloric reconstruction for severe vasomotor dumping after vagotomy and pyloroplasty. *Ann Surg* 1985; 202: 568−72.

Gastroenterostomy

Haile T. Debas MD
M. Galante Distinguished Professor of Surgery and Dean of the School of Medicine, University of California, San Francisco, California, USA

Gastroenterostomy is usually performed by the anastomosis of the stomach to the jejunum. Two types of anastomosis are possible: loop gastrojejunostomy and the Roux-en-Y gastrojejunostomy. In loop gastrojejunostomy no provision is made to exclude the regurgitation of bile, pancreatic and enteric secretions into the stomach. Roux-en-Y gastrojejunostomy, on the other hand, is designed to prevent the reflux of bile, pancreatic juice and succus entericus into the stomach. This is accomplished by creating a 40-cm long, isoperistaltic jejunal segment between the gastrojejunostomy and the jejunojejunostomy which returns bile and other secretions to the jejunum more distally. A Roux-en-Y gastrojejunostomy is performed to correct or prevent troublesome alkaline reflux gastritis and oesophagitis.

Indications

Anastomosis between the stomach and the small intestine is performed in four clinical settings: first, in surgery for peptic ulcer where gastrojejunostomy is used as a drainage procedure for truncal or selective gastric vagotomy or to restore gastrointestinal continuity after gastric resection (Billroth II anastomosis); secondly, in surgery for malignant disease either following palliative or curative subtotal gastrectomy or as a palliative bypass when the pylorus is obstructed and resection is impossible; thirdly, when the duodenum is obstructed, traumatized or resected; and, fourthly, when gastric bypass is used as a treatment for morbid obesity.

Gastroenterostomy may be constructed as a side-to-side anastomosis, or as a Roux-en-Y procedure. It may also be antecolic or retrocolic depending on whether the anastomosis is made to lie anterior to the transverse colon or behind it. The choice of the type of gastroenterostomy depends primarily on the surgical problem.

Gastroenterostomy in peptic ulcer surgery

The preferred type of gastroenterostomy in ulcer surgery is usually a retrocolic hook-up in which the stomach is anastomosed to a loop of jejunum behind the transverse colon. Since the advent of stapling instruments, and in the era where elective truncal vagotomy and gastrectomy are becoming rare, surgeons are constructing antecolic gastroenterostomies with increasing frequency. However, retrocolic rather than antecolic gastroenterostomy is preferred because fewer complications ensue (poor gastric emptying, afferent loop syndrome and volvulus[1]). Roux-en-Y gastrojejunostomy is rarely used in primary surgery for peptic ulcer disease. It is, however, employed in the management of postgastrectomy problems, particularly alkaline reflux gastritis[2] and dumping syndrome[3].

Gastroenterostomy in surgery for gastric malignancy

When the pylorus is obstructed with malignant disease and when resection is impossible, gastroenterostomy is occasionally performed to provide palliation. In this case, antecolic gastroenterostomy is preferred because the mesocolon may already be, or may in the future become, invaded with tumour. Antecolic gastroenterostomy is also preferred when subtotal gastrectomy is performed for gastric carcinoma for the same reason. Occasionally, radical gastrectomy may require removal of more than 75% of the stomach. In such a circumstance the surgeon should seriously consider performing total gastrectomy. However, if a decision is made to retain a small gastric pouch, Roux-en-Y gastroenterostomy may be more appropriate since this reconstruction will prevent the complication of bile reflux which occurs more frequently after extensive gastric resection.

Gastroenterostomy in duodenal obstruction or trauma

Palliative gastroenterostomy is frequently performed for actual or impending duodenal obstruction in patients with carcinoma of the pancreas and, less frequently, the duodenum or colon. In these circumstances, antecolic loop gastroenterostomy is the most expedient choice. In severe duodenal or pancreaticoduodenal trauma, gastroenterostomy may be required either because the duodenum has been resected or the pylorus intentionally closed with absorbable sutures or stapled across to divert gastric chyme to protect duodenal repair (duodenal diverticulization). Here, too, antecolic anastomosis is frequently selected.

Gastroenterostomy in gastric bypass surgery

After partition of the stomach in surgery for morbid obesity, the small proximal pouch is anastomosed to a Roux-en-Y[4] limb. The Roux-en-Y limb is brought up to the stomach through a defect created in the mesocolon.

Operations

Incision

The incision used is determined by the requirements of the primary operation. In peptic ulcer surgery and gastric bypass operation the incision is usually midline. In pancreaticoduodenal operations, however, the incision may be midline, right subcostal or double subcostal. When the operation is specifically performed to construct a gastroenterostomy, a supraumbilical midline incision is employed.

LOOP GASTROENTEROSTOMY

Retrocolic gastroenterostomy in peptic ulcer surgery

When the intact stomach is to be used for anastomosis, e.g. after truncal vagotomy, the most dependent portion, preferably just proximal to the muscular antrum, should be selected. The principles of the operation are that after the completion of gastroenterostomy: (1) the most dependent portion of the posterior wall of the stomach is anastomosed to the jejunum; (2) the afferent limb is as short as is comfortably possible (5–8 cm); (3) the anastomosis is retrocolic; and (4) the completed anastomosis lies infracolic.

Technique

1 The lesser sac is entered by dividing the gastrocolic omentum and the posterior wall of the stomach is exposed. The transverse colon is retracted out of the wound and transilluminated to visualize the middle colic vessels and their branches. An avascular portion of the mesocolon is selected, usually to the left of the middle colic vessels, and is opened with a scalpel or pair of scissors for a distance of 6–7 cm.

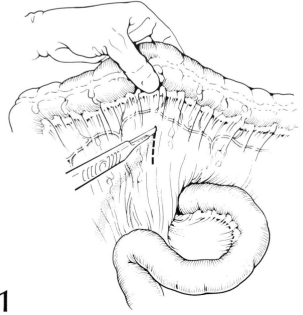

1

2 The site for anastomosis on the posterior wall of the stomach is selected and marked by applying two pairs of Babcock's forceps. Using several 3/0 silk sutures, the posterior edge of the window created in the mesocolon is approximated to the posterior wall of the stomach so that it lies at least 2 cm proximal to the gastrojejunostomy when it is completed. Next, a loop of jejunum is brought through the mesocolon for isoperistaltic anastomosis. The loop is selected so that the afferent limb is as short as possible, preferably no more than 5–8 cm.

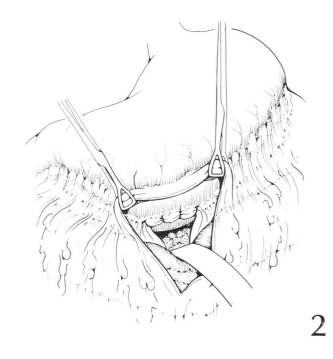

2

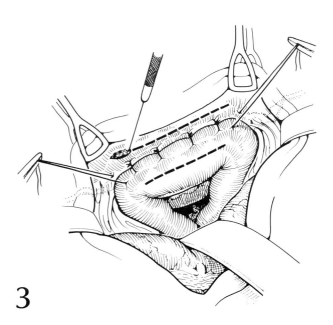

3

3 The anastomosis is begun by placing 3/0 silk sutures between the stomach and jejunum about 2 cm from the mesocolon previously sutured to the stomach. Corner sutures of 3/0 silk are first placed about 5–6 cm apart. The placement of these sutures will determine the size of the gastrojejunostomy. More interrupted sutures are then placed at 0.3–0.5-cm intervals. These seromuscular sutures must be deep enough to include the submucosa. This posterior row of sutures should be placed on the jejunum midway between the mesenteric and antimesenteric borders. All sutures are applied before they are tied. Once tied, the sutures are not cut until the openings on the stomach and jejunum are made. Before opening the stomach, nasogastric suction should be applied to empty it. The opening in the stomach is best made with cautery about 0.5 cm from the posterior row of silk sutures extending from one corner suture to the other. If large submucosal vessels are encountered, these are best secured by under-running them with 4/0 chromic catgut or Dexon sutures before cutting. As soon as the stomach is opened any fluid within it should be removed by suction. Next, the opening in the jejunum is made, again 0.5 cm from the previous suture line. Care must be taken not to damage the opposite wall of the jejunum. The jejunal opening should be slightly smaller than the gastric opening because the jejunal wall stretches and the opening gets larger during the performance of the anastomosis.

4 The posterior inner layer sutures can now be applied. Continuous absorbable 3/0 or 4/0 sutures (Dexon, Maxon or chromic catgut) are used, beginning at the middle of the incision and progressing laterally in both directions. These sutures are haemostatic and should encompass the full wall of both the stomach and jejunum. The suturing is carried onto the anterior wall, bringing the edges of the stomach and jejunum together. This suture will form the inner layer of the anterior portion of the anastomosis. It is often advantageous to use the Connell technique to simplify inversion of the mucosa when the anterior wall of the anastomosis is contructed.

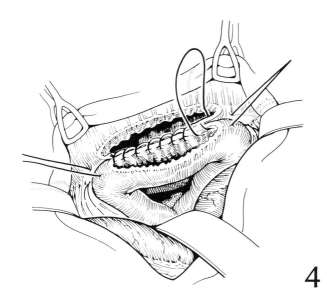

4

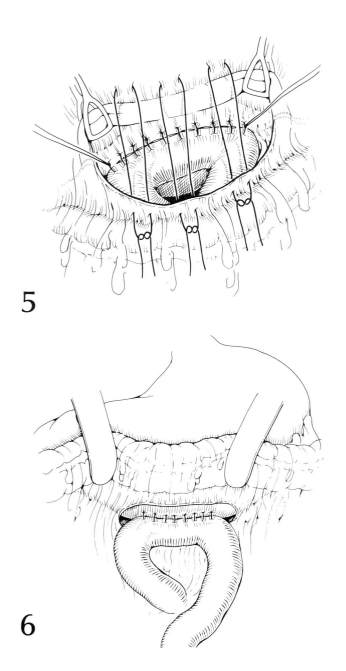

5

6

5, 6 Interrupted 3/0 silk sutures are next applied to complete the outer wall of the anterior portion of the gastroenterostomy. Finally, the anterior edge of the mesocolon is approximated to the stomach about 2 cm from the anastomosis. When these sutures are tied, the gastrojejunal anastomosis will come to lie in an infracolic position.

An alternative to the above approach where the gastrojejunocolic anastomosis is performed in the supracolic compartment and then reduced to the infracolic position is to bring the posterior wall of the stomach through the defect created in the mesocolon and to perform the anastomosis below the mesocolon.

Antecolic gastrojejunostomy

The construction of an antecolic gastrojejunostomy is similar to that of the retrocolic variety. The main difference is that the anastomosis lies in front of the transverse colon, and because of this the afferent loop of the jejunum must, of necessity, be longer. A site for the anastomosis is selected so that there is adequate space behind the anastomosis when it is completed for the transverse colon to distend as necessary. This point is usually 20–30 cm from the ligament of Treitz.

The anastomosis is performed in an identical manner to the retrocolic gastrojejunostomy. Both retrocolic and antecolic anastomoses can also be made using a stapler such as a GIA stapler. Stapled anastomoses are being used with increasing frequency, particularly in antecolic gastroenterostomy.

7–9 The sites for anastomosis on the stomach and jejunum are determined and the two organs are held together with either Babcock's clamps or, preferably, 3/0 silk traction sutures. Using electrocautery, an opening is made in the stomach large enough to allow insertion of one fork of the GIA instrument. A similar opening is made in the jejunum adjacent to the opening in the stomach and the other fork of the instrument inserted. The two forks are brought together and closed. The site for anastomosis is again inspected to ensure the instrument is approximated properly and no extraneous tissue is caught. The instrument is then fired. It applies two rows of staples on either side and cuts in between. The instrument is removed and the newly formed anastomosis examined for integrity and haemostasis.

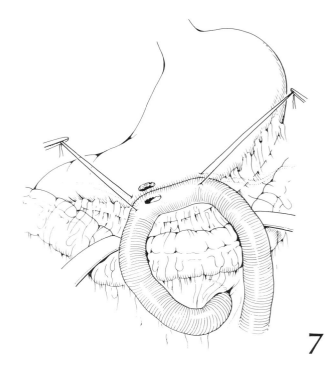

7

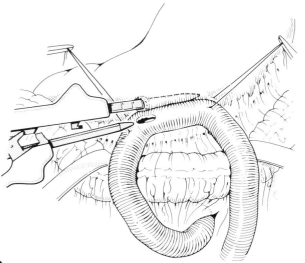

8

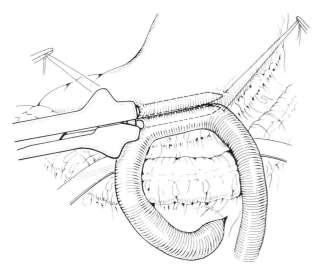

9

10 The stab wounds in the stomach and jejunum used to introduce the instrument are brought together with the application of the stapler and are closed using inverting sutures of 3/0 silk.

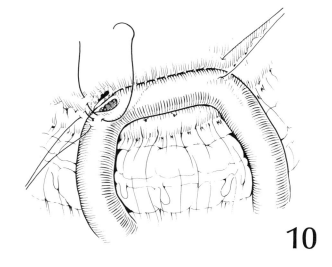

10

ROUX-EN-Y GASTROJEJUNOSTOMY

Indications

Roux-en-Y reconstruction is rarely used in primary surgery for peptic ulcer. It is employed in the following clinical situations: (1) following very high gastrectomy as may be required for a high-lying benign gastric ulcer or for gastric malignancy; (2) in patients with severe alkaline reflux following a previous gastrectomy; (3) in the treatment of dumping syndrome where a gastro-duodenal or a Billroth II anastomosis is converted to a Roux-en-Y gastrojejunostomy; and (4) in gastric bypass operation for morbid obesity[5].

Preoperative

When the indication is dumping syndrome or alkaline gastritis, the diagnosis must be firmly established. Dumping syndrome is diagnosed from typical clinical features including postcibal weakness, abdominal discomfort, tachycardia with palpitation, sweating and even flushing. These symptoms are frequently associated with urgent diarrhoea and constitute the 'early' dumping syndrome, occurring within the first 30–60 min of eating. The same patient may also have a 'late' dumping syndrome, where symptoms of hypoglycaemia occur 2–3 h after the ingestion of a meal. If necessary, the presence of dumping syndrome can be confirmed by showing rapid gastic emptying with radionuclide studies or by provoking the symptoms by asking the patient to drink 100 ml of 50% glucose in water. This will reproduce the early symptoms and, if the patient has late dumping syndrome, a fall of plasma glucose

below 50 mg/100 ml with concomitant increase in immunoreactive plasma insulin levels will be found 2–3 h after the ingestion of the meal. Unfortunately, the Roux-en-Y procedure is not always successful and sometimes replaces symptoms of stasis for those of dumping. There is no way to determine before operation which patients will develop stasis, although the longer the Roux limb the higher the incidence of dumping.

When a Roux-en-Y procedure is being contemplated to treat alkaline reflux, a firm diagnosis is necessary. Unfortunately, the diagnosis is very difficult to make. Endoscopy and biopsy should show the presence of severe gastritis and the absence of other lesions such as recurrent ulcer. Severe weight loss is common, and iron deficiency anaemia is seen in 25% of patients. If vagotomy and/or gastrectomy have been performed for ulcer disease, the presence of complete or near complete achlorhydria must be documented by gastric secretory tests. Two important clues include the presence of bilious vomiting and of heartburn unrelieved by antacids. The occurrence of bile reflux may also be demonstrated by measuring high concentrations of bile salts in the gastric aspirate or by scintigraphic studies using an intravenously administered radio-labelled substance normally excreted in the bile. The accumulation of radiolabel in the area of the stomach is evidence of bile reflux. Again, it should be pointed out that, despite all the best efforts of the surgeon, the diagnosis is difficult to establish.

Technique

Take-down of previous anastomosis

The operation is usually remedial, following previous gastrectomy. If the initial operation was a Billroth I gastrectomy, the anastomosis must be taken down. If the initial operation was a Billroth II, however, the anastomosis need not be taken down. Instead, the afferent limb may be divided with the GIA stapler and moved 40–45 cm down for jejunojejunal anastomosis.

11, 12 Traction sutures (3/0 silk) are applied at either edge of the anastomosis both on the stomach and the duodenal side. The anastomosis is divided with electrocautery. The duodenal stump is closed securely in two layers, an inner continuous layer of 3/0 absorbable suture and an outer layer of interrupted 3/0 silk. The opening in the stomach, which has been marked with traction sutures, is usually suitable, after minor preparation, for end-to-side anastomosis with the Roux-en-Y limb.

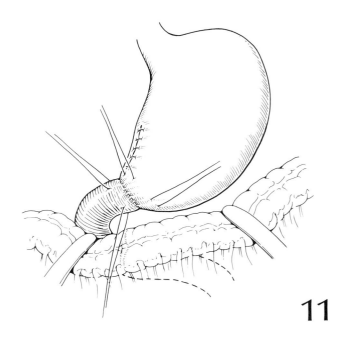

11

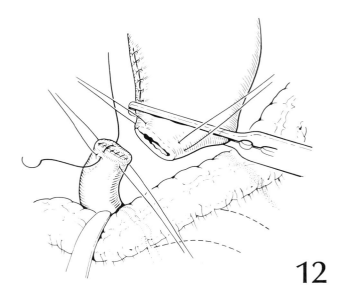

12

Division of jejunum

13 It is usually necessary to divide a few mesenteric vessels at the site of transection division and the adjacent avascular mesentery to the transverse arcade. The jejunum is divided with a GIA stapler (or clamps can be used). By always making this division distal to the previously placed 3/0 silk marking suture, the proximal end is never confused with the distal end. A row of 3/0 silk seromuscular sutures is used to invert the staple line on the distal end of the cut jejunum.

Selection of jejunal segment

14 A 40–45-cm Roux limb will be required. After delivering the transverse colon out of the abdominal wound, the jejunum is dissected free from any adhesions. The ligament of Treitz is identified and a point selected within 10–20 cm of the ligament for jejunal transection. Selection of this point depends on examination of the mesenteric vascular arcade, and the ease with which the distal resection line can be brought up to the stomach. This point is marked with a 3/0 silk suture on the antimesenteric side. Using a sterile ruler, 40–45 cm of the jejunum is measured distal to the suture. A second marking 3/0 silk suture is applied at this point.

By transilluminating the mesocolon an avascular area is selected to the left of the middle colic vessels. This is opened for a distance of 4–5 cm. The distal jejunum is now passed through the defect in the mesocolon for anastomosis with the stomach. Care must be taken not to twist the mesentery.

Anastomosis is made between the opening in the stomach and the side of the jejunum. Corner sutures of 3/0 silk are applied between the stomach and the jejunum such that the proximal suture is within 2 cm of the closed end of the jejunum to avoid creating a large blind pouch. A posterior row of 3/0 silk seromuscular sutures is applied and then tied.

The jejunum is now opened parallel to the gastric opening. The opening in the jejunum is made smaller than that in the stomach. The inner layer of continuous 3/0 Maxon (or other absorbable material) is started in the midpoint of the posterior wall using two sutures. The suturing is carried out towards each corner and onto the anterior wall. All layers of the jejunum and stomach are included. The anastomosis is completed with an anterior outer layer of inverting 3/0 silk sutures. The anastomosis should be 5–7 cm in width.

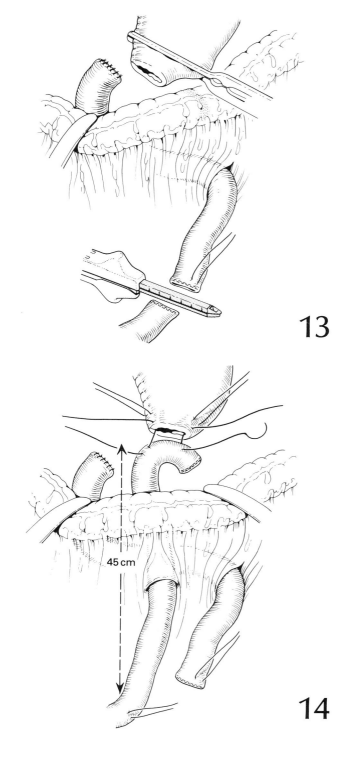

13

45 cm

14

Closure of defect in mesocolon

If the gastrojejunal anastomosis has been made to lie infracolic, the technique described for the construction of a retrocolic loop gastrojejunostomy is employed.

Often, however, the gastrojejunal anastomosis cannot be made to lie infracolic, either because the gastric remnant is small or adhesions prevent this from happening. In this case, the defect in the mesocolon is closed by interrupted sutures between the mesocolon and the Roux jejunal limb.

Jejunojejunal anastomosis

15 The proximal cut end of the jejunum is easily identified because of the traction suture on it. The second traction suture that marked a 40–50-cm segment is also identified. The proximal jejunum is anastomosed end-to-side to the jejunum at the level of the second traction suture. This creates effectively a 40–45-cm isoperistaltic Roux-en-Y limb of jejunum. The anastomosis is again performed in two layers with an inner layer of continuous absorbable suture and an interupted, inverting seromuscular layer of 3/0 silk. The posterior layer of interrupted silk sutures is first applied. The stapled end of the jejunum is then held with three Allis' clamps and, using electrocautery, the stapled edge is excised. The inner layer of continuous suture and the outer anterior layer of interrupted suture can then be inserted.

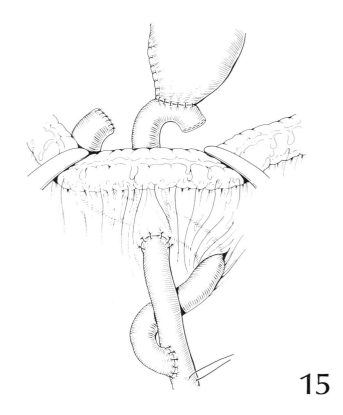

15

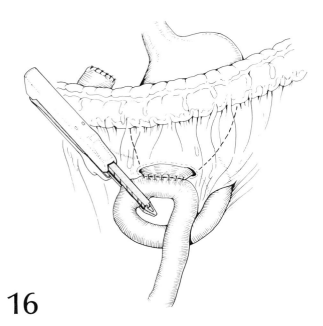

16

Creation of Roux-en-Y gastrojejunostomy after Billroth II gastrectomy

16 If the primary operation was a Billroth II gastrectomy, the original gastrojejunal anastomosis can be preserved. The anastomosis is identified and dissected so that the afferent and efferent limbs can be positively identified. The afferent limb is then transected with the GIA stapler just distal to the anastomosis. The gastric end of the transected jejunum is inspected and the staple line is inverted with interrupted 3/0 Lembert sutures.

17 Using a sterile ruler, a 40–45-cm length of jejunum is measured beyond the gastrojejunostomy and the point marked with a 3/0 suture. The divided end of the proximal jejunum (the afferent limb) is now anastomosed end-to-side to the jejunum at the previously selected site. The technique is identical to that described above.

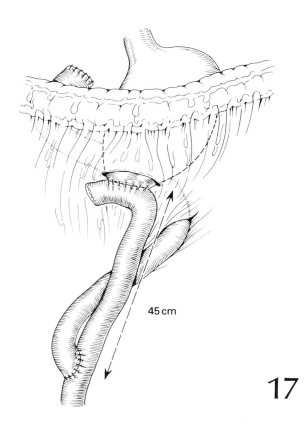

17

Postoperative care

Postoperative care is described in the chapter on pp. 39–44.

Complications

Early complications

Gastroenterostomy is associated with few specific complications in the early postoperative period. Suture line haematoma causing delayed gastric emptying can occur. This complication tends to occur more frequently after a stapled anastomosis. It is effectively prevented by the continuous haemostatic suture in a two-layer anastomosis. Problems in gastric emptying can also occur if the mesentery has been twisted or the operation has resulted in severe kinking of the jejunum. If a retrocolic loop gastrojejunostomy is not made to lie infracolic, the jejunal limb can become obstructed as it crosses the defect in the mesocolon. Small bowel herniation through this defect is also theoretically possible.

Late complications

Afferent limb syndrome
An afferent limb that is too long may develop a motility disturbance, causing improper emptying of the segment. Large volumes of bile accumulate in this reservoir. The segment tends to empty at once from time to time, causing a large volume of bilious fluid to enter the stomach. The patient becomes nauseated and vomits the fluid. The vomiting typically occurs in the morning.

The afferent limb syndrome is prevented by using a short afferent limb (less than 10–15 cm) between the ligament of Treitz and the gastrojejunal anastomosis. The treatment of the established syndrome is either to convert the anastomosis to a gastroduodenal (Billroth I) anastomosis or to revise it so that the afferent limb is shortened to 10 cm or less.

Jejunogastric intussusception
This rare but serious complication is well described in the literature[6,7]. It occurs only in loop gastroenterostomy. Irons and Lipin collected 100 cases from the literature in 1955. Either the efferent or afferent limb may intussuscept into the stomach. In 80% of cases the efferent limb is the intussusceptum. In most of the rest the afferent limb intussuscepts, and in rare cases both limbs may do so. The condition may produce an acute abdomen with high small bowel obstruction. Occasionally, however, a more chronic form of intermittent obstruction and occult bleeding results. A barium swallow will establish the diagnosis by demonstrating a filling defect in the stomach made up of coils of intestine. Treatment is surgical. Occasionally the intussusceptum is gangrenous and requires resection. If the intussusception is viable and can be reduced, however, several options exist. These include conversion to Billroth I anastomosis, resection of the anastomosis and creation of a new anastomosis with a shortened afferent limb, which is retrocolic if possible.

Twisted gastrojejunostomy

This rare complication is seen with antecolic loop anastomoses where a twisting of the gastrojejunal anastomosis around the vertical axis causes obstruction. It is conveniently treated by conversion to a retrocolic anastomosis or to Billroth I.

Alkaline reflux gastritis

This condition has been discussed above as an indication for Roux-en-Y gastrojejunostomy. Its true incidence is difficult to establish and the creation of Roux-en-Y gastrojejunostomy is associated with significant late failures.

'Roux syndrome'

Following Roux-en-Y gastrojejunostomy, some 10–30% of patients develop the 'Roux syndrome'. The longer the Roux limb, the higher the incidence. These patients are unable to tolerate oral intake, particularly of solids, and progressively lose weight. They have distressing bilious vomiting. Upper gastrointestinal contrast study, as well as endoscopy, shows a patent anastomosis with no gross abnormalities. However, radionuclide gastric emptying studies show severe impairment of emptying of both solids and liquids. The Roux limb of the jejunum appears to have no functional peristaltic activity; instead it appears to serve as an effective barrier to gastric emptying. Prokinetic agents such as metoclopramide and cisapride are of little benefit.

Treatment is surgical and requires conversion to Billroth I or II anastomosis.

References

1. Bushkin FL, Woodward ER. Alkaline reflux gastritis. In: Ebert PA, ed. *Postgastrectomy Syndromes. Major Problems in Clinical Surgery*, Vol. 20. Philadelphia: Saunders, 1976: 49–63.

2. Ritchie WP. Alkaline reflux gastritis: a critical reappraisal. *Gut* 1984; 25: 975–87.

3. Miranda R, Steffes BC, O'Leary JP, Woodward ER. Surgical treatment of the postgastrectomy dumping syndrome. *Am J Surg* 1980; 139: 40–3.

4. Alden JF. Gastric and jejunoileal bypass: a comparison in the treatment of morbid obesity. *Arch Surg* 1977; 112: 799–806.

5. Griffen WO Jr, Young VL, Stevenson CC. A prospective comparison of gastric and jejunoileal bypass procedure for morbid obesity. *Ann Surg* 1977; 1986: 500–9.

6. Irons HS, Lipin RJ. Jejuno-gastric intussusception following gastroenterostomy and vagotomy. *Ann Surg* 1955; 141: 541–6.

7. Waits JO, Beart RW Jr, Charboneau JW. Jejunogastric intussusception. *Arch Surg* 1980; 115: 1449–52.

Partial gastrectomy (and antrectomy) with a gastroduodenal anastomosis: Billroth I gastrectomy

Glyn G. Jamieson FRACS, FACS
Dorothy Mortlock Professor of Surgery, University of Adelaide, Department of Surgery, Royal Adelaide Hospital, Adelaide, South Australia, Australia

Haile T. Debas MD
M. Galante Distinguished Professor of Surgery and Dean of the School of Medicine, University of California, San Francisco, California, USA

History

In 1881 Theodore Billroth performed the first successful gastrectomy in a patient with distal gastric cancer. The operation was an extended pylorectomy, with the duodenum being anastomosed to the lesser curve of the stomach. He repeated this technique in his second patient, and then changed the anastomosis to the greater curve in his next three patients. Although only the first patient survived the operation, it is the technique practised in the last three that has come to be known as a Billroth I gastrectomy. Early in the 20th century, Shoemaker extended the resection to include all the distal stomach and much of the lesser curve of the stomach, in the operation known today as a Billroth I gastrectomy. Precise removal of the antrum may have been first performed by Edwards and Herrington in 1953, and it was certainly this group who popularized the technique with truncal vagotomy for duodenal ulcer disease.

Principles and justification

Indications

This operation is carried out much less often today than even 20 years ago, because of the decline in the need for peptic ulcer surgery and the change in incidence and site of gastric cancers from the distal stomach to the cardia region.

Nevertheless, gastric ulcer remains the peptic ulcer least successfully treated by acid-suppressant drugs, and distal gastrectomy with removal of the ulcer and a gastroduodenal anastomosis remains the gold standard of surgical treatment for gastric ulcer. The authors, however, believe that antrectomy rather than partial gastrectomy is all that is required.

Partial gastrectomy with duodenal anastomosis is virtually never indicated in the treatment of duodenal ulcer today.

In relation to gastric cancer, the debate continues over the extent of gastrectomy and of accompanying lymph node resection that should be carried out. Suffice it to say that many surgeons undertake the least possible operation that encompasses the gastric cancer primary, and for those surgeons a distal gastrectomy is the operation of choice for an antral cancer. Even here, however, surgeons are divided as to whether the anastomosis should be to the duodenum or to the jejunum, with the majority favouring the latter.

Preoperative assessment is considered in the chapter on pp. 39–44.

Operation

Incision

1 A midline incision is used to approach the stomach. The lesser sac is entered to the left of the midline outside the gastro-omental (epiploic) arcade. The gastrocolic omentum is divided, proceeding from right to left, until the left gastro-omental (epiploic) artery and one or two short gastric pedicles have been divided. In due course if there is any hint of tension on the anastomosis, additional short gastric vessels can be divided.

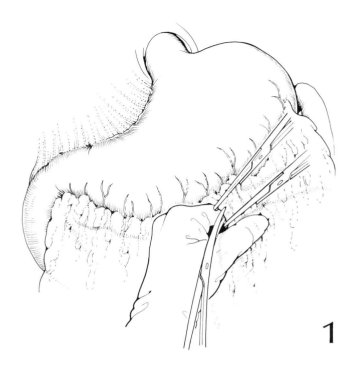

2 The gastrocolic omentum is now divided towards the duodenum; here the lesser sac is obliterated to a greater or lesser degree and it is necessary to recreate the separation between the gastrocolic ligament and the posterior wall of the lesser sac in order to remain separate from the middle colic vessels.

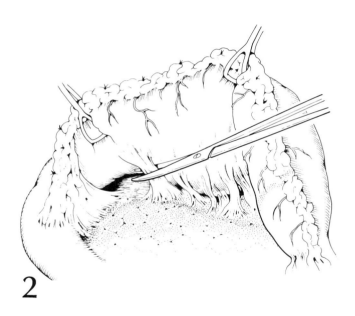

3 As the surgeon approaches the pylorus, the dissection is directed towards the duodenal wall so that the right gastro-omental (epiploic) artery is divided. The pylorus is recognized by a transverse vein running across it, and when picked up between finger and thumb, the pyloric ring of muscle is easily felt. The vessels between the head of the pancreas and the first part of the duodenum are small and easily torn and its is best to use fine artery forceps (mosquito forceps) to clip these vessels prior to division.

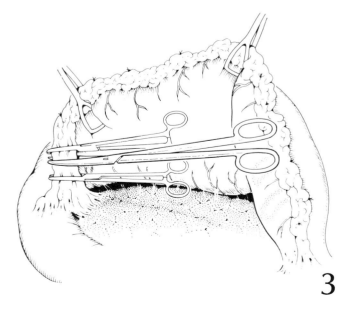

4 The first part of the duodenum immediately distal to the pylorus is completely mobilized and the right gastric artery is sought above and to the left of the pylorus. The right gastric artery is usually insubstantial, but occasionally can be of larger size. It is ligated and divided, and the filmy lesser omentum is divided up to the hepatic branch of the vagus, which is always easily identified as the structure limiting further cephalad dissection.

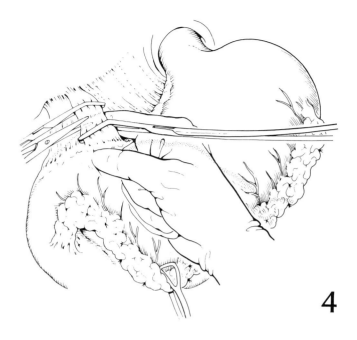

4

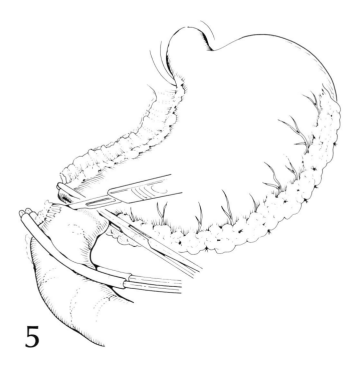

5

5 The duodenum is next divided between clamps applied immediately distal to the pylorus, with a crushing clamp on the gastric side and a soft bowel clamp applied several centimetres distally on the duodenal side. The division is performed with a scalpel to divide the intestine on the duodenal side of the crushing clamp.

6 The distal portion of the stomach can now be held skywards and any adhesions to the posterior surface of the distal stomach are divided. If the operation is being performed for gastric ulcer the point of division of the stomach on the lesser curve should include the ulcer, even if this lies quite close to the cardia (A–A). It is important to gently dissect the lesser omentum away from the stomach, immediately proximal to the ulcer. In order to do this, a pair of fine curved forceps can be of help, gently opening and closing the forceps next to the gastric wall in order to find a way through to the lesser sac. When this has been achieved, all the remaining tissue in the lesser omentum is divided. The determining factor for how high the lesser curvature of the stomach is resected is always the site of the gastric ulcer. How much of the greater curve is taken depends on whether a classic partial gastrectomy is to be undertaken (B–B) (and in the authors' view the only indications for this today would be in order to encompass a distal gastric cancer in a palliative procedure) or whether an antrectomy only is being undertaken, which is preferable for a gastric ulcer.

If a gastric ulcer is sited high on the lesser curve, it may be necessary to make a gastric division at right angles to the lesser curve for 2–3 cm. The gastric division then proceeds more nearly parallel to the proximal part of the lesser curve, and crosses the stomach to reach the greater curve. This resection line leads to the removal of about 25% of the stomach.

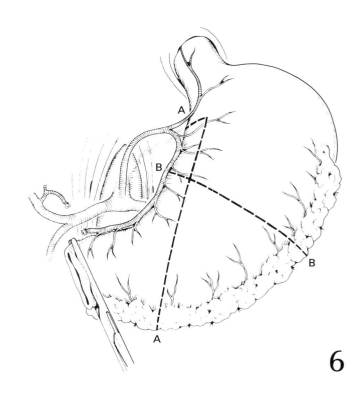

6

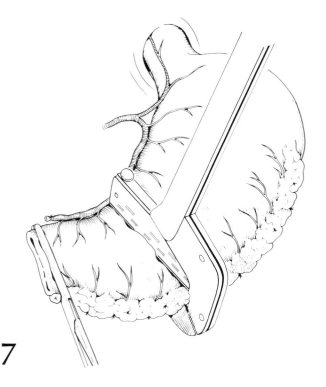

7

7 Removal can be accomplished by hand suturing of the divided stomach in two layers. This is time consuming, however, and the laxity of the gastric mucosa makes the suturing tedious at times. The authors prefer to use a transverse anastomotic stapler approximately 90 cm in length. If the resection is being carried out for a very distal tumour or ulcer, then the point of division is not much proximal to the 'crow's foot' on the lesser curve and vertically opposite this on the greater curve. There is no difficulty in encompassing the whole width of the stomach with a stapler at this point.

The staples on the greater curve side of this anastomosis are later excised in order to open a hole 3 cm in diameter for anastomosis of the stomach with the duodenum. If the ulcer is higher on the greater curve of the stomach, a transverse anastomotic stapler approximately 3.5 cm in length is used to make the right-angled limb and then the 90-cm stapler is used for the vertical limb.

8 On occasions the 90-cm stapler does not encompass the whole width of the stomach wall. In this instance the unstapled portion on the greater curve side is cut across and is later used for anastomosis with the duodenum.

It is a matter of preference whether the staple line is inverted by a running suture with one of the authors using this technique and the other not. The gastroduodenal anastomosis can be carried out in one layer, as described in the chapter on pp. 88–107, or in two layers as described below.

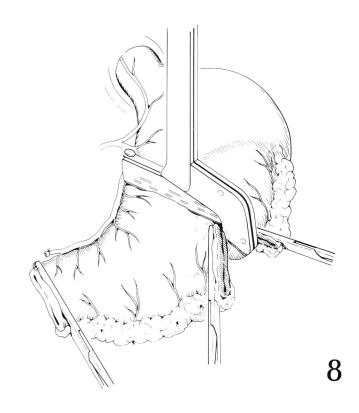

8

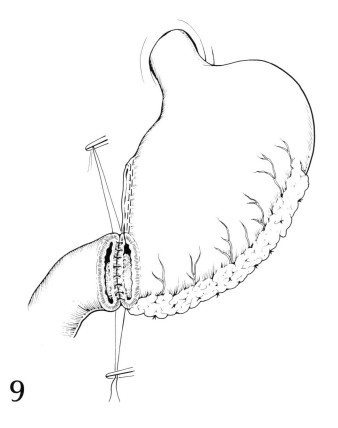

9

9 Stay sutures are placed at either end of the anastomosis and interrupted non-absorbable sutures, e.g. 3/0 silk or Prolene, are used to suture the posterior seromuscular layer of the stomach to the same layer of the duodenum.

10a, b A posterior all-coats running suture is then inserted using 3/0 polydioxanone or 3/0 chromic catgut. The authors begin this suture in the midline posteriorly, inserting two sutures – one to be brought clockwise and one to be brought anticlockwise. These sutures meet in the midline anteriorly. The anterior seromuscular coat is then closed using interrupted sutures as for the posterior wall. German surgeons at the turn of the century christened the three-way meeting point of the reconstructed lesser curve and the anterior and posterior wall of the gastroduodenal anastomosis as the *jammerecke* – the angle of sorrow! To prevent the angle of sorrow becoming a vale of tears, the authors insert a purse-string suture at the angle with the suture passing from the front wall of the anastomosis (stomach) to the front wall of the anastomosis (duodenum), to the back wall of the lesser curve (stomach), to the front wall of the lesser curve (stomach).

As mentioned previously, there should be no tension on the anastomosis; extra length for the stomach can always be obtained by further dividing short gastric vessels.

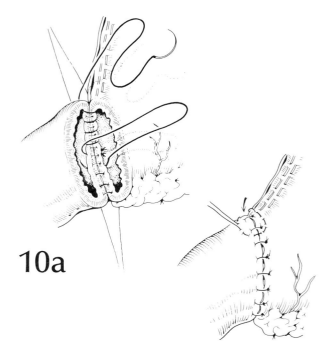

10a

10b

Wound closure

No drains are used and the wound is closed in a routine fashion.

Postoperative care

General postoperative care and the possible complications are considered in the chapter on pp. 39–44.

Illustrations by Raymond Evans

Partial gastrectomy with gastrojejunal anastomosis including Roux-en-Y reconstruction

Michael W. Mulholland MD
Associate Professor, Department of Surgery, University of Michigan, Ann Arbor, Michigan, USA

History

In 1881 Billroth performed the first successful partial gastrectomy for cancer. It was Shoemaker in 1911, however, who extended the indication for partial gastrectomy to include benign ulcer disease. For over 30 years thereafter subtotal gastrectomy became an important operation for peptic ulcer. Truncal vagotomy for peptic ulcer was reintroduced by Dragstedt in 1942, and truncal vagotomy with drainage or with partial gastrectomy became the most important ulcer operation in the 1950s and 1960s. In the subsequent three decades gastrectomy has been replaced by increasingly more selective types of vagotomy as the cornerstone in the treatment of duodenal ulcer. Gastric resection is now seldom employed as the sole operation for duodenal ulcer. Antrectomy combined with vagotomy is still a common procedure for duodenal ulcer in the USA. Gastric resection, however, is the standard procedure for benign gastric ulcers and gastric malignancies.

Principles and justification

Indications

Partial gastrectomy, performed so that the lesion is included, is utilized as treatment of benign gastric ulcer[1]. Partial gastrectomy in the form of antrectomy may be combined with truncal vagotomy in the operative treatment of duodenal ulcer disease, particularly when gastric outlet obstruction due to pyloric cicatrization has occurred[2]. Gastric malignancy confined to the distal stomach is another indication for partial gastrectomy. Occasionally, invasion of the stomach by malignant tumours originating in other organs, particularly the transverse colon, may require distal gastrectomy. Performance of gastrojejunal reconstruction in the form of a Roux-en-Y anastomosis is indicated in patients with alkaline reflux gastritis[3].

Preoperative

Preoperative preparation is dictated by the complication of the disease requiring gastrectomy for treatment. In the presence of pyloric obstruction, electrolyte abnormalities are common. Loss of gastric secretions high in hydrochloric acid through vomiting will lead to hypochloraemic alkalosis. Renal loss of potassium in attempts to retain hydrogen ions, together with potassium loss from vomiting, results in accompanying hypokalaemia. While prolonged preoperative nasogastric suction is not helpful in preventing postoperative gastric atony in patients with pyloric obstruction, vigorous attempts should be made to remove retained food and gastric bezoars before operation.

Anaemia and coagulation defects should be corrected before surgery. Because upper abdominal incisions may compromise pulmonary function, gastric surgery should not be performed in the presence of active pulmonary infection. Pulmonary physiotherapy and bronchodilators are often helpful; cigarette smoking should be stopped.

Patients undergoing gastric resection should receive preoperative systemic antibiotics. In the presence of pyloric obstruction or achlorhydria, the luminal flora of the stomach contains much higher numbers of enteric organisms and may resemble, qualitatively and quantitatively, the flora of the small intestine. A second or third generation cephalosporin usually provides sufficiently broad coverage.

Operation

Incision

1 A long vertical midline incision extending from the level of the xiphoid process to the umbilicus provides superior exposure of the upper abdomen for performance of partial gastrectomy.

Upon entering the peritoneal cavity, the round ligament may be divided to allow placement of retractors and to partially mobilize the left lobe of the liver.

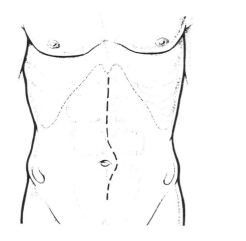

1

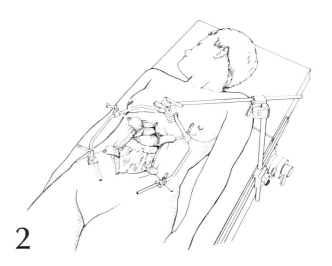

2

Retractors

2 Exposure of the upper abdomen is achieved using a Bookwalter retractor or other, similar, self-retaining device. The costal margins should be elevated and retracted superiorly. The left lateral segment of the liver does not need to be mobilized extensively; superior distraction with the retractor usually provides adequate exposure of the proximal stomach and the area of the left gastric artery. Placement of the patient in a mild degree of reverse Trendelenburg position is often helpful in improving exposure.

Anatomy

3 Performance of gastrectomy demands familiarity with the vascular anatomy of the stomach. Because of extensive intramural collateral vessels, the stomach may retain viability with only one major arterial supply intact. The first portion of the duodenum, in contrast, is much more susceptible to ischaemia produced by surgical devascularization. The vascular landmarks may be used to delineate various degrees of gastric resection. An approximately 50% resection of the stomach is achieved when the stomach is divided along a line from the mid point of the lesser curvature to a point half the distance from the pylorus to the gastro-oesophageal junction along the greater curvature. A 75% gastrectomy requires division of the stomach just distal to the first branch of the left gastric artery to the origin of the left gastroepiploic artery.

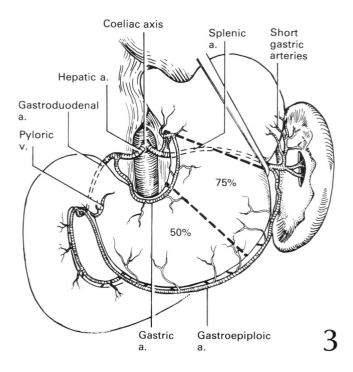

3

Division of gastrohepatic ligament

4 If the operation is performed for a neoplasm, possible posterior extension and fixation to the pancreas or to the middle colic vessels must be anticipated. The posterior wall of the stomach may be inspected by division of the relatively avascular superior portion of the gastrohepatic ligament.

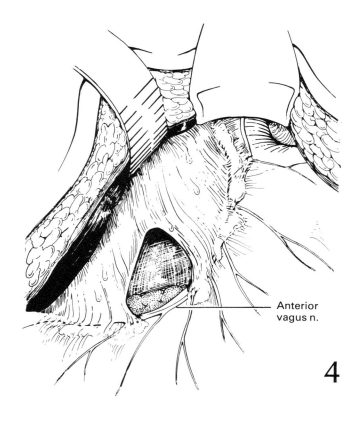

Anterior vagus n.

4

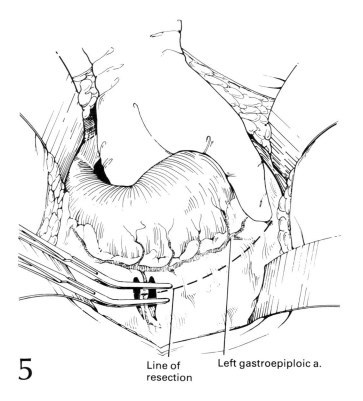

5

Line of resection   Left gastroepiploic a.

Mobilization of greater curvature

5 The gastrocolic ligament is divided, preserving the gastroepiploic vessels if the operation is performed for benign disease and omental resection is not required. Introduction of the surgeon's left hand through the incision in the gastrohepatic ligament can help to guide the dissection and to avoid damage to the middle colic vessels. The omentum receives its major blood supply from the right and left gastroepiploic vessels, and division of small vessels along the greater curvature will not lead to omental infarction.

Preparation of greater curvature

6 Division of the gastrocolic ligament for a 50% gastrectomy should proceed to a point midway between the pylorus and the gastro-oesophageal junction. This point often corresponds to the 'watershed' area between the right and left gastroepiploic vessels. The gastric wall should be cleared of adherent fat and areolar tissue in preparation for division and subsequent anastomosis. A suture, placed at the superior border of the cleared space, is helpful in marking the end of the dissection and as a means of applying traction to the proximal stomach after transection.

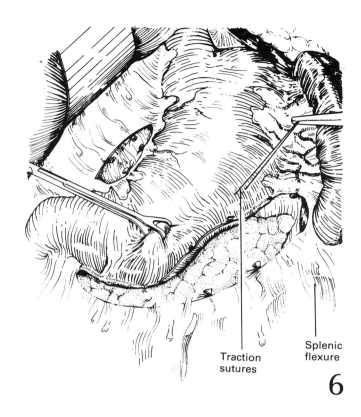

Traction
sutures

Splenic
flexure

6

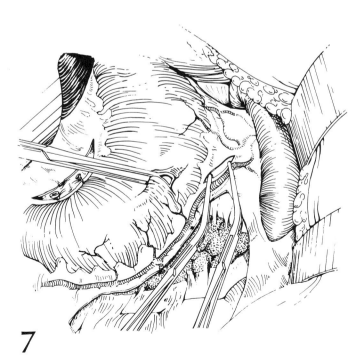

7

Division of left gastroepiploic vessels

7 Performance of a 75% gastrectomy may require division of the left gastroepiploic vessels or the lowermost short gastric vessels.

Ligation of right gastroepiploic vessels

8   Mobilization of the greater curvature is completed by division of the right gastroepiploic vessels. The stomach is retracted cephalad and the right gastroepiploic artery is identified at its origin from the gastroduodenal artery. The gastroepiploic artery is divided close to its origin, along with adjacent fibrous tissue.

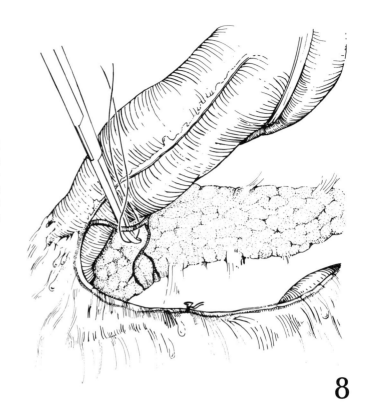

8

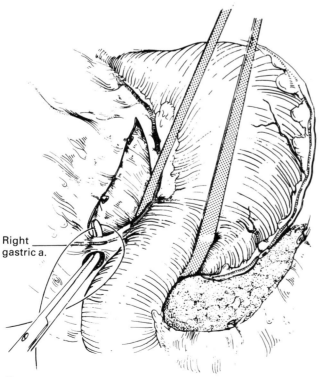

Right gastric a.

9

Ligation of right gastric vessels

9   As the dissection proceeds distally along the lesser curvature, the right gastric artery will be identified near the proximal duodenum. The artery should be ligated close to the duodenum. Care must be taken not to injure the common bile duct if inflammation caused by peptic ulceration has distorted the first portion of the duodenum.

Lesser curvature neurovascular arcade

10 The vascular arcade originating from the left gastric artery parallels the lesser curvature of the stomach. The left gastric vessels reach the stomach as paired branches supplying the anterior and posterior surfaces. The anterior and posterior arcades may be dissected separately; mass ligation, particularly in obese individuals, should be avoided.

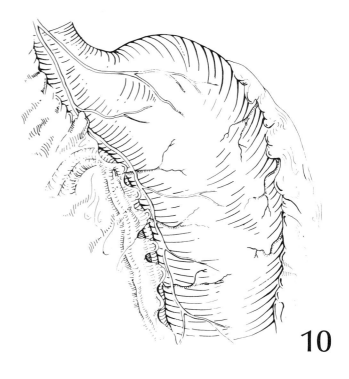

10

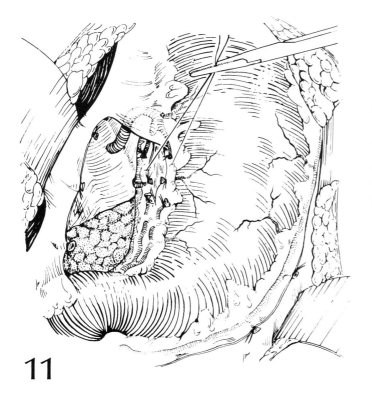

11

Preparation of lesser curvature

11 An area along the lesser curvature is prepared for division and subsequent closure analogous to the dissection performed along the greater curvature. A second traction suture should be placed to control the proximal stomach after transection.

Division of duodenum

12a–c Traction is applied to the stomach toward the patient's left. The duodenum is divided just distal to the pylorus and the ulcer, if present. Division may be accomplished either with a stapler or with clamps (*Illustration 12c*). Stapled transection has the advantages of ease and simultaneous closure of the duodenum.

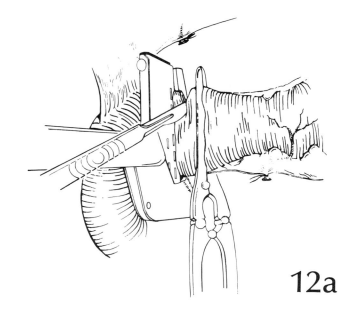

12a

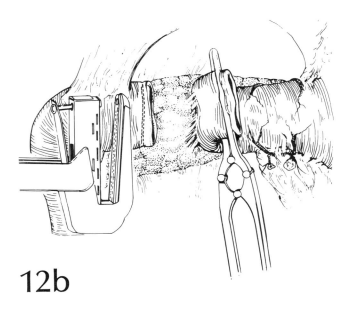

12b

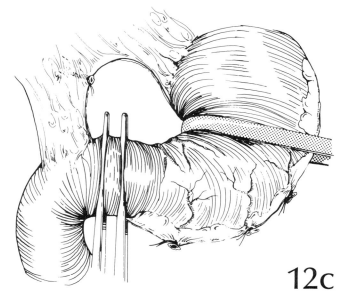

12c

Closure of duodenum

13a–d If the duodenum is divided using clamps, closure should be performed in two layers. The bowel clamp is replaced by Babcock's clamps, care being taken not to encompass an excessive amount of the duodenal wall. After placement of traction sutures superiorly and inferiorly, the cut edge of the duodenum is closed using interrupted absorbable sutures. Closure is completed by a second layer of interrupted seromuscular sutures, e.g. 3/0 silk. If the duodenum has been divided with a stapler the staple line is inverted with interrupted 3/0 silk sutures.

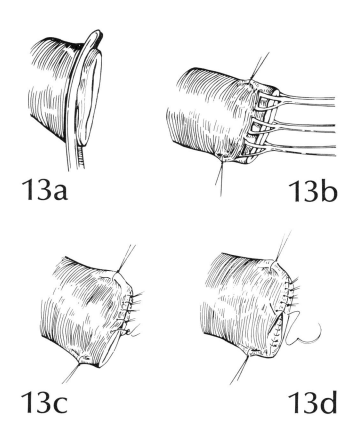

13a

13b

13c

13d

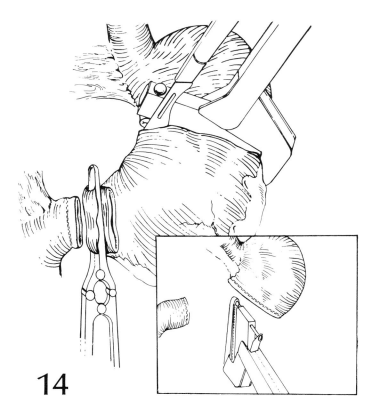

14

Proximal division of stomach

14 The use of surgical staplers greatly facilitates proximal division of the stomach. A TA-90 instrument can be used to close the proximal gastric pouch with a double row of staples: an occlusive clamp is placed distally to prevent escape of gastric contents during transection. Longer length GIA-type staplers may also be employed, using a second application if the stomach is too broad for division with a single load. Some oozing of blood may occur between staples. If this does not cease spontaneously, manual ligation should be performed or a running haemostatic suture applied.

Position of gastrojejunostomy

15 The gastrojejunal anastomosis may be constructed by bringing the jejunum to the gastric pouch either in front of the transverse colon or in a retrocolic position through the transverse mesocolon. In either case, a proximal loop of jejunum should be selected that will reach the stomach without tension and free of angulation. It is crucial that the afferent limb draining pancreatic and biliary secretions is not occluded due to excessive length or kinking.

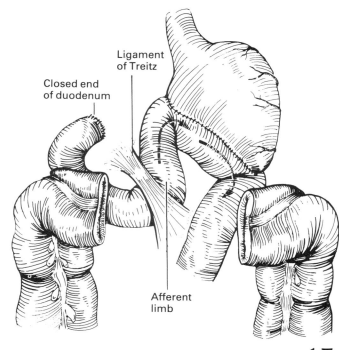

15

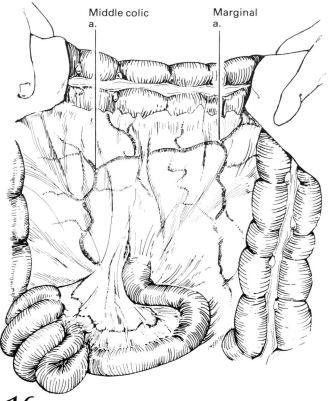

16

Incision in transverse mesocolon

16 If a retrocolic gastrojejunostomy is selected, an incision in the transverse mesocolon to the left of the middle colic vessels is performed. The transverse colon is placed on traction, exposing the course of the middle colic vessels and the marginal artery running parallel to the splenic flexure. The transverse mesocolon is incised in the clear area to the left of the middle colic vessels and an opening is created that will comfortably accommodate the jejunum.

Gastrojejunostomy: sutured technique

17 The gastrojejunal anastomosis may be performed with either a sutured or stapled technique. In the former, the staple line of the gastric transection is partially imbricated with interupted seromuscular sutures. The jejunal loop is delivered through the incision in the transverse mesocolon to approximate the gastric pouch. An appropriate length of stapled closure is excised with electrocautery after placement of interrupted sutures between the posterior gastric wall and the jejunum.

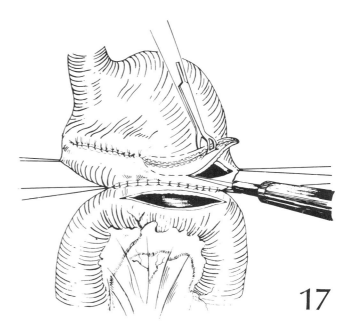

17

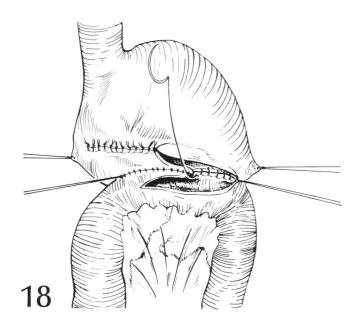

18

Posterior inner suture

18 The posterior layer of the anastomosis is reinforced with a running absorbable suture. The suture should include the full thickness of both the stomach and jejunum.

Anterior portion of anastomosis

19 The posterior running absorbable suture is continued anteriorly as a running Connell suture. The Connell stitch inverts the anastomosis in preparation for the second layer of interrupted seromuscular sutures.

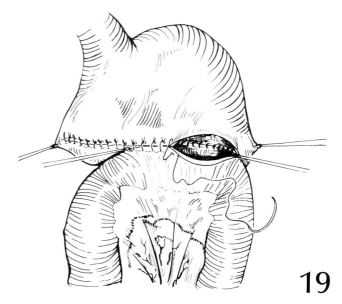

19

Completion of anastomosis

20 A second layer of non-absorbable interrupted sutures is placed to complete the anterior portion of the anastomosis.

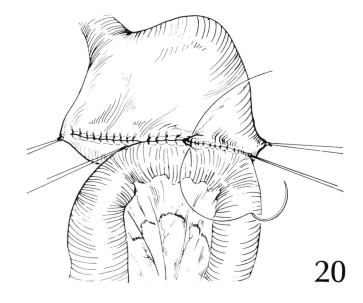

20

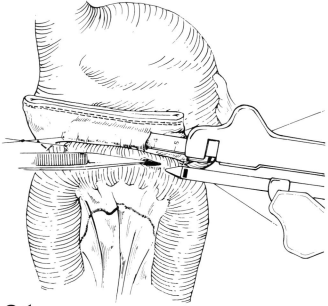

21

Stapled gastrojejunostomy

21 A stapled gastrojejunostomy may be performed with a GIA-type surgical stapler. The jejunum and stomach are approximated using traction sutures. A stab wound is made in the stomach using electrocautery so that an anastomosis will be created 2.5–3 cm from the line of gastric transection. Placement of the anastomosis in this position will ensure that the margin of gastric tissue between the anastomosis and the stapled closure has an adequate blood supply. A similar stab wound is made in the jejunum along its antimesenteric border, and both forks of the instrument are inserted.

Stapler application

22 The instrument is closed and fired, creating the anastomosis with two double, staggered, rows of staples. The instrument is removed and the staple line is inspected for haemostasis.

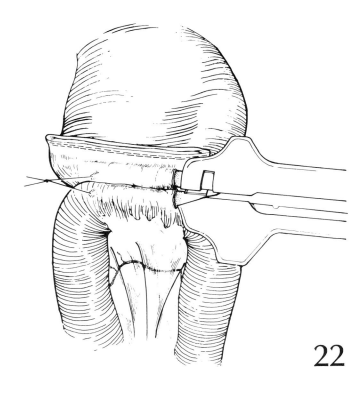

22

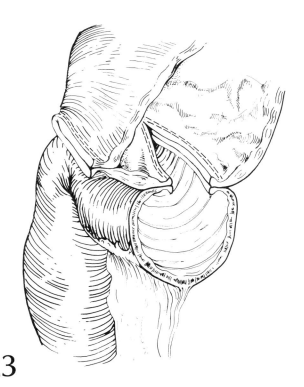

23

Anastomotic reconstruction

23 This view shows the geometry of the stapled gastrojejunal anastomosis.

Closure of stapler defect

24 Removal of the stapler reveals the presence of a (now common) hole used to introduce the instrument. This may be closed simply by placement of interrupted, inverting seromuscular sutures.

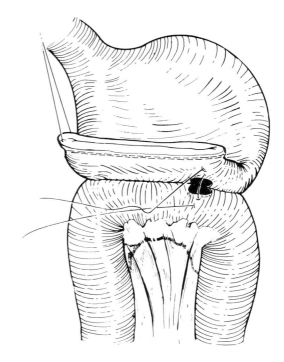

24

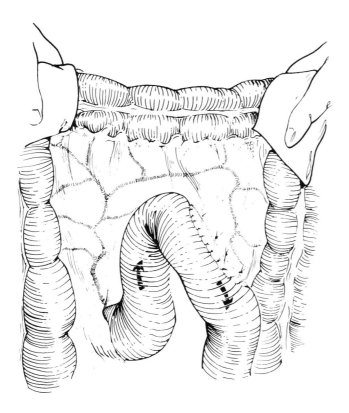

25

Closure of mesocolon

25 The potential hernia created by the incision in the transverse mesocolon should be repaired by sutures placed from the mesocolon to the gastric wall. The gastrojejunal anastomosis should lie inferior to the transverse mesocolon.

Roux-en-Y reconstruction

26 For a Roux-en-Y reconstruction, the stomach is mobilized and transected as previously described. The jejunum is transected distal to the ligament of Treitz so that the intestine distal to the transection may be approximated to the gastric remnant without tension. It is occasionally necessary to divide one of the jejunal arterial arcades to mobilize the intestine. The distal intestine is delivered through the incision in the transverse mesocolon and approximated to the posterior wall of the stomach using traction sutures.

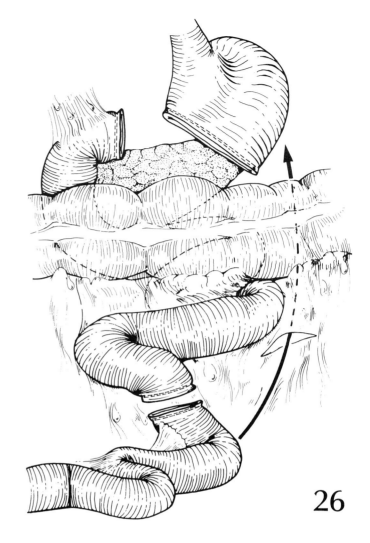

26

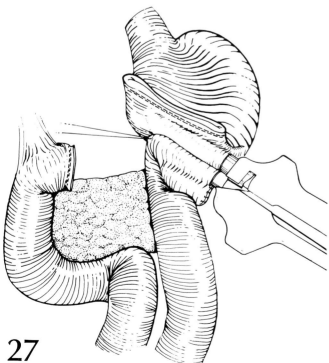

27

Gastrojejunal anastomosis

27 The gastrojejunal anastomosis may be performed in a manner analogous to that illustrated previously, using either staples or a sutured technique.

Enteroenterostomy

28 Intestinal continuity is restored by creation of an enteroenterostomy. In order to prevent reflux of biliary and pancreatic secretions into the gastric remnant, a jejunal limb of 40 cm is constructed. The small intestine should be measured along its antimesenteric border, with care not to unduly stretch it during this manoeuvre. As with the gastrojejunal anastomosis, the enteroenterostomy may be constructed by a sutured or stapled technique. For a stapled anastomosis, two small stab wounds are created in the antimesenteric borders of the small intestine. One fork of a GIA stapling device is placed in each intestinal lumen. The defect used for stapler introduction is closed with interrupted sutures after inspection of the staple line for haemostasis.

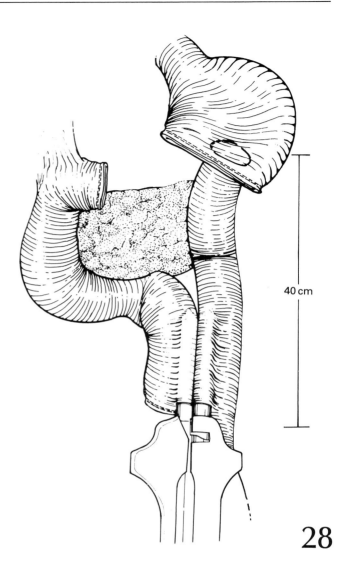

40 cm

28

Postoperative care

Postoperative care following partial gastrectomy includes the standard intravenous fluids, wound care and pulmonary toilet for major laparotomy. Nasogastric suction should be continued until ileus resolves. Perioperative antibiotics are administered in the first 24 h after the operation.

Complications

Haemorrhage may occur in the immediate postoperative period after partial gastrectomy, either into the peritoneal cavity or into the lumen of the intestine. Intraperitoneal haemorrhage can occur due to an improperly tied mesenteric, short gastric, or omental vessel, or because of an unrecognized injury to the spleen. Intraperitoneal haemorrhage, if rapid, presents as shock, and if less rapid as an unexplained fall in packed cell volume. Rapid haemorrhage requires immediate reoperation and control of the bleeding site.

Intraluminal haemorrhage occurs in the postoperative period in as many as 5% of cases of partial gastrectomy, most commonly from the operative suture line. Bleeding from the gastrojejunal suture line may be recognized intraoperatively by the anaesthetist if a properly functioning nasogastric tube is in place. Bleeding from the suture line that begins in the first few days after operation should be investigated endoscopically after evacuation of clots from the gastric remnant. Treatment of the bleeding vessel by endoscopic

electrocautery or heater probe application has greatly reduced the need for reoperation in this circumstance. Judicious application of insufflation and cautery must be performed, however, in the presence of fresh, partially healed suture lines.

Duodenal stump dehiscence is the most difficult complication following partial gastrectomy with gastrojejunal anastomosis, accounting for half of the operative deaths[4]. Duodenal dehiscence most commonly occurs within the first week after operation, with a peak incidence on the fifth day. Rapidly developing signs of peritonitis should alert the surgeon to this possibility.

Duodenal dehiscence may be caused by: (1) duodenal ischaemia caused by improper dissection of the first portion of the duodenum; (2) insecure closure of the duodenal stump due to technical error; (3) insecure closure of the duodenal stump due to scarring, oedema or tumour infiltration; (4) periduodenal infection or pancreatitis; or (5) duodenal distension caused by obstruction of the afferent limb of the gastrojejunostomy. Because prevention of duodenal dehiscence is preferable to its treatment, distal gastrectomy should be avoided when intraoperative assessment indicates that secure duodenal closure may not be possible. In these instances, an alternative operation, e.g. vagotomy and drainage, should be considered. If distal gastrectomy must be performed, protective decompressive duodenostomy may be used to avoid duodenal dehiscence or to establish a deliberate, controlled duodenal fistula rather than an uncontrolled leak[5]. A soft catheter (16-Fr Foley or Malecot) is inserted into the duodenal stump after placement of a purse-string suture. The area of the duodenal closure is drained with a closed drainage system (Jackson–Pratt drains).

Mechanical causes of gastric retention in the early postoperative period include anastomotic oedema or scarring, retrogastric hernia, hernia through the mesocolon and jejunogastric intussusception. Retrogastric hernia may occur after either antecolic or retrocolic gastrojejunal anastomosis. Because of greater length and mobility, the efferent limb usually herniates through the retrogastric hiatus created by formation of the anastomosis. This potential hernia can be eliminated by suturing either the efferent limb or the afferent limb to the posterior parietal peritoneum. Symptoms are not dramatic and include colicky abdominal pain and bilious vomiting. Contrast radiographic studies demonstrate the site of obstruction below the gastrojejunal stoma. Treatment is surgical.

Mechanical obstruction of the gastric outlet can also be caused by herniation of the gastrojejunostomy limbs through the mesocolonic defect created for a retrocolic anastomosis. The hernia occurs when either the mesocolon is not sutured to the gastric wall or when those sutures are disrupted. Symptoms are similar to those of retrocolic hernia, and upper gastrointestinal contrast studies are usually diagnostic. Prompt reoperation and reduction of the hernia is indicated because of the possibility of intestinal ischaemia. The mesocolon should be sutured circumferentially to the stomach above the gastrojejunostomy.

Jejunogastric intussusception involves the efferent loop in more than 75% of cases and presents in the early postoperative period with a syndrome of abdominal pain, nausea and vomiting. The complication may be diagnosed by contrast radiography or endoscopy. If spontaneous reduction is not prompt, operative repair should be undertaken because of the potential for small intestinal infarction.

References

1. Adkins RB, DeLozier JB, Scott HW, Sawyers JL. The management of gastric ulcers: a current review. *Ann Surg* 1985; 201: 741–51.

2. Mulholland MW, Debas HT. Chronic duodenal and gastric ulcer. *Surg Clin North Am* 1987; 67: 489–507.

3. Ritchie WP Jr. Alkaline reflux gastritis: late results of a controlled trial of diagnosis and treatment. *Ann Surg* 1986; 203: 537–44.

4. Ahmad W, Harbrecht PJ, Polk HC. Leaks and obstruction after gastric resection. *Am J Surg* 1986; 152: 301–7.

5. Rossi JA, Sollenberger LL, Rege RV, Glenn J, Joehl RJ. External duodenal fistula: causes, complications, and treatment. *Arch Surg* 1986; 121: 908–12.

Abdominal total gastrectomy without radical lymph node dissection

Lars Lundell MD, PhD
Associate Professor of Surgery, Department of Surgery, Sahlgren's Hospital, University of Gothenburg, Gothenburg, Sweden

Lars C. Olbe MD, PhD
Associate Professor of Surgery, Department of Surgery, Sahlgren's Hospital, University of Gothenburg, Gothenburg, Sweden

History

The object of performing a non-radical total gastrectomy is to remove as much of the tumour-involved tissue as possible without jeopardizing the safety of the operation and the postoperative recovery of the patient. There are, however, relatively few technical differences between the different surgical options in that even a palliative procedure is often best accomplished by having the dissection done in layers and anatomical planes which are usually taken advantage of when carrying out a more radical procedure.

When dealing with carcinomas of the stomach, which can be completely removed macroscopically with an adequate margin of uninvolved tissue, the authors routinely carry out a gastrectomy including a lymph node dissection and removal of the greater omentum. In gastric carcinomas involving the proximal part of the stomach a total gastrectomy is preferred, including a splenectomy. The reason for this approach is that this

dissection is the simplest to carry out and a dissection through tumour tissue should always be avoided to reduce postoperative complications.

There are, however, rare indications for a total gastrectomy due to benign disease (Ménétrièr's disease, haemorrhagic and/or phlegmonous gastritis, etc.), when there is no indication for lymph node dissection and splenectomy.

This chapter deals with total gastrectomy by the abdominal route and excludes carcinoma of the cardia which extends into the distal oesophagus. The jejunum is always used for the reconstruction.

Preoperative

The preoperative evaluation and preparation of the patients are similar to that described when performing a radical total gastrectomy (pp. 450–464).

Operations

TOTAL GASTRECTOMY

1 Access to the upper part of the abdomen is accomplished through a long upper midline incision with the patient in a reverse Trendelenburg position as described in the chapter on pp. 70–78.

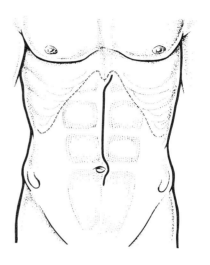

1

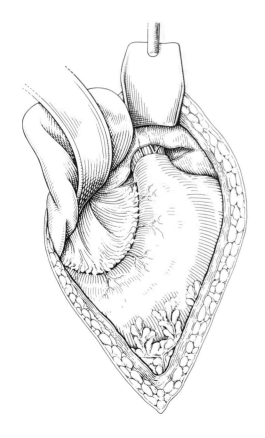

2 To facilitate access to the hiatus the left liver lobe is mobilized and retracted upwards to the right using a self-retaining retractor.

2

3 The resection is undertaken in a plane away from the tumour growth if possible. The greater omentum is dissected from the transverse colon in the bloodless line of Pauchet, using electrocautery. Lifting the omentum up allows adequate inspection and assessment of the tumour growth on the back of the stomach. This gives valuable information when assessing the strategy for the procedure. Occasionally the tumour may invade the middle colic artery which usually can be resected without problems, providing that the colic vascular arcade is left intact. Colonic resection should be avoided, if possible, due to the enhanced associated morbidity.

If the gastric carcinoma invades the pancreas, a pancreatic resection may be necessary, but this additional procedure is usually avoided in a palliative operation because it increases the postoperative morbidity.

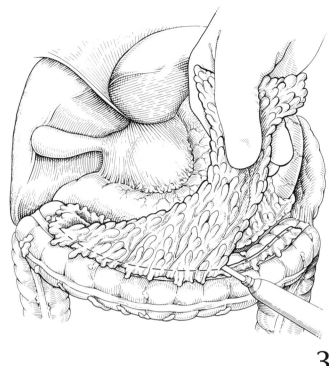

3

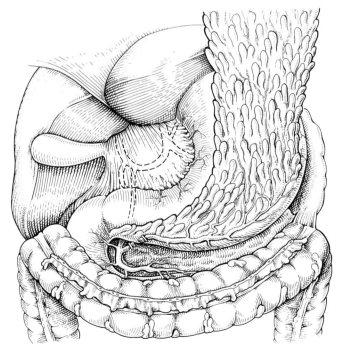

4

4 The entire omentum is included in the resection. After completion of this mobilization the site of division of the gastroepiploic artery can be exposed.

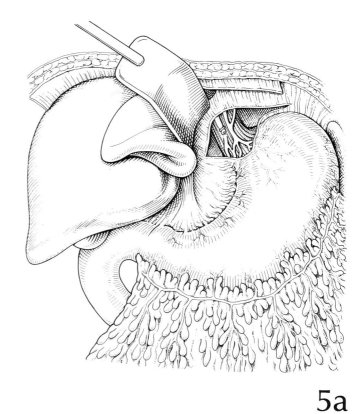

5a, b The alternative initial approach, which is applicable to tumours in the proximal part of the stomach, is to divide the peritoneum high up in the hiatus to determine the line of resection and division. Often parts of the crus have to be resected, but a plane of dissection can nearly always be found just anterior to the aorta in the hiatus. If the tumour is not fixed after these manoeuvres it can always be dissected out along the vascular planes.

5a

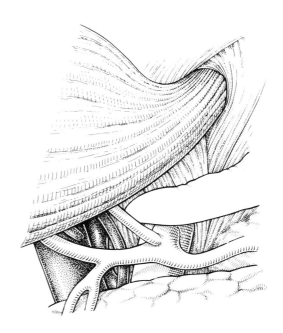

5b

6 As the next step it is convenient to mobilize the duodenum, a procedure that is easily and quickly performed in order to determine a safe line of division of the proximal duodenum which is especially important in carcinomas involving the distal part of the stomach. It is wise surgical practice to expose the structures in the hepatoduodenal ligament, particularly the common bile duct and the common hepatic artery.

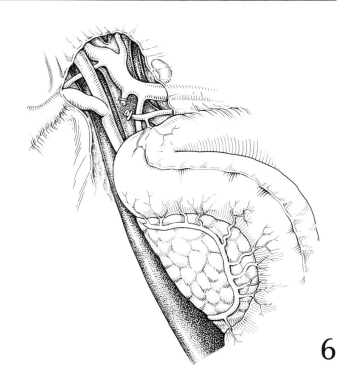

6

7a, b The duodenum is closed using staples and the staple line is covered by a suture line. This precaution is taken to prevent leakage of duodenal contents and does not significantly prolong the procedure. The gastric end of the duodenum can also be closed with staples.

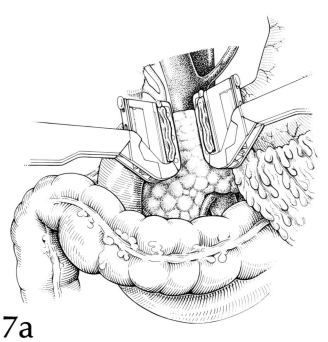

7a

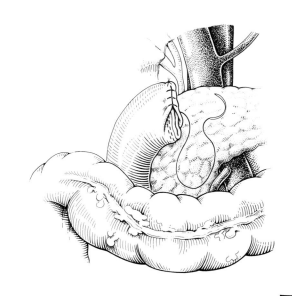

7b

8 The right gastric artery is divided close to its origin from the hepatic artery. The common hepatic artery is then traced by dissection in the adventitial plane towards the origin of the left gastric artery.

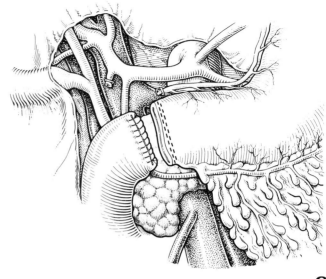

8

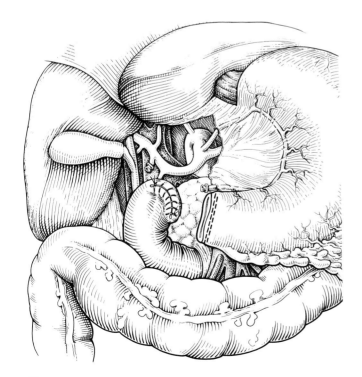

9

9 Turning the stomach to the left and dividing the connective tissue alongside the common hepatic artery exposes the coeliac axis. The origin of the left gastric artery is clearly seen after the coronary vein has been divided. The great advantage of dissecting in this plane is that it is essentially avascular and is very seldom invaded by tumour growth. The authors frequently use electrocautery along the great vessels, since many lymph vessels are divided. The left gastric artery is always ligated with double ligatures of unabsorbable material.

10 In obese patients it can be easier to approach the left gastric artery from the other side, i.e. after the spleen has been mobilized. The peritoneum behind the spleen is divided and the spleen is retracted to the right, exposing the splenic vessels which can be divided separately in the free space between the tail of the pancreas and the hilum of the spleen.

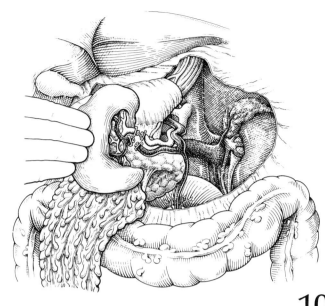

10

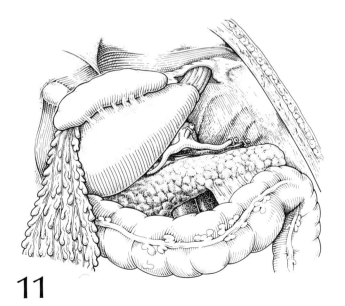

11

11 The coronary vein is also divided when the approach is from this side, after which the left gastric artery is secured at its origin.

LIMITED TOTAL GASTRECTOMY

12 The division of the gastrocolic omentum starts in the avascular area to the left side, caudad to the short gastric vessels, and may proceed outside or inside the gastroepiploic arch. Division of all the epiploic branches can be done using separate ligatures, forceps or clips working from left to right. If the dissection is performed outside the arcade, the omentum should be resected to avoid fat necrosis.

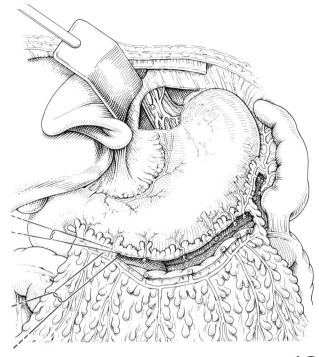

12

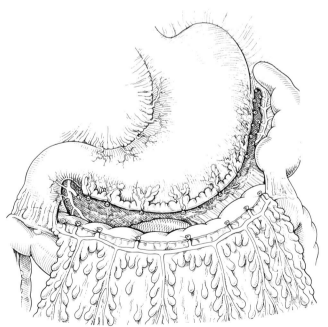

13

13 The gastroepiploic artery is exposed and divided behind the pylorus if the previous dissection has been performed outside the gastroepiploic arch.

14 The duodenum is mobilized to determine the line of transection, just distal to the pylorus. The use of staplers is recommended. The duodenal staple line is invaginated with a continuous suture line.

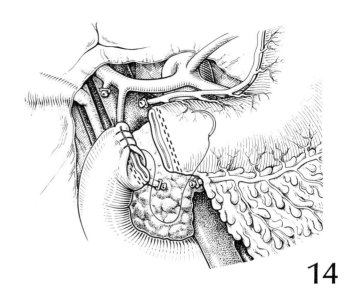

14

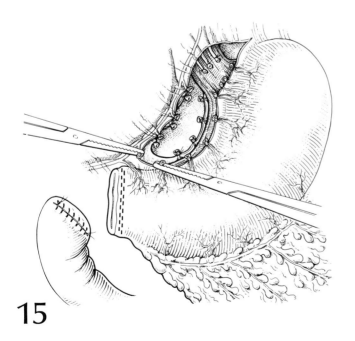

15

15 The dissection along the lesser curvature of the stomach is carried out close to the stomach wall using forceps or clips. It is recommended first to divide the anterior layer of the lesser omentum, and then the posterior layer.

16 Subsequently the distal oesophagus is mobilized and this dissection, which is similar to a proximal gastric vagotomy, preserves the vagal innervation to the extragastric part of the alimentary canal.

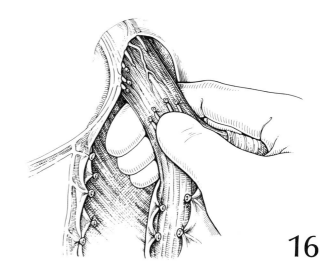

16

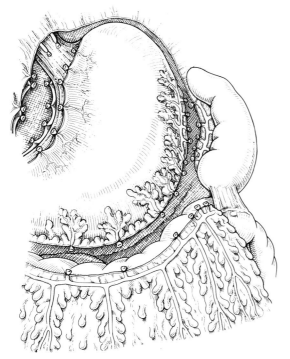

17

17 The short gastric vessels are divided between ligatures or clips.

Reconstruction

The most commonly used reconstruction after total gastrectomy, and also the simplest, is by end-to-end or end-to-side oesophagojejunostomy. The authors' experience with an end-to-side Roux-en-Y reconstruction and somewhat modified suture technique is very reassuring (120 consecutive cases without any clinically significant leakage).

A loop of the jejunum is identified just distal to the duodenojejunal flexure which has the appropriate anatomy of the vascular arcade. This procedure is described in the chapter on pp. 335–344.

18 For anatomical as well as practical reasons reconstruction after total gastrectomy should always be by the retrocolic route. An avascular area is located in the mesentery of the transverse colon and the mobilized loop of the jejunum is brought up to the divided end of the oesophagus. A vascular clamp can be applied to the oesophagus before transection. The transection is performed close to the clamp. The clamp holds the oesophageal stump in the correct position for placing the sutures, and the oesophageal mucosa sticks to the muscular layer after releasing the clamp.

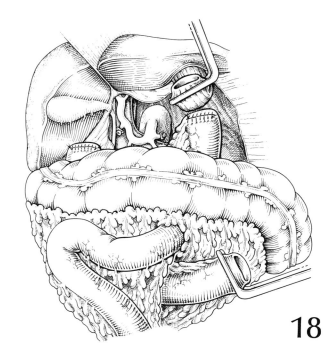

18

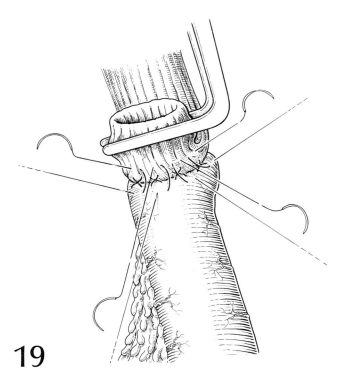

19

19 The blind loop of the jejunum is anchored to the posterior side of the distal oesophagus by two interrupted lines of sutures (synthetic absorbable material). Four sutures are carefully placed in each row. Each stitch in the oesophageal wall should be placed at an oblique angle to the oesophageal muscle fibres in order to maintain a firm hold on the tissue.

20 The redundant oesophagus contained in the clamp is removed and an incision is made in the anterior wall of the jejunal loop and a two-layer anastomosis is sutured using absorbable sutures. A nasogastric tube may be positioned through the anastomosis to minimize the risk of placing the sutures of the exterior front row too deep.

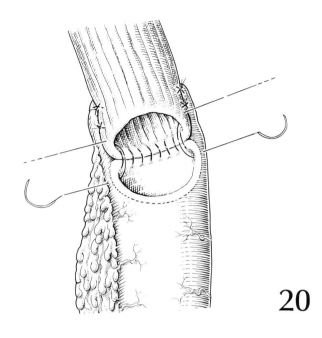

20

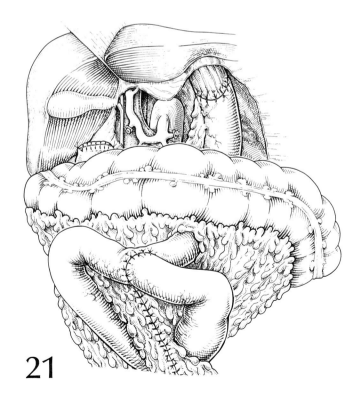

21

21 Below the transverse mesocolon and 50 cm distal to the oesophagojejunostomy, the duodenal end is sutured end-to-side to the Roux loop using a similar two-layer technique. Making the Roux loop so long virtually avoids alkaline reflux oesophagitis. To avoid internal herniations the authors always lay the mesentery of the loop, distal to the transverse colon, alongside the duodenal end of the jejunum.

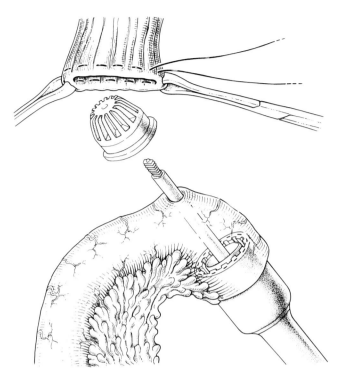

22a–c The use of EEA staplers may facilitate the construction of an anastomosis higher up in the hiatus. However, according to the authors' experience a hand-sewn anastomosis can virtually always be done even high in the hiatus.

22a

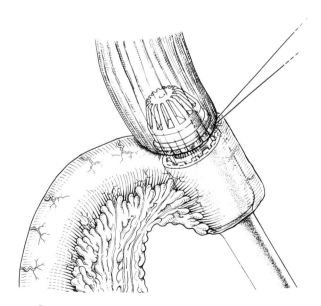

22b

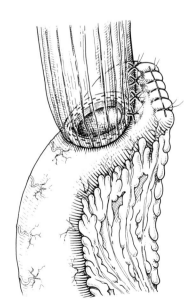

22c

al total gastrectomy without radical lymph node dissection** 449

Postoperative care

The rationale for and essentials of postoperative care, nutrition and analgesia are comprehensively covered in the chapter on pp. 39–44. The postoperative complication rate after these procedures has declined significantly over recent years but problems still remain when operating on older patients. Although the leakage rate from the oesophagojejunostomy has approached zero in specialized units, other problems persist and these are primarily respiratory, cardiovascular and infection related.

Patients are allowed to resume oral nutrition 3–4 days after surgery and shortly thereafter they are instructed by the nursing staff and by a dietician in order to accustom them to the novel anatomy of the alimentary tract and to avoid postoperative nutritional problems. This programme is continued on an outpatient basis for at least the first postoperative year.

Total gastrectomy with lymph node dissection

Jin-Pok Kim MD, FACS
Professor of Surgery, College of Medicine, Seoul National University Hospital, Seoul, Korea

Principles and justification

In contrast to the western world the incidence of gastric cancer is high in Korea and Japan and there is a relatively good 5-year survival rate. This has been attained by early diagnosis, aggressive surgical treatment and administration of postoperative adjuvant immunochemotherapy.

The site of proximal division of the stomach is very important. The proximal border of the tumour should be studied before and during operation using double contrast gastrofluoroscopy, gastroscopy with biopsy and cytology, ultrasonography of the stomach, computed tomographic scanning and gentle palpation. Total gastrectomy is indicated if the proximal distance from the cardia is less than 2 cm in patients with early cancer and less than 6 cm in those with infiltrative advanced cancer. Total gastrectomy is always indicated in cases of diffuse carcinoma (Borrmann type 4) regardless of its size. Total gastrectomy is also the method of palliation in patients who have an obstructing or bleeding tumour, provided that overt metastatic disease is not present and the primary tumour is not technically difficult to resect. For cancer in the fundus or along the greater curvature with direct infiltration into the distal pancreas, splenic hilum, mesocolon or transverse colon, or where there is a solitary direct extension into the left lobe of the liver, extended total gastrectomy including the distal pancreas, spleen, transverse colon or the left lobe of the liver is recommended.

Work by the Japanese Research Society and the Seoul National University Hospital Study for Gastric Cancer has shown that systematic lymph node dissection is the most essential part of resection of gastric cancer and is very effective for the treatment of lymph node metastasis.

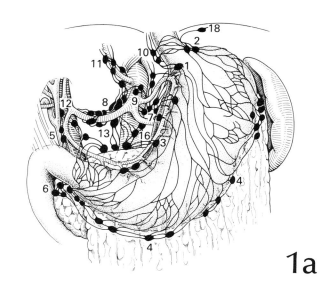

1a

1a, b

The lymph nodes around the stomach are numbered as follows; (1) right cardiac, (2) left cardiac, (3) lesser curvature, (4) greater curvature, (5) suprapyloric, (6) subpyloric, (7) left gastric artery, (8) common hepatic artery, (9) coeliac artery, (10) splenic hilum, (11) splenic artery, (12) hepatoduodenal ligament, (13) behind pancreas head, (14) the root of the mesentery, (15) middle colic artery, (16) para-aortic, (17) thoracic lower para-oesophageal and (18) diaphragmatic.

A curative resection is one in which patients without serosal involvement or peritoneal or hepatic metastases have undergone gastric resection with lymph node dissection which extends one level beyond the pathological level of lymph node involvement. A relative curative resection is one in which there is no serosal, peritoneal or hepatic metastasis and in which the level of pathological lymph node involvement is equal to the highest level of lymph node dissection.

Systematic regional lymph node dissection along the perigastric vessels, including the coeliac axis, common hepatic artery, proper hepatic artery, splenic artery and portal vein (so-called skeletonization) and retropancreatic lymph node dissection is the most important surgical procedure to accomplish true radical surgery.

Reconstruction after total gastrectomy is controversial. Among the various methods of reconstruction, loop oesophagojejunostomy with afferent loop occlusion and Roux-en-Y oesophagojejunostomy are the two most commonly used basic reconstructive methods. However, postoperative oesophageal reflux following loop oesophagojejunostomy and anastomotic leakage after Roux-en-Y oesophagojejunostomy have been annoying problems. The author has found that a simple loop oesophagojejunostomy with closure of the afferent loop to prevent the reflux of bile and pancreatic juice and a long jejunojejunostomy is a satisfactory reconstructive method without significant oesophageal reflux or leakage problems. With this technique oesophageal reflux is negligible and anastomotic leakage is very uncommon (1.6%).

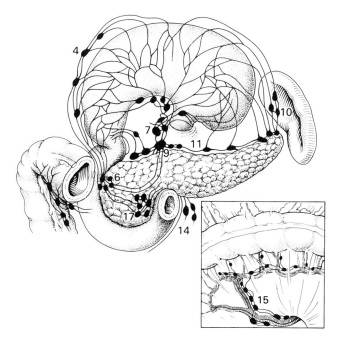

1b

Operation

Incision

2 A limited incision is made in the midline between the xiphoid and the umbilicus. If there are no contraindications for resection, a more liberal incision is made extending to the region of the xiphoid and down to the umbilicus. Examination of the liver, spleen, pancreas, large and small intestine, mesentery, ovary and rectal shelf is mandatory.

If the tumour has invaded the oesophagus above the gastro-oesophageal junction, a left thoracoabdominal incision through the seventh intercostal space should be considered (*see Illustration 24*).

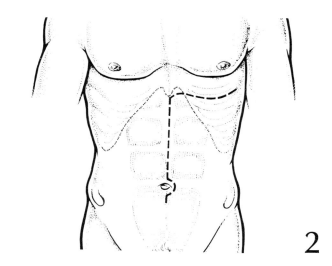

2

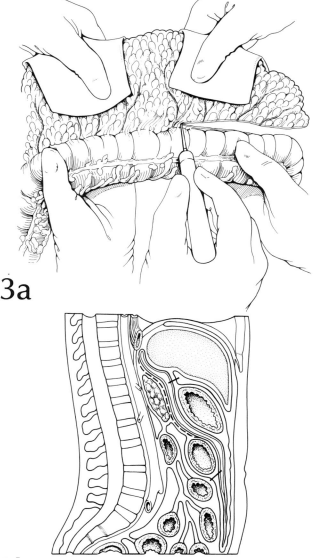

3a

Omentectomy

3 An abdominal pack is placed in the left subphrenic space to displace the spleen downwards to prevent its injury. The greater omentum is reflected upward, grasped with swabs and put on a stretch from the transverse colon to isolate an avascular plane. By sharp dissection with Metzenbaum scissors or electrocautery, the entire transverse colon, including the hepatic and splenic flexures, is freed from the omentum and retracted downward.

3b ⁼⁼ Dissection line

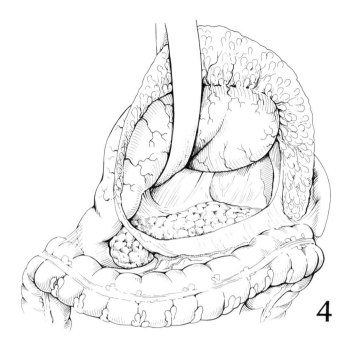

4 The lesser omentum is also divided alongside the liver surface. The stomach is then wrapped with abdominal gauze and lifted upward to visualize the gastroduodenal junction easily.

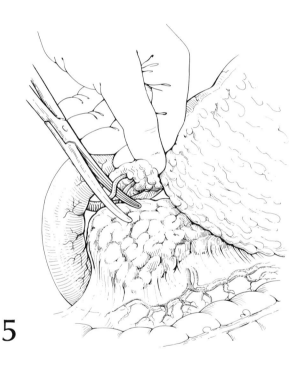

Dissection around duodenum

5 The right gastroepiploic vessels are ligated as far away from the inferior surface of the duodenum as possible to ensure that infrapyloric nodes and adjacent fat are removed. The right gastric vessels are sought along the superior margin of the first part of the duodenum, isolated by blunt dissection and ligated some distance from the duodenal wall. The posterior wall of the first part of the duodenum is freed from the adjacent pancreas.

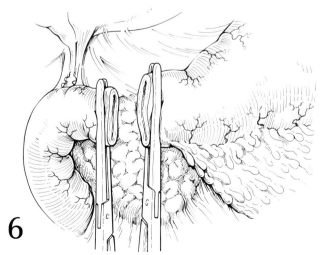

6 The duodenum is then divided between clamps and the distal margin sent for frozen section to make sure that it is free from tumour.

7a–d   The duodenal stump is closed with a continuous running suture under the clamp. When this has been completed the stump is plicated to reduce its diameter. Closure of the duodenal stump is completed with a continuous interlocking suture and the stump is oversewn using one layer of seromuscular interrupted sutures.

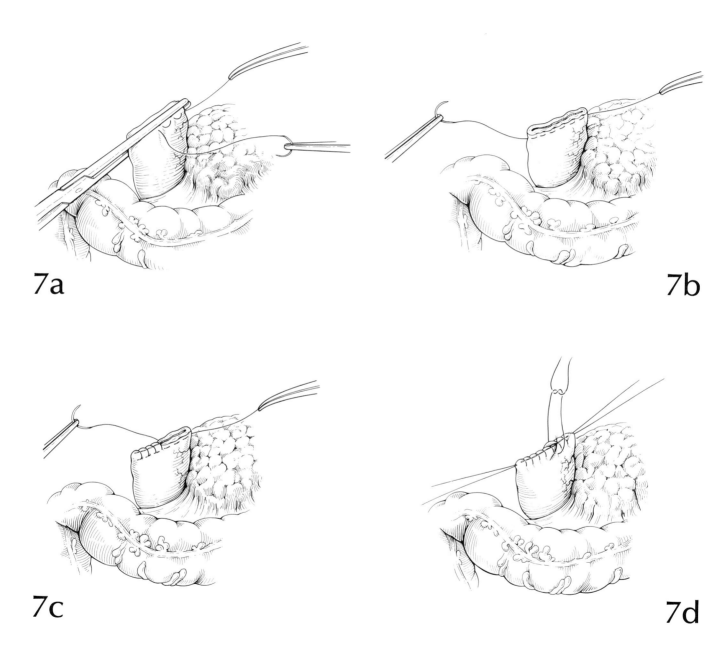

7a

7b

7c

7d

Lymph node dissection

8 The stomach is retracted upwards and the peritoneum along the upper border of the pancreas is divided. Lymph node dissection is started from the coeliac trunk, continuing along the left gastric artery, which is divided and ligated. The surrounding connective, nerve and lymphatic tissues are grasped with clamps and also divided. The left gastric vein, together with adjoining tissue, is removed as far distal as possible near to its junction with the portal vein.

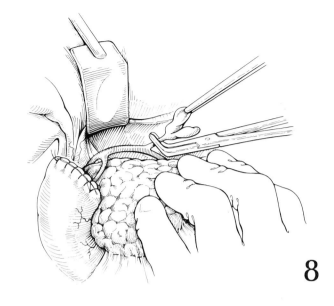

8

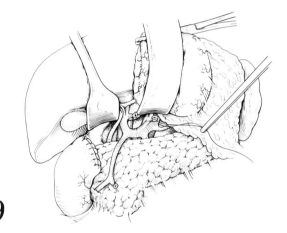

9

9 Dissection is continued in the adventitia of the common hepatic artery in the direction of the liver using scissors. Connective, nerve and lymphatic tissues are detached and removed. The hepatoduodenal ligament is freed of lymphatic and connective tissues when the hepatic artery has been dissected free and the lymph node groups adjoining the portal vein are excised. The remaining serosal leaf is incised with scissors as far toward the hepatic hilus as possible, grasped with clamps, and pulled or pushed in the direction of the duodenum together with the attached, generally delicate, connective and lymphoid tissue.

10 The index finger of the left hand is passed through the foramen of Winslow and behind the adjoining portal vein. Associated tissues are grasped with clamps and excised. The common hepatic artery is retracted downwards using a vein retractor and retropancreatic nodes are grasped with clamps alternately and excised. The splenic artery is exposed in its initial suprapancreatic course, and the adjacent connective and lymphatic tissue is removed.

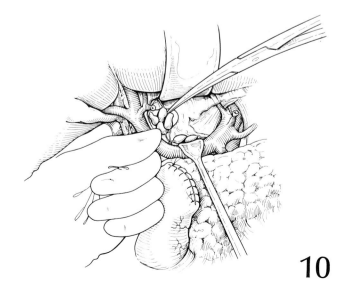

10

11 The lesser omentum is dissected downwards from the inferior margin of the liver and para-aortic lymph nodes are reflected along the side of the abdominal aorta and up to the diaphragmatic hiatus.

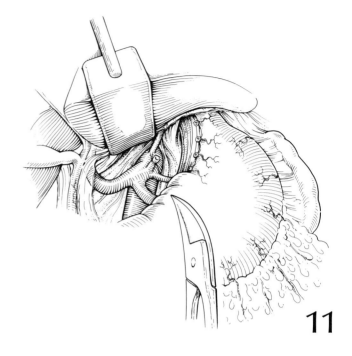

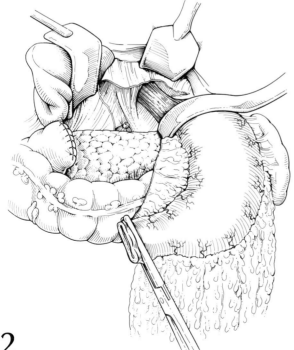

12 The node dissection or so-called 'skeletonization of major vessels' is now complete.

Dissection around spleen and oesophagus

13 The gastrosplenic ligament is divided up to the oesophagus and the left gastro-omental (epiploic) vessels are divided and ligated. The thickened portion of the gastrohepatic ligament which includes a branch of the inferior phrenic artery is divided up to the oesophagus. The oesophagus is mobilized by blunt dissection, the vagus nerves are identified and divided to release the oesophagus.

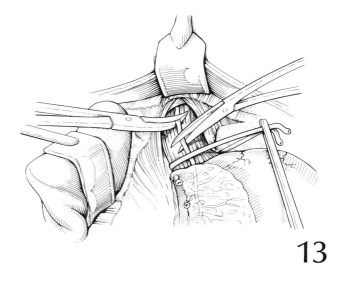

13

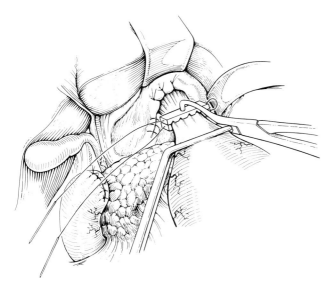

14

14 The oesophagus is then divided using a purse-string clamp on the proximal side and a crushing clamp on the distal side. A straight needle with 2/0 polypropylene is inserted in the purse-string clamp and the clamp removed. At this time the proximal margin of the oesophagus is sent for frozen section to make sure that the margin of excision is free from tumour. The oesophagus is now opened with a dilator.

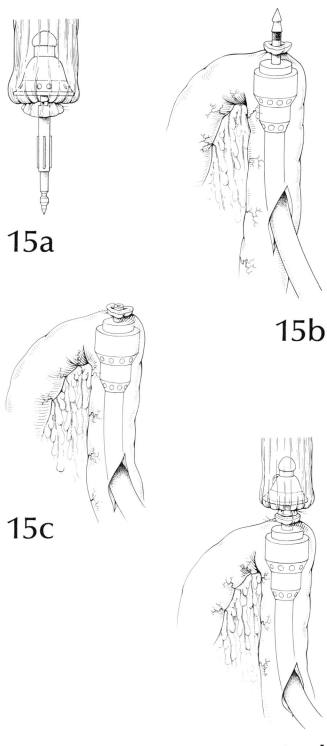

15a

15b

15c

15d

15a–d An EEA stapler is introduced through an opening which is made in the jejunum 40 cm distal to the ligament of Treitz. The trocar of the EEA is pierced through the jejunum and an end-to-side oesophagojejunostomy is made. A nasogastric Levin tube is inserted through the oesophagojejunostomy, and about 50 ml of methylene blue solution is injected through the tube to make sure that there is no leakage. If no leakage occurs, several anchoring sutures are placed around the oesophagojejunostomy site between the diaphragm and jejunum. A Kim's tie (*see Illustration 21*) is placed around the afferent loop close to the oesophagojejunostomy site with a strong silk suture.

Hand-sewn anastomosis (end-to-side loop)

16 The clamped oesophageal end and the jejunal loop are approximated and a posterior seromuscular layer of sutures with 3/0 silk is placed.

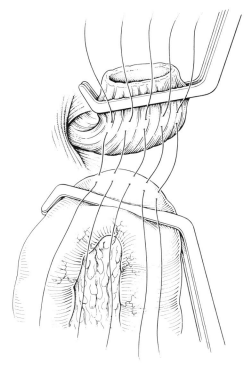

16

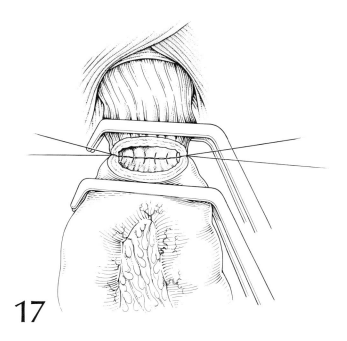

17

17 The jejunal loop is then opened and a continuous interlocking suture carried out.

18 Finally, the anterior wall is sutured using the same continuous interlocking suture.

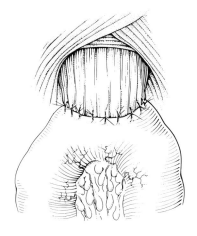

18

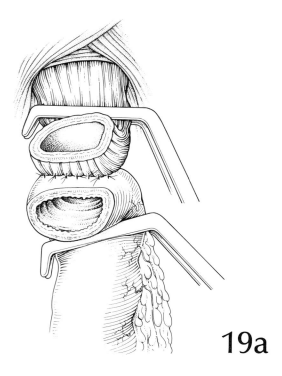

19a

19a, b An end-to-end Roux-en-Y anastomosis is hand-sewn.

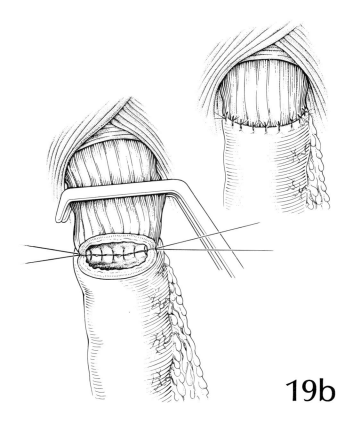

19b

Reconstruction of gastrointestinal continuity

20 The transverse colon is lifted upward and a cruciate incision is made in the avascular space of the mesocolon. Jejunum is brought through this opening. A tagging suture is made on the jejunum 10–20 cm distal to the ligament of Treitz.

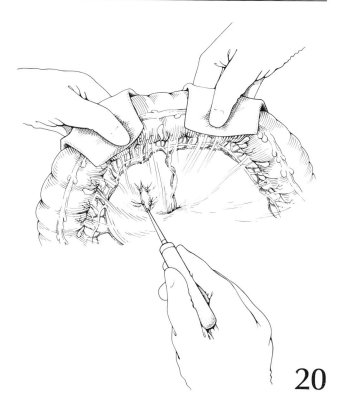

21 A Kim's tie is placed around the afferent loop close to the oesophagojejunostomy site with a strong silk suture.

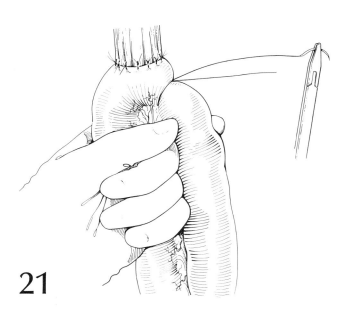

22 A side-to-side jejunojejunostomy is made between the limbs of the jejunum 20–30 cm distal to the oesophagojejunostomy site. Anchoring sutures are placed between the opening of the mesocolon and the jejunojejunostomy site.

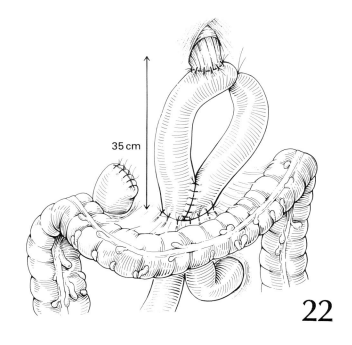

23a–c
Alternative reconstructions which can be used are end-to-end Roux-en-Y type (*Illustration 23a*) or end-to-side (*Illustrations 23b* and *23c*) oesophagojejunostomies.

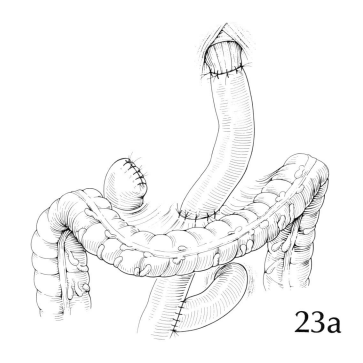

23a

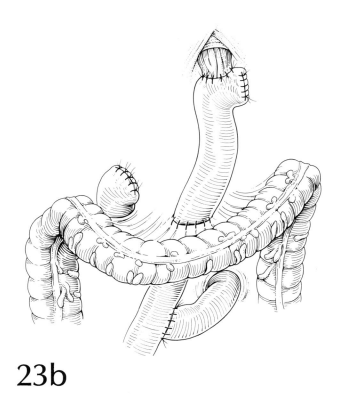

23b

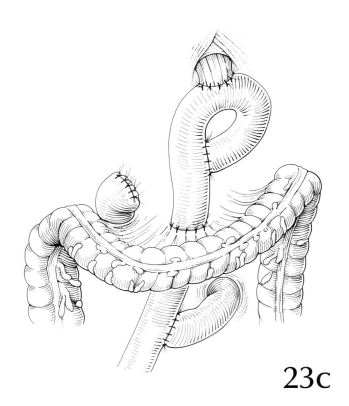

23c

24 If tumour has invaded the oesophagus for more than 5 cm above the gastro-oesophageal junction, a left thoracoabdominal incision through the seventh intercostal space is considered.

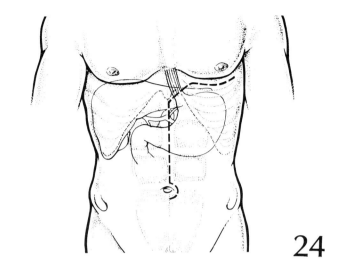

24

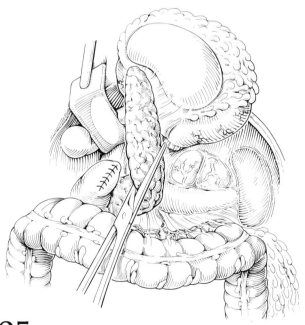

25

Combined resection of spleen and distal pancreas

25 The purpose of a combined resection of the spleen and distal pancreas is to remove all the lesions when direct invasion of the pancreas and retroperitoneum has occurred, a not infrequent finding in cases requiring total gastrectomy.

Postoperative care

To help attain minimal mortality and morbidity rates in patients undergoing total gastrectomy (1.5% and 8% respectively at Seoul National University Hospital), attention must be given to preoperative and postoperative management with such factors as nutrition and chest physiotherapy being addressed. To avoid sudden tension at the oesophagojejunostomy anastomosis, all patients are taught to undertake deep breathing without coughing and are encouraged to do this for the first 2 days after operation.

Constant nasogastric suction is instituted before operation and is maintained after operation until the seventh postoperative day. Methylene blue is then administered orally to see if there is any leakage through the drain. If there is no evidence of leakage the nasogastric tube is removed. The patient is placed on a postgastrectomy diet regimen that progresses gradually from bland liquids to eight small feeds per day.

Further reading

Kim J-P. Reconstructive surgery after gastrectomy in the stomach cancer patient. *Medical Postgraduates Korea* 1988; 16: 2–7.

Kim J-P. Current problems in gastric cancer surgery with special emphasis on immuno-chemo-surgery. *German J Gastroenterol* 1989; 24: 273–5.

Kim J-P, Jung S-E. Patients with gastric cancer and their prognosis in accordance with number of lymph node metastases. *Scand J Gastroenterol* 1987; 22(Suppl 133): 33–5.

Maruyama K, Okabayashi K, Kinoshita T. Progress in gastric cancer surgery in Japan and its limits of radicality. *World J Surg* 1987; 11: 418–25.

Yehuda GA, Gershon E. Trends and controversies in the management of carcinoma of the stomach. *Surg Gynecol Obstet* 1989; 169: 371–85.

High lesser curve gastrectomy with oesophagojejunogastric reconstruction

Attila Csendes MD, FACS
Professor of Surgery, University of Chile, Department of Surgery, University Hospital, Santiago, Chile

Italo Braghetto MD
Associate Professor of Surgery, University of Chile, Department of Surgery, University Hospital, Santiago, Chile

Owen Korn MD
Instructor of Surgery, University of Chile, Department of Surgery, University Hospital, Santiago, Chile

In 1965 Johnson classified gastric ulcers into three types according to blood group characteristics, clinical features and gastric acid secretory pattern[1]. The authors have described type IV gastric ulcer, which is very common in Chile and which corresponds to the high or subcardial gastric ulcer[2-4]. Type IV ulcers are defined as those ulcers located less than 4 cm from the squamocolumnar junction. They are characterized by a frequent association with type O blood group[5], by low basal and stimulated acid secretion[6], by a high incidence of upper gastrointestinal bleeding[7], by slower emptying of liquids[8] and by a high incidence of deep penetration[4]. These high gastric ulcers can be classified into two subgroups, according to their location:

1. Subcardial ulcers found 2–4 cm from the gastro-oesophageal junction. These account for 90% of all type IV gastric ulcers[9].
2. Juxtacardial or cardial ulcers, which are those located within 2 cm of the squamocolumnar junction. These account for about 10% of type IV ulcer.

Traditionally, high-lying ulcers have been treated by four-quadrant biopsy and distal gastrectomy without removal of the ulcer; the Kerling–Madlener procedure. However, many of the juxtacardial ulcers encountered by the authors have been penetrating ulcers that extend beyond the gastric wall. The authors have devised an operation that accomplishes resection of the ulcer, distal gastrectomy, and gastrointestinal reconstruction using a Roux-en-Y jejunal limb to accomplish oesophagojejunogastrostomy.

Principles and justification

The main goals for definitive surgical treatment of patients with gastric ulcer are: (1) resection of the ulcer; (2) resection of the area with chronic atrophic gastritis; (3) reduction of acid secretion; and (4) improved gastric emptying[1, 10]. These goals are accomplished adequately when a partial distal or subtotal gastrectomy is performed. This surgical procedure is easily performed with a low rate of operative mortality (0.8%) when the ulcer is located in the antrum or corpus of the stomach. However, when the ulcer is located in the upper third of the stomach, at or in the vicinity of the cardia, surgical resection can be hazardous and ulcer removal can involve a difficult dissection with a high rate of mortality[9].

In the last 15 years nearly 1000 patients with gastric ulcer have undergone surgery. Of these, 290 patients had type IV gastric ulcers including 27 in whom the gastric ulcers were within 2 cm of the squamocolumnar junction. For these juxtacardial ulcers a special surgical technique has been devised that accomplishes all the goals described above[11-13].

Preoperative

Each patient undergoes all the necessary general laboratory examinations. Barium study of the upper gastrointestinal tract is important, but it is endoscopy that provides the crucial information. Endoscopy has to be performed with great care and multiple biopsies must be obtained to rule out adenocarcinoma. The patient is fasted for a minimum of 12 h and is given a first generation cephalosporin within 2 h of surgery.

General anaesthesia is always used.

Operation

The patient is placed on the operating table in the Grassi position, with the head elevated 20° in order to obtain a caudal displacement of supramesocolic organs. An upper midline incision is employed. A special sternum-elevating retractor, similar to that employed for antireflux surgery or for total gastrectomy, is used.

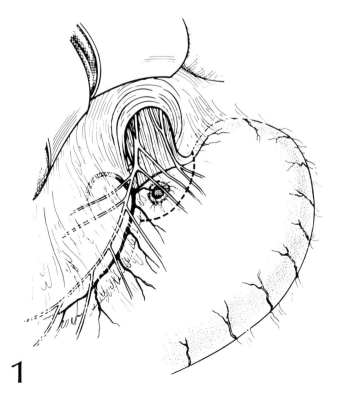

1

1   After careful abdominal exploration the stomach is retracted caudally. These high gastric ulcers are almost always located on the posterior wall of the stomach, near the lesser curvature in the vicinity of the cardia. They have usually penetrated beyond the gastric wall, so good exposure of this area, including the ulcer, is essential to perform an adequate resection.

2 The first step consists of the dissection of the angle of His and section of the upper two or three short gastric vessels in order to expose the abdominal portion of the oesophagus and the greater curvature. Both vagal trunks are then divided in order to elongate the distal oesophagus.

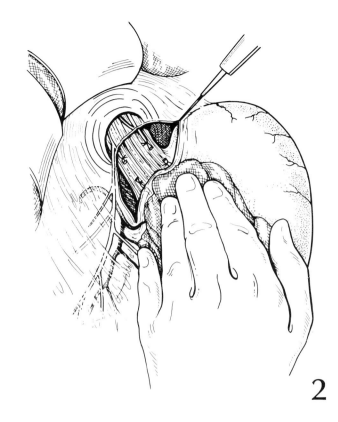

2

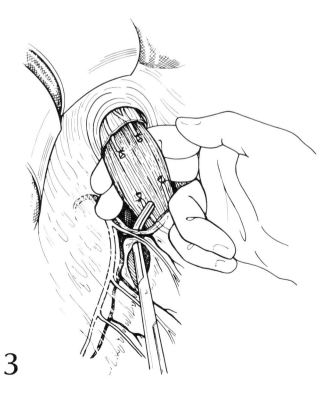

3

3 Further lengthening of the abdominal oesophagus is obtained by applying traction on a Nelaton catheter.

It is essential to cut the left gastric artery near its origin from the coeliac trunk to avoid the inflammatory process in the area that often involves the branches of the left gastric artery. These three manoeuvres – dissection of the angle of His, section of the vagal trunks and division of the left gastric artery – greatly facilitate exposure of the posteriorly placed high gastric ulcer.

4 A subtotal gastrectomy with 75% resection of the stomach is then performed. The duodenum is divided 1 cm distal to the pylorus and closed using a stapler device or a hand-sewn, double layer closure.

The goal of the operation is to remove the high-lying gastric ulcer, resecting more of the posterior wall of the stomach in a manner similar to Pauchet's technique.

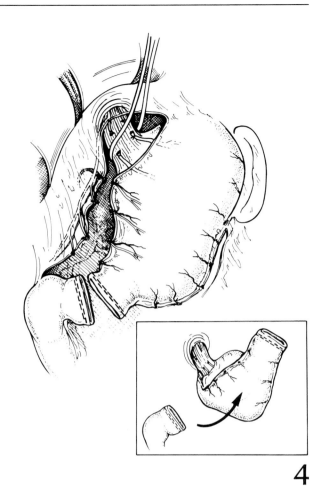

4

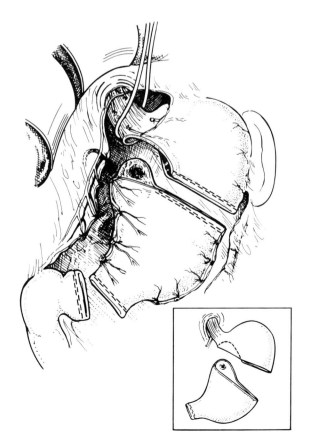

5

5 At the greater curvature nearly 25% of its proximal portion is preserved and the stomach is cut between straight nippers. Towards the lesser curvature gastric resection is performed in an open manner, using electrocautery and resecting more of the posterior than the anterior wall.

The resection includes the adjacent portion of the oesophageal mucosa at the cardia. This means the lesser curvature is completely resected. Reconstruction of the gastrointestinal tract is accomplished using a 60-cm long Roux-en-Y jejunal limb. The end of the Roux limb is closed and passed retrocolic for anastomosis to the cut edges of the oesophagus and stomach.

6 The anastomosis starts about 3 cm from the closed end of the jejunal limb, suturing first the posterior layer, and then the anterior layer by a continuous single layer suture of 3/0 polyglactin (Vicryl).

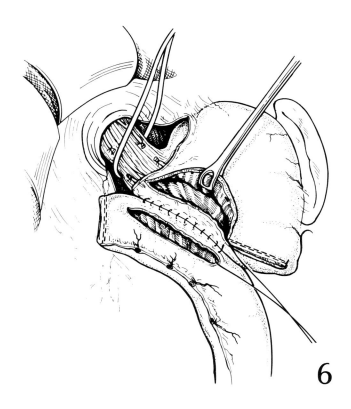

6

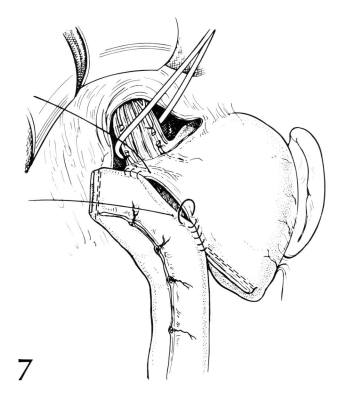

7

7 About 5–8 cm of the greater curvature is closed in order to avoid a Pólya type of anastomosis. At the conclusion of the anastomosis, methylene blue is injected under pressure through the nasogastric tube in order to check the integrity of the suture line.

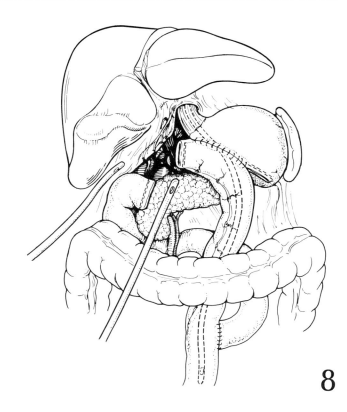

8 Two drains are left, one at the site of the oesophagogastrojejunostomy and the other at the duodenal stump.

Salient points of technique

1. Mobilization of the cardia containing a high-lying posterior ulcer is accomplished by: (a) dissection of the angle of His with division of the uppermost two or three short gastric vessels; (b) bilateral truncal vagotomy; and (c) division of the left gastric artery at its origin beyond the inflammatory process that often involves branches of the left gastric artery.
2. Resection of the distal 75% of the stomach with removal of the ulcer requires: (a) excision of more of the posterior than the anterior wall of the cardia; and (b) resection of the adjacent wall of the oesophagus.
3. Restoration of gastrointestinal tract is achieved using: (a) a 60-cm long, retrocolic Roux-en-Y jejunal limb; and (b) creation of an oesophagojejunal–gastric anastomosis.

Postoperative care

No oral intake is allowed for 10 days. The patients receive parenteral hyperalimentation or enteral feeding through a nasojejunal tube inserted during operation. Antibiotics are given for 1–2 days after surgery. If a septic complication occurs (such as pulmonary infection, subphrenic collections, etc.), however, broad-spectrum antibiotics specific to the cultured organisms are used whenever possible. On the 10th postoperative day a Hypaque or Gastrografin study is undertaken to examine the integrity of the anastomosis. If no leak is demonstrated, oral feeding is started.

Outcome

The main indications for surgery in the 27 patients with juxtacardial gastric ulcers treated by the authors are shown in *Table 1*. Refractory ulcer with no healing or intractable pain was the main indication for surgery in 59% of cases, while in the rest massive or repeated upper gastrointestinal haemorrhage led to a decision to operate. The mean duration of ulcer pain was 6.5 (range 2–11) years. All patients were submitted to endoscopy (*Table 2*). The mean distance between the squamo-columnar junction and the proximal border of the ulcer

was 10 mm and the mean diameter of the ulcer was 18 mm (range 10–32 mm). A mean of five biopsies was taken in each case. The postoperative course of these 27 patients is shown in *Table 3*. There was no postopera-

Table 1   Surgical indications in 27 patients with high juxtacardial ulcer

Refractory ulcer (no healing)	16
Upper gastrointestinal haemorrhage	11
Massive	8
Repeated	3

Table 2   Endoscopic findings in 27 patients with high juxtacardial ulcer

Squamocolumnar junction	40.5 cm from incisor
Location of the ulcer	41.5 cm from incisor
Mean size	18 mm
Biopsies	5.2 per patient

Table 3   Postoperative course in 27 patients with high juxtacardial ulcer

Mortality	0
Uneventful recovery	23
Acute bronchitis	2
Wound infection	1
Type I fistula	1
Mean postoperative stay	17 days

Table 4   Late follow-up of 27 patients with high juxtacardial ulcer

Visick I	21
Visick II	3
Visick III	1
Dead	2
Oesophagitis	0
Incisional hernia	3

tive mortality. Four patients (15%) developed some morbidity after surgery. Only one patient developed a leak with localized fistula formation, type I. All patients were followed for a mean of 6.5 (range 3–10) years. Two patients died as a result of carcinoma of the gallbladder and pancreas 3 and 5 years, respectively, after surgery. Twenty-one patients (78%) were classified as Visick I, three cases as Visick II and one case as Visick III due to the development of late dumping and steatorrhoea (*Table 4*). None of the 14 cases examined endoscopically after surgery had oesophagitis. Three patients developed incisional hernia requiring operative correction.

References

1. Johnson HD. Gastric ulcer: classification, blood group characteristics, secretion patterns and pathogenesis. *Ann Surg* 1965; 162: 996–1004.

2. Csendes A, Miranda M, Rappoport J *et al.* Clinical features and results in 809 patients with gastric ulcer submitted to surgery. *Rev Med Chile* 1982; 34: 35–40.

3. Csendes A, Smok G, Medina E. Frequency of high gastric ulcer in Chile. Another type of ulcer? *Rev Med Chile* 1983; 111: 883–8.

4. Csendes A, Braghetto I, Smok G. Type IV gastric ulcer: a new hypothesis. *Surgery* 1987; 101: 361–6.

5. Csendes A, Medina E, Angel Ulloa EO, Obard E. Distribution of blood group ABO and Rh in patients with gastric ulcer, duodenal ulcer, gastric cancer and controls. *Rev Med Chile* 1975; 103: 470–3.

6. Csendes A, Larach J, Carvajal C. Chronic gastric ulcer, basal and stimulated gastric acid secretion according to the location of the ulcer. *Rev Med Chile* 1977; 105: 1–3.

7. Csendes A, Elizalde I, González P *et al.* Different parameters that are important in the evolution of patients with upper gastrointestinal bleeding. *Rev Med Chile* 1983; 111: 676–83.

8. Csendes A, Henriquez A, Eguigurren AL. Gastric emptying studies with the double sampling technique in patients with gastric and duodenal ulcer. *Rev Chilena Cir* 1978; 30: 361–4.

9. Csendes A, Braghetto I, Calvo F *et al.* Surgical treatment of high gastric ulcer. *Am J Surg* 1985; 149: 765–70.

10. Calvo F, De La Cuadra R, Csendes A *et al.* Results in patients with high gastric ulcer submitted to conservative or alternative operations. *Rev Chilena Cir* 1985; 37: 27–35.

11. Csendes A, Lazo M, Braghetto I. A possible surgical solution for cardial or juxtacardial gastric ulcer. *Rev Chilena Cir* 1977; 29: 8–11.

12. Csendes A, Lazo M, Braghetto I. A surgical technique for high (cardial or juxtacardial) benign chronic gastric ulcer. *Am J Surg* 1978; 135: 857–8.

13. Csendes A, Velasco N, Braghetto I *et al.* Subtotal gastrectomy with esophago-gastro-jejunostomy for cardial or juxtacardial gastric ulcer. *Rev Chilena Cir* 1983; 35: 29–36.

Miscellaneous gastric resections

David Fromm MD
Penberthy Professor and Chairman, Department of Surgery, Wayne State University, Detroit, Michigan, USA

Ulcerative and neoplastic lesions of the stomach are usually treated by formal subtotal gastrectomy or antrectomy. Occasionally, however, either because of the nature of the lesion or because of the patient's poor condition, segmental gastric resection is employed. Very uncommonly, proximal gastrectomy may be required for benign lesions of the stomach. In this group of highly selected patients, it may be physiologically advantageous to maintain a normally functioning antrum and pylorus by preserving the vagal innervation of the distal stomach and using a segment of isoperistaltic jejunum to restore gastrointestinal continuity. In this chapter segmental gastric resection and gastric resection with preservation of innervation will be discussed.

Segmental resections

Principles and justification

A grossly or biopsy-proven benign tumour of the stomach is the most common indication for segmental resection. A focal resection is also sometimes indicated for a patient with a bleeding gastric ulcer who remains unstable after control of the haemorrhage. Traumatic injuries and local invasion by non-gastric malignancies are among other indications.

Preoperative

If the patient has been on medication that suppresses acid secretion or has significant amounts of blood in the gastric lumen, serious consideration should be given to the observation that luminal bacterial counts increase along with the increase in pH.

Operation

If a nasogastric tube is not in place, it is inserted and kept on suction to minimize spill from the gastric lumen.

Incision

A midline or left paramedian incision is preferable to a transverse or oblique incision that denervates abdominal musculature.

Exposure of the upper abdomen

1 The falciform ligament is divided so that a fixed retractor can be placed under the lower sternum, which can now be pulled anteriorly and towards the patient's head without injuring the liver. Adhesions between the liver and anterior parietal peritoneum, if present, are divided before retraction of the sternum. The edges of the abdominal incision are retracted laterally.

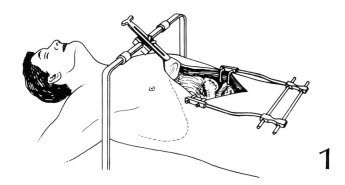

1

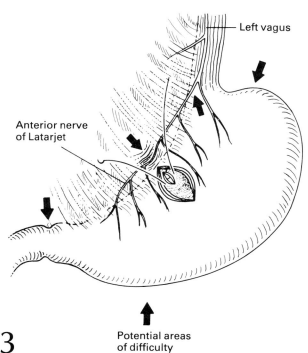

2

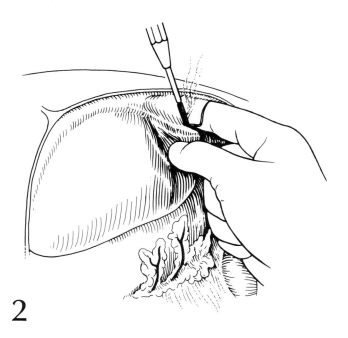

3

Potential areas
of difficulty

Exposure of the stomach

2 If the lesion to be resected lies high on the lesser curve, the left triangular ligament is divided and the left hepatic lobe is folded posteriorly and retracted to the right.

If the lesion lies posteriorly, the lesser sac is entered by dividing the gastrocolic omentum, taking care not to injure potentially adherent middle colic vessels. The gastropancreatic membrane is divided as necessary for exposure.

Areas of potential trouble

3 If the lesion approximates the lesser curve, consideration should be given to excising the lesion without injury to the nerves of Latarjet, lest antral function becomes impaired. Another problem area lies high along the greater curve, where retraction can result in avulsion of the highest short gastric vessels, which can be difficult to control. This is avoided by first sacrificing the vessels. Local resection of a proximal, or high lying, lesser curve lesion near the cardio-oesophageal junction can compromise the junctional lumen if the resulting defect is closed longitudinally rather than transversely. Resections involving a portion of the pylorus are also best closed transversely to avoid luminal compromise. The long-term effects of excising the gastric pacemaker, which in man lies in the mid-body along the greater curve, 5–7 cm distal to the cardia[1], are not clear. Transection of the gastric body, thereby isolating the distal stomach from its natural pacemaker, results in the appearance of a new pacemaker in the distal stomach but with a slower frequency.

Postoperative care

There is nothing specific about the postoperative care. A nasogastric tube is seldom necessary once the patient leaves the operating room.

Resection with preservation of innervation

Principles and justification

Gastric resection with preservation of vagal innervation to the antrum is of potential benefit for selected patients. Patients requiring proximal gastrectomy for benign conditions such as a broad area of polyps or Ménétrièr's disease, or a sleeve resection of mid-stomach which rarely is required for trauma, can maintain near normal antral emptying of solids if vagal innervation of the antrum is preserved. Gastro-oesophageal continuity is maintained by interposing a 15-cm segment of isoperistaltic jejunum in order to prevent significant oesophageal reflux[2].

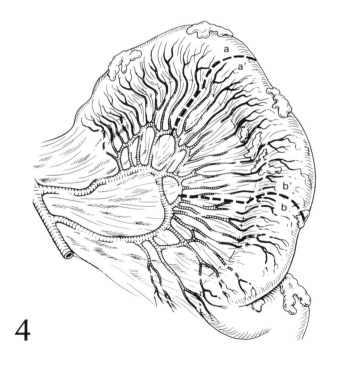

4

Operation

Incision and exposure

Incision and exposure are as described previously.

Preservation of antral vagal innervation

Proximal gastric vagotomy is performed first in order to avoid injury to the vagus nerves and their branches.

Proximal gastrectomy

The lesser curve has already been freed of its vascular and mesenteric attachments as a result of the proximal gastric vagotomy. After dividing the gastrocolic omentum at the site of gastrectomy, the omentum is divided towards the left, sacrificing the left gastroepiploic and short gastric vessels. Once the proximal stomach is mobilized from its posterior attachments, the oesophagus is divided about 1–2 cm proximal to the cardio-oesophageal junction and the stomach is transected at the proximal antral border, which is then closed.

Isolation of the jejunal segment

4   The proximal jejunum is divided at a point distal to the ligament of Treitz where the vasa recti become longer. The mesentery is divided to the peripheral arcade, which may have to be divided in the case of a short mesentery. The jejunum and mesentery are similarly divided 15 cm distally.

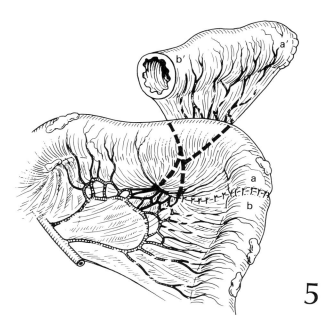

5 An anastomosis is performed between the most proximal and distal segments of jejunum. The proximal end of the isolated jejunal segment is closed, because it is easier to do an end-to-side oesophageal to jejunal anastomosis. Avoidance of an end-to-end anastomosis minimizes the chances of proximal jejunal ischaemia, as it is usually necessary to divide vasa recti in order to straighten out the proximal end of the jejunum for anastomosis to the oesophagus.

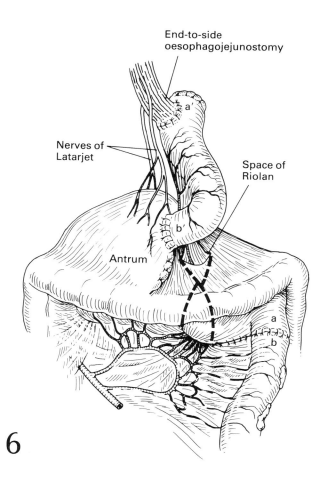

6 The jejunum is led through the space of Riolan in such a way that the closed proximal end points to the left. This results in a partial, non-occlusive twist of the mesentery. The distal end of the interposed jejunum is anastomosed to the anterior wall of the antrum about 2 cm distal to the proximal antral suture line.

Depending on the clinical circumstances, a feeding jejunostomy may be desirable, in which case the jejunostomy catheter is placed distal to the jejunojejunostomy.

Postoperative care

Postoperative care is as described previously. Again, a nasogastric tube is seldom necessary following jejunal interposition.

References

1. Hinder RA, Kelly KA. Human gastric pacesetter potential. Site of origin, spread, and response to gastric transection and proximal gastric vagotomy. *Am J Surg* 1977; 133: 29–33.

2. Lenzi V, Fromm D. Preservation of the distal part of the stomach by esophagoantral jejunal interposition. *Surg Gynecol Obstet* 1989; 168: 175–6.

Bleeding gastric or duodenal ulcer

John E. Meilahn MD
Assistant Professor of Surgery, Department of Surgery, Temple University School of Medicine, Philadelphia, Pennsylvania, USA

Wallace P. Ritchie Jr MD PhD
Professor and Chairman, Department of Surgery, Temple University School of Medicine, Philadelphia, Pennsylvania, USA

Of the estimated 4 000 000 people in the USA with peptic ulcer disease, about 100 000 bleed each year. The attendant mortality rate has remained relatively constant at 6–10% during the past 30 years, despite numerous advances in therapy. Predictors of increased chance of death from an episode of ulcer haemorrhage include an age of over 60 years, multiple organ system disease, transfusion of 5 or more units of whole blood or its equivalent, the recent stress of operation, trauma or sepsis, and the performance of emergency surgery to control haemorrhage (in these patients mortality rates range from 15 to 25%). The mortality rate in patients undergoing emergency surgery is twice as high for bleeding gastric ulcer as it is for bleeding duodenal ulcer.

Duodenal ulcer: background

Although the number of elective operations for duodenal ulcer disease has declined dramatically in recent years (due, at least in part, to the widespread use of H_2 antagonists and other agents), the rate of hospitalization for duodenal ulcer haemorrhage has been relatively stable over the past several decades (25 per 100 000 US population). It is important to note that nearly 70% of these patients will stop bleeding spontaneously without the need for surgical or endoscopic intervention.

Predictors of continued bleeding or rebleeding

A subset of patients with upper gastrointestinal haemorrhage carry a major risk for rebleeding, and therefore for emergency surgery. These include patients who present with shock and acute anaemia because of the magnitude of their blood loss, those with a documented coagulopathy, those in whom bleeding occurs while the patient is already hospitalized for a related or unrelated condition, those in whom endoscopy reveals active bleeding or oozing, and those in whom a visible vessel or sentinel clot is demonstrated, whether bleeding or not (50–100% rebleeding rate). The location of the ulcer also influences the risk of rebleeding, specifically ulcers located deep on the posterior and inferior wall of the duodenum in close proximity to the gastroduodenal artery, and those gastric ulcers which are high on the lesser curvature in close proximity to the left gastric artery.

Aims of surgery

Surgical intervention is used to arrest acute bleeding either by resecting the ulcer or by direct suture of the bleeding point to control the major arterial branches adjacent to the ulcer. In addition, a procedure designed to decrease gastric acid production should be added to allow healing of the ulcer and to prevent rebleeding. This usually involves some form of vagotomy to limit parietal cell innervation, or antrectomy to ablate gastrin production, or both. For gastric ulcer, control of the ulcer diathesis may require antrectomy to remove the portion of stomach at highest risk for ulcer formation.

Gastric ulcer: background

Gastric ulcer is a chronic disease characterized by cyclical exacerbations with significant recurrence rates even while the patient is receiving medical treatment. Unlike duodenal ulcer disease, it is not usually associated with hypersecretion of acid; rather its pathogenesis is probably multifactorial, including increased duodenogastric reflux, gastric stasis, decreased gastric mucosal blood flow, use of non-steroidal anti-inflammatory drugs, and hereditary factors. It is thought that the resistance of the gastric mucosa to injury is impaired so that subsequent exposure to both acid and pepsin results in ulceration. Hospital admissions for perforated gastric ulcers have been stable (one per 100 000 US population), but those for bleeding gastric ulcers have recently increased dramatically[1] (from 14 to 28 per 100 000 between 1980 and 1985).

While up to 70% of gastric ulcers may heal spontaneously at 12 weeks, healing may be enhanced by medical management, including the use of H_2 antagonists (up to 89% healing), antacids (up to 79% healed, but with significant side effects), sucralfate (up to 75% healing), omeprazole or misoprostol. However, relapse is common, even with intially successful therapy. Between 7 and 20% of patients on H_2 antagonists may experience recurrence at 1 year. Without maintenance therapy, up to 80% recur within the same time period.

Types of gastric ulcer

Type I gastric ulcers are the most common type of gastric ulcer with an incidence ranging from 60 to 70%. They are usually located in the antrum near the zone of transition between the proximal acid-secreting mucosa and the distal antrum, but are often located near the lesser curvature. This zone moves proximally with age. Acid secretion is usually low.

Type II gastric ulcers are those found with a simultaneous duodenal ulcer or scar. Pre-existence of the duodenal ulcer may have contributed to partial gastric outlet obstruction and to formation of the gastric ulcer. Acid production is higher than in type I ulcers and is more characteristic of typical duodenal ulcer disease. These ulcers account for 10−20% of all gastric ulcers.

Type III gastric ulcers (20% incidence) are located within 3 cm of the pylorus (prepyloric), and are almost always associated with increased acid production.

Csendes and colleagues[2] from Chile have proposed the existence of a fourth type of gastric ulcer (type IV) which is found in the upper third of the stomach less than 5 cm from the gastro-oesophageal junction. This type of ulcer was found in 27% of patients in the study and a 75% incidence of blood group O and a 64% incidence of presentation with haemorrhage was noted. Acid secretion was low, comparable to that found with type I ulcers. In the USA and Europe this group comprises less than 5% of all gastric ulcers.

Relationship to non-steroidal anti-inflammatory drugs

Since a single ingestion of aspirin can cause gastric subepithelial haemorrhage within 1 h, and regular intake can commonly cause gastric erosions, it is not surprising that chronic use of non-steroidal anti-inflammatory drugs leads to frank gastric ulceration in up to 25% of patients, with a special predilection for the antrum. The use of H_2 receptor antagonists along with non-steriodal anti-inflammatory drugs in arthritic patients does appear to reduce the incidence of duodenal ulcers in these individuals and also reduces the incidence of gastric mucosal haemorrhage. This latter effect is probably of minor clinical significance, and, in any case, H_2 antagonists have little effect on prevention of gastric ulcers in users of non-steroidal anti-inflammatory drugs. Sucralfate or omeprazole may be more effective in this setting.

Concurrent use of misoprostol, a prostaglandin analogue, has been shown to reduce gastric ulcer formation (from 22% to 6% in one recent prospective study). Since the complications of gastric ulcer, including bleeding, may present without significant warning, especially in elderly patients with arthritis or a history of peptic ulceration and who take non-steroidal anti-inflammatory drugs, this group of patients should be considered for active prophylaxis.

Competing therapies

Surgeons have come to rely on preoperative oesophago-gastroduodenoscopy to diagnose both the cause and location of an upper gastrointestinal bleed. The use of the endoscope has been extended to include immediate treatment of the bleeding ulcer in selected patients. As already noted, if successful, endoscopic haemostasis may allow avoidance of surgery altogether in high-risk patients, or may permit the performance of a definitive operation under elective conditions.

Endoscopic haemostasis is generally unsuccessful in those patients with ulcers which bleed massively or in those which are relatively inaccessible to the endoscopist because they are located in a scarred duodenal bulb or have thick overlying clot. If the ulcer is actively but not massively bleeding, or if it bears the stigmata of recent haemorrhage, including the presence of a visible vessel or clot, endoscopic haemostasis may be attempted provided that surgical back-up is promptly available if the attempt fails. Intervention is also justified in the non-bleeding ulcer in which a visible vessel is seen, because, in this setting, in-hospital rebleeding rates are as high as 50−80%. Ulcers which have a clean base, or which have a flat pigmented spot indicative of old haemorrhage, represent a low risk for rebleeding and do not require attempts at endoscopic haemostasis[3].

Endoscopic injection or sclerosis

This method was initially used to control variceal bleeding and its use has since been extended to control bleeding gastric and duodenal ulcers. Enthusiasm for the approach is due to its relatively low cost, ease of availability and application, and apparent effectiveness in several controlled trials. Absolute ethanol, polidocanol with adrenaline (epinephrine), or adrenaline alone have all been injected around the ulcer base, into a visible vessel if present. These treatments have been applied both to actively bleeding gastroduodenal ulcers and to those demonstrating the stigmata of recent haemorrhage. With the latter, the injection itself may cause immediate bleeding in up to 30% of cases; this is usually readily controlled by immediate continued injections.

Initial success in arresting haemorrhage has been reported in up to 90% or more of cases. Rebleeding may occur in 10–30% of these, with the higher rates observed when the ulcer is actively bleeding before therapy. It has been noted that injection therapy may be less efficacious in ulcers which are greater than 2 cm in size and in those which produce torrential bleeding, especially in the duodenum. The long-term effects of sclerosant injection on the gastroduodenal wall have not been well studied.

Endoscopic cautery

Monopolar electrocoagulation with or without simultaneous water irrigation has been used to achieve immediate haemostasis in patients with bleeding ulcers. However, the depth of tissue penetration and injury is difficult to control, and the end of the probe may require frequent cleaning, making this modality less attractive than injection.

On the other hand, bipolar electrocoagulation produces a well-defined current pathway and controlled subsequent tissue coagulation, minimizing the possibility of transmural injury. The current modification of this concept is the bipolar circumactive probe (BICAP), which uses six equally spaced electrodes, allowing coagulation independent of tip orientation. A central water channel enables irrigation of the bleeding area. The 50-W probe is pressed against the ulcer to coapt the underlying artery and current applied to coagulate the ulcer base and feeding vessel. The BICAP is available in two sizes (3.2 mm and 2.4 mm) to allow passage through the endoscope, and is both portable and relatively easy to use.

Recent prospective studies involving either actively bleeding gastric or duodenal ulcers or those with a non-bleeding visible vessel demonstrate initial immediate haemostasis with BICAP therapy in 91–100% of cases, with rebleeding rates of 6–20%. The large majority of rebleed episodes were treated with surgery.

It should be noted that delayed perforation of duodenal ulcers after treatment with the BICAP has been reported.

Endoscopic heater probe

The heater probe has an aluminium tip containing an internal heater coil which is controlled by an external power source which regulates both the amount of energy and the duration of the applied pulse. The tip of the probe is covered with polytetrafluoroethylene to minimize adherence to tissues and is heated to 250°C, thus transferring heat energy to tissues by thermal conduction. Heater probes are available in sizes 2.4 and 3.2 mm (10-Fr), and are used by pressing the probe firmly against the bleeding point with subsequent application of multiple pulses to a preset energy (20–40 J), producing coaptive coagulation. The probe may be applied around the ulcer base, and also to the bleeding point. It may be applied to the ulcer tangentially as well as *en face*.

The heater probe has been used successfully to control actively bleeding ulcers, although occasional difficulty has been noted in proper positioning of the probe in the duodenum, especially if scarring and deformity are present. A recent prospective trial with actively bleeding gastric and duodenal ulcers noted immediate haemostasis in 83% of patients, with the remainder requiring immediate surgery. In patients whose ulcers were initially controlled, 11% experienced a rebleed and also required surgery. Attempts to treat four rebleeding duodenal ulcers with a second heater probe application resulted in anterior duodenal perforation in two patients. Another prospective study, including non-bleeding ulcers with a visible vessel as well as actively bleeding gastric and duodenal ulcers, reported a rebleeding rate of 28%, with one duodenal perforation during initial heater probe treatment.

Laser

Both argon and neodymium–yttrium–aluminium–garnet (NdYAG) lasers are suitable for use with the flexible endoscope. The argon laser wavelength (440– 520 nm) corresponds to that of maximal absorption of haemoglobin, so that tissue penetration is low, achieving only superficial coagulation. Although immediate haemostasis can be achieved, rebleeding rates appear to be higher than those seen with the NdYAG laser, which has been widely investigated and has been shown to be effective. The NdYAG laser, with a wavelength of 1064 nm (near infrared), demonstrates deeper tissue penetration and coagulation than the argon laser, and has superior efficacy in preventing rebleeding. The equipment, however, is extremely expensive, immobile, not widely available and is relatively difficult to learn to use properly.

To control oozing or bleeding, the laser is manoeuvred as close to an *en face* position as possible, about 1–1.5 cm from the ulcer. Multiple pulses are applied circumferentially around the base of the ulcer, beginning at the periphery and then moving closer to the centre. A visible vessel is not directly coagulated since this may cause bleeding. Anatomical characteristics which may prevent laser use include duodenal deformity or a poorly accessible gastric ulcer high on the lesser curvature.

Controlled trials demonstrate that the NdYAG laser is effective in controlling both actively bleeding ulcers and those with the stigmata of recent haemorrhage, including a visible vessel. However, rebleeding rates have been reported to be high after treatment of actively bleeding ulcers with a visible vessel (up to 60%) and during the operator's learning phase (rebleeding rate of 57% compared with 14% after experience has been gained).

Principles and justification

Indications

Traditional indications for operation for bleeding gastric or duodenal ulcers include: massive bleeding on presentation with exsanguination and hypotension; ulcers which continue to bleed over time so that frequent transfusion is necessary to maintain a stable haematocrit (generally the need for more than 1 unit of whole blood every 6–8 h constitutes an indication for surgery); and ulcers which, after initial cessation of bleeding, rebleed while the patient is still hospitalized. The advent of various endoscopic methods of treatment has changed the indications for surgery in those centres in which such expertise exists. This is particularly true in elderly patients in whom emergency surgery has a high mortality rate. Success in achieving haemostasis endoscopically may lead either to surgery in an elective setting or to no surgery at all if subsequent medical management is effective in healing the ulcer. The danger in relying exclusively on non-operative endoscopic therapy is that patients who fail then come to surgery in a more unstable state with a higher transfusion requirement, and hence a higher rate of surgical mortality.

Greater urgency is attached to modest bleeding in situations where blood availability for transfusion is limited, either because of local conditions or difficulty in cross-matching individual patients with preformed antibody. Transfusions may not be possible in the face of patient refusal because of religious beliefs. In these situations, early operation may be warranted.

Bleeding duodenal ulcers

The majority of bleeding duodenal ulcers are located along or near the posterior aspect of the duodenal bulb, where the gastroduodenal artery travels from the superior to the inferior border of the duodenum. The typical penetrating posterior ulcer erodes into a branch of this large artery or into the artery itself, with the vessel partially exposed at the ulcer base. The vessel acquires a hole in the side, resulting in either active bleeding through the hole or clot extrusion from the visible vessel.

Ulcers based posteriorly are fed by a rich gastroduodenal arterial supply, and direct suture control of both superior and inferior aspects is necessary. In addition, the transverse pancreatic artery connects to the medial aspect of the gastroduodenal artery behind the duodenum. Thus, suture control of the medial aspect of a duodenal ulcer is also frequently necessary.

Post-bulbar ulcers are located lateral to the gastroduodenal artery and may impinge closely upon the ampulla of Vater. In this instance, it is essential to appreciate the position of the common bile duct to avoid its compromise by improper suture placement.

Oversewing with truncal vagotomy and pyloroplasty

Control of bleeding from a duodenal bulb ulcer can often be accomplished quickly by longitudinal division of the anterior proximal duodenum with extension across the pylorus onto the stomach. This approach readily exposes the bleeding ulcer and permits digital compression of the bleeding point. The ulcer may then be oversewn superiorly, inferiorly and along its medial aspect. After haemostasis has been achieved, closure is performed using the Weinberg modification of the Heineke–Mikulicz pyloroplasty. Definitive control of the ulcer diathesis is accomplished by truncal vagotomy of both anterior and posterior branches, resulting in a decrease in acid production of about 50%. Since the procedure can be done relatively quickly, it has special applicability in elderly patients. Mortality rates are related to age and associated risk factors, ranging from 2% to 17%; the incidence of rebleeding ranges from 4% to 22% and may be reduced by the effective placement of multiple deep sutures during oversewing as described.

Oversewing with vagotomy and antrectomy

When bleeding has been controlled by direct pressure and suture through an anterior duodenotomy with extension onto the stomach, partial distal gastric resection, including the antrum, may be performed with reconstruction via a Billroth I gastroduodenostomy or, preferably in the author's opinion, as a Billroth II gastrojejunostomy. Anterior and posterior truncal vagotomy must be added to this procedure. Such an approach results in a decrease in acid production of about 90%, with ulcer recurrence rates as low as 1%. Mortality rates range from 11% to 21%, and are greatly influenced by the risk status of the patient. Using the APACHE II scoring system to stratify patients, it has been found that patients with a score of greater than 10 are at high risk compared with patients with a score of 10 or less. For these high-risk patients[4], truncal vagotomy with antrectomy for bleeding duodenal ulcer has a mortality rate of 33%, while truncal vagotomy with drainage has a significantly lower mortality rate of about 17%.

Oversewing with duodenotomy and parietal cell vagotomy

In selected young patients who are considered to be stable and at low risk, the bleeding duodenal ulcer may be visualized by a longitudinal duodenotomy and oversewn. The duodenotomy may then be closed longitudinally. If the pylorus is not divided and the patient remains haemodynamically stable, a parietal cell vagotomy may then be performed. The procedure generally requires a relatively prolonged operating time (up to, or more than, 3 h). In a recent retrospective review of 52 low-risk patients (median age 47 years, with mean preoperative transfusion requirement of 5 units and only two patients in shock), duodenotomy and parietal cell vagotomy was performed with no post-operative deaths[5]. It should be noted that only 12 of these patients were bleeding actively at the time of operation. Duodenal ulcer recurrence was reported to be 12% at 3 years, with half of these presenting with rebleeds.

Transection of the pylorus was not required in any of these patients to visualize the bleeding ulcer, and may be avoided altogether if ulcer location has been determined by adequate preoperative endoscopy. However, division of the pylorus for ulcer localization or for exposure to allow oversewing does not necessarily preclude subsequent parietal cell vagotomy as the pylorus may be reconstructed longitudinally in the line of the incision.

Giant duodenal ulcer

Patients with giant duodenal ulcers (diameter of 2 cm or more) present with bleeding as the most common indication for emergency operation. These ulcers are more likely to rebleed on medical therapy, and demonstrate higher mortality rates compared with smaller duodenal ulcers. Since they represent a more severe form of the ulcer diathesis, consideration should be given to a more extensive surgical procedure to prevent recurrence. If the intraoperative haemodynamic status permits, resection with antrectomy and truncal vagotomy should be performed.

Oversewing of the ulcer with truncal vagotomy and pyloroplasty may be performed in less stable patients. If the duodenum is heavily scarred and non-pliable, pyloroplasty may not be possible. Instead, antrectomy should be performed with reconstruction as a Billroth II gastrojejunostomy. Closure of the duodenal stump may be difficult if fibrosis is present. The anterior wall of the duodenum, if pliable, can be sutured onto the posterior wall and the distal edge of the ulcer crater using the Nissen method, avoiding suture placement into the common bile duct. Alternatively, if the anterior wall is too stiff to allow closure, a jejunal serosal patch may be fashioned to close the duodenal stump with either a loop of jejunum or a Roux-en-Y limb. It must be emphasized that attempts to resect the ulcer bed under these conditions are fraught with extreme hazard.

Procedure of choice

Although oversewing of the bleeding ulcer with subsequent vagotomy and antrectomy has been shown to be effective in the prevention of recurrent ulcer bleeding and may be undertaken with low mortality rates in the selected low-risk patient, most surgeons favour truncal vagotomy and pyloroplasty after suture control of bleeding for the usual duodenal bulb ulcer, despite a somewhat higher risk of rebleeding. The procedure is straightforward and can be speedily performed with lower mortality rates in elderly high-risk patients. However, when a giant duodenal ulcer is encountered or when extensive duodenal scarring and deformity is present, resection combined with antrectomy and vagotomy may be preferable.

Bleeding gastric ulcers

The lesser curvature of the stomach is supplied by both right and left gastric arteries, while the greater curvature is supplied by both right and left gastro-epiploic arteries and the short gastric vessels. Each artery divides into anterior and posterior branches which perforate the muscular layers to supply the submucosal plexus which serves as the blood supply for the gastric mucosa. Because of the rich collateral blood flow represented by the submucosal plexus, the stomach can have multiple feeding arteries ligated without compromising its viability. The submucosal plexus is more vestigial along the lesser curvature, so that mucosal ischaemia can occur in this area if the lesser curvature is extensively devascularized (as in parietal cell vagotomy). This is uncommonly seen clinically. Previous or concomitant splenectomy with sacrifice of the left gastroepiploic artery may place a proximal gastric remnant at risk of ischaemia if the left gastric artery is taken simultaneously. This situation is also rare. More common (10% of patients) is the aberrant left hepatic artery which arises from the left gastric artery. Care must be taken to preserve this hepatic blood supply when dissecting close to the lesser curvature.

Many bleeding gastric ulcers penetrate only to the submucosa and have little or no scar tissue in their base. Submucosal vessels found bleeding may have a diameter of the order of 0.5 mm and usually travel across the base of the ulcer. Larger more chronic ulcers have usually penetrated the muscularis propria. In these, a serosal artery, typically with a diameter of 0.9 mm or more, may loop up to the base of the ulcer. In both types, the bleeding vessel may protrude above the floor or be flush with it, with localized aneurysmal dilatation and rupture at the point of bleeding.

Oversewing alone

Simple oversewing for bleeding gastric ulcer has traditionally been performed only in very high-risk patients thought to be poorly suited for more definitive therapy. In non-randomized studies, a mortality rate of 10% and a recurrence rate of 14% has been noted. In actuality, recurrence rates are probably much higher. If this approach is elected, multiple intraoperative ulcer biopsies are essential to exclude carcinoma. Postoperative use of H_2 receptor antagonists is also recommended. In general, if patients develop a bleeding complication while on H_2 blockers or during concurrent use of non-steroidal anti-inflammatory agents which must be continued, this procedure should not be used. In the authors' opinion, it is rarely appropriate under any circumstances.

Oversewing or excising the ulcer with vagotomy and pyloroplasty

Because of the relatively high mortality rates (10–40%) for emergency partial gastrectomy in the elderly, some surgeons oversew the ulcer or resect it by wedge resection if anatomically possible. This approach is then combined with truncal vagotomy and pyloroplasty. Mortality depends on the underlying status of the patient. For high-risk patients (APACHE II score of over 10), the mortality rate from truncal vagotomy and drainage was 9% in a recent series compared with a 22% mortality rate for patients undergoing distal gastrectomy. Therefore, this procedure may be appropriate in the elderly high-risk patient, even though ulcer recurrence rates range from 8% to 25%.

Distal gastrectomy including the ulcer

Ulcer recurrence is minimized by distal gastrectomy to include the antrum and ulcer. This procedure removes the ulcer and enables thorough histological examination to rule out carcinoma. It also removes the gastric

ulcer-prone antrum near the antral–corporal border and eliminates the antrum as a source of gastrin. Billroth I gastroduodenostomy is usually possible and is preferable to Billroth II reconstruction. Truncal vagotomy is not felt to be necessary for the usual type I gastric ulcer, since it may predispose to gastric stasis in about 10% of patients and to severe diarrhoea in about 1%. However, vagotomy should be added for a type II ulcer (those found in association with duodenal ulcer) or type III ulcer (prepyloric), since these are usually associated with acid hypersecretion.

For elective operations, mortality rates are as low as 1–2%, with recurrence rates of about 2%. Mortality rates increase to 10–40% in emergency cases, with higher rates found in elderly patients with multiple associated medical problems.

Gastric ulcer with non-steroidal anti-inflammatory drugs

Because the antrum is at risk for ulceration in patients taking non-steroidal anti-inflammatory drugs, distal gastrectomy including the bleeding ulcer should be performed. Gastric erosions are commonly present and should be resected with the ulcer and antrum if possible.

Giant gastric ulcer

These ulcers are defined as those with a diameter equal to, or greater than, 3 cm. Patients having this condition require emergency operation for haemorrhage more frequently than those with smaller ulcers, massive bleeding being present in up to 50% of instances. Additional gastric ulcers may coexist. Unusual complications such as gastrocolic or duodenal–gastric fistulae have been noted. Biopsy should always be performed, since up to 10% of these ulcers are malignant, especially those over 5 cm in diameter. Non-operative therapy for uncomplicated giant ulcer has been reported to be effective, but, as noted, bleeding occurs frequently. Under these conditions, partial gastrectomy including the ulcer with a Billroth I gastroduodenostomy is the procedure of choice.

High-lying gastric ulcer

Total gastrectomy or proximal partial gastrectomy are both associated with high mortality rates, and are completely inappropriate for these ulcers. Wedge resection alone carries a recurrence rate of 33–48% and is often difficult. Non-resective procedures for haemorrhage are followed by high rates of rebleeding. A reasonable approach to high-lying ulcers is as follows: bleeding is controlled by immediate gastrectomy and oversewing. If the ulcer is located high on the posterior wall, Pauchet's procedure can be used (a distal gastrectomy with excision of a tongue of the lesser curvature, including the ulcer). If the ulcer penetrates into adjacent organs and cannot be resected, bleeding is controlled, the ulcer base is biopsied, and if benign, left *in situ*. A distal gastrectomy (not including the ulcer) is then performed (the Kelling-Madlener procedure) and a Billroth I gastroduodenostomy is created. This procedure is associated with a very low recurrence rate (0% in two studies), but a mortality rate of up to 15% has been noted in the elderly. Oversewing or excision with vagotomy and pyloroplasty may be considered, but these procedures have been associated with a rebleeding rate of up to 18%. When the ulcer is less than 2 cm from the oesophagogastric junction, resection using Csendes' procedure (Roux-en-Y oesophagogastrojejunostomy) may be performed with very low recurrence rates (none reported by Csendes)[2], but with significant mortality rates in the elderly, bleeding patient.

Procedure of choice

Distal gastric resection including the ulcer with Billroth I gastroduodenostomy is the procedure of choice for the usual bleeding type I gastric ulcer located in the antrum or distal body. A truncal vagotomy should be added for coexistent duodenal ulcer disease or for prepyloric gastric ulcers. Ulcer oversewing with biopsy or excision in conjunction with truncal vagotomy and pyloroplasty should be used only in high-risk and unstable patients because of the risk of rebleeding.

Preoperative

When the patient presents with upper gastrointestinal haemorrhage, assessment and correction of hypovolaemia, shock and tachycardia should be performed urgently. Initial resuscitation includes maintenance of the airway and breathing with supplemental oxygen. Intubation should be considered for the severely compromised patient. Cardiac monitoring and a 12-lead electrocardiogram should be performed to assess rate, rhythm and ischaemia.

Volume resuscitation via two large-bore peripheral intravenous catheters should be started. In the elderly, a central venous catheter should be inserted for volume replacement and its position confirmed by chest radiography.

Immediate laboratory studies should include haemoglobin or haematocrit, platelet count, electrolytes, creatinine and coagulation factors, including prothrombin time and partial thromboplastin time. At least 6 units of blood should be typed and cross-matched, and the patient transfused to, and kept at, a haematocrit of at least 30% and checked frequently.

A large-bore nasogastric tube should be placed to assess ongoing bleeding and to enable lavage and clot evacuation for subsequent endoscopy. Urine output should be assessed frequently by continuous bladder catheterization as a guide to volume resuscitation. Unless immediate transport to surgery is required, upper endoscopy should be performed to locate the source of the bleeding, to achieve endoscopic haemostasis if available and appropriate, and to guide the surgeon should laparotomy be necessary. The patient should be monitored and cared for in the intensive care unit with continuous systemic arterial pressure monitoring. As laboratory studies become available, coagulopathy should be corrected with either fresh frozen plasma or platelets.

If the patient continues to bleed massively with hypotension, preoperative endoscopy may not be possible; immediate operation should be undertaken. Intravenous antibiotics should be given before operation (for example, a broad-spectrum cephalosporin), but aminoglycosides should be avoided because of potentially compromised renal blood flow.

Anaesthesia

The bleeding patient brought for operation as an emergency requires general anaesthesia with endotracheal tube placement. A nasogastric tube should be placed before induction of anaesthesia to empty the stomach. Cricoid pressure during paralysis and intubation should be performed to prevent aspiration of the gastric contents. A neuromuscular blocking agent should be given to allow complete relaxation of the abdominal wall for maximal exposure.

If the patient has been fully resuscitated and is stable, conventional anaesthetic induction may be possible with thiopentone and the subsequent use of inhalational agents. Both thiopentone and inhalational anaesthetic agents are vasodilatory and their use may be inadvisable in the unstable patient with active bleeding. Instead, induction can be accomplished with either ketamine or etomidate which lack hypotensive side effects. A neuromuscular blocking agent is essential, and amnesic effects can be realized with hyoscine (scopolamine) or a benzodiazepine. If the patient then becomes stable, either an inhalational agent can be started in low doses or narcotics can be used, with a synthetic agent such as fentanyl preferred over morphine because of its better amnesic effects and fewer haemodynamic side effects.

Operations

BLEEDING DUODENAL ULCER: OVERSEWING, TRUNCAL VAGOTOMY AND PYLOROPLASTY

Incision and exposure

The patient is placed supine with both arms extended on arm boards. Following a prescrub, a prep solution such as povidone-iodine 10% is applied from the nipples to the pubic symphysis and the abdomen is draped. An upper midline incision is preferred as it allows extension both upward beside the xiphoid and downward around the umbilicus to permit adequate exposure.

1 The round and falciform ligaments are divided between clamps. Retraction of both costal margins upward is readily accomplished with bilateral retractors mounted on an 'upper arm'; a Balfour retractor is then placed to open the bottom of the incision. Alternatively, a large ring-type retractor such as a Bookwalter also provides excellent exposure. Laparotomy pads are placed to pack the transverse colon downward and are held in place with retractors, exposing the stomach and duodenum.

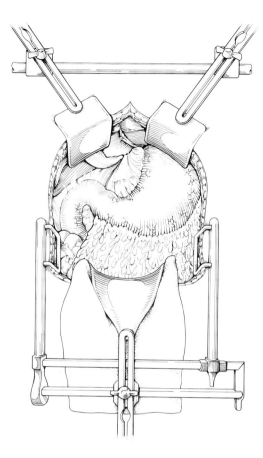

1

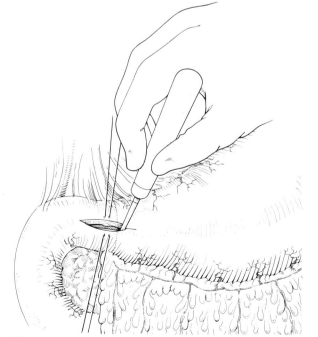

2

Duodenotomy

2 The pylorus is identified by inspection, using the prepyloric vein of Mayo running transversely on the anterior pylorus as a reference, and by palpation of its thickened ring. The approximate location of the common bile duct is noted so that injury during dissection can be avoided. Division of some of the lateral duodenal retroperitoneal attachments facilitates both duodenal exposure and the subsequent pyloro-plasty. If the bleeding ulcer has been localized to the duodenal bulb by endoscopy, two 3/0 sutures are placed near the centre of the pylorus and held with haemostats for retraction. A longitudinal pylorotomy is made with electrocautery and extended onto the duodenum until the bleeding ulcer is visualized. Proximal extension onto the stomach for a total length of about 6 cm is then performed. Evacuation of blood and clot is performed with suction and manual extraction, avoiding mech-anical injury to the duodenal mucosa.

Suture ligation

3a, b The ulcer base is examined to determine the location of vessels or the precise point of active bleeding. Immediate haemostasis can be effected by direct digital compression of the bleeding point. This also permits effective resuscitation by the anaesthetist. The bleeding point can be oversewn in a figure-of-eight manner using a 2/0 silk suture on a half-round needle. The gastroduodenal artery can then be suture-ligated both above and below the ulcer, and a U stitch placed to control bleeding from the medial aspect of the ulcer. In placing deep sutures, the location of the common bile duct should be noted and efforts made to ensure that it is not injured. After suture control of haemorrhage, irrigation and suction is used to clear the remaining duodenum and distal stomach of blood; a thorough search for other ulcers or causes of bleeding should be undertaken.

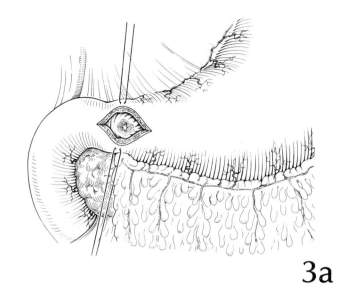

3a

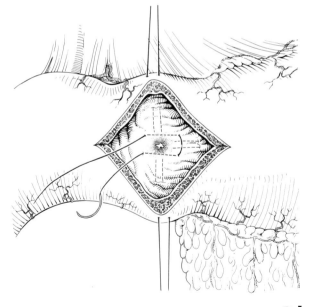

3b

Pyloroplasty

4 The longitudinal incision is then closed transversely as for a Heineke–Mikulicz pyloroplasty, with the previously placed pyloric sutures used for superior and inferior traction. Interrupted 3/0 silk sutures on a tapered needle are placed using a modified Gambee stitch. All sutures are placed before tying. The superior and inferior ends of the closure will 'dog ear' as the sutures are tied. Additional interrupted simple sutures may be placed to approximate the serosa closely, although few are usually needed. If the bleeding ulcer is located on the anterior wall, it may be excised as the duodenotomy is performed, and closure can also be performed as for a transverse pyloroplasty. If the ulcer is more distally located with a longer duodenotomy, or if duodenal stenosis is present distal to the pylorus because of scarring, closure utilizing a two-layer Finney pyloroplasty can be performed.

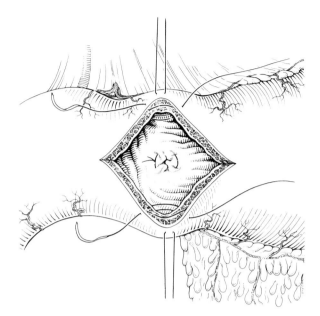

4

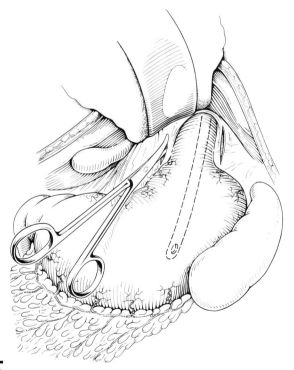

5

Oesophageal exposure

5 Attention is then turned to the distal oesophagus for truncal vagotomy. A long retractor is placed under the left lateral segment of the liver down to the diaphragm to elevate the liver anteriorly, exposing the distal oesophagus. The oesophagus is readily identified by palpation of the nasogastric tube. Downward traction of the stomach is maintained by pulling on the nasogastric tube along the greater curvature, taking care to avoid injury to the spleen. If the liver precludes adequate visualization of the oesophagus, the left triangular ligament may be divided and the left lateral segment can be folded to the right behind the retractor. The peritoneum to the right and left of the oesophagus is opened with scissors. With the surgeon standing on the right of the patient, the index finger of the right hand is passed behind and around the oesophagus from left to right using blunt dissection anterior to the aorta. The finger is passed out through the lesser omentum to the right of the oesophagus, using scissors to assist if necessary. A Penrose drain may be passed around the oesophagus at this point to assist with downward retraction.

Posterior vagal trunk

6,7 The posterior (right) trunk of the vagus is identified as a cord behind the oesophagus which can be pushed by the finger to the right to allow visualization. Skeletonization with a nerve hook or right-angled clamp can verify its structure. The trunk should be clipped superiorly and inferiorly, and a section between clips should be removed for gross inspection and subsequent microscopic verification.

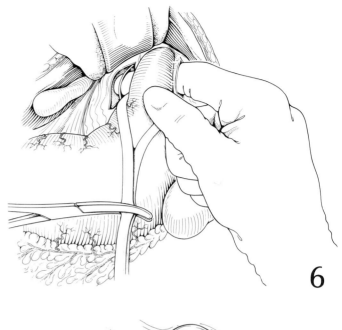

6

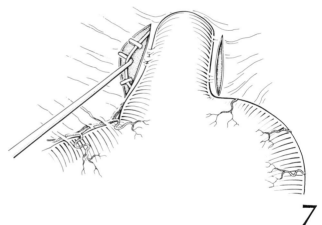

7

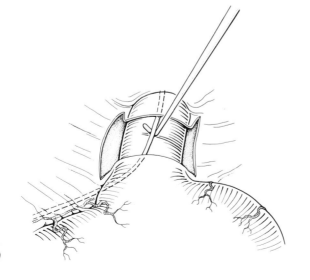

8

Anterior vagal trunk

8 The anterior (left) trunk should then be located in the areolar tissue anterior to the oesophagus by palpation for the cord and direct inspection. It may be necessary to divide this areolar tissue successively to identify the nerve, which should then be clipped and sectioned as for the posterior trunk. The oesophagus should be cleaned of tissue over a distance of 4 cm above the gastro-oesophageal junction to verify that no vagal branches persist.

BLEEDING GASTRIC ULCERS: DISTAL GASTRECTOMY WITH GASTRODUODENOSTOMY

Ulcer exposure

The patient is positioned and draped as described for bleeding duodenal ulcer, with the upper midline incision preferred. Details of retraction and placement of laparotomy packs are the same as shown in *Illustration 1*.

9 After exposure of the stomach, a longitudinal gastrotomy is made in the antrum using electrocautery and either narrow Deaver retractors or Babcock clamps are placed on each edge for elevation and exposure. Blood and clots within the stomach are evacuated with suction and manual extraction, and saline is used for irrigation. Narrow Deaver retractors may be placed within the gastrotomy to expose the gastric mucosa adequately in the search for the bleeding ulcer. Once located, haemostasis is achieved by direct digital compression and subsequent oversewing of the bleeding point using multiple 3/0 silk sutures. If malignancy is suspected, biopsy and frozen section should be performed. A thorough exploration of the abdominal cavity to exclude unsuspected disease should also be undertaken.

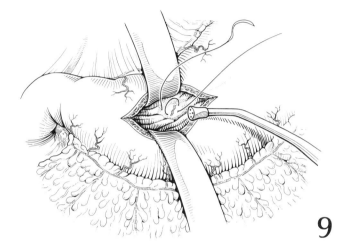

9

Gastric mobilization

10 The ulcer location is noted relative to the planned line of excision for antrectomy as the ulcer should be excised with the specimen. The antrum begins approximately 8–10 cm proximal to the pylorus along the lesser curvature, or at the incisura angularis. Along the greater curvature, it begins at a point about one-eighth the distance from the pylorus to the oesophagus. To ensure adequate distal resection, the line of gastric resection extends from the mid point of the greater curvature to a point on the lesser curvature just proximal to the incisura angularis. Silk sutures (3/0) are placed on both greater and lesser curvatures at these points and held on haemostats. The transverse colon is retracted inferiorly and the gastrocolic omentum is divided at the mid point of the greater curvature next to the stomach. Individual branches of the right gastroepiploic artery are taken between 3/0 silk ties, dissecting distally towards the pylorus. Dissection is kept close to the stomach to avoid injury to the middle colic vessels, which may be adherent. The posterior wall of the stomach is freed of adherent tissue to permit a finger to be placed under the stomach and to tent up the gastrohepatic ligament along the lesser curvature. If the ulcer has penetrated posteriorly, it may be adherent to the pancreas, and dissection will be proximal to this. If the stomach cannot be mobilized from the pancreas, then the posterior wall can be incised with electro-

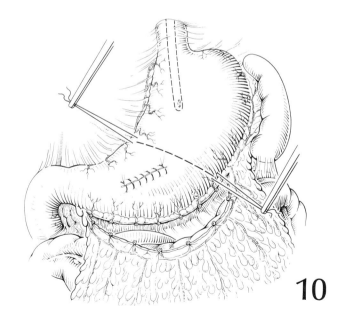

10

cautery around the ulcer base, leaving it *in situ*. The gastrohepatic omentum can then be divided distally, and the right gastric artery ligated between 2/0 silk ties. The left gastric artery need not be divided since the stomach is usually transected distal to it. If an aberrant left hepatic artery is present (10% incidence), it should be preserved.

Duodenal mobilization

11 Mobilization of the duodenum is necessary and is accomplished by the Kocher manoeuvre, in which the second portion of the duodenum is retracted medially and the lateral peritoneal and retroperitoneal attachments are divided. Blunt finger dissection behind the duodenum and head of pancreas is helpful in elevation. The duodenum should be mobilized from the area distal to the common bile duct down through the proximal third portion, taking care not to injure the superior mesenteric vein which travels across the anterior aspect of the third portion of the duodenum. As the Kocher manoeuvre is performed, the inferior vena cava, which lies posteriorly, should not be injured.

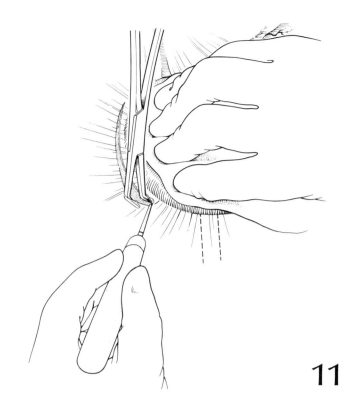

11

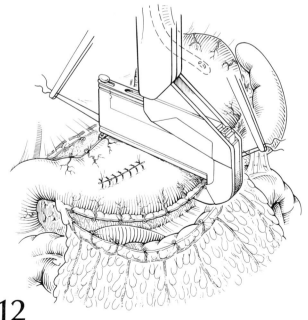

12

Division of stomach

12 The stomach may be transected at this point using a TA 55 or TA 90 stapler passed from the greater to the lesser curvature. Considerable embarrassment is avoided if the nasogastric tube is positioned proximal to the stapler before using it. Kocher clamps applied to the stomach distal to the stapler prevent gross spillage when a knife is used to divide the stomach along the distal side of the stapler.

Division of duodenum

13 Upward and medial traction on the distal stomach remnant allows dissection of the pylorus and proximal duodenum on their superior, posterior and inferior aspects. The duodenum should be mobilized to a point about 3 cm distal to the pylorus. The gastroduodenal artery should be preserved. A GIA stapler can then be passed from the inferior to superior aspect of the duodenum, and used to divide it just distal to the pylorus, allowing removal of the distal stomach and some proximal duodenum.

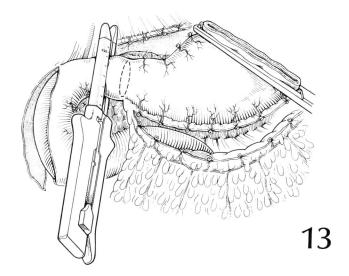

13

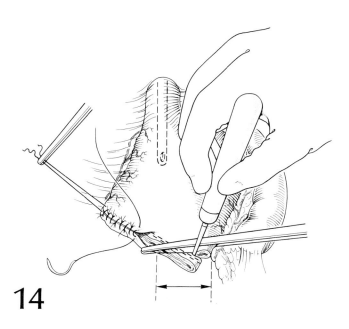

14

Preparation of gastric remnant

14 The proximal stomach and duodenal stump can then be approximated to assess the need for further dissection to remove tension from the anastomosis. If satisfactory, the width of the duodenum is superimposed on the distal stomach on a line at right angles to the greater curvature. The staple line superior to this anastomotic site is oversewn with interrupted 3/0 silk Lembert sutures. A bowel clamp is applied to the distal stomach, and electrocautery is used to resect the bottom corner of the stomach over the length corresponding to the width of the duodenum.

Gastroduodenal anastomosis: back row

15 The stomach and duodenal stump are approximated and 3/0 silk corner sutures are placed and held with haemostats. The corner suture at the superior aspect should be placed through both the front and back walls of the stomach as well as the duodenum. After turning both stomach and stump to expose their back walls, a back row of interrupted seromuscular 3/0 silk sutures is placed and tied. Electrocautery is used to resect the staple line across the duodenal stump, opening the lumen.

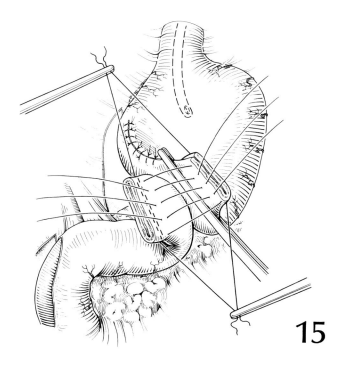

15

Anastomosis: inner layer

16 Beginning at the superior corner, a 3/0 polyglactin (Vicryl) suture is passed through the mucosa and serosa of both the stomach and the duodenum and tied. The short end is held on a haemostat, and the inner layer of the anastomosis is begun with a continuous, locking posterior suture. At the inferior corner the same suture is used to begin a Connell stitch to close the inferior half of the front wall. Before the front wall is completed, a second 3/0 polyglactin suture is placed adjacent to the first one at the back wall through the full thickness of stomach and duodenum and tied. It is then run as a Connell stitch along the remainder of the front wall to meet the first polyglactin suture and tied, thus inverting the front wall. The clamp is then removed from the stomach.

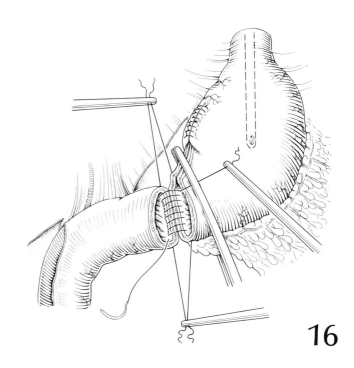

16

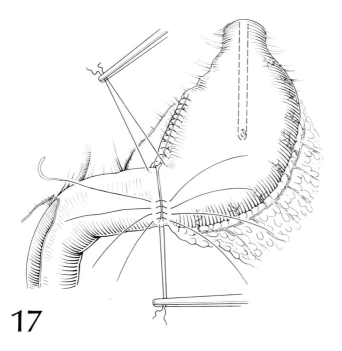

17

Anastomosis: front row

17 Both corner sutures are tied. A row of interrupted Lembert 3/0 silk sutures is placed to complete the outer layer of the front wall. The anastomosis is examined thoroughly to assess the need for additional Lembert sutures. The abdomen is irrigated with warm saline; some surgeons use an antibiotic such as cephazolin dissolved in the irrigant. Adjacent omentum can be placed over the anastomosis and tacked in place. If the gastric ulcer was either type II or III, truncal vagotomy should be added as in *Illustrations 5–8*.

Postoperative care

The patient may be cared for after operation in the intensive care unit or the recovery room with transfer to the ward determined by age, associated medical problems and intraoperative stability. Ventilatory support should be continued as necessary. Cardiac monitoring should be performed with a 12-lead electrocardiogram and compared with that obtained before operation. Serial creatine phosphokinase enzyme fractions should be obained if evidence of intraoperative or postoperative cardiac ischaemia exists. The haematocrit should be serially checked, with transfusions as necessary to maintain a level of at least 30. A full set of serum electrolyte levels should be measured. If dissection near the common bile duct has been performed, daily liver function tests should be done.

Nasogastric suction should be continued to monitor daily output, presence of blood, and to monitor and correct gastric pH to greater than 5.0. Administration of intravenous H_2 antagonists should be used to control gastric pH, with adjunctive use of antacids if necessary. Urinary catheterization should be continued to assess hourly urine output and to aid intravenous fluid therapy. In the elderly, a central venous catheter is advisable to monitor central venous pressure and to enable timely replacement of electrolytes such as potassium. If there is evidence of cardiac dysfunction, a Swan–Ganz catheter should be inserted to monitor cardiac output, left ventricular filling pressures, and systemic vascular resistance, and to guide the use of vasoactive agents if those are required.

Coagulation abnormalities or platelet deficiencies should be corrected as necessary. Several doses of antibiotics should be given after operation because of the clean-contaminated nature of the procedure with intragastric blood being an excellent culture medium.

Total parenteral nutrition should be considered for the high-risk patient. Subcutaneous heparin should be avoided, but sequential calf compression devices may be used to reduce the incidence of deep venous thrombosis.

Outcome

Acute complications

Complications following truncal vagotomy include ischaemia of the distal oesophagus when more than 4 cm has been skeletonized, or iatrogenic perforation if extensive dissection of vagal fibres has been undertaken with excessive enthusiasm. Left pneumothorax may result from finger dissection posterior to the oesophagus. Splenic injury may result from excessive traction on the stomach, omentum or splenic flexure of the colon. Complications of parietal cell vagotomy include ischaemia of the lesser curvature of the stomach after devascularization (incidence less than 1%) and postoperative intra-abdominal bleeding (about 1%).

If the ulcer has not been resected (as in vagotomy and pyloroplasty for bleeding posterior duodenal ulcer), early rebleeding may occur in 5–8% of patients[6]. Wound infections are more common after operation for gastrointestinal haemorrhage. Complications from gastroduodenostomy include gastric outlet obstruction from anastomotic narrowing, requiring anastomotic revision. Other complications include anastomotic leakage, bleeding from either intraluminal or extraluminal sources, and postoperative pancreatitis.

Postvagotomy and postgastrectomy syndromes

The dumping syndrome has been described either early or late after eating, but the early syndrome is much more common, occurring in up to 25% of patients after pyloroplasty or resection. With rapid travel of gastric contents into the duodenum, cramping and diarrhoea may result, with additional vasomotor symptoms of pallor, faintness and perspiration. Most patients can be managed with dietary changes.

Postvagotomy diarrhoea is often unassociated with eating and may occur at night. While cholestyramine may be helpful in the majority, truly refractory diarrhoea is found in only about 1% of patients.

Alkaline reflux gastritis with relatively constant epigastric pain and bilious emesis may be helped with H_2 antagonists or cholestyramine but, if these are unsuccessful, conversion to a Roux-en-Y gastrojejunostomy may be required to divert alkaline secretion from the stomach.

Options for patients with recurrence

Many patients with recurrences can be successfully managed medically; as with the original case, haemorrhage, perforation, obstruction or intractability may demand surgical correction. Recurrent ulcer disease should prompt investigation for gastrinoma, hyperparathyroidism, retained antrum in the case of a duodenal stump, or for antral gastric cell hyperplasia. Recurrent gastric ulcer should be biopsied to exclude a carcinoma. If no obvious cause is found and surgical intervention is deemed necessary, then antrectomy is usually performed if truncal vagotomy or parietal cell vagotomy was performed initially. If antrectomy was the initial procedure, then a subtotal gastrectomy with vagotomy or revagotomy should be considered.

References

1. Kurata JH, Corboy ED. Current peptic ulcer time trends: an epidemiologic profile. *J Clin Gastroenterol* 1988; 10: 259–68.

2. Csendes A, Braghetto I, Calvo F *et al*. Surgical treatment of high gastric ulcer. *Am J Surg* 1985; 149: 765–70.

3. Laurence BH, Cotton PB. Bleeding gastroduodenal ulcers: non-operative treatment. *World J Surg* 1987; 11: 295–303.

4. Schein M, Gecelter G. APACHE II score in massive upper gastrointestinal haemorrhage from peptic ulcer: prognostic value and potential clinical applications. *Br J Surg* 1989; 76: 733–6.

5. Miedema BW, Torres PR, Farnell MB, van Heerden JA, Kelly KA. Proximal gastric vagotomy in the emergency treatment of bleeding duodenal ulcer. *Am J Surg* 1991; 161: 64–8.

6. Hunt PS, McIntyre RLE. Choice of emergency operative procedure for bleeding duodenal ulcer. *Br J Surg* 1990; 77: 1004–6.

Bleeding oesophageal and gastric varices: shunts

Marshall J. Orloff MD
Professor of Surgery, School of Medicine, University of California, San Diego, California, USA

Mark S. Orloff MD
Assistant Professor of Surgery, University of Rochester School of Medicine and Dentistry, Rochester, New York, USA

Bleeding from oesophageal and/or gastric varices is responsible for more deaths than all other causes of gastrointestinal haemorrhage combined. Prospective studies have shown that once bleeding has occurred the patient is almost certain to bleed again and, ultimately, to die unless effective treatment is provided. Variceal bleeding is caused by portal venous hypertension. Clinically important portal hypertension exists when the difference between portal and inferior vena caval pressures (called the *corrected* portal pressure) exceeds 150 mm saline (11 mmHg). The elevated pressure in the portal venous system is almost always the result of obstruction to portal blood flow, usually within the liver (90–95% of patients), but occasionally at an extrahepatic site (5–10% of patients). The only definitive treatment of portal hypertension and bleeding from gastro-oesophageal varices is decompression of the portal system by a bypass shunt between the portal and systemic circulations.

Principles and justification

Indications

The most frequent indication for portasystemic shunt is bleeding gastro-oesophageal varices, usually caused by cirrhosis of the liver. Other (uncommon) indications are Budd–Chiari syndrome, intractable ascites, severe hypersplenism, and two rare metabolic disorders unassociated with portal hypertension: glycogen storage disease and type II hyperlipoproteinaemia. There are three circumstances in which portasystemic shunt has been used in patients with gastro-oesophageal varices due to portal hypertension caused by liver disease.

Prophylactic shunt

Prophylactic shunt has been advocated to prevent bleeding in patients with demonstrable oesophageal varices who have never bled. However, there is nothing to suggest that the mere demonstration of varices permits a prediction regarding the likelihood of variceal rupture, and recent statistics indicate that no more than one-half of patients with oesophageal varices who have no history of bleeding will subsequently develop variceal haemorrhage. Thus, one-half or more of patients subjected to prophylactic portacaval shunt undergo an operation to prevent a complication that would not have developed. Not surprisingly, three prospective, controlled clinical trials of prophylactic portacaval shunt reported from 1968 to 1972 demonstrated that it did not prolong life. There is no indication that the prophylactic operation is worthwhile.

Elective therapeutic shunt

Elective therapeutic shunt is indicated in patients who have recovered from an episode of bleeding oesophageal varices unless they have little chance of surviving the operation because of hepatic decompensation[1]. There are no clearcut criteria for determining which patients have less chance of surviving with operative treatment than with non-operative therapy, which almost invariably is unsuccessful. The presence of persistent jaundice, intractable ascites, repeated bouts of encephalopathy, advanced muscle wasting and a poor appetite indicate that surgery is unlikely to succeed. Because of the high mortality rate associated with the first episode of variceal haemorrhage, only 25–35% of bleeding cirrhotic patients survive the bleeding episode *and* recover sufficient hepatic function to become eligible for elective therapeutic portacaval shunt.

Emergency therapeutic shunt

This is indicated at the time of bleeding in most patients with liver disease and variceal haemorrhage[2]. Prospective studies over the past 30 years have demonstrated that the emergency operation is applicable to the vast majority of bleeding cirrhotic patients and provides by far the best chance of long-term survival and useful life[3–5]. The only type of patient in whom emergency portacaval shunt may not be of value is the one who presents with concurrent bleeding, intractable ascites, severe jaundice, hepatic encephalopathy and severe muscle wasting, and even some of these patients have survived for more than 5 years after undergoing emergency portacaval shunt.

Preoperative

Diagnosis of bleeding gastro-oesophageal varices due to liver disease

In most patients who enter the hospital with upper gastrointestinal haemorrhage the diagnosis of bleeding oesophageal varices depends on affirmative answers to three questions. Does the patient have liver disease? Does the patient have portal hypertension and oesophageal varices? Are the varices the site of the bleeding, rather than some other lesion such as duodenal or gastric ulcer, gastritis or hiatus hernia?

Information sufficient to answer these questions usually can be obtained within a few hours of admission to the hospital by means of an organized diagnostic plan that usually includes the first four steps described below.

History and physical examination

A history of chronic alcoholism, hepatitis, jaundice, previous bleeding episodes, melaena, abdominal swelling, oedema and mental abnormalities, and the absence of symptoms of peptic ulcer suggest chronic liver disease. The most important physical findings are hepatosplenomegaly, spider angiomas, palmar erythema, collateral abdominal veins, muscle wasting, jaundice, ascites, oedema and neurological signs such as tremor and asterixis. However, in many patients not all these classic signs are present.

Nasogastric aspiration and stool examination for blood

Confirmation of gastrointestinal bleeding by aspiration of the stomach through a nasogastric tube and by gross and chemical examination of the stool is an essential early measure and should be considered part of the physical examination. A nasogastric tube should be inserted in all patients. In an acutely bleeding patient, lack of blood in the nasogastric aspirate rules out variceal bleeding.

Blood studies

Blood samples for typing, cross-matching and for studies are drawn immediately on admission. The initial studies include a complete blood count, liver function tests (prothrombin, bilirubin, alkaline phosphatase, albumin, globulin, glutamic oxalacetic transaminase, glutamic pyruvic transaminase), urea nitrogen, electrolytes, pH, blood gases, blood alcohol, and arterial blood ammonia. It is not unusual for there to be only slight abnormalities of the routine liver function tests in the presence of advanced cirrhosis.

Oesophagogastroduodenoscopy

With the development of the flexible fibreoptic oesophagogastroscope, endoscopy has become a well tolerated, relatively simple procedure that can be performed rapidly at the bedside in the emergency room. It is the best diagnostic measure for determining with certainty the presence or absence of gastritis and of Mallory–Weiss syndrome, and it makes the diagnosis of oesophageal varices possible with a high degree of confidence.

Other studies

Additional studies are occasionally required. However, if there is uncertainty about the diagnosis after endoscopy, a barium contrast upper gastrointestinal series may be obtained. Radiographic studies are directed at determining the presence or absence not only of oesophageal varices, but also of other lesions such as a duodenal ulcer, gastric ulcer or hiatus hernia. The literature contains many statements that suggest that oesophageal varices are demonstrated in only 50–60% of patients who have them. Our experience indicates that a skilful and interested radiologist can accurately demonstrate varices at the time of bleeding in more than 90% of patients.

When there is uncertainty about the presence of portal hypertension, hepatic vein catheterization may be performed to determine wedged hepatic vein pressure, free hepatic vein pressure and inferior vena caval pressure. Hepatic venography is usually added to the studies, although it is not essential and does not yield information as important as that obtained from the pressure measurements. The main purpose of venography is to determine the direction of flow in the portal vein. Wedged hepatic vein pressure accurately reflects portal pressure in the common forms of cirrhosis and establishes the diagnosis of portal hypertension with certainty.

Angiographic studies are not usually required for diagnosis of variceal haemorrhage in patients with liver disease. However, in the small number of patients with normal liver function who are suspected of having extrahepatic portal obstruction, splanchnic angiography provides crucial information about the site of obstruction and patency of the portal venous system. Percutaneous selective catheterization and visualization of the splenic artery or superior mesenteric artery usually provides delayed visualization of the portal vein and its collateral connections, a technique known as *indirect portography*. *Percutaneous splenoportography*, which provides visualization of the portal venous system by direct injection of contrast media into the spleen, is an alternative procedure that carries a slightly higher risk.

Preparation of patient

Certain general principles of treatment apply to all patients with liver disease and bleeding varices, regardless of the specific therapeutic measures used to control portal hypertension.

Stopping the haemorrhage

Temporary haemostasis can be obtained in most patients by systemic intravenous administration of vasopressin (posterior pituitary extract). The agent is administered intravenously over a period of 15–20 min in a dose of 20 units diluted in 200 ml solution, or it may be administered as a continuous infusion at a dosage rate of 0.2–0.4 units/min. Systemic intravenous administration of vasopressin is as effective as continuous infusion of vasopressin into an indwelling catheter inserted in the superior mesenteric artery, and is both simpler and less hazardous. All of the authors' patients with bleeding oesophageal varices are given vasopressin soon after admission, and this has largely replaced oesophageal balloon tamponade as our means of obtaining immediate control of haemorrhage. However, in the few patients who do not respond to vasopressin (approximately 5%), the Sengstaken–Blakemore oesophageal balloon tube, or one of its variants, is used for temporary haemostasis.

Prompt restoration of the blood volume

Vigorous replacement of blood loss is an essential initial step in therapy. Large-bore intravenous catheters should be inserted in each arm at the start of therapy. Combined administration of packed red blood cells and fresh frozen plasma is used because of the serious defects in coagulation associated with liver disease. Bleeding cirrhotic patients usually have thrombocytopenia in addition to abnormalities of the protein blood clotting factors. Platelet packs are administered when the peripheral platelet count falls below 30 000/mm³.

Prevention of portasystemic encephalopathy

Although the nervous disorders associated with liver disease are diverse and poorly understood, the encephalopathy observed in patients with bleeding oesophageal varices sometimes appears to be the result of the absorption of large quantities of ammonia directly into the systemic circulation via portasystemic collaterals. For this reason, measures directed at destroying ammonia-forming bacteria and eliminating all nitrogen from the gastrointestinal tract are initiated promptly. These include removal of blood from the stomach by lavage with iced saline through a nasogastric tube, instillation of cathartics (60 ml magnesium sulphate), neomycin (4 g) and lactulose (30 ml) into the stomach, and thorough and repeated cleansing of the colon with enemas containing neoymcin (4 g in 250 ml of water). The fear that insertion of a nasogastric tube will perforate the varices is unfounded, and such a tube should be placed at the start of the diagnostic examination. Although ammonia-binding agents such as sodium glutamate and arginine and ion exchange resins have been used, there is no evidence that agents of this sort have been of value.

Support of the failing liver

Parenterally administered hypertonic glucose solutions containing therapeutic doses of vitamins K, B and C are included in the initial treatment regimen. Appropriate amounts of electrolytes are added to the parenteral fluids. In general, administration of sodium is avoided because patients with advanced cirrhosis usually have an increase in total body sodium and a tendency to retain salt and water.

Correction of hypokalaemia and metabolic alkalosis

Most of the many bleeding cirrhotic patients studied by the authors have been found to have significant hypokalaemia and a metabolic alkalosis before or immediately after surgery. The deleterious effects of hypokalaemia are well known. In addition, alkalosis has a number of harmful consequences that include: (1) interference with the release of oxygen to the tissues by shifting the oxyhaemoglobin dissociation curve to the left; (2) in combination with hypokalaemia, precipitation of cardiac arrhythmias, particularly in patients taking digitalis; (3) potentiation of ammonia toxicity by elevating the tissue concentration of ammonia and increasing the passage of ammonia across the blood–brain barrier; and (4) production of tetany by lowering the level of ionized calcium in extracellular fluid. Correction of hypokalaemia and metabolic alkalosis is undertaken soon after admission to the hospital and consists of parenteral administration of large quantities of potassium chloride. Administration of potassium is usually required for several days, occasionally in amounts as high as 500 mmol per day.

Frequent monitoring of vital functions

The usual techniques used to determine the magnitude of bleeding and adequacy of blood volume replacement include measurements of vital signs, urine output by way of an indwelling catheter, central venous pressure via a polyethylene catheter threaded through an arm cutdown into the superior vena cava, haematocrit and rate of blood loss by continuous suction through a nasogastric tube. Serial measurements of arterial pH and blood gases are facilitated by insertion of an indwelling catheter into the radial artery, which also makes possible continuous recordings of blood pressure. Because of the systemic circulatory abnormalities and hyperdynamic state that frequently exist in bleeding cirrhotic patients, we have added serial determinations of cardiac output by the dye dilution technique using indocyanine green to our monitoring regimen, and occasionally perform measurements of pulmonary artery wedge pressure by percutaneous insertion of a Swan–Ganz pulmonary artery catheter.

Choice of portasystemic shunt

Because the portal venous system contains no valves it can be decompressed at various points, provided the anastomosis with the low-pressure systemic venous system is of sufficient size to accommodate a large flow of blood. The portasystemic shunts most commonly used for relief of portal hypertension are shown, together with some brief comments on each.

End-to-side portacaval shunt

1   This anastomosis accomplishes splanchnic decompression by shunting all splanchnic venous blood into the inferior vena cava and, at the same time, it decompresses the liver sinusoids by eliminating the contribution of portal venous blood to hepatic inflow and pressure. However, it rarely lowers hepatic sinusoidal pressure to normal, and sinusoidal hypertension often persists because hepatic arterial blood continues to encounter difficulty in leaving the liver through the obstructed hepatic venous outflow system.

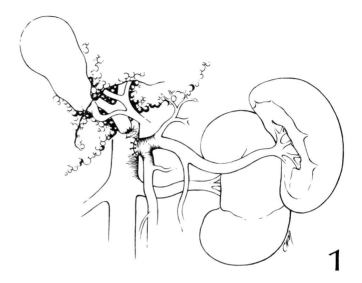

Side-to-side portacaval shunt

2   This other type of direct anastomosis between the portal vein and inferior vena cava produces splanchnic decompression equivalent to the end-to-side anastomosis, but it accomplishes significantly greater hepatic decompression by allowing egress of liver blood in a retrograde direction through the portal vein into the low-pressure vena cava. The side-to-side shunt converts the portal vein into an outflow tract, and portal blood does not continue to perfuse the liver in substantial amounts, if at all.

Although the two types of direct portacaval shunt produce similar splanchnic decompression and are equally effective in relieving and preventing variceal haemorrhage, the overall haemodynamic effects of the two procedures are distinctly different. Hence, there has been a continuing controversy regarding the comparative advantages and disadvantages of the end-to-side and side-to-side anastomoses. In a series of studies, we have compared the effects of the two types of shunt on hepatic blood flow, liver function, liver morphology and ammonia tolerance in dogs with experimental cirrhosis; and on hepatic function, ammonia tolerance, the 5-year incidence of encephalopathy and the 5-year survival rate in cirrhotic humans who were operated on for bleeding oesophageal varices[6]. There were no significant differences between end-to-side and side-to-side portacaval shunt in any of the parameters that were evaluated. We have concluded that there is no demonstrable advantage of one type of direct portacaval

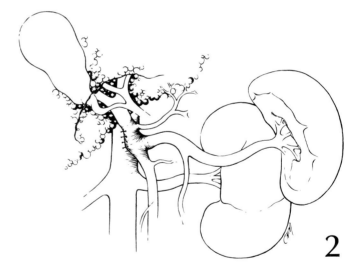

shunt over the other in most circumstances. The one exception may be the patient with severe hepatic outflow obstruction manifested by a pressure on the hepatic side of a clamp occluding the portal vein higher than the free portal pressure. Such patients may have a reversal of portal flow, and they have been known to develop intractable ascites following an end-to-side portacaval shunt, which eliminates the portal vein as an outflow tract and, thereby, may increase sinusoidal hypertension. Although clear documentation of this phenomenon does not exist, a side-to-side portacaval shunt would seem to be the procedure of choice in such cases.

Mesocaval shunt

3 This operation consists of an anastomosis between the upper end of the divided inferior vena cava and the side of the superior mesenteric vein. In principle, it is haemodynamically similar to the side-to-side porta-caval shunt. In patients with extrahepatic portal hypertension caused by occlusion of the portal vein this type of shunt is very effective; however, in adult cirrhotic patients it is doubtful that this procedure represents a first choice. Cirrhotic patients have a tendency to retain salt and water, and division of the inferior vena cava may lead to intractable oedema of the lower extremities.

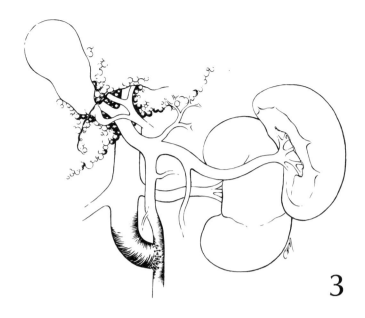

3

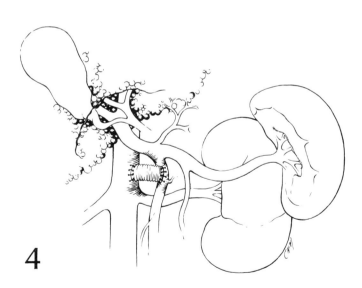

4

Interposition mesocaval H graft shunt

4 The use of H grafts between the intact portal or superior mesenteric vein and inferior vena cava, introduced 35 years ago, attracted renewed interest in the 1970s. Synthetic prostheses of Dacron and Teflon, autogenous jugular vein and homologous vena cava have been used for this purpose. The interposition mesocaval or portacaval H graft is a relatively minor technical variation of the direct side-to-side portacaval shunt and, despite claims to the contrary, the two procedures are haemodynamically identical. The major advantage claimed for the H graft procedure is that it is technically less difficult to perform than conventional shunts. The major potential disadvantage is the possibility of thrombosis, particularly of the synthetic prostheses.

Short-term results of interposition shunts with synthetic grafts involving a collective total of some 240 patients have been reported from 10 centres. The operative mortality rate in this heterogeneous collection of patients has been about 15%, which is no different from that associated with conventional portacaval shunts. The short-term incidence of thrombosis has ranged from 5 to 20% which is unacceptable when compared with the less than 2% long-term occlusion rate of direct portacaval anastomoses in experienced hands.

Splenorenal shunt (conventional)

5 The conventional splenorenal anastomosis is a variant of the side-to-side, in-continuity shunt. It utilizes tributaries of the portal vein and vena cava which are of smaller size than the parent vessels. It is followed by a lower incidence of protein-related portasystemic encephalopathy than the direct porta-caval anastomosis because it shunts a small volume of nitrogen-containing portal blood into the systemic circulation. At the same time, it does not decompress the portal bed as effectively as the direct portacaval shunt, is associated with a significant incidence of variceal rebleeding and has a high incidence of thrombosis. In the author's opinion it is the procedure of choice only in rare instances when severe and intractable hypersplenism complicates portal hyperten-sion and requires splenectomy.

The most commonly used type of splenorenal shunt involves removal of the spleen and anastomosis of the end of the splenic vein to the side of the left renal vein. However, a central side-to-side splenorenal shunt can be performed in continuity, without splenectomy. It has been proposed that the latter operation permits continued portal venous perfusion of the liver, but it is doubtful that such is the case because the principles that govern the haemodynamics of the valveless system dictate that flow is in the direction of the area of lowest pressure, i.e. the splenorenal anastomosis. When sple-norenal shunt is indicated, the authors use the central side-to-side anastomosis with preservation of the spleen whenever it is technically possible.

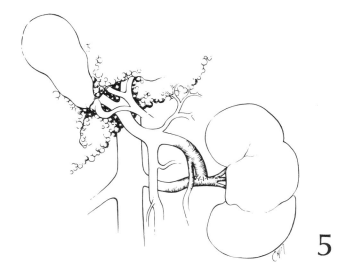

5

Selective distal splenorenal shunt

6 This procedure is designed selectively to decom-press oesophageal varices while at the same time preserving blood flow to the liver and avoiding systemic shunting of intestinal blood. The operation involves anastomosis of the splenic stump of the divided splenic vein to the intact left renal vein, and is combined with gastrosplenic isolation aimed at diverting the gastro-oesophageal venous flow through the shunt. Gastro-splenic isolation is accomplished by ligation of the coronary vein, right gastric vein and right gastroepiploic vein and division of the gastrohepatic, gastrocolic and splenocolic ligaments. The operation is applicable to a relatively small segment of the bleeding cirrhotic population which does not have ascites, has good liver function and is eligible for elective treatment. It is technically the most difficult of all the shunt proce-dures. Since its introduction 25 years ago, selective distal splenorenal shunt has been used widely and the results have led to the following impressions when compared with direct portacaval shunt performed electively in similar patients: (1) distal splenorenal shunt appears to be associated with a higher operative mortality rate and higher incidences of shunt occlusion, persistence of varices and recurrent varix haemorrhage; (2) the 5-year survival rate does not appear to be different; (3) the incidence of encephalopathy during the first few years postoperatively appears to be slightly lower and encephalopathy tends to be milder. However, with passage of time the incidence of encephalopathy appears to increase along with evidence of development of collateral vessels connecting the portomesenteric and gastrosplenic sides of the portal circulation, and evidence of loss of portal perfusion of the liver. Furthermore, there appears to be a substantial incidence of late thrombosis of the portal vein, which eliminates the possibility of continued portal perfusion of the liver.

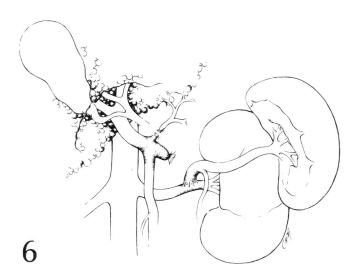

6

Operation

DIRECT PORTACAVAL ANASTOMOSIS

Anaesthesia

During the past 35 years we have systematically evaluated a variety of anaesthetic regimens and have come to the conclusion that the technique of 'balanced anaesthesia' gives the best results. This technique entails giving a nitrous oxide–oxygen mixture by endotracheal inhalation with intravenous administration of an analgesic such as meperidine and a muscle relaxant. Parenteral fluid therapy consists of a solution of 10% dextrose in water in addition to transfusion of packed red blood cells and fresh frozen plasma to replace blood loss. Because patients with liver disease usually have an excess of total body sodium and water, solutions containing sodium are avoided. However, potassium is added to the parenteral fluids to repair the almost invariable deficit in body potassium. Performance of an emergency portacaval shunt usually requires 2.5–4 h and transfusion of 2–6 units of packed red blood cells.

Position of patient

7 The patient is placed on the operating table with the right side elevated at an angle of 30° to the table. The costal margin is at the level of the flexion break of the table, the right arm is suspended from an ether screen with towels, and the left arm is extended on an arm board cephalad to the ether screen. Monitoring and sampling devices include

1. Nasogasric tube placed on intermittent suction.
2. Naso-oesophageal temperature probe for continuous recording of body temperature.
3. Left radial artery catheter for continuous recording of arterial blood pressure via a transducer and polygraph.
4. Large-bore intravenous catheter inserted percutaneously or through a cutdown in the left arm or neck for administration of blood transfusions and parenteral fluids.
5. Large-bore intravenous catheter inserted into the superior vena cava percutaneously or through a cutdown in the right arm or neck for continuous recording of central venous pressure (via a transducer and polygraph), blood sampling and administration of parenteral fluids.
6. Blood pressure cuff on the right arm for intermittent determination of arterial blood pressure as a reserve alternative to direct intra-arterial recording.
7. Three ECG leads on chest for continuous recording of electrocardiogram.
8. Indwelling Foley bladder catheter attached by tubing to a collecting bag at the head of the table for continuous monitoring of urine output.
9. Ground plate for electrocautery fixed to the right thigh.

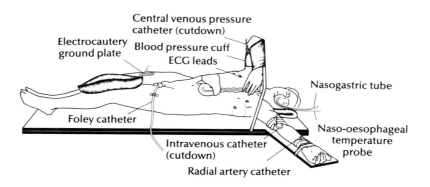

7

8 The initial position of the patient is shown from the right side of the table where the operating surgeon stands. The right side of the body is elevated at an angle of 30° by two sandbags placed underneath the patient. The patient is secured to the table by a large strap placed over a towel across the iliac crest. A large pillow is positioned between the lower extremities.

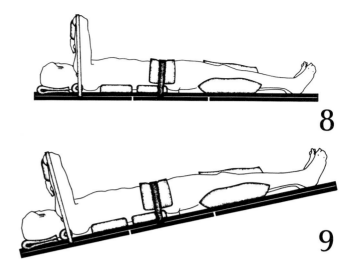

8

9 The head-down position is next adopted in preparation for breaking the table.

9

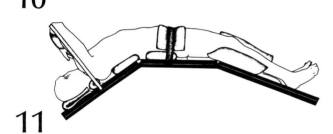

10

10 The table is then 'broken' at the level of the costal margin. The objective is to widen the space between the right costal margin and right iliac crest so that the operation can be performed easily through a right subcostal incision.

11

11 The final step involves breaking the table at the level of the knees by dropping the leg support section about 20°.

Incision

12 A long right subcostal incision extending from the xiphoid to well into the flank is made two fingers' breadths below the costal margin. We have used this incision in every operation during the past 30 years; it is associated with many fewer postoperative complications than the previously popular thoracoabdominal incision. The skin is incised superficially with the scalpel and the other layers with the electrocautery, which greatly reduces the blood loss and shortens the operating time. When the electrocautery is used it is usually unnecessary to clamp any blood vessels with haemostats. The right rectus abdominis, external oblique and transversus abdominis muscles are completely divided and the medial 3–4 cm of the latissimus dorsi muscle is often incised. The peritoneum often contains many collateral blood vessels and is incised with the electrocautery to obtain immediate haemostasis.

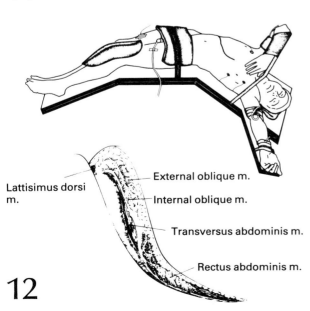

Lattisimus dorsi m.

External oblique m.

Internal oblique m.

Transversus abdominis m.

Rectus abdominis m.

12

Exposure of operative field

13 The operative field is exposed by retraction of the viscera with three Deaver retractors positioned at right angles to each other. The inferior retracts the hepatic flexure of the colon toward the feet, the medial displaces the duodenum medially and the superior retractor retracts the liver and gallbladder toward the head. The posterior peritoneum is often intensely 'stained' with portasystemic collateral vessels.

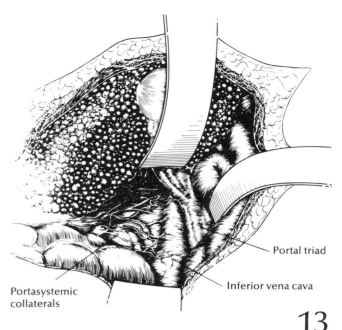

Portal triad

Inferior vena cava

Portasystemic collaterals

13

Incision of posterior peritoneum by an extended Kocher manoeuvre

14 The posterior peritoneum overlying the inferior vena cava is incised with the electrocautery by an extended Kocher manoeuvre just lateral to the descending duodenum. The peritoneum is often greatly thickened and contains many collateral blood vessels. Bleeding usually can be controlled with the electrocautery but sometimes requires suture ligatures.

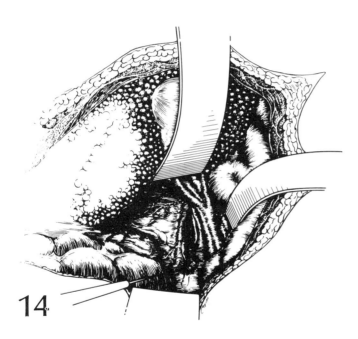

14

Exposure of anterior surface of inferior vena cava

15 The medial retractor is repositioned to retract the head of the pancreas as well as the descending duodenum medially, thereby exposing the inferior vena cava which lies behind the duodenum. The inferior retractor is repositioned to retract the right kidney as well as the hepatic flexure of the colon towards the feet. The anterior surface of the inferior vena cava is cleared of fibroareolar tissue by sharp and blunt dissection.

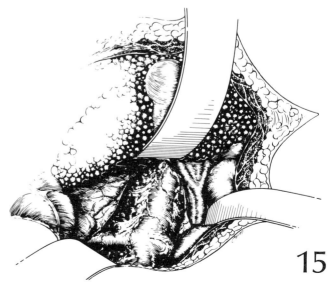

15

Isolation of inferior vena cava between renal veins and liver

16 The inferior vena cava is isolated around its entire circumference by blunt and sharp dissection from the entrance of the right and left renal veins below to the point where it disappears behind the liver above, and it is surrounded with an umbilical tape. To accomplish the isolation several tributaries often must be ligated in continuity with fine silk ligatures and then divided. These include the right adrenal vein, one or two pairs of lumbar veins that enter on the posterior surface, and the caudal pair of small hepatic veins that enter on the anterior surface of the vena cava directly from the liver.

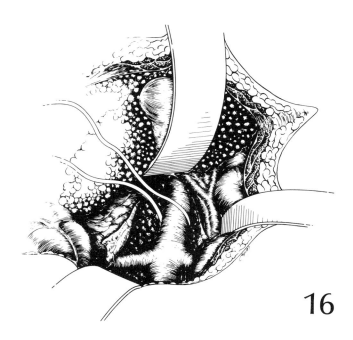

16

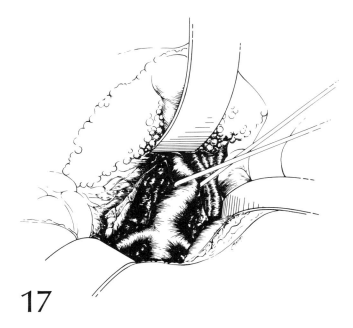

17

17 When the inferior vena cava has been mobilized completely it can be lifted up towards the portal vein. Failure to isolate the vena cava circumferentially is one major reason for the erroneous claim that the side-to-side portacaval shunt often cannot be performed because the portal vein and inferior vena cava are too widely separated.

Exposure of portal vein

18 The superior retractor is repositioned medially so that it retracts the liver at the point of entrance of the portal triad. The portal vein is located in the posterolateral aspect of the portal triad and is approached from behind. The fibrofatty tissue on the posterolateral aspect of the portal triad, which contains nerves, lymphatics and lymph nodes, is divided by blunt and sharp dissection. This is a safe manoeuvre because there are no portal venous tributaries on this aspect of the portal triad. As soon as the surface of the portal vein is exposed, a vein retractor is inserted to retract the common bile duct medially.

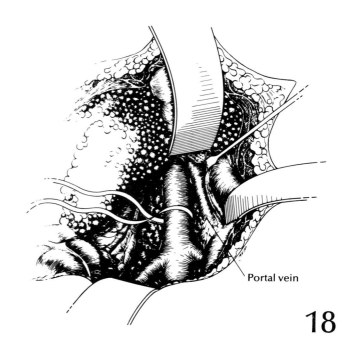

Portal vein

18

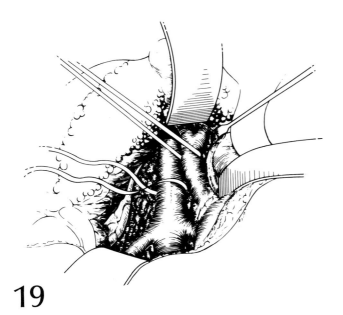

19

19 The portal vein is mobilized circumferentially at its mid portion and is surrounded with an umbilical tape. It is then isolated up to its bifurcation in the liver hilum. Several tributaries on the medial aspect are ligated in continuity with fine silk and divided.

Mobilization of portal vein behind the pancreas

20 Using the umbilical tape to pull the portal vein out of its bed, the portal vein is cleared to the point where it disappears behind the pancreas. The tough fibrofatty tissue that binds the portal vein to the pancreas must be divided. Several tributaries that enter the medial aspect of the portal vein, and one tributary that enters the posterolateral aspect are divided. It is usually not necessary to divide the splenic vein. Wide mobilization of the portal vein is essential for performance of a side-to-side portacaval anastomosis. Failure to mobilize the portal vein behind the pancreas is a second major reason for difficulty in accomplishing the side-to-side shunt.

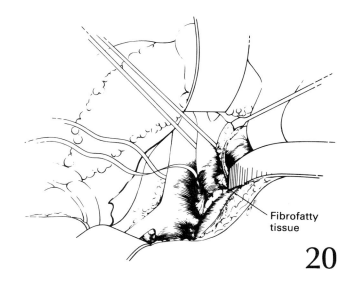

Fibrofatty tissue

20

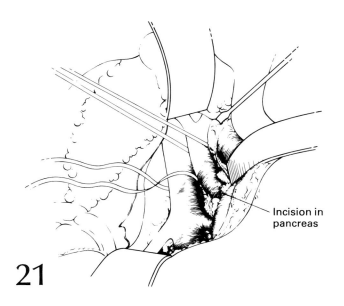

Incision in pancreas

21

21 In some patients it is necessary to divide a bit of the head of the pancreas between right-angled clamps to obtain adequate mobilization of the portal vein. Bleeding from the edges of the divided pancreas is controlled with suture ligatures. Division of a small amount of the pancreas is a very helpful manoeuvre and we have never observed postoperative complications, such as pancreatitis, from its performance.

Determination of adequacy of mobilization of inferior vena cava and portal vein

22 To determine the adequacy of mobilization of the inferior vena cava and portal vein, the two vessels are brought together by traction on the umbilical tapes that surround them. It is essential to determine that the two vessels can be brought together without excessive tension. If this cannot be done it is almost always because the vessels have not been adequately mobilized, and further dissection of the vessels should be undertaken. Resection of part of an enlarged caudate lobe of the liver, recommended by some surgeons to facilitate bringing the vessels together, is associated with many difficulties and, in our opinion, is neither necessary nor advisable.

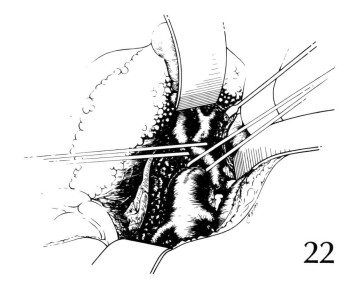

22

Measurement of venous pressures

23a–e Pressures in the inferior vena cava and portal veins are measured with a saline (spinal) manometer by direct needle puncture. For all pressure measurements, the bottom of the manometer is positioned at the level of the inferior vena cava, which is marked on the skin surface of the body with a towel clip. All portal pressures are *corrected* by subtracting the inferior vena caval pressure from the portal pressure. A corrected free portal pressure of 150 mm saline or higher represents clinically significant portal hypertension, and most patients with bleeding oesophageal varices have a corrected free portal pressure of 200 mm saline or higher. The pressure measurements include:

1. IVCP – inferior vena caval pressure (*Illustration 23b*);
2. FPP – free portal pressure (*Illustration 23c*);
3. HOPP – hepatic occluded portal pressure, obtained on the hepatic side of a clamp occluding the portal vein (*Illustration 23d*);
4. SOPP – splanchnic occluded portal pressure, obtained on the intestinal side of a clamp occluding the portal vein (*Illustration 23e*).

In normal humans HOPP is much lower than FPP, and SOPP is much higher. In patients with portal hypertension, the finding of a HOPP that is higher than the FPP suggests the possibility that blood flow in the portal vein is reversed because of severe hepatic outflow obstruction.

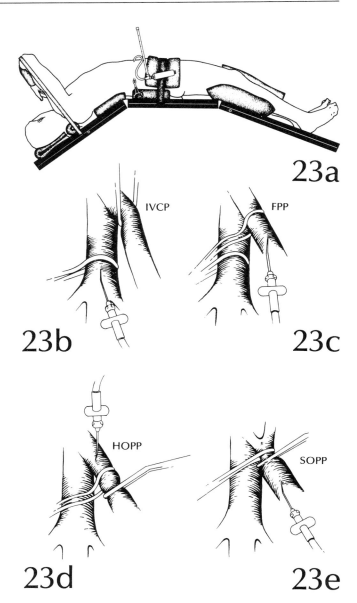

23a

IVCP   FPP

23b   23c

HOPP

SOPP

23d   23e

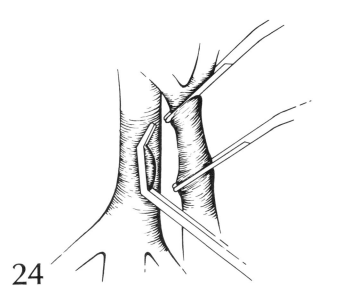

24

Side-to-side portacaval anastomosis

24 A Satinsky clamp is placed obliquely across a 5-cm segment of the anteromedial wall of the inferior vena cava in a direction parallel to the course of the overlying portal vein and the vena cava is elevated towards the portal vein. A 5-cm segment of the portal vein is isolated between two angled vascular clamps and the portal vein is depressed towards the vena cava, bringing the two vessels into apposition.

25 A 2.5-cm long strip of the inferior vena cava and a 2.5-cm long strip of the portal vein are excised with scissors. It is important to excise a longitudinal segment of the wall of each vessel rather than simply to make an incision in each vessel. A retraction suture of 5/0 silk is placed in the lateral wall of the vena caval opening and is weighted by attachment to a haemostat to keep the vena caval orifice open. The clamps on the portal vein are momentarily released to flush out any clots and then the openings in both vessels are irrigated with saline.

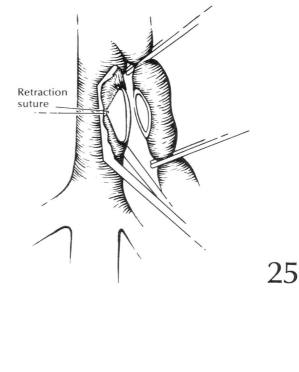

Retraction suture

25

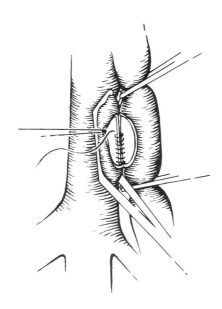

26

26 The anastomosis is started with a posterior continuous over-and-over suture of 5/0 vascular suture material. The posterior continuous suture is tied at each end of the anastomosis.

27 The anterior row of sutures consists of an everting continuous horizontal mattress stitch of 5/0 vasuclar suture material started at each end of the anastomosis. The suture started at the inferior end of the anastomosis is discontinued after three or four throws and is deliberately left loose so that the interior surface of the vessels can be visualized as the anastomosis is completed. In this way inadvertent inclusion of the posterior wall in the anterior row of sutures is avoided. The suture started at the superior end of the anastomosis is inserted with continuous tension until it meets the inferior suture, at which point the inferior suture is drawn tight and the two sutures are tied to each other. Before drawing the inferior suture tight, the clamps on the portal vein are momentarily released to flush out any clots, and the anastomosis is thoroughly irrigated with saline.

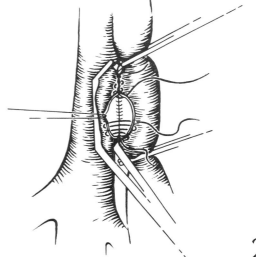

27

28 Upon completion of the anastomosis a single interrupted tension suture is placed just beyond each end of the anastomosis to take tension off the anastomotic suture line. The clamp on the inferior vena cava is removed first, the clamp on the hepatic side of the portal vein is removed next, and finally the clamp on the intestinal side of the portal vein is removed. Bleeding from the anastomosis infrequently occurs; it can be controlled by one or two well placed interrupted sutures of 5/0 vascular suture material.

Pressures in the portal vein and inferior vena cava must be measured after the anastomosis is completed. Usually the postshunt pressures in the portal vein and vena cava are identical. A pressure gradient of > 50 mm saline between the two vessels indicates an obstruction in the anastomosis, even when no obstruction can be palpated. In such circumstances, the anastomosis should be opened to remove any clots and, if necessary, the entire anastomosis should be taken down and redone. It is essential that there be no more than a 50-mm saline gradient between the portal vein and inferior vena cava to achieve permanently adequate portal decompression and to avoid ultimate thrombosis of the shunt. Only two of the shunts performed by the authors during the past 33 years have closed (both of them end-to-side anastomoses).

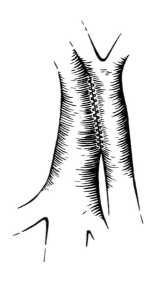

28

End-to-side portacaval anastomosis

The end-to-side portacaval anastomosis is a satisfactory alternative to the side-to-side shunt in most cases, and some surgeons believe that it is somewhat less difficult to perform. It is not essential to isolate the inferior vena cava around its entire circumference, and it is often not necessary to clear as long a segment of the portal vein as in the lateral anastomosis.

29 The Satinsky clamp on the inferior vena cava is placed obliquely on the anteromedial wall in the direction that will receive the end of the portal vein at an angle of about 45°. A 2-cm long strip of the inferior vena cava is excised and a retraction suture is placed in the lateral wall. The portal vein is doubly ligated with a free ligature and a suture ligature of 2/0 silk just before its bifurcation in the hilum of the liver. An angled vascular clamp is placed across the portal vein near the pancreas, and the portal vein is divided obliquely just proximal to the ligation site.

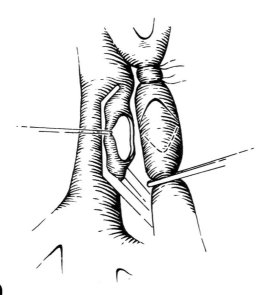

29

30 In order to maximize the size of the anastomosis, the portal vein is transected tangentially so that the anterior wall is longer than the posterior wall at the transected end. After transection the clamp on the portal vein is momentarily released to flush out any clots before starting the anastomosis. This manoeuvre is repeated just before the final sutures in the anterior row of the anastomosis are placed.

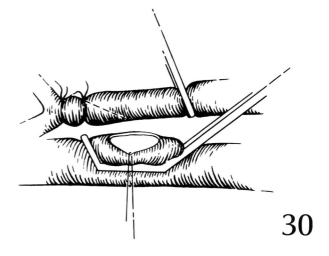

30

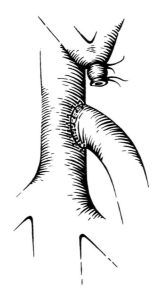

31

31 The end-to-side anastomosis is performed with a continuous, over-and-over 5/0 vascular suture in the posterior row and a second 5/0 vascular suture in the anterior row. It is important that the portal vein describes a smooth curve in its descent toward the vena cava and that it is attached to the vena cava at an oblique angle. Twisting and kinking of the portal vein are the most common causes of a functionally unsatisfactory anastomosis. After the anastomosis is completed, pressure measurements are performed according to the guidelines described for the side-to-side shunt.

Liver biopsy

32 A wedge liver biopsy is always obtained. The wedge of liver is excised with the scalpel and the excision site is cauterized with the electrocautery. No sutures are required in this rapid and effective method of liver biopsy which has been used in over 3000 patients without complications.

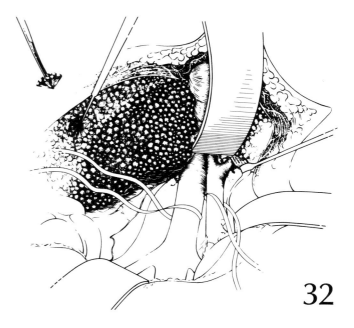

32

Wound closure

33 The peritoneum is closed with a continuous locking suture of 1 chromic catgut. The muscles are closed in layers with interrupted sutures of 2/0 braided stainless steel wire or 1 Tevdek. The subcutaneous tissues are approximated with interrupted sutures of 3/0 chromic catgut, and the skin edges are approximated with stainless steel staples. No drains are used. Drainage of the peritoneal cavity often leads to continuous and substantial losses of ascitic fluid and creates problems in fluid and electrolyte balance.

Summary of important technical features

1. The position of the patient on the operating table is crucial and can make the difference between an easy and difficult operation.
2. A long right subcostal incision is associated with many fewer postoperative complications than a thoracoabdominal incision and is much to be preferred.
3. Use of the electrocautery throughout the operation substantially reduces the operating time and the blood loss.
4. Bleeding from the many portasystemic collateral vessels is best managed by pressure with gauze sponge packs, particularly as most of the bleeding stops as soon as the portacaval anastomosis is completed and the portal hypertension is relieved. Attempts to control each of the bleeding collaterals with ligatures and sutures prolong the operation and increase the blood loss. The objective is to decompress the portal system as rapidly as possible.
5. Circumferential mobilization of the inferior vena cava between the entrance of the renal veins and the liver is essential for the side-to-side anastomosis and is neither hazardous nor difficult to perform. Apposition of the two vessels is greatly facilitated by elevation of the vena cava towards the portal vein.
6. Mobilization of a long segment of portal vein, which includes division of the tough fibrofatty tissue that binds the portal vein to the pancreas and sometimes includes division of a bit of the head of the pancreas, is essential for the side-to-side anastomosis and sometimes for the end-to-side anastomosis.
7. Resection of an enlarged caudate lobe of the liver to facilitate apposition of the two vessels is hazardous and unnecessary.
8. Pressures in the inferior vena cava and portal vein should always be measured after completion of the portacaval shunt. A pressure gradient of greater than 50 mm saline is unacceptable and requires revision of the anastomosis.

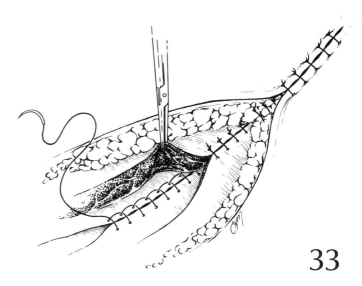

33

Postoperative care

Patients with liver disease who bleed from oesophageal varices are among the most seriously ill patients in any hospital, regardless of the specific therapy used to control the bleeding. In those who undergo emergency portacaval shunt, the expertise of the postoperative care is a major factor in determining survival. All such patients should be admitted to an intensive care unit with equipment and personnel geared to managing the complicated problems associated with hepatic disease. A description of specific prophylactic and therapeutic aspects of postoperative care follows.

Monitoring

Careful monitoring of vital signs, central venous pressure, urine output, arterial pH, arterial and alveolar gases, fluid balance, body weight and abdominal girth is essential. Serial electrocardiograms and determinations of cardiac output and peripheral resistance are often very helpful. Measurement of pulmonary artery wedge pressure with a Swan–Ganz catheter is occasionally indicated. Serial measurements of liver function, of the formed elements in the blood (including platelets), of blood coagulation, of serum electrolytes, and of renal function, must be performed.

Parenteral fluid therapy

Patients with liver disease are often waterlogged before the onset of bleeding from varices, and they have a markedly impaired capacity to excrete water loads. The bleeding episodes and the operation intensify renal sodium and water retention and exaggerate the already existing fluid intolerance. Parenteral fluid therapy should be calculated to maintain such patients on the dry side. Fluid losses are replaced by a solution of 10% dextrose in water containing all the B group vitamins and vitamins C and K. The total volume usually amounts to 1500–2000 ml/day, based on daily losses of 500 ml of nasogastric aspirate, 500–1000 ml urine, 800–1000 ml insensible water, and a gain of 250–500 ml from endogenous water formation. Sodium is given only to replace nasogastric losses, which rarely exceed 30–40 mmol/day. Parenteral potassium therapy is started as soon as the urine output is adequate and is given in whatever amounts are necessary to maintain the serum potassium concentration at 4–5 mmol/l. The usual requirement is 150–200 mmol/day but may be as high as 500 mmol/day. If a metabolic alkalosis develops, it usually responds to repletion of potassium with large quantities of parenteral potassium chloride. In addition to crystalloid fluid therapy, colloid therapy is often necessary to replace continuing losses of blood and plasma. Transfusions of packed red blood cells are given for blood loss or a haematocrit below 30%. Type-specific, single-donor plasma, fresh-frozen plasma, or salt-poor concentrated albumin is given for losses of fluid into the operation site and peritoneal cavity (acute ascites), as determined by the combined measurements of abdominal girth, central venous pressure, urine output, body weight and a haematocrit showing haemoconcentration.

Pulmonary therapy

Pulmonary complications, particularly infection and wet lung, are a major cause of morbidity and mortality in patients with cirrhosis and bleeding varices. In about 5% of our cases it has been necessary to maintain the patient on a respirator for several days after surgery. In such cases mechanical ventilatory support usually can be provided through an endotracheal tube that may be left indwelling for 48–72 h. Occasionally it is necessary to perform a tracheostomy for ventilation and tracheo-bronchial toilet, but it should be recognized that complications of tracheostomy, particularly bleeding, are more frequent in cirrhotic patients. Portable chest radiographs are obtained daily in patients on respirators or those having pulmonary problems. The decision to taper off and then discontinue mechanical ventilatory support is based on measurements of arterial blood and alveolar gases, ventilatory volumes, chest radiographs and physical findings.

All patients not on a respirator are given continuous oxygen therapy by nasal catheter or mask for 5–7 days postoperatively because of the frequent cardiovascular abnormalities and arteriovenous shunting that exist in cirrhosis. From the start, all patients receive intensive respiratory therapy that consists of intermittent tracheobronchial aspiration, postural drainage, chest physiotherapy, intermittent positive pressure respiration, frequent turning, encouragement to cough and to breathe deeply, and the use of blow bottles and a humidifier. Diuretics may be of value in the treatment of pulmonary oedema caused by left heart failure or infection.

Hyperdynamic circulation

Numerous studies have shown that patients with cirrhosis and portal hypertension frequently have a hyperdynamic state that consists of a decrease in vascular tone and peripheral resistance, an increase in cardiac index, an increase in venous oxygen saturation with widespread peripheral arteriovenous shunting, and marked pulmonary arteriovenous admixture. These abnormalities are sometimes intensified by bleeding from oesophageal varices or performance of a portacaval shunt, and high output cardiac failure may develop, particularly in older patients and those with far advanced liver disease. It is for this reason that we perform serial measurements of cardiac output in all patients both before and after surgery. Patients with hyperdynamic state (cardiac output ≥ 6 l/min) are digitalized immediately after surgery before there are any signs of cardiac failure. Vigorous correction of hypovolaemia is undertaken simultaneously. Once blood volume is restored, fluids are restricted to avoid circulatory overload, and diuretics are used if there are any signs of overhydration. Inotropic drugs are used when appropriate.

Delirium tremens

Alcoholic cirrhotic patients frequently have delirium tremens following haemorrhage alone or in combination with a portacaval shunt or other operation. There is not always a close temporal correlation between alcohol withdrawal and the development of this serious disorder; we have observed postoperative delirium tremens weeks or months afer ingestion of alcohol was stopped. Delirium tremens by itself, in the absence of bleeding or an operation, is associated with a mortality rate of 10–15%; when added to the stress of haemorrhage or major surgery, the mortality rate climbs to 50–60%. Initial treatment consists of administration of a central nervous system depressant. The authors prefer intramuscular magnesium sulphate in doses of 2 g every 2–4 h. If magnesium sulphate therapy is not rapidly effective, diazepam is added in a dose of 5–10 mg intramuscularly every 6 h.

Supportive treatment in the form of parenteral fluids containing concentrated glucose and vitamins, antipyretic agents and pulmonary therapy is important. This hyperactive, hypermetabolic disorder must not be confused with hepatic encephalopathy, because the use of a central nervous system depressant in hepatic encephalopathy may be lethal. Intravenous alcohol is a severe hepatotoxin, and there is no basis for its use in cirrhotic patients with postoperative delirium tremens. Parenteral paraldehyde has no advantages over other hypnotic drugs and, in the authors' opinion, should not be used because of the frequent soft tissue abscesses and noxious odour it produces.

Hepatic failure

The majority of patients appear to be in surprisingly good condition immediately after an emergency portacaval shunt. However, by the second or third postoperative day there is evidence of some deterioration of liver function in most patients. Usually the liver dysfunction stabilizes and then improves, but in some patients it progresses to hepatic coma and the full syndrome of hepatic failure, with jaundice, severe abnormalities of blood coagulation, ascites and renal insufficiency. Liver failure is the most frequent cause of death in cirrhotic patients who bleed from oesophageal varices, whether or not they have had a portacaval shunt.

It should be emphasized that the hepatic coma that occurs during the immediate postoperative period is due to liver cell failure and is *not* related to ammonia intoxication or systemic shunting of nitrogenous substances absorbed from the intestines. Unfortunately, there is no specific therapy for hepatic failure, and all that can be done is to provide parenteral nutritional support and symptomatic therapy of the individual abnormalities that arise. There is no evidence that exchange transfusion, haemodialysis or extracorporeal perfusion of the blood through a pig, baboon or human liver is of value in this situation. Spontaneous recovery sometimes occurs.

Because it is rarely possible to remove all of the blood from the gastrointestinal tract before surgery, neomycin therapy (1 g every 6 h via the nasogastric tube), or lactulose (30 ml every 6 h via the nasogastric tube), cathartics (60 ml magnesium sulphate per day via the nasogastric tube) and a daily neomycin enema (4 g in 250 ml of water) are continued for 3 days following surgery. If continued beyond 3 days, troublesome diarrhoea usually follows. With this regimen, significantly elevated blood ammonia levels or signs of nitrogen-related encephalopathy rarely occur within the first postoperative week.

Gastric acid hypersecretion

Inconclusive evidence suggests that, following portacaval shunt, gastric acid hypersecretion develops and is associated with an increased incidence of peptic ulcer. To protect against this potential complication, nasogastric suction is continued for 3–4 days after surgery and the patient is given ranitidine parenterally. As soon as the nasogastric tube is removed, the patient is started on hourly antacid therapy until the oral dietary intake is good and then the antacid schedule is changed to between meals and at bedtime. An antacid that does not contain sodium is used. Antacid and ranitidine therapy are discontinued 3 months after surgery.

Renal failure

Two common forms of renal dysfunction follow variceal haemorrhage and portacaval shunt. The first is *acute tubular necrosis* which results from a period of hypotension and consequent renal ischaemia. It is manifested by oliguria, uraemia, hyperkalaemia, a low, fixed urine specific gravity and osmolality, substantial quantities of sodium in the urine, and a urine sediment containing casts and red blood cells. Treatment consists of stringent fluid restriction, measures to reduce serum potassium, and, if necessary, haemodialysis.

The second renal disorder is *spontaneous renal failure* associated with hepatic decompensation, the so-called 'hepatorenal syndrome'. It is more insidious in onset than acute tubular necrosis and is manifested initially by progressive uraemia without striking oliguria. In contrast to acute tubular necrosis, the urine specific gravity is variable and ranges up to 1.020. There is almost no sodium in the urine, the osmolality of the urine is high and the urine sediment is normal. There is no specific treatment for spontaneous renal failure and therapy is directed at reversing the hepatic decompensation, minimizing dilutional hyponatraemia and correcting problems as they appear. There is no indication for the use of diuretics and, in fact, they may intensify the renal abnormality. Numerous vasoactive agents have been used for the purpose of improving renal blood flow, but none has influenced the outcome significantly. Haemodialysis has created more problems than it has solved. The mortality rate of the combined syndrome of hepatic and renal decompensation is very high.

Infection

Substantial evidence indicates that patients with cirrhosis have a high incidence of infection, perhaps because of their debilitated general condition. Surprisingly, wound and intraperitoneal infections following emergency portacaval shunt have been uncommon in our experience, but pulmonary infections have been common and urinary tract infections not infrequent. We routinely give prophylactic antibiotics immediately before and for 3 days after operation. Furthermore, appropriate antibiotics are given for proven infections, always on the basis of bacterial cultures and antibiotic sensitivity tests. We routinely obtain cultures of tracheal aspirates and urine during the early postoperative period to avoid delays in therapy should infection develop.

Nutrition

Nutritional therapy is very important in liver disease. Oral diet is started as soon as the patient tolerates removal of the nasogastric tube for 24 h, usually on the fifth or sixth postoperative day. Initially a bland diet containing 2 g sodium, 4000 cal (16.8 kJ), high carbohydrate, regular fat and 20 g protein is introduced. There is no basis for restricting fat and doing so only serves to make the diet unpalatable. The protein content of the diet is increased in 20 g increments every 2 days up to 80 g and the patient is carefully observed for signs of portasystemic encephalopathy. If the patient tolerates 80 g of protein per day, he or she is discharged on a diet containing 60 g protein, 2 g sodium after receiving a diet list and specific instructions from a dietician. Sodium restriction is continued for life. Daily therapeutic doses of vitamins B and C are added to the diet.

Alcoholism

Perhaps the major factor that determines long-term survival following portacaval shunt is abstinence (or failure to abstain) from alcohol. It is vitally important that a frank discussion be held with the patient regarding the extreme dangers of further ingestion of alcohol. The help of psychiatrists and social workers should be obtained while the patient is in hospital and continued after discharge. It is incumbent upon the surgeon to exploit the special relationship with the patient in a long-term effort to cure the underlying cause of the patient's liver disease.

Follow-up

A life-long programme of follow-up evaluation and treatment is a crucial part of the care of cirrhotic patients who have undergone portacaval shunt. The liver disease cannot be cured, but it can be stabilized to the point of permitting a long and productive life in reasonable comfort. After discharge from the hospital, outpatient visits are scheduled every other week for the first month, monthly for the remainder of the first postoperative year and every 3 months thereafter for the remainder of the patient's life. At each clinic visit the patient is seen by a dietician who reviews in detail the 60 g protein, 2 g sodium diet. Dietary control of protein intake has a profound influence on the incidence of portasystemic encephalopathy. Also at each clinic the patient is counselled about abstinence from alcohol.

The aspects of follow-up that are of critical importance for survival and a life of acceptable quality are dietary control of protein intake to prevent portasystemic encephalopathy; abstinence from alcohol to prevent hepatic failure; outpatient visits at least every 3 months for life.

Outcome

Between 1958 and 1990 1451 portasystemic shunts for portal hypertension have been performed by the authors, all but 43 of which were for variceal haemorrhage[7, 8]. In 162 of these patients the shunt was performed electively for bleeding gastro-oesophageal varices due to extrahepatic portal obstruction in the absence of liver disease. There were no operative deaths and the 5-year survival rate was 98%. None of the patients developed portasystemic encephalopathy. An additional 824 patients were referred to us from other hospitals after they recovered from bleeding gastro-oesophageal varices due to liver disease, and they underwent elective therapeutic portacaval shunts. The results of elective shunt in these highly selected patients are shown in *Table 1*. The remaining patients with variceal bleeding in our series underwent emergency therapeutic portacaval shunt for acute haemorrhage.

Table 1 Follow-up data on 824 patients with liver disease who underwent elective therapeutic portacaval shunt for variceal bleeding

	No. of patients	Percentage of group
Total group	824	100
30-day mortality	13	1.6
5-year survival	558	68
Variceal rebleeding	3	0.4
Shunt patency	824	100
Encephalopathy at any time	142	17

Between 1963 and 1990 the authors conducted a prospective study of emergency portacaval shunt in 391 unselected patients, most of whom had alcoholic cirrhosis[3-5]. The study had two important features that distinguished it from all others that have been reported to date: (1) the patients were *unselected*, which means that all were included and no patient with variceal bleeding was excluded from emergency shunt; and (2) the shunts were *emergency* operations performed in the face of acute bleeding *within 8 h* of admission of the patient to the emergency room. The patients have been divided into an 'early' group of 180 patients operated on from 1963 to 1977, and a 'recent' group of 211 patients operated on from 1978 to 1990. The 10-year follow-up rate is 97%. The results are shown in *Table 2* and *Figure 1*.

All of the patients had cirrhosis proven by biopsy, gastro-oesophageal varices proven by endoscopy or radiography, and portal hypertension proven by direct pressure measurements at operation. On admission, half of the patients had jaundice and ascites, one-third had portasystemic encephalopathy or a past history of same, 36% had severe muscle wasting, and 88% had a hyperdynamic cardiovascular state. Emergency porta-

Table 2   Results of emergency portacaval shunt in 391 patients with bleeding gastro-oesophageal varices due to cirrhosis

	Early group (1963–1977)	Recent group (1978–1990)
Number of patients	180	211
Blood transfusions before and during operation: mean units (range)	10.2 (2–37)	9.2 (0–42)
Permanent control of bleeding (%)	98	100
Early survival – 30 days and left hospital (%)	58	85
5-year survival (%)	38	74
Actuarial 10-year survival (%)	30	68
Shunt patency long-term (%)	99	100

caval shunt promptly stopped the variceal bleeding in all patients, and permanently prevented recurrent haemorrhage in all but four (99%). Fifty-eight per cent of the early group of 180 patients and 85% of the 211 patients in the recent group survived 30 days and left the hospital alive. Five-year survival rate increased from 38% in the early group to 74% in the recent group. Actuarial 10-year survival increased from 30% in the early group to 68% in the recent group. Long-term shunt patency has been demonstrated by yearly angiography or Doppler ultrasonography in all but two patients, both of whom were in the early group and had end-to-side shunts. The long-term survival rate of emergency shunt in the recent group of unselected patients, all patients included, is at least as high as the survival rate of elective portasystemic shunt in highly selected patients reported by us and other surgeons (*Figure 1*).

Data on the quality of life after 5 years in survivors of emergency portacaval shunt are shown in *Table 3*. One-third of the patients had portasystemic encephalopathy before the shunt. After the shunt, 32% of the early group and 17% of the recent group have had encephalopathy at some time, but recurrent encephalopathy requiring dietary protein restriction and medication occurred in only 7.6% of the patients. The low incidence of recurrent encephalopathy was the result of continuing emphasis on dietary protein control during life-long follow-up. Abstention from alcohol was sustained throughout the follow-up period in 48% of survivors in the early group and 69% in the recent group. After 5 years, liver function had improved in 70% of the recent group, was unchanged in 18%, and was worse in 12%, all of whom had resumed alcohol consumption. The general health of survivors in the early and recent groups, respectively, was excellent or good in 62 and 77%, fair in 28 and 15%, and poor in 9 and 8%, all but one of whom had resumed heavy alcoholism. After 5 years, 28% of the eligible workers in the early group and 52% of those in the recent group were gainfully employed or were women doing full-time housekeeping.

Table 3   Quality of life after 5 years in 224 survivors of emergency portacaval shunt

	Early group (n = 68)	Recent group (n = 156)
Encephalopathy		
Preoperative	32	33
Postoperative		
Recurrent	7	8
Single episode	25	9
Alcohol use		
Abstention	48	69
Occasional	24	16
Regular	27	15
Liver function		
Improved	44	70
Unchanged	33	18
Worse	22	12
General health		
Excellent/good	62	77
Fair	29	15
Poor	9	8
Work status		
Retired	22	20
Employed or housekeeping	28	52

All values are percentages

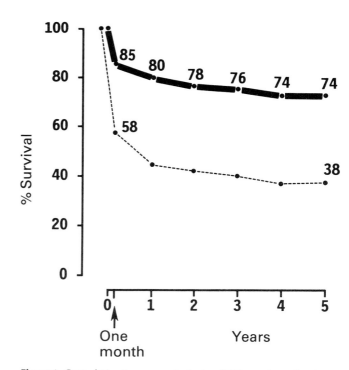

Figure 1 *Cumulative 5-year survival rate of 391 unselected patients with cirrhosis who underwent emergency portacaval shunt. The 'early' group (-----) contained 180 patients operated on during 1963–1977, and the 'recent' group (–·–·–) contained 211 patients operated on during 1978–1990*

Table 4 Results of emergency portacaval shunt in 94 patients with Child's class C cirrhosis and bleeding gastro-oesophageal varices

	Percentage of patients
Early survival – 30 days and left hospital	80
5-year survival	64
Permanent control of bleeding	100
Shunt patency long-term	100
Encephalopathy	
Preoperative	71
Postoperative	
Recurrent	9
Single episode	9
Abstention from alcohol	69
Child's class after 1 year	
A	21
B	73
C	5

Recently the results of a prospective study of 94 unselected class C patients of the quantitative Child–Turcotte classification who underwent emergency portcaval shunt from 1978 to 1990 for acutely bleeding gastro-oesophageal varices have been reported[9]. All reports of Child's class C patients have described a very high mortality rate during the acute bleeding episode and a negligible long-term survival rate regardless of treatment. Of the 94 patients 97% has ascites, 86% had jaundice, 71% had encephalopathy on admission or in past history, 96% had severe muscle wasting, 100% had a serum albumin level of 29 g/l or less, 98% had a hyperdynamic cardiovascular state, 16% had delirium tremens on admission, and all had biopsy-proven cirrhosis which in 93% was caused by alcoholism. *Table 4* shows the results of emergency portacaval shunt in these very sick cirrhotic patients. Of the 94 patients 75 survived more than 30 days and left the hospital alive, an early survival rate of 80%; 5-year survival rate was 64%. Variceal bleeding was promptly and permanently controlled in all patients. Yearly Doppler ultrasonography or angiography demonstrated shunt patency in all patients. As a result of life-long follow-up with emphasis on dietary protein control and abstinence from alcohol, recurrent encephalopathy occurred postoperatively in only 9% of patients, compared with 71% preoperatively, and 69% of survivors abstained from alcohol. Liver function tests after 1 year showed improvement in 82%, no change in 15%, and worsening in 3%. It is noteworthy that 73% of survivors had converted to Child's class B, and 21% had converted to class A 1 year after emergency shunt.

In conclusion, these studies have shown that emergency portacaval shunt, by preventing death from variceal haemorrhage, results in prolonged survival and a life of acceptable quality in many cirrhotic patients, including those in Child's class C. The results are attributable to rapid diagnosis, prompt operative portal decompression, an organized system of care, and rigorous life-long follow-up that emphasizes dietary protein control and abstinence from alcohol.

References

1. Orloff MJ. Portal venous hypertension. In: Wilson SE, Veith FJ, Hobson II RW, Williams RA, eds. *Vascular Surgery: Principles and Practice.* New York: McGraw-Hill, 1987: 768–800.

2. Orloff MJ, Duguay LR, Kosta LD. Criteria for selection of patients for emergency portacaval shunt. *Am J Surg* 1977; 134: 146–52.

3. Orloff MJ. Emergency surgical treatment of bleeding esophagogastric varices in cirrhosis. In: McDermott WV, ed. *Surgery of the Liver.* Boston: Blackwell Scientific Publications, 1989: 327–50.

4. Orloff MJ, Bell RH Jr, Hyde PV, Skivolocki WP. Long-term results of emergency portacaval shunt for bleeding esophageal varices in unselected patients with alcoholic cirrhosis. *Ann Surg* 1980; 192: 325–40.

5. Orloff MJ. Emergency portacaval shunt: a comparative study of shunt, varix ligation, nonsurgical treatment of bleeding esophageal varices in unselected patients with cirrhosis. *Ann Surg* 1967; 166: 456–78.

6. Orloff MJ, Chandler JG, Charters AC et al. Comparison of end-to-side and side-to-side portacaval shunts in dogs and humans with cirrhosis and portal hypertension. *Am J Surg* 1974; 128: 195–201.

7. Orloff MJ. Effect of side-to-side portacaval shunt on intractable ascites, sodium excretion, and aldosterone metabolism in man. *Am J Surg* 1966; 112: 287–98.

8. Orloff MJ, Orloff MS, Daily PO. Long-term results of treatment of Budd–Chiari syndrome by portal decompression. *Arch Surg* 1992; 127: 1182–8.

9. Orloff MJ, Orloff MS, Rambotti M, Girard B. Is portal-systemic shunt worthwhile in Child's class C cirrhosis? Long-term results of emergency shunt in 94 patients with bleeding varices. *Ann Surg* 1993; 216: 256–68.

Bleeding oesophageal and gastric varices: stapling procedures

George W. Johnston MCh, FRCS
Honorary Professor, Queen's University Belfast, and Consultant Surgeon, Royal Victoria Hospital, Belfast, UK

History

Since Boerema and Crile first described direct ligation of oesophageal varices by a transthoracic approach there have been many modifications of the method. Japanese surgeons, disillusioned by the results of shunt surgery, employed transthoracic paraoesophageal devascularization and oesophageal transection combined with an abdominal component consisting of splenectomy and devascularization of the upper stomach together with vagotomy and pyloroplasty[1]. This extensive operation has never gained popularity in the West, and even in Japan thoracotomy is now included less frequently. The advent of mechanical staplers has renewed interest in the transection–devascularization procedures.

Principles and justification

Portal hypertension in itself does not require treatment and there is, as yet, insufficient evidence to support prophylactic therapy for oesophageal varices which have not bled. When varices do bleed the clinician is presented with a life-threatening situation, not only because of haemorrhage but because of the risk of liver failure in cirrhotic patients with limited liver reserve. Where efficient emergency sclerotherapy is available only a small proportion of patients require urgent surgery, either in the form of a portal systemic shunt or a devascularization–transection procedure. Burroughs and colleagues consider that if two attempts at sclerotherapy fail to control acute bleeding, one should proceed to emergency transection[2]. Where sclerotherapy is unavailable, emergency transection–devascularization is a viable alternative. Even if the initial bleeding episode is controlled by acute sclerotherapy, consideration has to be given to the prevention of recurrent bleeding whether by chronic injections, portal systemic shunt, or some form of oesophageal transection–devascularization procedure. Perhaps transection–devascularization is the preferred option in countries where compliance with a chronic injection programme is poor or where the risk of encephalopathy after the shunt procedure is high. A recent three-centre controlled trial demonstrated similar survival following either transection or repeated sclerotherapy[3].

Preoperative

Emergency oesophageal transection carries a high rate of mortality in these seriously ill patients and should be avoided in most patients with Child's grade C disease. Even in the elective situation the operation should probably be confined to those with Child's grade A and B disease. All patients should have documented varices which have bled. Where doubt exists about the source of bleeding, ultrasonographic examination is useful to assess splenic size when the organ is not palpable or percussible (one cannot have bleeding varices without splenomegaly). The aetiology of the liver disease should be established where possible by liver function tests, serological, immunological and histological examination. Coagulation studies are essential and replacement therapy should be employed where indicated. One dose of an intravenous cephalosporin is indicated at the time of surgery because of the necessary gastrotomy in these immunocompromised patients.

Anaesthesia

Halothane is probably best avoided for medicolegal rather than good scientific reasons. The volume distribution of most non-depolarizing muscle relaxants is increased, thereby giving rise to relative resistance but a longer duration of action. Obviously good hydration with adequate diuresis is desirable to reduce the risk of the hepatorenal syndrome, but overloading should be avoided in those patients with a high risk of postoperative ascites. Care is required with postoperative analgesia because of the impaired detoxication rate of the liver.

Operations

CONTROL OF OESPHAGEAL VARICES USING A CIRCULAR STAPLER

Position of patient and incision

The patient is placed supine on the operating table and a midline epigastric incision used in most patients. Where splenectomy is considered necessary because of hypersplenism a left subcostal incision gives better exposure. Exploration of the abdomen is carried out to confirm the diagnosis and exclude other disease. In portal hypertension the spleen is always enlarged and can be damaged by careless retraction. The hard, cirrhotic liver can also cause difficulties of access to the lower oesophagus.

Exposure of the left gastric pedicle

1 The most important route transmitting the high portal pressure to the oesophageal varices is the left gastric or coronary vein. This vessel requires ligation and can be approached either through the gastrohepatic omentum or via a window in the gastrocolic omentum. The latter route gives excellent access to the lesser sac and also to the splenic artery, should one wish to carry out a splenic artery ligation for hypersplenism in patients where the spleen is not being removed.

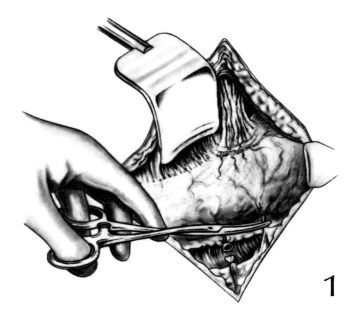

1

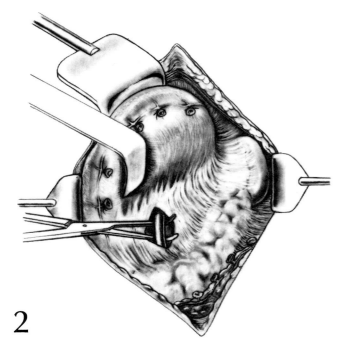

2

Ligation of the left gastric pedicle

2 The mobilized stomach is retracted upwards and adhesions in the lesser sac are divided until the left gastric pedicle is reached at the upper border of the pancreas. Even in portal hypertension these adhesions are generally not very vascular and diathermy is sufficient to control bleeding. The pedicle of the left gastric vessels is cleared sufficiently to allow vision of the main left gastric vein. It is not necessary to dissect out the individual vein, as this can give rise to unnecessary bleeding. The group of vessels present in the pedicle can be ligated in continuity using a non-absorbable suture placed by fine right-angled forceps. A number of ligatures should be applied. The largest size of metal Ligaclip should also be used as it provides a useful marker in later radiology.

Mobilization of the oesophagus

3 Attention is now turned to the region of the gastro-oesophageal junction. In portal hypertension the peritoneum on the front of the oesophagus generally contains multiple spidery venules. In spite of this extra vasculature it is usually possible to visualize the 'white line' underneath the peritoneum marking the position of the phreno-oesophageal ligament. A transverse incision is made in the peritoneum at this level, bleeding from the small peritoneal vessels being controlled by diathermy. When the phreno-oesophageal ligament has been exposed it is brushed upwards with a small gauze dissector. This exposes the oesophagus and the large perioesophageal collateral veins which lie deep to the peritoneum. The lateral and posterior aspects of the lower oesophagus are mobilized under direct vision using gauze dissection, bringing into view the large collateral channels which run with the posterior vagus nerve. This mobilization should not be done blindly, particularly if there is perioesophagitis as a result of previous injection sclerotherapy or secondary to previous reflux oesophagitis.

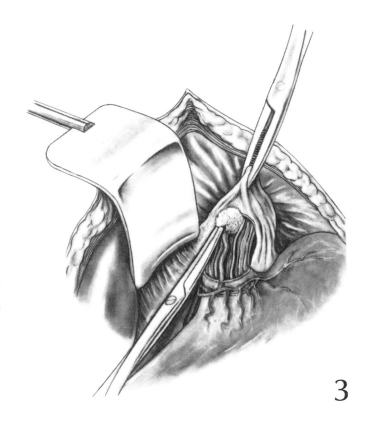

3

Devascularization of the lower oesophagus

4 There are usually one or two large collateral channels which run with the anterior vagus and a number of even larger vessels with the posterior vagus. It is usually possible to free these vessels from the vagal nerves which are then protected in Silastic slings. At this stage it is useful to place a rubber catheter sling around the oesophagus, excluding the vagal nerves. The anterior collateral veins are divided between ligatures. With the fingers of the right hand positioned behind the oesophagus the posterior veins are displaced forwards to facilitate their separation from the posterior vagus and subsequent division. It is permissible to sacrifice one of the vagi, usually the anterior, if there is significant difficulty in separating it from the venae comitantes. Some operators consider that these portoazygos collaterals should be preserved. In any case, it is essential to free the oesophagus from these large extrinsic vessels for a distance of about 6–8 cm.

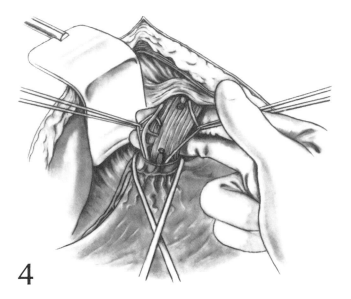

4

Division of perforating veins

5 Perforating branches passing directly into the oesophagus from the venae comitantes require individual ligation or diathermy coagulation. Usually there are only one or two perforating branches on the front of the oesophagus but three or four such veins usually penetrate the oesophagus from the posterior vessels. It is often stated that dissection around the hiatus carries a high risk of serious haemorrhage in patients with portal hypertension but this is rarely the case. However, mobilization of the oesophagus can be more difficult in patients with perioesophagitis.

The extent of devascularization of the upper stomach depends on whether or not it is considered necessary to undertake a splenectomy. In Western society hypersplenism is not a major problem and splenectomy is indicated in a minority of patients only. If the spleen is not being removed, perhaps it is wiser not to divide the short gastric vessels since one can easily encounter troublesome bleeding, particularly if these vessels are very short.

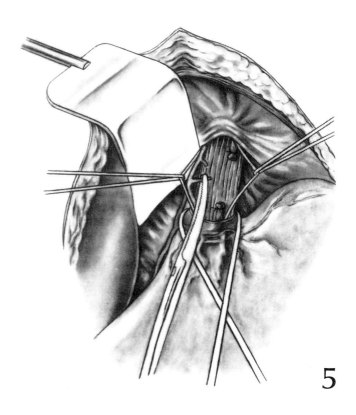

5

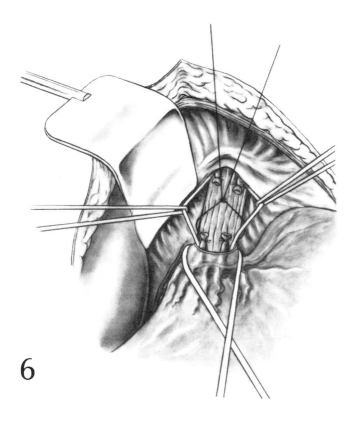

6

Placement of encircling ligature

6 A 0 linen or silk ligature is passed around the now cleared oesophagus and loosely tied. It is important to place this ligature in position before the insertion of the stapling device; with the rigid gun in position it is technically more difficult and increases the risk of damage to the oesophageal wall. Again it is important to ensure that both vagal nerves lie outside the encircling ligature.

Insertion of stapling gun

7 A small gastrotomy is made in a relatively avascular part of the anterior wall of the stomach and an obturator sizer is passed into the oesophagus to determine the largest size of gun head that can be slipped into the oesophagus without risk of damage. The correct size of EEA stapler (usually no. 28 or 31) or ILS stapler (usually 29 or 32) is selected. The closed gun is advanced via the gastrotomy into the lower oesophagus, making sure that neither the encircling ligature nor the sling around the oesophagus impede the passage of the gun up the lumen.

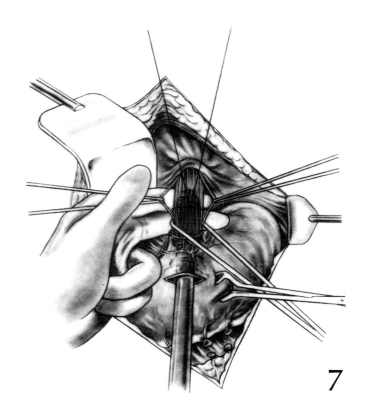

7

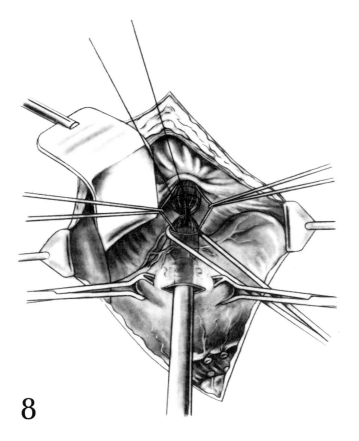

8

Technique of transection

8 When the gun has been advanced into the oesophagus for 5–6 cm, a 3-cm gap is opened up in the head and the instrument is drawn back down the oesophagus until the lowest part of the gap lies immediately above the gastro-oesophageal junction. Light traction is applied to the oesophageal sling while the assistant carefully maintains the gun in the correct position. The encircling ligature is tightened around the stem of the gun into the gap between the anvil-carrying nose cone and the staple-carrying cartridge immediately above the cardia. It is important to remove the rubber sling from around the oesophagus at this point before the head of the gun is tightened, otherwise one risks entrapment of the sling, thereby interfering with stapling. The head of the gun is closed and the trigger pulled to complete the anastomosis.

Confirmation of a satisfactory transection

9 The head of the gun is opened and the instrument drawn through the newly completed anastomosis. A complete 'doughnut' indicates a satisfactory transection. A finger is gently introduced through the gastrotomy to confirm a satisfactory suture line and to direct a nasogastric tube into the stomach for postoperative decompression. The gastrotomy wound is closed in two layers. Since a vagotomy has not been carried out, a gastric drainage procedure is not required. The abdomen is closed without drainage.

Modifications of circular stapler technique

Simple transection

In a patient with acute bleeding the operating time can be reduced by doing a simple transection alone without any devascularization. However, the risk of rebleeding may be greater although there is no controlled trial to prove this.

Addition of splenectomy

In Western society hypersplenism is rarely a significant problem. In areas where schistosomiasis is prevalent, however, massive splenomegaly is often present and splenectomy should therefore be considered almost as a routine. Splenic artery ligation alone can be useful in non-schistosomiasis patients in helping to lower portal pressure, at least on a temporary basis.

Addition of vagotomy and drainage

Although this is part of the Sugiura operation, there is no logical justification for the procedure as a routine. If there is a concomitant peptic ulcer, however, the gastrotomy for the introduction of the gun should be made in the most dependent part of the stomach and this opening subsequently used for a gastrojejunostomy in conjunction with vagotomy.

Transection of the mucosa only

Since full thickness oesophageal transection removes a portion of the lower oesophageal sphincter, Hirashima and colleagues[4] advocate mucosal transection only,

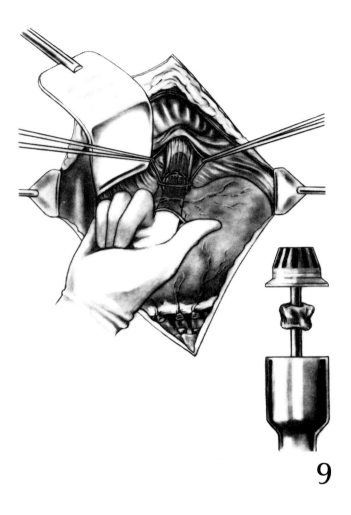

9

leaving the muscle intact. A longitudinal incision is made in the muscle layer of the distal oesophagus and a mucosal cuff isolated circumferentially using scissor dissection. A ligature is placed around the mucosa inside the oesophageal muscular tube. When the stapling gun is inserted only the mucosal flange is resected, leaving the muscular mechanism intact. The oesophageal muscle coat is then sutured over the mucosal staple line.

Addition of an antireflux procedure

Vankemmel advocates a cardioplasty using a linear stapler to provide a valvular flange in the fundus[5]. He claims that this 'gastro-oesophageal dam' minimizes gastro-oesophageal reflux. Some advocate the use of a Nissen fundoplication. This is technically easy if the spleen has been removed or the short gastric vessels divided, but is somewhat more difficult if the fundus has not been mobilized, since one cannot safely pull down on the recently sutured oesophagus.

CONTROL OF GASTRO-OESOPHAGEAL VARICES USING A LINEAR STAPLER

Transabdominal subcardiac linear stapling for oesophageal varices

Although the technique of managing bleeding varices using linear staplers is described in the literature supplied by the manufacturers of stapling instruments, very few patients have been reported and there is little evidence of the long-term effectiveness of the technique. Subcardiac linear stapling does not attack the site of bleeding in 90–95% of patients, i.e. the lower 3–5 cm of the oesophagus, and thus late rebleeding rates are high. The technique, however, has merit in a few well defined situations in patients with acutely bleeding varices:

1. Where there is a fixed hiatus hernia which causes difficulty in mobilization of the oesophagus.
2. Where the oesophagus is likely to be friable in a patient bleeding within a few days of recent sclerotherapy, particularly if there have been a number of episodes of sclerotherapy.
3. Where there is gross perioesophagitis related to previous repeated sclerotherapy, making mobilization of the oesophagus dangerous.

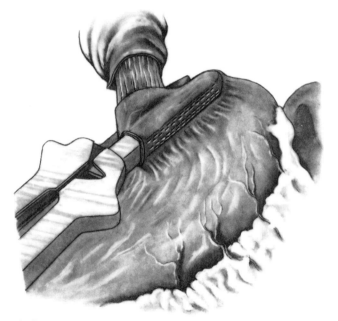

10

10 The stomach is exposed and the region of the gastro-oesophageal junction identified. A small gastrotomy is made on the lesser curvature of the stomach, 2 cm below the cardia, and the bleeding from the edges of the wound controlled. An SGIA 50 stapler, which contains no blade, is used. One limb is inserted inside the stomach via the gastrotomy and advanced to the top of the fundus. The second limb is placed on the anterior gastric wall on the serosal aspect and the gun closed and fired. Four lines of staples are inserted into the anterior gastric wall. The identical procedure is carried out on the posterior gastric wall and the gastrotomy closed. Nasogastric aspiration is advisable for a few days.

Cardiofundectomy for gastric varices

Although gastric varices account for well under 10% of all variceal bleeding, they are a particularly difficult problem. Sclerotherapy is technically difficult and often ineffectual. Direct suturing gives temporary control but rebleeding is common. Even portal systemic shunts do not always stop bleeding from gastric varices. Yu and colleagues have described an oblique cardiofundectomy for the control of bleeding gastric varices[6].

11 Initially the oesophagus and upper stomach are devascularized and Yu and colleagues also advise splenectomy. This gives easy access for the TA90 stapler, applied obliquely across the fundus of the stomach from halfway down the greater curvature to within about 2 cm of the gastro-oesophageal junction. The gun is fired and the redundant fundic area with its tortuous varices excised and the gun removed. It is wise to add a continuous seromuscular suture of 2/0 polyglactin (Vicryl) to ensure complete haemostasis. Nasogastric aspiration is advised for a few days.

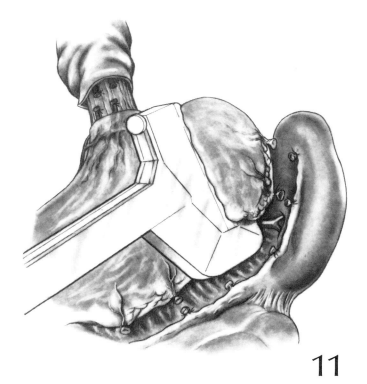

11

Postoperative care

Following transection nasogastric aspiration continues for 24–48 h after surgery and oral fluids are withheld until the 5th postoperative day. There is no indication for radiological studies before starting oral fluids. In some patients increasing ascites may be a problem postoperatively and the cautious use of diuretics is required. On returning to solid food the patients are warned that they may experience some temporary dysphagia. With modern staplers only about 5% require later oesophageal dilatation.

Outcome

Since January 1976 the author has performed 136 stapled oesophageal transections with devascularization. Only 27 were done as emergencies, the remainder being performed electively, often during the same hospital admission but usually within a few weeks of the onset of bleeding. In addition to oesophageal transection and subdiaphragmatic devascularization, 26 patients had splenectomy and 12 had splenic artery ligation because of hypersplenism. There were 22 operative deaths in the series, 10 of these occurring in patients with Child's grade C disease. There were eight deaths in the 27 patients undergoing emergency transection, giving an emergency mortality of 30%

compared with a 13% mortality rate for the 109 patients undergoing an elective procedure. No patient developed a suture line leak. However, two patients did have oesophageal leaks; both occurred about 2 cm above the anastomosis and were thought to be related to intraoperative dilatation before transection. One of these patients died from mediastinitis and the other survived following simple suture. Fifteen patients in the series required oesophageal dilatation because of stricture formation. Of the 114 patients who survived to leave hospital, 42 have had recurrent haemorrhage in a follow-up period extending from 3 months to 16 years. Often recurrent haemorrhage was of a minor nature and only 7 of the 42 patients died as a result of bleeding. Where recurrent varices were identified as the cause, post-transection sclerotherapy was used in 28 of the patients. The overall 5-year and 10-year cumulative survival rates for the whole series were 46% and 27%, respectively. Forty-seven patients remain alive at the time of review and the majority are well and free of jaundice, ascites or encephalopathy.

References

1. Sugiura M, Futagawa S. A new technique for treating oesophageal varices. *J Thorac Cardiovasc Surg* 1973; 66: 677–85.

2. Burroughs AK, Hamilton G, Phillips A, Mezzanotte G, McIntyre N, Hobbs KEF. A comparison of sclerotherapy with staple transection of the esophagus for the emergency control of bleeding from esophageal varices. *N Engl J Med* 1989; 321: 857–62.

3. Triger DR, Johnson AG, Spencer EFA *et al*. A controlled trial comparing endoscopic sclerothrapy with oesophagogastric devascularisation and transection in the long term management of bleeding esophageal varices. *Gut* 1990; 31: A592.

4. Hirashima T, Hara T, Benitani A, Juan I-K, Sato H. A new stapling technique in esophageal mucosal transection. *Jpn J Surg* 1982; 12: 160–2.

5. Vankemmel MH. Highly selective portal decompression for bleeding esophageal varices. *Int Surg* 1985; 70: 125–8.

6. Yu T-J, Cheng K-K, Lai S-T *et al*. A new operation for the management of gastric varix bleeding. *Chinese Med J (Taipei)* 1989; 43: 49–56.

Bleeding: three miscellaneous conditions

Glyn G. Jamieson FRACS, FACS
Dorothy Mortlock Professor of Surgery, University of Adelaide, Department of Surgery, Royal Adelaide Hospital, Adelaide, Australia

Mallory–Weiss tear

A Mallory–Weiss tear is a split in the oesophagogastric mucosa in the region of the gastro-oesophageal junction. It is unusual for surgery to be necessary, but if it is indicated the most important aspect of the operation is adequate exposure of the gastro-oesophageal junction. This is most certainly achieved by complete mobilization of the area.

1 The dissection of the lesser curvature side of the gastro-oesophageal junction is identical to the most caudad dissection of a proximal gastric vagotomy. All connections between the anterior and posterior trunks of the vagus nerves and the lesser curve are divided between ties, for both the anterior and posterior leaf of the lesser omentum. The dissection slopes across the gastro-oesophageal junction to reach the left side of the oesophagus.

The vagi are then swept away to the right and approximately 5 cm of oesophagus is mobilized; the fundus of the stomach round to the spleen and the connections in the bare area posteriorly are also divided.

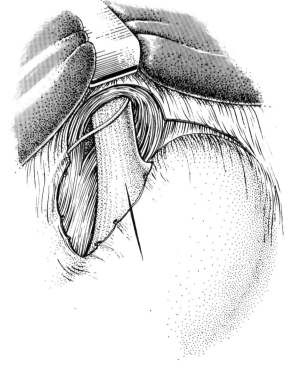

1

2 A vertical incision is made through the stomach immediately caudad to the gastro-oesophageal junction. The mucosal split is identified and quite often can be closed with several absorbable synthetic sutures, without the need to extend the incision into the oesophagus. The incision is then closed, using the surgeon's preferred method of closure.

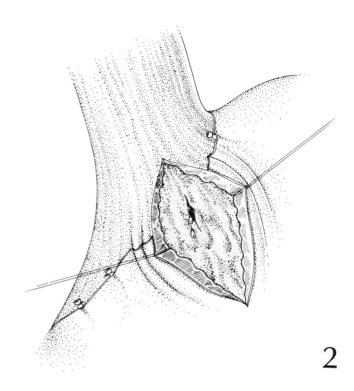

2

Dieulafoy's lesion

In this situation, bleeding occurs from an artery technically known as calibre persistent artery of the stomach. The main difficulty lies in finding the lesion. It usually occurs in the proximal stomach and is associated with a pinhead-sized bleeding point. The only way to find it is to make a generous gastrotomy and pack the stomach with gauze to obtain a completely dry field. Once discovered, under-running the lesion may not be sufficient treatment, and it is probably best to excise the area locally and close it from within the stomach.

Watermelon stomach

This is sometimes also known as antral vascular malformation, as it afflicts the antrum often immediately proximal to the pylorus. It may be caused by chronic prolapse of the antral mucosa through the pylorus and is sometimes associated with portal hypertension. The antrum shows linear raised red streaks. It is one of the conditions for which conservative operations may be appropriate, as the most that is required is a distal antrectomy. Distal antrectomy with preservation of an innervated pylorus is an attractive method of treatment for this condition, although it must be acknowledged that such an operation has not yet established a place as a useful alternative to the more conventional antrectomy, which removes the pylorus.

High gastrostomy with peritoneal cuff

D. Gavriliu
Professor at UNEX-AZ SRL, Universitatea Romana de Stünte si Arte and Professor at Ecologic University, Bucharest, Romania

Principles and justification

This procedure is little used in modern practice but, in certain cases, a gastrostomy is useful for gastrointestinal access.

Indications

The introduction of percutaneous endoscopic gastrostomy placement has lessened the necessity for formal gastrostomy procedures.

This external digestive stoma has many advantages and causes negligible discomfort if performed correctly, with the use of a small incision, a peritoneal cuff to prevent leakage of gastric contents into the retro-aponeurotic space, and positioning the stoma high on the lesser curvature of the stomach.

The advantages include easier intragastric feeding (which is preferable to intravenous feeding) and an increase in gastric size if a gastric tube needs to be constructed later. This procedure also allows the possibility of simultaneous gastric drainage and jejunal feeding, if necessary.

The author has used this gastrostomy temporarily about 10 000 times on patients threatened with starvation before replacement of the oesophagus was performed.

Operation

Incision

1a, b A midline incision 6 cm long is made below the xiphoid process. The anterior aspect of the stomach is grasped near the lesser curvature at the highest point that can be brought outside the wound. The mushroom of a No. 44 Pezzer catheter should be cut away and the catheter introduced into the stomach through a small stab wound in the centre of a purse-string suture placed around the edges of the gastric wound to ensure haemostasis and inversion of the mucosa.

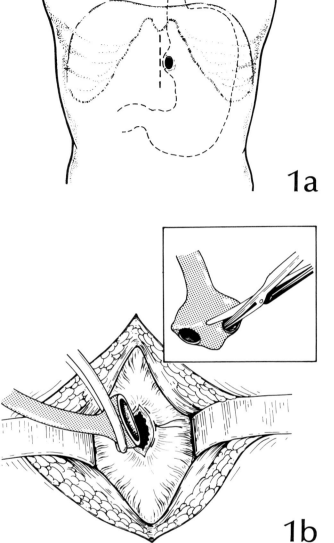

1a

1b

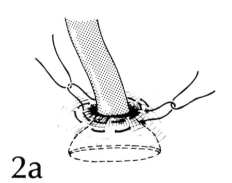

2a

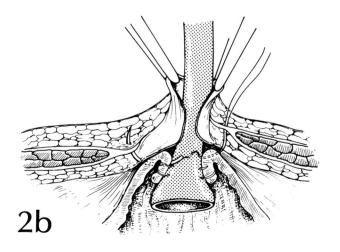

2b

2a, b The purse-string suture is tied. The peritoneum is grasped with forceps and pulled outside the wound over the skin. The gastrostomy is fastened to the abdominal wound by two stitches placed close to the catheter, above and below it. These fastening stitches pass though the aponeurosis of the rectus sheath, through the base of the peritoneal flap, and through the structures of the opposite edge of the wound, in the same way but in a reverse order.

3 When both stitches placed above and below the catheter have been tied, the peritoneal cuff is complete.

Wound closure

The rest of the wound is closed in the usual way using a layer of Vicryl stitches to suture the peritoneum and rectus aponeurosis and a second layer of stitches to fasten the edges of the skin. No drain is required. The peritoneal flaps adhere and seal off in 24 h to close the aperture.

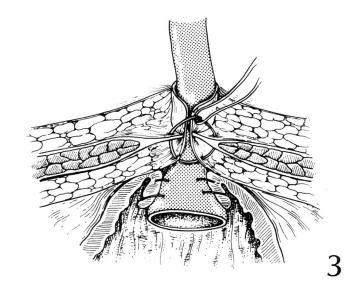

3

Outcome

The resultant peritoneal cuff prevents spillage of gastric contents into the subaponeurotic tissues by excluding the layers of the abdominal wall from possible gastric contamination. It also enhances closure of the gastrostomy once the catheter is removed.

Illustrations by Diane Kinton

Perforated peptic ulcer

F. J. Branicki DM, FRCS
Department of Surgery, University of Queensland, Royal Brisbane Hospital, Queensland, Australia

Principles and justification

Perforated peptic ulcer may be suspected following the sudden onset of abdominal pain in a patient presenting with signs of peritoneal irritation, even in the absence of a history of peptic ulceration. A diagnosis of visceral perforation may be substantiated by the presence of free gas on plain abdominal radiographic examination and this is evident in up to 92% of patients with perforated duodenal ulcer; it is possible to detect as little as 1 ml of free gas on scrutiny of erect and supine films. Voluminous free gas is usually evident following gastric perforation.

Conservative management

Prospective trials have shown that three risk factors merit consideration: (1) a history of concomitant medical illness (diabetes mellitus, cardiovascular disorders, pulmonary disease, etc.); (2) history of duration of perforation greater than 24 h; and (3) hypotension (systolic blood pressure < 100 mmHg) on presentation[1]. Any one risk factor militates against any form of definitive surgery for perforation in the absence of haemorrhage. In the presence of all three risk factors surgery is very often associated with a fatal outcome – open surgical intervention in such a patient is obviously inappropriate and conservative, non-operative management is advisable. The use of combination antibiotic therapy, total parenteral nutrition in the fasted patient undergoing continuous gastric decompression, and the possibility of percutaneous drainage under image guidance of intra-abdominal infected collections which may become apparent, hold the best prospects for survival in the moribund patient.

A perforated duodenal ulcer may seal spontaneously with fibrin, omentum or by contact with adjacent organs. Conservative management may be advocated[2], particularly if abdominal symptoms and signs on serial physical examination are improving. When conservative treatment is contemplated a Gastrografin swallow should be performed soon after admission to determine whether any free extravasation of contrast material is evident. A conservative management regimen, without resort to surgery for perforated duodenal ulcer, has been shown in a randomized trial to carry a mortality rate comparable with simple closure, although the subsequent duration of hospital stay was greater in the non-operated group[2]. If abdominal signs do not improve within 6 h of first assessment on admission, surgery is recommended.

It is unwise to adhere to a non-operative management plan if free leakage of contrast medium into the peritoneal cavity is seen, laparotomy then being advisable unless the patient has all three risk factors for mortality following simple closure of the perforation[1] and is moribund.

Surgical management

The consensus among general surgeons is that surgical intervention is necessary in most patients with gastroduodenal perforation, but there is less accord with regard to the desirability of definitive antiulcer surgery in an emergency setting. The advent of satisfactory medical therapy for peptic ulcer has led many surgeons to advocate simple closure with antiulcer medication and subsequent maintenance therapy and lifelong treatment may be sensible in patients with concurrent medical disorders. Simple closure is safe in even relatively inexperienced hands but carries the disadvantage that, in the absence of long-term antiulcer treatment, recurrence is a major cause of morbidity in patients with acute[3] or chronic[1] duodenal ulceration. There is evidence to support an individualized management policy, with definitive surgery in the form of highly selective vagotomy following simple closure and lavage being recommended for the low-risk patient[3].

Perforated duodenal ulcer

No human data have confirmed that mediastinitis is a cause for concern following mobilization of the oesophagus to facilitate vagotomy in a contaminated peritoneal cavity; nevertheless, a definitive antiulcer procedure is not recommended for the surgeon who lacks expertise in gastric surgery. There is, however, general agreement that perforation associated with overt gastric haemorrhage does require definitive antiulcer surgery rather than simple closure alone. Postoperative gastrointestinal haemorrhage may arise from a suture line, from the primary ulcer or from a second 'overlooked' lesion. Simple closure of a small anterior/superior perforation of a duodenal ulcer may not enable adequate inspection of the posteromedial duodenal wall. Postoperative haemorrhage is a well recognized risk in patients with so-called 'kissing' duodenal ulcers, subjected to simple closure of a perforated anterior ulcer without recognition of a second posterior lesion. Endoscopic documentation of antecedent ulceration at multiple sites is usually lacking and the operating surgeon usually has no knowledge of the likelihood of ulceration at several sites, before or even during laparotomy, when such a possibility is often not even considered. An awareness of ulcer disease previously diagnosed at endoscopy and the nature and extent of recent active lesions is of value when surgical strategy is under deliberation.

Occasionally at operation a duodenal ulcer may be found to have already spontaneously closed, being sealed by omentum or fibrin. In these circumstances, unless the site of the perforation is thoroughly inspected, it is impossible to determine the exact nature of the perforation and the strength of the fibrin seal, which may be very thin and tenuous. A greater degree of confidence as to outcome may be obtained by taking down the seal and closely inspecting the perforation site before proceeding with simple closure, with or without definitive surgery. In addition, real concerns exist as to the safety of omental patch repair for closure of a perforation greater than 2 cm in diameter, some form of excisional surgery being preferred. Options for excisional surgery include vagotomy and antrectomy with gastroduodenal or gastrojejunal reconstruction or Pólya gastrectomy. Simple closure of even small perforations is not generally recommended; sutures may cut out and the defect increase in size – omental patch repair is generally the procedure of choice, with or without definitive surgery.

In the author's experience, there has been no hospital fatality from definitive surgery in patients without any of the three identifiable risk factors already mentioned[1] who were managed by omental patch repair and highly selective vagotomy. The only major mobidity encountered, requiring a lengthy hospital stay, occurred in a patient who developed a biliary fistula, subsequently demonstrated to arise from the site of duodenal closure. This highlights the need to seal the leaking duodenum adequately.

Perforated gastric ulcer

When perforated gastric ulcer is encountered at laparotomy, there is always the concern that the ulcer may be malignant, because even frozen section may fail to confirm underlying malignant disease. Gastric ulcers are often larger than duodenal ulcers and simple closure may give rise to further leakage. With the exception of high-risk surgical candidates, perforated gastric ulcer is best managed by gastrectomy: there is little place for ulcer excision alone and suture closure of the defect. When operative and/or histological findings suggest that a gastric perforation is likely to be neoplastic in origin, it is preferable to perform a gastric resection along the lines practised for malignancy proven preoperatively at endoscopic biopsy. Despite the fact that perforation of a gastric neoplasm is associated with intraperitoneal seeding of malignant cells, a radical gland dissection is justifiable in the absence of disseminated macroscopic disease, provided that the patient's general condition is satisfactory. Gastric resection, deferred for 1 week following patch repair of a perforated gastric neoplasm, is preferred in the patient deemed to be unfit for the procedure at first presentation.

Perforated stomal ulcer

Simple closure alone is advisable in the high-risk surgical candidate with perforated stomal ulcer. In fit patients definitive treatment is recommended but complete vagotomy following an incomplete procedure in the past is not for the inexperienced surgeon. Indeed, a gastric resection may be accomplished with greater ease and safety. The choice of procedure will depend on the patient's general condition and the exact nature of previous surgery. Multiple sites of ulceration may be identified in a patient found at laparotomy to have perforation of a single ulcer. If the patient's general condition permits, some form of definitive therapy is advisable, particularly if the need for non-steroidal anti-inflammatory drugs (NSAIDs) is ongoing.

Preoperative

Once a diagnosis of perforated peptic ulcer has been made on clinical and/or radiological grounds, effective analgesia is prescribed. A vented nasogastric tube of large calibre is inserted to enable continuous decompression of the stomach. Shaving of the abdominal skin is unnecessary in many patients, and may be deferred until anaesthesia has been induced. An intravenous infusion is established and occasionally rapid correction of extracellular fluid deficit is necessary in the hypotensive patient. Although most patients are afebrile on admission, broad-spectrum antibiotic therapy (e.g. cephalosporin and metronidazole) is commenced before surgery if gross contamination is suspected. In patients presenting with hypotension, an indwelling urethral catheter is passed to enable urinary output to be monitored, preoperatively and at least hourly in the postoperative period. In most patients over 60 years of age preoperative prophylaxis against venous thromboembolism is wise (heparin, 5000 units twice daily) unless there is evidence of concomitant overt haemorrhage or if multiple sites of ulceration are suspected.

Anaesthesia

Surgery is usually performed under general anaesthesia. Thoracic epidural anaesthesia provides adequate analgesia in the immediate postoperative period, and is particularly useful for patients with pulmonary disease.

Operations

Incision

The incision of choice for upper abdominal emergency surgery is a midline incision. An upper midline incision gives adequate exposure for simple closure of a perforation and/or definitive surgery. Open operation for visceral perforation requires access sufficient to enable adequate peritoneal lavage with (preferably) Hartmann's solution which, in contrast to normal saline, does not interfere with macrophage function in the first 24 h after surgery.

In patients presenting late with a large perforation, gross contamination of the abdominal cavity often requires the removal of fluid collections and also of food debris. A decision to proceed with definitive surgery requires the midline skin incision to be extended superiorly. A paraxiphoid extension of the incision is particularly important in obese patients, in whom access to the oesophageal hiatus may be otherwise poor. In addition, it is sometimes necessary to continue the incision inferiorly beyond the umbilicus. This distal extension may be made during the course of the procedure should access prove inadequate. The author's preference is to use an Upper Hand (Hepco) retractor. With the use of self-retaining retractors for each costal margin it is usually unnecessary for an assistant to have to retract costal margin or liver during the performance of a highly selective vagotomy or gastric resection.

It is salutary to recall that patients presenting with features of perforated peptic ulcer may, at first sight, have no gross abnormality apparent on opening the abdominal cavity. It is particularly important to open the lesser sac, aspirate any contents in its deepest recesses in the left upper quadrant, and inspect with great care the posterior gastric wall superiorly. Unless such attention to detail is paid, a small perforation with minimal contamination in the lesser sac may be overlooked.

SIMPLE CLOSURE OF PERFORATED DUODENAL ULCER

At laparotomy the diagnosis is confirmed and free gastroduodenal contents are aspirated with a sump sucker inserted in subphrenic, subhepatic, paracolic, infracolic and pelvic compartments. Repeated peritoneal lavage is usually withheld until the perforation has been closed or the lesion excised.

The stomach can be retracted to the left in a gauze swab held by the assistant; in obese individuals the duodenum may be brought to a more accessible position by manipulating the nasogastric tube until it lies close to the anterior gastric wall adjacent to the greater curvature of the stomach and then holding the nasogastric tube by a Babcock's clamp, over a gauze swab, to facilitate safe gastric retraction without fear of slippage. The Babcock's clamp is sited just proximal to the pylorus. The position of the Babcock's clamp may be adjusted during the procedure to provide optimal access and avoid damage from prolonged application to the gastric wall.

1 Most duodenal perforations are less than 1 cm in size and are amenable to expeditious omental patch repair. Application of an omental patch requires prior placement of a series (three or four only for small ulcers) of interrupted absorbable sutures. For small perforations the sutures may be placed directly through the wall to the lumen of the duodenum to emerge on the far side of the ulcer for retrieval.

In larger ulcers, suture placement requires retrieval from within the site of perforation before passage within the lumen to the opposite side. This is cumbersome and is not recommended. Dissolution of absorbable sutures must also be borne in mind and it is advisable not to place the sutures through the open lumen but to take transverse seromuscular bites of the viscus on either side of the ulcer. Arterial haemostats may be placed on the end of each suture before tying each one over an omental patch. It is not usually necessary to fashion an omental frond as a redundant portion of omentum which does not need division is available.

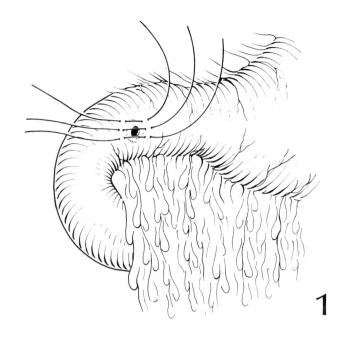

1

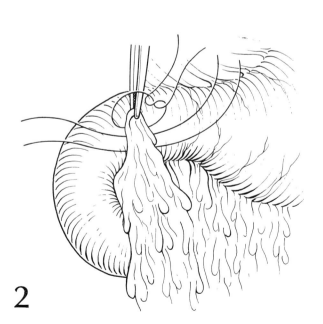

2

2 A seromuscular suture is placed through the duodenum superior to the perforation and is passed through the apex of the selected area of omentum. This suture is the first to be tied and fixes the apex of the omentum to a site beyond the ulcer, obscuring the site of perforation from view.

3 The sutures are released in turn from the haemostats and are then tied, without tension, to avoid the possibility of ischaemia in the patch or cutting out of the sutures.

Interrupted non-absorbable sutures are then placed to join the patch and the duodenal wall to isolate the site of perforation and make it watertight. This is particularly important when the perforation is larger than usual and excisional surgery is considered inadvisable in view of the patient's poor general condition.

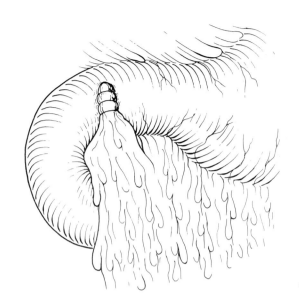

3

PERFORATED DUODENAL ULCER WITH OBSTRUCTION

A combination of significant duodenal obstruction and perforation is unusual. A chronically stenosed fibrotic duodenum is unlikely to perforate spontaneously at this stage in the natural history of the disease but occasionally, intraoperative concern is raised that omental patch repair will be followed by postoperative gastric outlet obstruction. However, oedema and inflammatory damage in the duodenal wall adjacent to a perforated ulcer are responsible for the appearances and these often subside in the postoperative period. Gastroenterostomy or gastric resection are usually unnecessary, except to treat the small perforation which occurs within ulceration which is almost circumferential in nature. In these circumstances a patch repair may be followed by progressive stenosis as ulceration heals postoperatively on medical management. If circumferential ulceration is suspected at the time of perforation then vagotomy and antrectomy are advocated, but the latter procedure should be avoided in patients over 60 years of age as it may be associated with functional gastric outlet obstruction, in the absence of mechanical hold-up, and may take up to 6 weeks to resolve. In the elderly, who tolerate prolonged hospitalization less well, a Pólya gastrectomy is preferable.

PERFORATED DUODENAL ULCER WITH HAEMORRHAGE

While posterior duodenal ulcers are more likely to bleed than anterior ulcers, large anterior ulcers may occasionally present with features of overt haematemesis and/or melaena and free perforation. Simple ulcer closure is inappropriate and some form of

definitive surgery is required. Plication following adequate luminal exposure and subsequent truncal vagotomy and pyloroplasty or gastroenterostomy is inappropriate for the large (>2 cm) anterior ulcer. Excisional surgery is advocated in these circumstances; truncal vagotomy and antrectomy are associated with the lowest rate of ulcer recurrence and provide for a larger gastric remnant, and therefore are advocated in preference to Pólya gastrectomy in younger patients.

In the patient with a combination of free perforation and haemorrhage arising from a small anterior ulcer of the duodenum, ulcer excision with subsequent pyloromyotomy to include the defect and pyloroplasty closure is recommended, followed by truncal vagotomy. Personal experience has led to the view that the more time-consuming procedure of highly selective vagotomy is not justifiable as definitive surgery in most patients presenting with bleeding peptic ulcer, particularly in the elderly if there has been evidence of shock on presentation. Patients presenting with haemorrhage often have concomitant medical illness in concert with haemorrhagic instability. Accordingly, the more expeditious procedure of truncal vagotomy and pyloroplasty is advised for bleeding duodenal ulcer with ulcer excision/plication, the use of highly selective vagotomy being confined to relatively fit younger patients[4].

DEFINITIVE OPERATION FOR PERFORATED DUODENAL ULCER

There is little doubt that, for the patient with a long history of protracted peptic ulcer disease or those in whom gastrointestinal bleeding/perforation has occurred in the past, definitive surgery is the preferred option. Experience in Hong Kong, where peptic ulcer disease reaches almost epidemic proportions, has shown that even patients with acute ulceration presenting with perforation fare better in the long term with definitive antiulcer surgery in the form of omental patch repair and highly selective vagotomy[3]. However, this report documents the results obtained by a small group of surgeons with particular experience of the procedure in an elective setting and it would be inappropriate to recommend highly selective vagotomy in combination with patch repair on a widespread basis to surgeons with little or infrequent practice of the technique.

Highly selective vagotomy has a greater role to play in the management of perforated duodenal ulcer than is currently promoted. This view implies a thorough training in operative technique, which can give good results even without intraoperative testing. In the absence of familiarity with the procedure, a truncal vagotomy and pyloroplasty with closure of the defect is advocated. Recurrent perforation with localized abdominal signs occurring in the days following patch repair may be treated conservatively in the absence of haemodynamic instability, but haemodynamic instability or generalized peritonitis merits surgical intervention, either further omental patch repair or gastric resection with truncal vagotomy and antrectomy or Pólya gastrectomy.

PERFORATED GASTRIC ULCER

Optimal treatment of a perforated benign gastric ulcer is dependent on its location. Prepyloric ulceration is amenable to truncal vagotomy and antrectomy in patients under 60 years. For patients with ulceration at the angulus incisura or on the lesser curvature, Billroth gastrectomy with gastroduodenal reconstruction is preferable. Gastric ulcers are often large, and closure is more difficult, with a propensity for early reperforation. Simple closure is advisable for patients presenting with risk factors previously described for duodenal ulcer[1] or when a small ulcer perforation is suspected to be drug related (e.g. NSAID ingestion). Simple closure of a gastric ulcer may be accomplished in much the same manner as for duodenal ulcer, although division of the gastrocolic or gastrohepatic omentum may be required to provide adequate access.

PERFORATED STOMAL ULCER

Stomal ulcer perforation is often dealt with by simple closure. Subsequently the acid secretory status of the patient may be investigated with appropriate decisions for management strategy. If, however, the patient is considered to be in a satisfactory condition, some form of definitive procedure is preferable, either omental patch repair combined with vagotomy or gastric resection. If the previous operation was a partial gastrectomy, truncal vagotomy is the procedure of choice and will obviate the hazards of a further gastric

resection. Perforation of stomal ulcer is rare following vagotomy and gastroenterostomy but the services of an accomplished gastric surgeon are required for completion of a previously inadequate vagotomy or, perhaps, gastric resection.

Postoperative care

Following simple closure of a perforated duodenal ulcer, peritoneal lavage with at least 3 litres of Hartmann's solution should be performed and should be continued until the aspirated intra-abdominal fluid is no longer turbid. Intra-abdominal drainage is unnecessary in the majority of patients: it is prudent, however, to drain the right subhepatic space with a large-bore drain, if closure of a large perforated ulcer has been performed in a patient unfit for excisional surgery. A drain should be chosen so that, should leakage around the patch occur, it will excite an inflammatory reaction to produce a conduit for a fistulous track on withdrawal. In this situation latex rubber is preferred.

Gastrointestinal haemorrhage should be investigated with upper endoscopy, which can be safely performed, despite suture lines and air insufflation, 2–3 days following surgery. The identification of a bleeding site suitable for therapeutic endoscopic measures with, for example, adrenaline 1:10 000 injection is the goal for the control of continued or recurrent haemorrhage. Endoscopic application of diathermy near a suture line is best avoided early in the postoperative period because of the possible risk of disruption with anastomotic leakage.

Future developments

The adoption of laparoscopic techniques for oversewing of duodenal ulcer perforation[5] is certain to become more widespread. The use of definitive laparoscopic antiulcer surgery, posterior truncal vagotomy and anterior seromyotomy has been described in an elective setting for the treatment of duodenal ulceration[6]. It is likely that definitive antiulcer laparoscopic surgery in combination with patch repair will be introduced in the immediate future. In the high-risk patient the use of laparoscopic techniques must be monitored with suitable randomized trials to evaluate long-term efficacy.

References

1. Boey J, Choi SKY, Poon A, Alagaratnam TT. Risk stratification in perforated duodenal ulcers: a prospective validation of predictive factors. *Ann Surg* 1987; 205: 22–6.

2. Crofts TJ, Park KG, Steele RJ, Chung SS, Li AK. A randomized trial of nonoperative treatment for perforated peptic ulcer. *N Engl J Med* 1989; 320: 970–3.

3. Boey J, Branicki FJ, Alagaratnam TT *et al*. Proximal gastric vagotomy. The preferred operation for perforations in acute duodenal ulcer. *Ann Surg* 1988; 208: 169–74.

4. Branicki FJ, Coleman SY, Fok PJ *et al*. Bleeding peptic ulcer: a prospective evaluation of risk factors for rebleeding and mortality. *World J Surg* 1990; 14: 262–70.

5. Nathanson LK, Easter DW, Cuschieri A. Laparoscopic repair/peritoneal toilet of perforated duodenal ulcer. *Surg Endosc* 1990; 4: 232–3.

6. Katkhouda N, Mouiel J. A new technique of surgical treatment of chronic duodenal ulcer without laparotomy by videocoelioscopy. *Am J Surg* 1991; 161: 361–4.

Illustrations by Gillian Oliver

Surgical management of duodenal diverticula

Haile T. Debas MD
M. Galante Distinguished Professor of Surgery and Dean of the School of Medicine, University of California,
San Francisco, California, USA

Sam H. Carvajal MD
Research Fellow, Department of Surgery, University of California, San Francisco, California, USA

Principles and justification

Duodenal diverticulum was first described by Chomel[1] in 1710, but the first demonstration in a living person did not occur until the advent of fluoroscopy in 1913. Forsell and Key were the first to operate on the anomaly in 1915, and by 1940 Morton[2] was able to collect 49 cases of surgical removal from the world literature.

The incidence of duodenal diverticula is approximately 1–5% on radiological examination and 10–15% at post-mortem examination. Fewer than 1% of patients with duodenal diverticula require surgical management. Because the symptoms are often non-specific, it is difficult to ascribe a patient's symptoms to a radiologically demonstrated diverticulum. In addition, the abnormality frequently coexists with biliary tract disease or diverticulosis coli. Diverticulectomy can be difficult, is associated with high mortality rates, and must not be undertaken electively unless clear evidence exists that the diverticulum is the culprit.

The location of the diverticulum is of critical significance in surgical treatment. The majority of duodenal diverticula (62%) occur in the second portion of the duodenum. Of these, 90% are in close relationship to the ampulla of Vater. Occasionally the ampulla of Vater enters the fundus or the base of the diverticulum. Approximately 30% of diverticula are found in the third portion, and 8% in the fourth portion. Nearly 90% of diverticula present on the medial aspect of the duodenum. Multiple diverticula are present in 10–15% of patients with the condition.

Asymptomatic diverticula require no treatment. Surgical treatment is indicated when complications arise. The complications may be grouped as follows.

1. Inflammation: diverticulitis with or without perforation.
2. Stasis leading to bacterial overgrowth resulting in malabsorption of vitamin B_{12}, and diarrhoea caused by deconjugation of bile salts.
3. Obstruction of: common bile duct resulting in obstructive jaundice and cholangitis; pancreatic duct leading to intermittent acute pancreatitis; duodenum, either by extrinsic compression or due to an intraluminal diverticulum.
4. Haemorrhage.

Preoperative

1 Duodenal diverticulum is best demonstrated on barium examination of the stomach and duodenum. The major problem is assigning the patient's symptoms to the diverticulum, particularly when the patient presents with chronic upper abdominal pain, flatulence, weight loss or melaena. To establish that the diverticulum is the cause of the clinical problem is easier in the emergency situation when the patient presents with perforation, obstruction or haemorrhage. The retention of barium for 6 h or more within the diverticulum is indicative of stasis. Most patients are investigated for biliary tract disease and are found to have gallstones. A dilated common bile duct found on endoscopic retrograde cholangiopancreatography (ERCP) or at operation is significant, especially if there is no choledocholithiasis. If surgical resection of the diverticulum is the treatment of choice, ERCP should be performed to determine the relationship between the diverticulum and the ampulla of Vater.

If the patient is haemorrhaging, oesophagogastroduodenoscopy is necessary. It is often difficult to establish the site of bleeding, particularly if the diverticulum is in the third or fourth portion of the duodenum. If the patient is bleeding briskly (>0.5 ml/min), selective mesenteric angiography may demonstrate the bleeding site and the extravasated contrast medium may even outline the diverticulum. When the presenting symptomatology is that of upper abdominal perforated viscus, emergency laparotomy is necessary. If peritoneal signs are equivocal, a Gastrografin swallow may be necessary to make the diagnosis of perforated duodenal diverticulum. If the clinical picture is that of upper abdominal sepsis, computed tomography is the most useful test to demonstrate abscess or phlegmon.

Whether in the emergency or elective setting, a second generation cephalosporin or even more expanded antibiotic coverage will be necessary immediately before surgery.

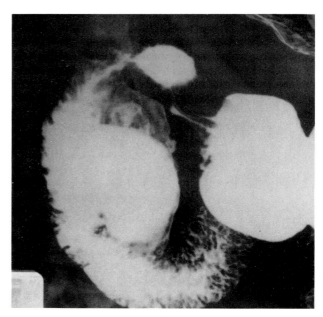

1

Operations

Exposure

A midline incision from the xiphoid to just below the umbilicus is employed. Thorough abdominal exploration to exclude other pathology is performed, and attention is focused on the duodenum. If perforation has occurred, a mass, phlegmon, or even retroperitoneal air may be appreciated close to the retroperitoneal duodenum.

2, 3 Exposure of a diverticulum in the second portion of the duodenum is best accomplished by the Kocher manoeuvre. A diverticulum in the third or fourth portion of the duodenum is best exposed by dividing the lateral peritoneal attachment of the ascending colon and reflecting the right colon and the mesentery of the small intestine to the left. The ligament of Treitz may need to be taken down.

If the diverticulum is not immediately obvious, the nasogastric tube should be advanced into the duodenum, a non-crushing clamp applied to the duodenum distal to the suspected site of the diverticulum and air insufflated.

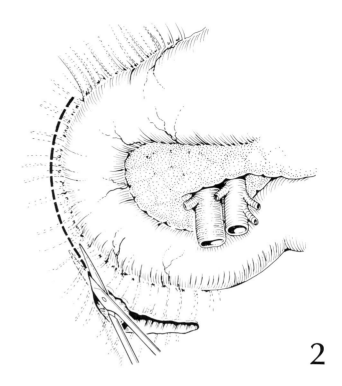

2

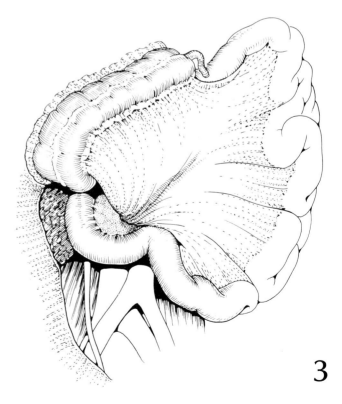

3

DIVERTICULECTOMY

The definitive treatment is excision of the diverticulum. The surgeon needs to establish early in the operation the relationship of the diverticulum to the ampulla of Vater and the pancreas. Simple diverticulectomy may be unsafe if the ampulla of Vater opens into the diverticulum. In this situation the ampulla may require reimplantation into the duodenum after diverticulectomy. It is wise to obtain an operative cholangiogram early in the operation to define the ampullary anatomy. Diverticulectomy may also be unsafe in the presence of a severe inflammatory mass involving the duodenum and the head of the pancreas. In this situation, bypassing the mass may be a safer option. However, even when the diverticulum has perforated, it can often be dissected out. The base is often remarkably free of inflammation, allowing diverticulectomy to be accomplished safely.

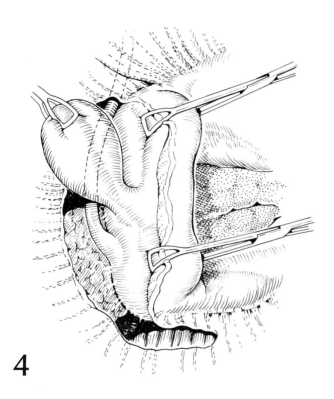

4

Simple extraduodenal diverticulectomy

4 Simple diverticulectomy is most appropriate when the diverticulum originates either from the lateral or posterior aspect of the duodenum. Adequate exposure is obtained and the relationship between the diverticulum and the ampulla of Vater is defined. The fundus of the diverticulum is then picked up with Babcock clamps.

5 The diverticulum is dissected bluntly to its base, where the pulsion diverticulum will be found to emerge through the muscular coat of the duodenum. A clamp is applied to the base of the diverticulum about 1 cm from the duodenum. The diverticulum is then amputated. The mucosa is closed with a running 3/0 absorbable suture. A second layer of interrupted 3/0 silk sutures is used to approximate the seromuscular layer. Closed drainage of the retroperitoneum is accomplished using a soft drain. It is important that the drain does not lie against the duodenal closure. The abdomen is thoroughly irrigated with saline and closed after bringing the drain out laterally through a stab wound in the right upper quadrant.

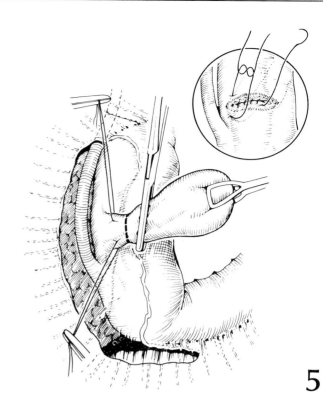

5

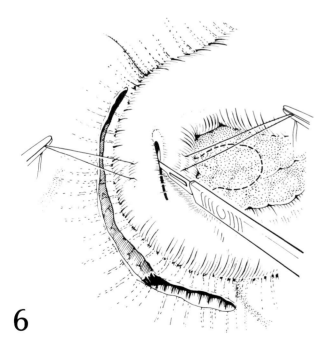

6

Transduodenal diverticulectomy

This approach is indicated when the ostium of the diverticulum is close to the ampulla or when the diverticulum arises from the medial aspect of the duodenum and is embedded in the pancreas. In the latter case, the procedure is not suitable if severe inflammation is present.

6 Two 3/0 traction stay sutures are applied on either side of the midline of the anterior duodenum at the level of the diverticulum. The duodenum is incised longitudinally with either diathermy or scalpel for 3–4 cm.

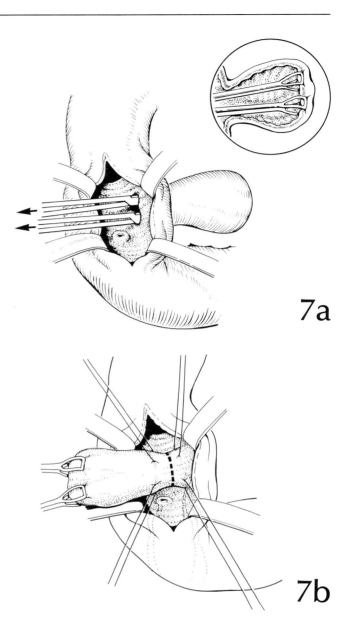

7a

7b

7a, b The ostium of the diverticulum should be evident and its relationship to the ampulla is examined. Two Babcock clamps are inserted into the diverticulum via the ostium and the fundus is grasped. With gentle and continuous traction on the two Babcock clamps, the diverticulum is inverted into the lumen. It may sometimes be necessary to perform minor dissection at the junction of the diverticulum and pancreas to free the fundus. However, this dissection should be kept to a minimum. Four 3/0 silk stay sutures are then applied to the base of the diverticulum and the diverticulum is amputated, leaving enough mucosa at the base for closure.

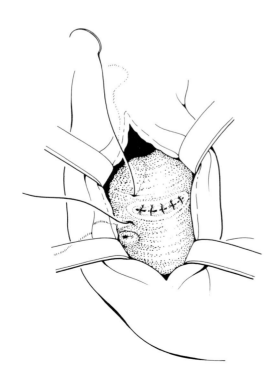

8

8 Interrupted sutures of 3/0 silk are used to approximate the muscle layer. It is best to place all sutures first and tie them at the end. The mucosal layer is closed with a continuous 3/0 absorbable suture (e.g. polyglyconate). Following this, the duodenotomy is closed transversely in two layers: an inner continuous suture of 3/0 polyglyconate and an outer layer of interrupted 3/0 silk. The retroperitoneum around the duodenum should be drained with a closed system.

Diverticulectomy with reimplantation of the ampulla of Vater

This procedure should be undertaken rarely since the morbidity and mortality rates are high. Before performing this operation, the surgeon should consider other options such as Roux-en-Y duodenojejunostomy as recommended by Critchlow *et al.*[3], or extended sphincteroplasty. Recently, the authors had to perform this operation on a patient with severe recurrent acute pancreatitis because the patient had non-dislodgeable food concretions in the diverticulum and the ampulla of Vater entered the fundus of the diverticulum.

The duodenum should be mobilized thoroughly using a Kocher manoeuvre. If the gallbladder is present, it is removed. An operative cholangiogram is performed through the cystic duct to delineate the relationship of the ampulla of Vater and the diverticulum further. The diverticulum is then dissected by retracting the duodenum to the left. The diverticulum should be mobilized as much as possible from this approach, and completely if possible. Sometimes, however, the lateral and posterior dissection will need to be complemented with a medial dissection to free the diverticulum from the adjacent pancreas. The surgeon should be prepared to abandon the procedure if the dissection is hazardous. Also, the surgeon must not hesitate to perform anterior duodenotomy for transduodenal diverticulectomy if the dissection or the anatomy is difficult.

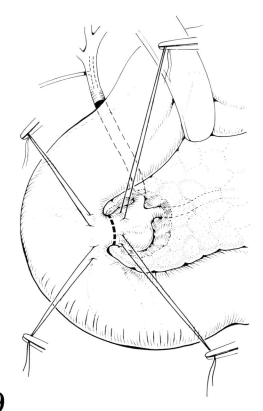

9 Once the diverticulum is dissected to its fundus circumferentially, diverticulectomy is possible. Two 3/0 silk traction sutures are applied approximately 2 cm distal to the base. Another two 3/0 silk traction sutures are applied to the duodenal wall, one at the superior edge and the other at the inferior edge of the diverticular ostium. The diverticulum is then opened 1 cm from its base to empty the contents. It is then divided circumferentially, leaving approximately 0.5 cm of mucosal edge on the duodenal side.

9

10   Attention is then focused on the detached diverticulum. The diverticulum is excised, leaving a fundal circumference of approximately 2 cm. The surgeon must decide whether it would be possible to implant the fundus at the ostium. This is likely to be difficult, in which case the cut edge of the mucosa at the base of the diverticulum is closed with a continuous 3/0 absorbable suture such as polyglyconate. The seromuscular layer around the ostium of the diverticulum is then closed with 3/0 interrupted silk sutures.

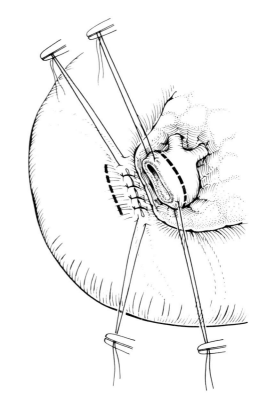

10

11   A comfortable site for implantation is then selected, typically further anteriorly on the anteromedial aspect of the duodenum. A longitudinal duodenotomy of 2–3 cm in length is performed between two 3/0 traction sutures. The implant is then sutured to the duodenal wall with closely applied interrupted 3/0 silk sutures. These sutures must go through the full thickness of the duodenum and the diverticular wall.

The posterior part of the anastomosis is performed first. At this stage, an 8-Fr plastic catheter is inserted into the pancreatic duct and secured at the papilla with a single 3/0 chromic suture. The tube is then brought out through the duodenum 5–6 cm distal to the implant and is secured at its exit point from the duodenum with another 3/0 chromic suture. This tube will be brought out through a stab wound in the abdominal wall at the end of the procedure. If possible, a tongue of omentum is mobilized to cover the implantation.

Three additional procedures are necessary to obtain control in the event of a complication. An appropriate sized T-tube is inserted into the common bile duct. This not only allows diversion of bile, but also provides access for postoperative radiological evaluation. A Stamm-type tube gastrostomy is also constructed in the

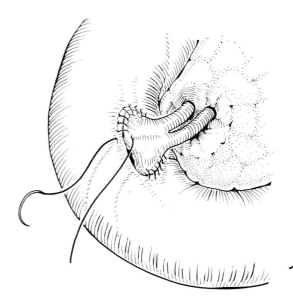

11

event that prolonged gastric suction is needed. Finally, a feeding tube jejunostomy is constructed. The peri-duodenal retroperitoneum and the subhepatic space are drained with soft drains connected to closed suction systems. The abdomen is then closed with the T-tube, pancreatic duct tube, gastrostomy tube and jejunostomy tube exteriorized through stab wounds in the anterior abdominal wall.

PROCEDURES THAT DO NOT REQUIRE DIVERTICULECTOMY

Because the mortality rate of diverticulectomy is as high as 20% in some series, some surgeons have advocated procedures that do not involve the diverticulum directly. These procedures include: extended sphincteroplasty, which is designed to alleviate biliary (and pancreatic) obstruction; and bypass procedures such as Billroth II gastrectomy and Roux-en-Y duodenojejunostomy, which are designed to remove the diverticulum from the food stream.

Extended sphincteroplasty

This procedure, as advocated by Kaminsky et al.[4], achieves three goals: first, a constant flow of bile is established through the diverticulum to decrease stasis; second, the neck of the diverticulum is opened, further improving drainage; and third, there are improved pressure changes that favour keeping the common bile duct open.

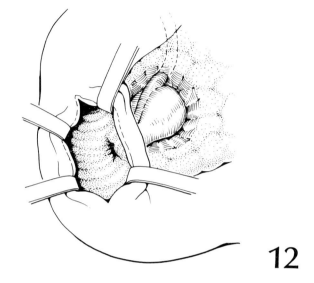

12

12, 13
The procedure is performed through an anterior duodenotomy. The anatomy of the juxtapapillary diverticulum must be clearly defined by cholangiography if necessary. Following identification of the papilla, two fine haemostats are applied as in routine sphincteroplasty, and the sphincter is divided between them. This procedure also divides the common wall between the diverticulum and the bile duct, thus establishing flow and relieving stasis in both the duct and the diverticulum. Sphincteroplasty is completed by using interrupted 3/0 silk sutures, placed with precision, particularly at the apex.

The duodenotomy is closed in routine fashion. It should be noted that there is little experience with this procedure.

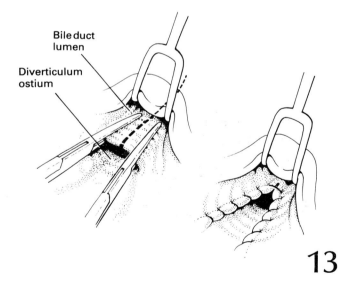

Bile duct lumen

Diverticulum ostium

13

Duodenojejunostomy[3]

The purpose of this procedure is to remove the diverticulum from the food stream, thereby resolving the problems of recurrent cholangitis and pancreatitis caused by food stasis in the diverticulum.

The abdomen is opened using an upper midline incision. The duodenum is mobilized by the Kocher manoeuvre. Cholecystectomy is performed and a cholangiogram obtained if ERCP has not been performed before operation. Choledochostomy is performed above the duodenum between two 4/0 silk stay sutures. A 3-mm Baker dilator or a 10-Fr rubber catheter is passed into the duodenum to ascertain the status of the papilla of Vater. This procedure can sometimes be performed via the cystic duct, obviating the need for choledochostomy.

14 The first portion of the duodenum is then dissected. Pancreaticoduodenal vessels are divided between clamps and tied with 4/0 silk, beginning 2–3 cm distal to the pylorus for a distance of approximately 2 cm. The duodenum is transected at this point and the distal end closed in two layers, with an inner layer of 3/0 absorbable sutures (e.g. polyglyconate) and an outer layer of interrupted 3/0 silk sutures.

15 The jejunum is divided approximately 30 cm distal to the ligament of Treitz, and the distal end brought through the transverse mesocolon for a two-layer anastomosis to the proximal duodenum. The proximal end of the transected jejunum is anastomosed end-to-side to the jejunum 45 cm distal to the duodenojejunal anastomosis. The Roux-en-Y technique is described in greater detail in the chapter on pp. 403–413.

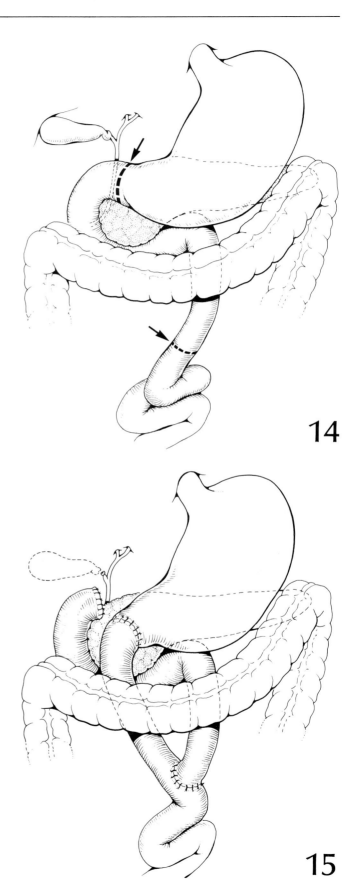

14

15

Postoperative care

General postoperative management is similar to that described in the chapter on pp. 39–44. Only that which is specific to this condition will be discussed here. All patients should be given antibiotics for 48 h.

Three specific complications must be watched for: (1) leakage from the duodenal closure; (2) biliary or pancreatic fistula; and (3) postoperative pancreatitis. In the hope of minimizing the occurrence of the last two complications, the long-acting analogue of somatostatin, octreotide, is used throughout the operative period (100 μg subcutaneously on call to the operating room and 100 μg every 8 h after the operation for 5 days). Octreotide therapy is probably most useful in operations in which the pancreas is dissected or the ampulla is instrumented.

Nasogastric suction is maintained until gastrointestinal function returns as evidenced by the passage of flatus. At that time a Gastrografin study of the duodenum is obtained through the nasogastric tube. If this demonstrates no leak, the nasogastric tube is removed and a fluid diet is started. If, on the other hand, a leak is demonstrated, the choice is immediate reoperation or expectant treatment by institution of total parenteral nutrition (TPN). The size of the leak, the adequacy of drainage and the clinical picture determine which option to choose.

Daily serum amylase and white blood cell determination are necessary to diagnose postoperative pancreatitis. Minor elevations of serum amylase are not significant, but if the patient complains of excessive abdominal pain and the return of gastrointestinal function is delayed, particularly in the presence of fever, computed tomographic scan of the abdomen should be obtained to determine whether acute pancreatitis or a periduodenal abscess has developed. Pancreatitis is best treated conservatively with the institution of TPN. An abscess may be amenable to percutaneous drainage. An associated duodenal fistula must be sought either by a sinogram or examination of the upper gastrointestinal tract with a water-soluble contrast medium.

The postoperative course of patients with diverticulectomy and ampullary implantation is particularly complex. The T-tube and the pancreatic duct tubes should be left to gravity drainage. Fluid and electrolytes lost should be replaced. As soon as gastrointestinal function returns, feeding via the jejunostomy can begin. On about the tenth postoperative day, a T-tube cholangiogram and a Gastrografin study through the gastrostomy tube are obtained. If there is no leak and the patient's clinical course has been satisfactory, the T-tube is clamped and the pancreatic duct tube is removed. The retroperitoneal drains are removed on the next day. The patient can now take clear fluids by mouth. The gastrostomy, jejunostomy and T-tubes can then be removed by the 11th or 12th day after surgery, and the patient discharged from hospital. Alternatively, the patient may be discharged with these tubes clamped; they are removed at the first postoperative outpatient visit.

References

1. Cattell RB, Mudge TJ. The surgical significance of duodenal diverticula. *N Engl J Med* 1952; 246: 317–24.

2. Morton JJ. Surgical treatment of primary duodenal diverticula. *Surgery* 1940; 8: 265–74.

3. Critchlow JF, Shapiro ME, Silen W. Duodenojejunostomy for pancreaticobiliary complications of duodenal diverticulum. *Ann Surg* 1985; 202: 56–8.

4. Kaminsky HH, Thompson WR, Davis B. Extended sphincteroplasty for juxtapapillary duodenal diverticulum. *Surg Gynecol Obstet* 1986; 162: 280–1.

Gastric operations in obesity surgery

Edward E. Mason MD, PhD, FACS
Professor Emeritus, Department of Surgery, University of Iowa College of Medicine, Iowa City, Iowa, USA

Cornelius Doherty MD, FACS
Assistant Professor, Department of Surgery, University of Iowa College of Medicine, Iowa City, Iowa, USA

History

Gastric restriction surgery for obesity began in 1966 with the empirical use of gastric bypass, an analogue of Billroth II gastric resection (an operation that had the unwanted effect of causing patients with duodenal ulcer to remain below their desired weight). In order to simplify gastric restriction operations for severe obesity and to decrease their side effects, increase their safety, and improve lifelong weight control, the operation used today – vertical banded gastroplasty with a 5-cm circumference collar and a measured pouch averaging 13 ml – has evolved.

Principles and justification

Operations for treatment of obesity, beginning with intestinal bypass, were based on a general principle of doing no harm. It was apparent that severe obesity required a lifelong effective operation, as the basic underlying cause was not changed by any of the operations used. It had to be permanent, but also reversible if the patient could not tolerate the operation or required a normal digestive tract at some time later in life. Resection of stomach or intestine, either at the primary operation or as a treatment for complications, was to be avoided. One operation per patient per life was an important goal. Revisions and conversions of failed gastric bypass to vertical banded gastroplasty have been used during the learning phase. The lessons learned have been incorporated into the primary operation in order to minimize the need for subsequent operations.

The use of gastroenterostomy and exclusion was studied in animals before gastric bypass was introduced in 1966 to ensure that it would not produce stomal ulcers. There is always a low risk of stomal or duodenal ulcer after an exclusion operation, and this has been one of the reasons for replacing gastric bypass with vertical banded gastroplasty, beginning in November 1980.

Roux-en-Y gastric bypass and vertical banded gastroplasty were recognized as acceptable operations in March 1991 by a panel assembled by the National Institutes of Health at a consensus development conference on gastrointestinal surgery for treatment of severe obesity. At the University of Iowa Hospitals and Clinics, both operations have been used as primary procedures and in the correction of deficiencies of operations that failed or developed complications. As a result of this experience, bypass operations are no longer used. Both operations succeed or fail on the basis of the size of the pouch and outlet and the ability of the patient to make use of the restriction in size of meal.

Many patients who had gastric bypass failed to maintain a lowered weight. Such patients now have their operation converted to a vertical banded gastroplasty. The only way that a bypass operation can be made more effective in weight reduction and control than a well measured and properly constructed vertical banded gastroplasty is to extend the length of bypassed small intestine. This increases the risk of complications of the bypass, which is already significantly greater than for a gastroplasty. The risks of a bypass operation are with the patient for a lifetime. The main justification for use of any bypass operation is to obtain greater weight loss over a longer time. The early dumping that occurs with bypass of pyloric muscle does allow some patients to lose more weight early and without as small a pouch as is used with vertical banded gastroplasty. If the bypassed intestine is extensive, a larger pouch and outlet are mandatory so that the patient can overeat meat and protein-rich foods to compensate for malabsorption and prevent depletion of body proteins. The exact pouch volume and lengths of intestine needed in a bypass operation are unpredictable, which adds to the risk and the need for further surgery.

The more complex the primary operation, the more operations the patient will need in a lifetime for treatment of complications. These include occasional closed segment obstructions, bleeding duodenal and stomal ulcers, iron deficiency anaemia, osteopenia and, if the bypass is extensive, protein malnutrition. Vertical banded gastroplasty, by contrast, is a simple operation that carries less risk for the long effective life that these operations must have. It may require revision if the primary pouch is too large or if the partition fails. These revisions, however, are minimized by appropriate quality control at the time of the primary operation.

The operative mortality has been reduced by an order of magnitude, from 5% for the original gastric bypass to 0.3% for vertical banded gastroplasty during the first decade of its use. Leak risk has been reduced from 6% to 0.6%. Wound infection rate is now 1.6% and the infections are usually minor. Long-term risks of iron deficiency anaemia and osteopenia from loss of duodenal absorption of iron and calcium after gastric bypass have been eliminated by the purely restrictive operation of vertical banded gastroplasty.

The limitations of gastric restriction operations apply to vertical banded gastroplasty and to those forms of gastric bypass with a limited bypass of intestine. To increase weight loss in larger numbers of patients increases the risks during the remaining life of the patient. Thus, a realistic goal of weight reduction is an important starting point in determining the operation that will be used. Surgeons who use bypass operations do so to increase the weight loss. As the standard bypass operation does not bring most patients to a normal weight, there is too often a conversion to a more radical bypass of intestine with consequent increase in risk of malabsorption complications, stomal ulcer, duodenal ulcer (unless the distal stomach is removed) and closed segment obstruction with serious to lethal consequences if it is not promptly diagnosed and treated by operation. Furthermore, the complications are likely to occur where there is no surgeon available who is experienced in the care of these patients. The simplest operation is a pure vertical gastroplasty that restricts food intake. Such an operation is the least likely to lead to further and more radical operations, with ultimately irreversible changes in the digestive tract.

Indications

The justification of operative treatment of severe obesity rests on the presence of a body weight high enough to impair the ability to work, play and be comfortable with the normal acts of daily living. In addition, there must be an implied or apparent impairment of health or a decrease in life expectancy. This is the basis for the guideline of at least 45 kg over estimated ideal weight. Surgical treatment of severe obesity by an operation is also justified by the absence of any effective non-operative treatment. Diet is effective only temporarily or in a controlled environment. It should not be necessary for a patient to have documented proof of failure of dietary treatment before an operation can be used, because there are no documented safe and effective lifelong non-operative treatments. Finally, it is necessary to have available a safe and effective operation that will improve the quality of life, decrease the risk of complications, and increase longevity for the majority of patients who are treated.

Preoperative

Assessment and preparation

The prospective patient should be judged by an experienced clinician to have a low probability of success with non-operative treatment. There should be either a failure of dietary treatment or a reluctance on the part of the patient to enter into a non-operative treatment programme. The patient should be well informed and motivated. Television tapes and booklets are an excellent means of educating patients as to what to expect in the hospital, after an operation and how to eat to obtain optimum benefit from the operation. The risk and restriction imposed by the operation must be understood. Proper motivation should be to improve health and quality of life. Patients should be aware that they must participate in their lifelong care and that a normal weight cannot be reached without maximum effort on their part. The patient's goals should be realistic in not expecting a normal weight and in not thinking that further operations can accomplish additional weight loss after they have reached a maximum weight reduction with the primary operation. The patient should understand that the operation does not cure their disease and that they must continue lifelong follow-up.

Risk–benefit assessment must be done for each patient. The patient should be an acceptable operative risk, which may mean that some patients will need a period of hospitalization for supervised dietary weight reduction and physical rehabilitation to eliminate retained fluid, improve cardiac and pulmonary function, and improve general physical reserve. The operation can usually be performed when the cardiorespiratory function is improved to the extent that the patient can maintain nearly normal blood gas levels on room air without assistance from a respirator. It is possible to operate safely on patients who require nasal continuous positive airways pressure if the heart and lungs are functioning normally. The ability of the patient to participate in lifelong follow-up is a desirable guideline but cannot always be assured. In certain instances, exceptions must be made because of the severity of the obesity and the need to improve patient care. For example, patients with low intelligence or well controlled schizophrenia, for whom weight reduction by operation can be of great help in further care, may not be able to assure continued compliance with lifelong follow-up. In addition, other exceptions may be made to some of the above guidelines when, for example, a lower weight is a sufficient indication for operation if there is a life-threatening or health-threatening condition that would benefit from weight maintenance at a lower level. Degenerative joint disease or diabetes that is difficult to control because of the inability of the patient to follow a diabetic diet are examples of situations in which an operation might be considered for a patient whose weight is less than 45 kg above the estimated ideal.

Anaesthesia

The heavier the patient, the more desirable it is that the anaesthetist has experience working with severely obese patients. These patients have a limited ability to restore normal blood gas levels and need to have their airways protected and to remain well oxygenated. Relaxation is even more important with the difficulty in exposure that is often encountered. The agents and the technique used should allow early ambulation and deep breathing. The severely obese achieve the best aeration of their blood when upright, and they do poorly with atelectasis, which is even more likely because of the compression of the lung by external weight as well as by their increased blood volume.

Operation

The surgeon of choice for either Roux-en-Y gastric bypass or vertical banded gastroplasty is one who has made a commitment to the treatment of these patients, is performing the selected operation frequently, and is evaluating results over the years. These operations may not accomplish their purpose if performed only occasionally or by surgeons who do not measure the pouch or understand the many details of the operation that help to make the operation both safe and effective. Vertical banded gastroplasty is recommended at the University of Iowa Hospitals and Clinics as the simplest and safest operation. It requires a pouch measuring 10–16 ml in volume and is constructed with a stapler that fires four rows of staples from a single cartridge, with the rows 1 mm apart. It can produce weight control that is nearly equal to that of Roux-en-Y gastric bypass if the pouch is measured and small. Gastric bypass is less dependent on intraoperative measurements and may provide better early weight loss because of the dumping symptoms with sugar-rich foods. It allows the patient to eat foods that are more fibrous and are not as well chewed. Over time, however, the pouch, stoma and adjacent jejunum stretch after Roux-en-Y gastric bypass, with a progressive increase in the amount of food that can be eaten at one time and, in a significant number of patients, a loss of weight control.

Position of patient

Positioning of the patient on the operating table should be performed while the patient is awake to avoid unnecessary lifting, and the gown should be untied and out from under the patient. An upright foot board is placed so that the patient will not slide when the table is tilted into the reverse Trendelenburg position. Padded straps are placed across the legs near the knees to keep the knees from bending when the table is tilted up. The arms are suspended with skin traction from upright holders attached to the table so that the arms and drapes will move with the patient. After the self-retaining retractor is in place, the table is tilted sufficiently into the reverse Trendelenburg position that gravity assists in retraction of the viscera from the upper abdomen.

Incision

1   Vertical banded gastroplasty is performed through a midline upper abdominal incision, distracting the subcutaneous fat. The incision in the linea alba provides maximum strength of closure at the completion of the operation.

A plastic wound protector is used to keep the wound edges moist and free of lint. A self-retaining retractor is anchored to the table over the drapes and is used to retract the edges of the wound and to hold the left lobe of the liver up under the diaphragm. The suspensory ligament of the liver is not divided. The operation is carried out from the lesser curvature and with most of the critical manoeuvres performed while the fingers of the surgeon's left hand are in the lesser sac to maintain proper orientation for guiding tubes and staplers safely in the area of the oesophagus, stomach and pancreas. The greater curvature of the stomach and spleen are avoided. No vessels supplying the stomach are divided.

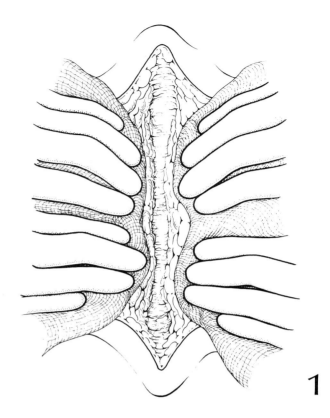

1

Hand position

Six landmarks assist the surgeon during encirclement of the abdominal oesophagus and during placement of a second sling around the lesser omentum. These are the oesophageal diaphragmatic hiatus, the oesophagus with an indwelling 32-Fr Ewald tube, the angle of His, the lesser sac, the crow's foot of the anterior nerve of Laterjet with accompanying vessels, and the folded edge of the lesser curvature of the stomach. Except for the crow's foot, these are all identifiable by palpation. The sense of touch adds greatly to visual identification of landmarks in this operation, as some areas behind the

oesophagus and stomach cannot be seen but must be safely dissected. The surgeon also makes use of bimanual examination and dissection, and at several steps in the operation makes use of the kinesthetics of holding or performing a manoeuvre while the opposite hand provides countertraction or holds an instrument in order to provide additional spatial orientation. The Ewald tube is passed by the anaesthetist through the mouth early in the operation, while the surgeon monitors the position of the tube along the lesser curvature.

Preparation of stomach for stapling

2 The cardia is left attached posteriorly, and the dissection is carried out above it. The dissection is directed into the posterior mediastinum above the left gastric artery and into the area encompassed by the oesophageal hiatus. This is safely accomplished by grasping the oesophagus with the indwelling Ewald tube and elevating it with the left hand, while the index finger of the right hand opens up the area behind.

When the dissection meets tissue that is too tough to easily separate, a shift of hands allows the right hand to hold the oesophagus while the left index finger explores the posterior mediastinal tissues. This technique of 'walking' around the back of the oesophagus with the index fingers protects the oesophagus from injury. The blunt dissection is kept within the oesophageal hiatus posteriorly and is directed cephalad, because the diaphragm forms an arching roof to the abdomen and it is important to avoid the attachments of the cardia posteriorly.

3 Once the oesophagus has been encircled by the surgeon's dissecting fingers it is held in the left hand, with the left index finger approximated to the thumb, while a Harrington–Mixter clamp is inserted with the right hand so that the point is on the left index finger. The tip of the instrument can then be safely guided around the back of the oesophagus while being held firmly against the surgeon's finger. A Penrose drain is then inserted into the jaws of the Harrington–Mixter clamp under direct vision and pulled around the oesophagus.

The second step in preparation of the stomach is carried out through the area between the lesser curvature and the liver, where the pancreas can almost always be seen covered by a diaphanous membrane. The membrane is avascular and is gently wiped away as the surgeon inserts the fingers of the left hand into the lesser sac from the lesser curvature aspect, below the left gastric artery, and to the patient's left of the porta hepatis. The smooth posterior wall of the stomach is then explored, freeing it from any avascular fine attachments that may exist between the stomach and pancreas. There may be an extension of the membrane that covered the pancreas posterior to the stomach, and this membrane should be wiped away so that the stomach can be spread out and its smooth posterior wall examined.

With the 32-Fr Ewald tube positioned along the lesser curvature in the lumen of the stomach, the lesser curvature is elevated to demonstrate the crow's foot. Although this is made up of fibres of the anterior branch of the nerve of Latarjet, it is best identified from the accompanying vessels. There is almost always a spur on the crow's foot which is located at about the point

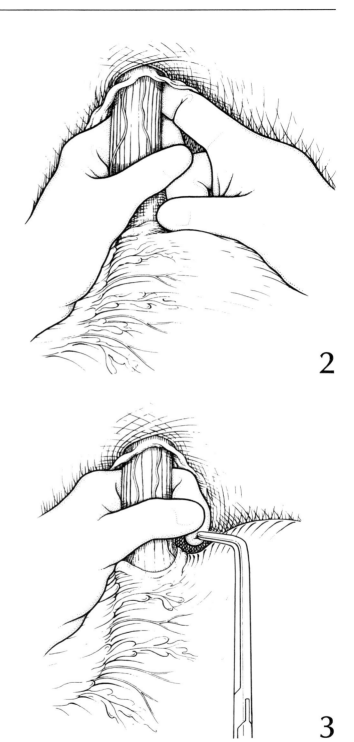

where the outlet of the pouch should be. It is usually better to go orally than aborally to this branch, if such a choice must be made regarding the location of the outlet of the pouch. The pouch should not be more than 9 cm long and preferably about 7 cm. Measurement with a ruler from the angle of His may help in deciding on the location of the opening.

4a, b

An opening must be made near the lesser curvature, and this is accomplished without dividing any vessels by compressing the anterior and posterior parietal peritoneal surface of the lesser omentum at the chosen level. The folded edge of the lesser curvature can be felt and will slide out of the pinching thumb and index finger so that when the tip of an Adson haemostat is inserted through these tissues, the stomach is not injured.

The site should be located where there are no obvious small vessels and a few millimetres away from the edge of the stomach, so that a small branch of the artery or vein will not be avulsed. There is not much room here, but little is required. A second Penrose drain is picked up with the Adson haemostat and brought around the lesser omentum. No vessels have been divided during the dissection up to this point in the preparation of the stomach for stapling.

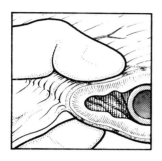 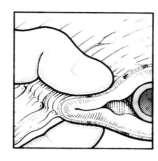 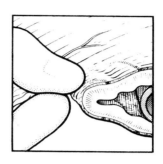

4a

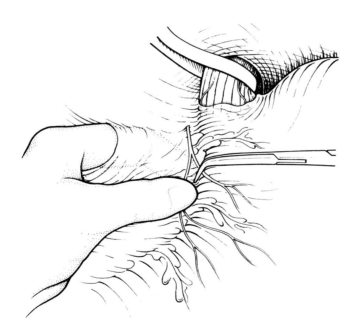

4b

Gastric stapling

5 The anvil of a 25-mm circular EEA stapler is placed between the first and second fingers of the left hand and held up against the posterior wall of the stomach in the lesser sac and near the Ewald tube, which is held along the lesser curvature to help in placement of the window. The surgeon's thumb feels and stabilizes the anvil by palpation through the anterior wall of the stomach. The anvil is adjusted so that it is opposite the lower Penrose drain, where the drain passes through the lesser omentum, near the lesser curvature. There must be enough stomach wall between the prospective EEA window and the lesser curvature so that, when the EEA stapler is closed, the stomach will not be pulled out of the clamp. This is not the time for calibration of the pouch. The lesser curvature of the stomach must not be pulled too tightly around the Ewald tube. There should not be so much redundant stomach, however, that the wall of the stomach will be pleated beneath the collar. There should be enough room from the fundus to empty into the antrum, past the greater curvature side of the window. The lesser omentum should not be caught between the anvil and the posterior wall of the stomach.

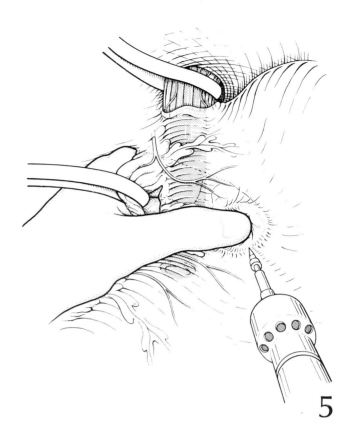

5

6 The yellow plastic pointed tip that has been snapped onto the end of the shaft of the stapler is now placed where the centre of the anvil has been felt and is directed at right angles to the surface of the anterior stomach wall, through the stomach, and into the central hole of the anvil. As the pointed tip comes through the back wall of the stomach and enters the central hole in the anvil, the stomach wall becomes gripped between the tip and the anvil. The surgeon then allows the anvil to fall back into the palm of the hand and slides the thumb and fingers of that hand to a position around the tip (as one would hold a strawberry to be enjoyed) and the stomach is pushed further up onto the shaft. Thus, there is no danger of injury to the pancreas, and the shaft of the stapler is moved far enough through the stomach so that the posterior stomach wall will remain on the shaft as the tapered point is angled off and the anvil is attached.

It is important that the shaft of the stapler is not moved laterally during these manoeuvres, because such movement will enlarge the opening made by the stapler shaft in the stomach wall, allowing leakage of gastric contents and increasing the chance of incomplete rings of staples. The stapler is closed, fired and removed, and the two rings of stomach inspected for completeness. If there are spurting bleeders in the cut edge of the window, these are secured with figure-of-eight sutures, placed between the staples and the cut edge, so as not to distort the position of the staples.

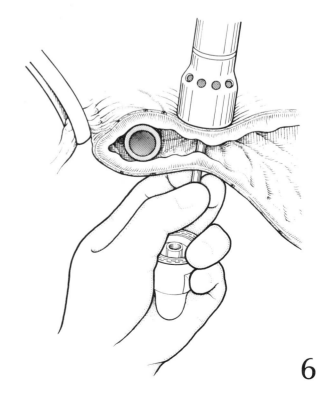

6

7 The index finger of the left hand is now placed into the lesser sac from the lesser curvature through the area over the pancreas, and the stapled window is palpated. The finger is then slid cephalad on the smooth posterior surface of the stomach towards the angle of His. The Ewald tube acts as a landmark, and the Penrose drain around the abdominal oesophagus shows exactly where the gastro-oesophageal angle is located.

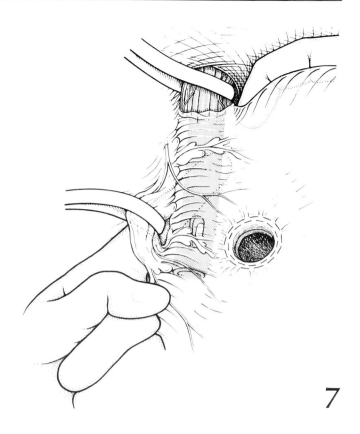

7

The index finger of the right hand is simultaneously slid up on the anterior surface of the stomach toward the same target area. In the region of the angle, the stomach is no longer smooth because it is covered with connective tissue posteriorly, and there is a small anterior fat pad. A bimanual blunt dissection is carried into the angle, in the same fashion as the dissection of the abdominal oesophagus, using one hand to hold the stomach safe from injury while the opposite index finger develops a passage. When the dissection becomes difficult, the opposite index finger is used at a more dorsal level to continue the dissection, 'walking' the fingers past the gastro-oesophageal junction and over the angle of His, into the lesser sac.

Once this channel is open, the stomach is grasped in the left hand, with the index finger and thumb approximated over the angle. The point of the Harrington–Mixter clamp is placed by the surgeon's right hand with the point of the clamp on the left index finger and carefully guided over the angle of His and into the lesser sac. The assistant then passes the closed end of a 26-Fr rubber Robinson catheter down into the surgeon's left palm and into the groove between the first and second fingers, where it is carefully manoeuvred by the surgeon's left hand into the opened Harrington–Mixter clamp. The point of the clamp remains against the surgeon's index finger to protect the posterior wall of the stomach from injury. The Robinson catheter is then pulled around the angle and left in position. The tip of the freed Harrington–Mixter clamp is then guided from anterior into the stapled window and out of the opening between the lesser omentum and liver and used to pull the back end of the Robinson catheter out

through the window. The end of the Penrose drain that encircles the lesser omentum is similarly pulled through the window so that it is now around the outlet of the pouch. The tip of the Harrington–Mixter clamp is always guided by the surgeon on the tip of the opposing index finger when the clamp is out of direct line of vision.

The toe of a four-row vertical stapler (TA-90B) is inserted into the back end of the Robinson catheter, which is used to guide the stapler through the previously stapled window, the lesser sac and beyond the angle of His. The surgeon's left hand in the lesser sac assists the positioning of the stomach in the stapler. The window can usually be lifted gently around the heel of the stapler to help stretch the stomach out in the clamp.

8 The next manoeuvre seems awkward until learned, but moves the toe of the stapler safely beyond the stomach and holds it there, while the pin is inserted. In this manoeuvre the surgeon uses the left index finger from the patient's left of the clamp and follows the Robinson catheter around to where the anvil is felt, and then lifts the angle of His over the toe of the stapler and into the clamp. The left index finger is then used to hold the stomach in the clamp, while the Robinson catheter is removed with a large curved clamp which is used to grasp the catheter just beyond the toe of the stapler and is then levered over the end of the staple cartridge to dislodge the catheter from the toe of the anvil. With the stomach held in the clamp by the left index finger, the pin is placed in the four-row vertical stapler, thus avoiding injury to the stomach by the pin at the angle.

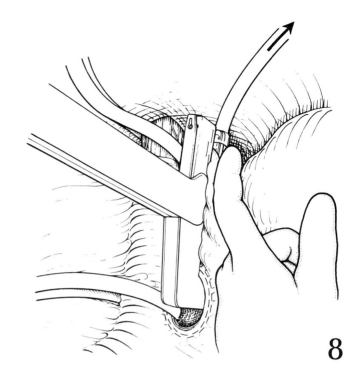

8

9 The stomach is pulled through the vertical stapler to obtain a small pouch by holding the stapler up with the left hand while the stomach is pulled through the jaws of the clamp and over the anvil with the right hand.

The majority of surgeons do not measure the pouch and are unaware of how difficult it is, in some patients, to obtain a small pouch. Pouches average 13 ml in volume and should not be larger than 16 ml when measured with the clamp in place. It is not unusual for a surgeon who is inexperienced with the operation to require several measurements and readjustments of the stomach in the clamp to achieve the required small pouch. Even with experience it is common to be surprised by a measured pouch that is larger than optimum and must be made smaller before the staples are fired. Measurement at the primary operation will save many patients another operation for inadequate weight control, reflux, vomiting, or various combinations of these undesirable outcomes. Some surgeons have given up the use of vertical banded gastroplasty because of this avoidable sequence of events and a failure to realize that too large a pouch was the basis for their dissatisfaction with the operation.

Calibration of the pouch is accomplished by a slide of the stomach over the anvil, coordinated under the operator's watchful eye. The open stapler is lifted with the surgeon's left hand while the right hand gently pulls the stomach down over the anvil. An unfolded lap pad is placed close to the clamp on the anterior wall of the stomach to provide needed traction for the fingers that are placed close to the anvil on the lap pad. Downward pressure on the stomach, while the stapler is lifted, pulls the pouch containing the 32-Fr Ewald tube towards the clamp. The surgeon has control of the stapler and can close it with the left hand at that point where the pouch is thought to be of a properly small and uniform width.

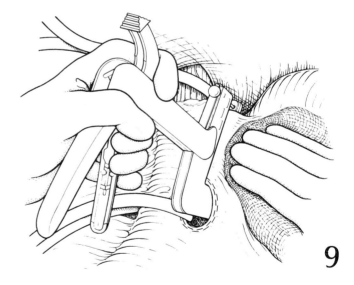

9

The desired shape of the vertical pouch is neither a light bulb with an expanded upper end nor an hourglass, but a cylinder that has a uniform, narrow width. The upper end of the stapler should extend to, or even cephalad to, the angle of His, to ensure that there is no defect in the upper end of the staple line. It must not be positioned with the upper end angled out onto the fundus. Quality control requires measurement of pouch volume at a hydrostatic pressure of 70 cm. The 32-Fr Ewald tube is positioned so that the rounded end of the tube is at the constricted lower end of the pouch. The vertical stapler is not fired until the desired pouch volume is achieved.

Pouch measurement

10 The Ewald tube is always positioned so that the end is beyond the outlet when the vertical stapler is positioned so that the outlet will not be compromised. The first step in measuring the pouch is therefore to move the Ewald tube back into the lower end of the pouch. The Penrose drains are tightened and clamped at both ends of the pouch.

The Ewald tube is filled with saline from an open syringe attached to the upper end of its extension. The tube with its extension must be long enough to reach from the stomach to at least 70 cm above the stomach (ear level). The operating table should be level during measurement. This will also relieve any congestion that has developed in the lower extremities from the reversed Trendelenburg position. Keeping the tube on a slant with no redundant loops will help displace any contained air with saline, which is required in order that an accurate measurement can be obtained. The non-sterile tube is managed by the circulating nurse. The surgeon can help to evacuate air from the pouch by compressing it. This also provides the surgeon with information about the approximate size of the pouch and whether there is free communication between the pouch and the syringe.

A 70-cm suture is held at the ear and the other end at the meniscus and a reading is taken where the meniscus is located on the calibrations of the syringe. The syringe is then lowered to the ear level and a second reading taken. The difference plus 8 ml for the volume of Ewald tubing that is in the pouch represents the volume of the pouch. Readings are taken until two duplicate measurements are obtained. If the pouch is 17 ml or greater in volume, the syringe is lowered so as to not trap air, the

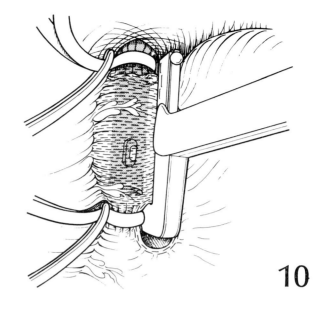

10

vertical stapler is opened and the stomach pulled over further. During this manoeuvre, the Ewald tube is positioned through the outlet of the pouch and after the stapler is closed the tube is pulled back to within the pouch for further measurement. With experience, a small pouch can be obtained and measured in only a few minutes. Even if a longer time is required, it will save some patients another operation and is therefore well worth the time required to obtain an accurate measurement. The pin should be completely removed before the vertical stapler is opened in order to avoid laceration of the anterior wall of the stomach. When the stapler is opened, the stomach, colon, or other tissue should not be pinched in the portion of the stapler between the frame and the cartridge holder.

Placement of Marlex mesh

11 Marlex mesh is cut to 7 × 1.5 cm from a piece of mesh 3 × 10 cm which has two non-stretching selvedges and is oriented with the weave, so that it will stretch under tension along the cut edge. It will not stretch across the width or on the remaining selvedge. The mesh is marked near one end and at 5 cm from the first mark, so that the final collar will be 5 cm in circumference when the material is not under tension. It is placed without twist or cuff while held in a Harrington–Mixter clamp, with the cut edge of the mesh orally and the selvedge aborally. This provides compliance of the collar with the pouch during expansion after a meal, facilitated by the stretch of the cut edge near the pouch. The selvedge, away from the pouch, will not stretch. Thus, a potential funnel into the outlet is created in order to avoid pressure of the oral edge of the collar on the wall of the pouch at the outlet at times when there is a full pouch. The object is not obstruction but a prevention of progressive dilatation of the outlet of the pouch. The overlapping Marlex is sewn with the first calibration stitch of polypropylene through the two marks, followed by two more stitches. These are arranged serially along the middle of the overlapped ends of the mesh so that the upper edge can expand with the pouch as it expands with a meal.

The sutures are prevented from entering the wall of the stomach by placement of the handle of a forceps between the collar and the stomach while the second and third sutures are placed. Thus, luminal bacteria will not have a ready pathway to the mesh along the non-absorbable sutures that coapt the overlapping ends of the mesh.

The window allows positioning of the collar and maintains this position as the collar is infiltrated with connective tissue. The collar becomes a new layer on the outer surface of the stomach at the outlet of the pouch, and thus stabilizes the outlet at a circumference with an inside diameter of about 11 mm. The actual diameter depends also on how much stomach wall is included under the collar and the compressibility of this tissue during the passage of pouch contents into the distal stomach. The objective of gastric reduction operations is to stabilize the outlet at approximately 11 mm inside diameter, but not to create obstruction. If there is a cuff on the collar after it is sewn in place, this should be effaced by grasping one edge with a haemostat for countertraction while the cuff is unfolded

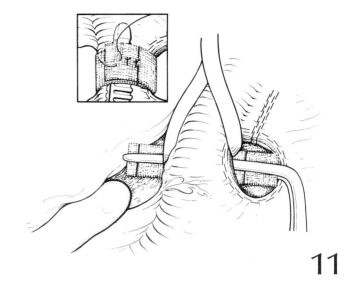

11

with a right-angled haemostat. The collar can be rotated on the outlet of the pouch to get at the back wall if the cuff is located there. Once the collar is free of cuff it will remain flat.

The entire stomach is distended with air under sterile saline to check for leaks. During this the Penrose drain is tightened around the oesophagus, and the antrum and duodenum are invaginated into the pyloric ring with the left index finger and thumb to keep the air in the stomach. The right hand is used to monitor the pressure by palpation so as to not overdistend the stomach with air. If bubbling is seen, the abdominal saline is aspirated until the site can be identified, and sutures are placed to close the leak. Leaks are occasionally observed, but if present are usually in the cut edge of the stapled window. Finally, the Ewald tube is advanced into the main stomach and the air aspirated. The Ewald tube is then removed. No nasogastric tube is used. The passage of the Ewald tube through the outlet of the pouch is a final check on the adequacy of the lumen of the pouch outlet. In fact, it always does pass easily.

Wound closure

12 Early in the history of vertical banded gastroplasty it was observed that although Marlex mesh is inert, infiltration with connective tissue occurs, and this tissue can adhere to the left lobe of the liver if the mesh is not covered by omentum. Such adherence may cause obstruction by kinking of the outlet of the pouch. Therefore, the greater omentum is sewn to the lesser omentum with three sutures to cover the Marlex mesh. Omentum is brought up from wherever it is most redundant, taking care not to pull omental attachments from the capsule of the spleen.

Closure is performed using 1 Maxon as a running suture in the fascia. The subcutaneous tissues are irrigated with sterile saline until all loose particles of fat have been washed out. Haemostasis is complete at the time of opening of the abdomen, but is confirmed at the time of closure. No drains or sutures are used in the subcutaneous space. The skin is approximated with stainless steel skin staples.

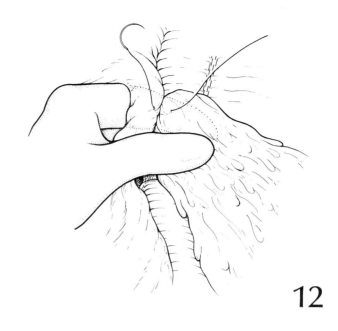

12

Postoperative care

Heavy patients experience compression of the lungs from the weight of fat on the chest and on the abdomen, forcing the diaphragm to rise. There is also an increase in blood volume, which compresses the alveoli from within. A semi-upright position takes away some of this compression excess, both externally and internally, and improves the patient's ability to breathe. Oxygen saturation is monitored with oximetry and appropriate analyses of arterial blood during the early recovery period. Oxygen is administered by respirator, nasal tongs, or not at all, depending on the results of the early arterial blood gas analyses. Most patients are extubated before they leave the operating room. As soon as possible patients are asked to walk, and this is repeated several times the first night and frequently thereafter. No nasogastric tube is used. Clear liquids are commenced the first morning after operation, and pureed food the second morning. Patients use a medicine cup to drink and eat out of, to remind them not to take too much at any one time. They are usually discharged on the fourth or fifth day after operation. They are given small multivitamin capsules and advised not to take any irritating drugs such as aspirin (or most of the substitutes for aspirin). Paracetamol (acetaminophen) is allowed. They are asked to avoid any large pills that might block the pouch and cause vomiting. Some pills can be crushed, and liquid medications can be used. Any patient with heartburn should be questioned about medications being taken.

Outcome

Approximately 80% of morbidly obese patients (weighing 160–225% of estimated ideal at the time of operation) are successful in maintaining a loss of at least 25% of their excess weight at 5 years. Failure was due to inadequate weight loss in 13.9% or revision in 6.1%. These are minimal figures for success, as the patients evaluated were from the earliest years of experience with the operation, and there have been some additional changes in the operative technique during the last decade. Fifty-one percent of morbidly obese patients sustained a loss of more than 50% of their excess weight at 5 years. The superobese patients (those with an operative weight of more than 225% of ideal) were 75% successful at 5 years. They also had a 6% reoperation rate during the 5 years which assigned them to the failure group. There was a marked decrease in the need for medications for diabetes and hypertension in all of the successful patients. Death from complications of obesity have been reduced and operative mortality has been maintained at a level of 0.3%. As a result, the risk of death for all patients after vertical banded gastroplasty during the last 10 years has not been significantly different from the risk for a comparable group of people, matched for sex and age, derived from the United States Census for 1984.

Further reading

Gastrointestinal surgery for severe obesity: proceedings of a National Institute of Health Consensus Development Conference. *Am J Clin Nutr* 1992; 55(suppl).

Mason EE. Vertical banded gastroplasty for obesity. *Arch Surg* 1982; 117: 701–6.

Mason EE, Maher JW, Scott DH, Rodriguez EM, Doherty C. Ten years of vertical banded gastroplasty for severe obesity. *Probl Gen Surg* 1992; 9: 280–9.

Mason EE, Renquist KE, Jiang D. Perioperative risks and safety of surgery for severe obesity. *Am J Clin Nutr* 1992; 55: 573S–6S.

Scopinaro N, Gianetta E, Friedman D, Traverso E, Adami GF, Vitale B. Biliopancreatic diversion for obesity. *Probl Gen Surg* 1992; 9: 362–79.

Yale CE. Choice of operation for morbid obesity. *Probl Gen Surg* 1992; 9: 406–10.

General techniques in abdominal laparoscopic surgery

Allan E. Siperstein MD

Department of Surgery, Mount Zion Medical Center of University of California, San Francisco, USA

Laparoscopic surgery promises to be a major revolution in the field of general surgery. It is now realized that the pain and other inflammatory mediators resulting from a large abdominal incision, rather than the intra-abdominal dissection, are the major determinants of speed of perioperative recuperation. The advantages of minimally invasive surgery are well known in other surgical disciplines such as gynaecology and orthopaedics, and general surgeons have been relatively slow in adopting this technology. Several years ago, laparoscopic cholecystectomy was considered to be a clinical curiosity and its acceptance by the surgical community was delayed, in part because of its radical departure from standard surgical practice and in part because it was developed outside major academic centres. A variety of complex general surgical procedures, including colonic resection, gastric resection, Nissen fundoplication, adrenalectomy and even Whipple procedures have now been successfully performed laparoscopically, and it is felt by many in the field that in the future the majority of cases will be performed laparoscopically, including operations such as hepatic resection and vascular anastomoses.

Factors driving the rapid advancement in laparoscopic surgery are rapid recovery and discharge of the patient from hospital. There appear to be fewer wound problems, especially with infection and dehiscence, as the small portals of entry result in far less tissue devascularization. There is also considerable drive from the patients to have their procedures performed laparoscopically because of the decreased perioperative pain, an earlier return to work and a better cosmetic result. Reports of higher complication rates with laparoscopic surgery, especially among surgeons with more limited experience, are cause for concern. As the surgeon's experience increases, the complication rate decreases significantly to the point where currently the rate of complications of laparoscopic cholecystectomy may be the same as, or lower than, that for open cholecystectomy.

This chapter will review the major techniques common to laparoscopic surgery. Previously, emphasis has been placed on reinventing operations so that they may be undertaken laparoscopically. Now there is more emphasis placed on applying the tried and established methods of open surgery to laparoscopic procedures. Although much of the instrumentation may be different, the honoured principles of gentle tissue handling, careful dissection, exposure and haemostasis apply equally to both open and laparoscopic surgery.

Equipment

Video cameras

1 The technical advance that made laparoscopic surgery practical, although it had been in theory possible for many decades, was the advent of the single chip camera. This was small enough to be used practically in the operating room.

Previously, laparoscopic procedures, mostly diagnostic, had been widely performed; however, the surgeon had to look directly through the laparoscope so that only one person at a time in the operating room could view the field. This made it possible for a single operator to perform only diagnostic laparoscopy and simple tissue manipulation and biopsy. Beam splitters were developed that allowed two surgeons to look through the same laparoscope simultaneously, but these were cumbersome and reduced the brightness of the field considerably. With the advent of the video camera attached to the end of the laparoscope, it is now possible for all personnel in the operating room to view the operative field comfortably.

Laparoscopic surgery also represents a new era of technical and electronic complexity in the operating room, requiring a variety of electronic equipment, including cameras, light sources, insufflators, television monitors and often video cassette recorders and video printers. This equipment is delicate, expensive and requires considerable training in its use and maintenance. As all personnel are able to view the operative field equally well, this has resulted in a different level of interaction between the surgeons and the nursing staff. Once the nurses are trained in the step-by-step conduct of the procedure, they are better able to anticipate the instrument needs of the surgeon.

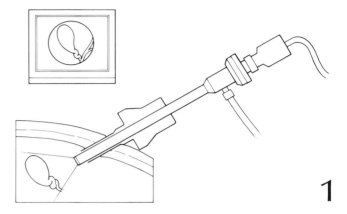

1

Instruments

2a–i Laparoscopic surgery presents several major limitations not present in open surgery. A more limited array of instruments is available, but new instrumentation is evolving rapidly, with many new and innovative products being brought to market. Currently there is a variety of instruments, such as straight and curved dissectors, scissors, cautery devices, bowel graspers, and more that are of a design very similar to that used in open surgery. A major limitation placed on the surgeon is the restricted degree of freedom of instrument movement imposed by working through ports placed through the abdominal wall. The surgeon is able to move the instrument in and out of the port, rotate it along the axis of the port and pivot it around its fixed point in the abdominal wall. This is considerably more limiting than the movements possible by the human arm and hand, and requires new skills so that instrument movement is not clumsy. The laparoscopic surgeon manipulates a three-dimensional world on a two-dimensional television monitor and therefore lacks binocular vision. Depth perception is considerably impaired, often resulting in repetitive motions of underpointing or pastpointing. As the surgeon's hands are no longer able to manipulate tissue directly, there is severely diminished tactile feedback. By probing the tissues with an instrument the surgeon is able to gain some idea as to how rigid or mobile a structure is but this sense is obviously severely impaired.

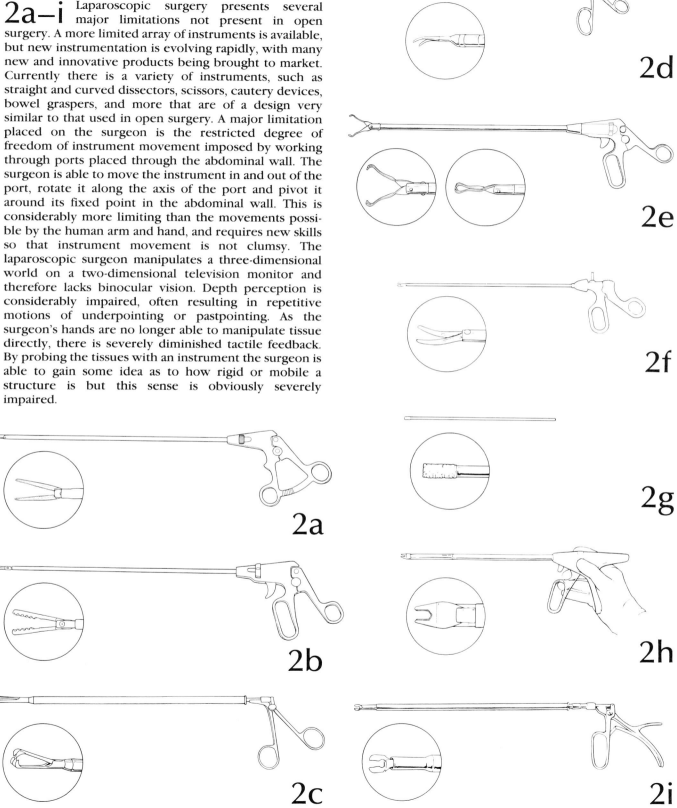

2a

2b

2c

2d

2e

2f

2g

2h

2i

Operative techniques

Abdominal procedures

3 A prerequisite for performing a laparoscopic procedure is creation of a potential working space within the abdominal cavity as well as the use of trochars to provide a portal for entry. This is most commonly done by insufflating the peritoneal cavity with carbon dioxide gas to a pressure of 15 mmHg. Insufflators now exist that automatically sense the intra-abdominal pressure and deliver carbon dioxide gas at a controlled rate until the desired pressure is established.

4 To create a pneumoperitoneum, the most common technique is to create an infraumbilical incision where the abdominal wall is thin. It is then important that the abdominal wall is pulled upwards, usually with towel clips, to create a negative intra-abdominal pressure so that a specially designed Veress needle can be passed into the abdominal cavity. The needle itself is designed with a spring-loaded blunt tip that retracts into the shaft of the needle when pushed against the tissues. This exposes the sharp tip of the needle which may be felt to pop twice as it crosses first the fascia and then the peritoneum. The spring-loaded blunt tip then slides forward, protecting the viscera from the sharp needle tip. The purpose of pulling up on the abdominal wall is both to put the fascia under tension and to create a negative intra-abdominal pressure so that when the needle enters the peritoneal cavity, air begins to enter the peritoneum through the needle, further helping to keep the needle tip away from the viscera.

Various methods have been described to try to improve the safety of this technique. The patient is placed in a Trendelenburg position so that the viscera moves cephalad and the needle is directed towards the pelvis to minimize the chance of entering the aorta or vena cava. It is most important, however, to appreciate the tactile feedback from the Veress needle such that advancement is stopped once the needle is felt to enter the peritoneal cavity. The major contraindication to use of the Veress needle is previous abdominal surgery in the area where the needle is to be placed, as the viscera may have adhered to the abdominal wall.

Once the tip of the needle is felt to be within the peritoneal cavity, it is essential to perform a saline drop test. A syringe with saline is affixed to the needle; the most important part of this test is actually drawing back on the syringe to make sure that neither the bowel nor a blood vessel has been entered. A small amount of saline is then gently injected, feeling that there is no undue resistance. Finally, the syringe is taken off the Veress needle and the small amount of saline left in the hub of the needle is seen to drop freely into the peritoneal cavity. At this point it is safe to attach the hose from the insufflator to the Veress needle and begin insufflation

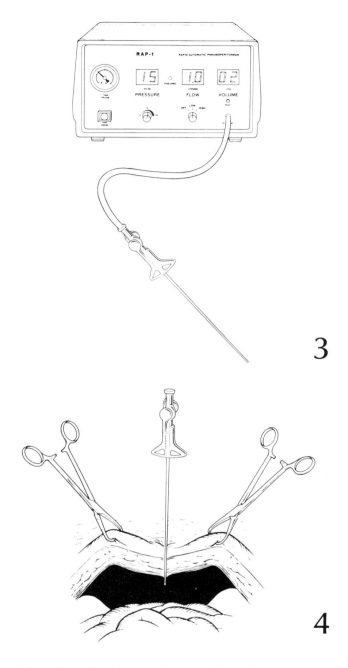

with carbon dioxide at a low rate for at least the first litre. The abdomen should be percussed at this point to ensure that a pneumoperitoneum is being established. While gas is being introduced, it is important to see that the abdomen is distending symmetrically, otherwise the tip of the needle may have inadvertently entered the viscera. To reduce potential complications further, all patients should have nasogastric tubes and Foley catheters placed before the beginning of the procedure so that these structures are maximally decompressed. During the process of insufflation it is best to keep the Veress needle still to minimize the chance of bowel laceration.

Placement of trocars

5 Once pneumoperitoneum has been established to 15 mm pressure, a 10-mm diameter laparoscopic trocar for the camera is placed through the infraumbilical incision. Most of the designs today consist of a sharp metal point for cutting through the abdominal wall and some mechanism to prevent the point from cutting the viscera once it has entered the abdominal cavity. After the Veress needle has been withdrawn, the trocar is pushed with constant pressure, sometimes with a slight twisting motion, to advance it through the abdominal wall. It is important to apply most of the force through the wrist rather than the shoulder. In addition, the other hand should grip the shaft of the trocar to prevent sudden overadvancement of the trocar into the underlying structures once it has cut through the abdominal wall. Again, tactile feedback is important to place these trocars safely. The sudden decrease in resistance as the trocar goes through the abdominal wall and the subtle click of the safety shield coming into place should alert the surgeon that the tip of the trocar has entered the peritoneal cavity. The centre core of the trocar is then removed, leaving a thin tube through the abdominal wall with some type of valve arrangement to retain the pneumoperitoneum when no instrument is in the trocar.

6 Alternative methods exist for obtaining access to the abdominal cavity. Hasson has developed a blunt-tipped trocar that bears his name.

It is inserted by performing a small, usually infraumbilical, cut down so that the peritoneal cavity can be entered directly. Once this has been done, the blunt-tipped trocar is passed under direct vision into the abdominal cavity, and as a slightly larger skin incision must be made, sutures are used to approximate tissue and to hold the trocar in place. The method is indicated in patients who have had previous surgical incisions near the intended site of trocar placement. In fact, this method offers several advantages and should be considered for routine use. As the abdominal cavity is entered directly and without sharp instruments, the risk of bowel or vessel injury is minimized. In addition, as the diameter of this trocar is much larger than that of the Veress needle, the pneumoperitoneum may be established much more rapidly, allowing the laparoscope to be introduced into the abdomen and the procedure started before the full pneumoperitoneum has been established. Many patients have a small umbilical hernia and this pre-existing fascial defect is easily and quickly entered with the Hasson trocar.

Other alternative methods to pneumoperitoneum establishment have been described using so-called gasless laparoscopy where the potential space in the peritoneal cavity is created by lifting up on the abdominal wall with a device placed within the peritoneal cavity. One potential advantage of such an

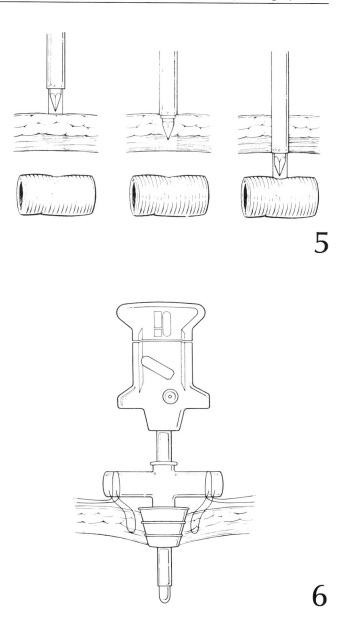

5

6

approach is that there is no risk of gas embolization in the creation of the pneumoperitoneum. Another is that trocars may be used without the valves or reducers which are necessary for an airtight fit in conventional laparoscopy. What has limited the widespread acceptance of such devices is the fact that they create less space within the abdominal cavity. The technique may be suitable for more limited procedures.

To access the thoracic cavity, no gas needs to be instilled. In fact, this should in general be avoided because of the risk of gas embolism. A small incision is made between the ribs and a valveless trocar may be placed directly into the thoracic cavity. Double-lumen endotracheal tubes are used and the lung on the operated side is allowed to deflate.

Laparoscopes

7a–d The laparoscope consists of a metal rod usually 10 mm in diameter with a viewing port as well as another channel for illuminating the field via a fibreoptic cable connected to a light source. The camera is clipped to the back of the laparoscope, thus allowing the image to be displayed on a television monitor. The simplest laparoscopes to use are the 0° or end-viewing design in which the field of view is directly ahead of the scope. An alternative design is for the field of view to be angled at 30° or 45° from the axis of the laparoscope. The advantage of this configuration is that the laparoscope may be moved in an arc allowing two sides of a given structure to be observed. With the 0° laparoscope it is possible only to move nearer to or farther from an object but not to change the angle of view. With more complex laparoscopic procedures it is highly desirable to be able to view a given structure from different angles during the course of dissection. Although the field of view is generally small, it is highly magnified, allowing fine structures, even small blood vessels, to be identified.

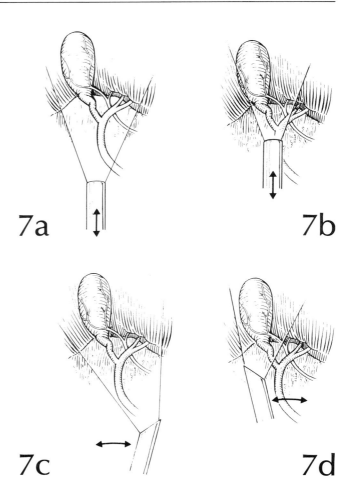

7a

7b

7c

7d

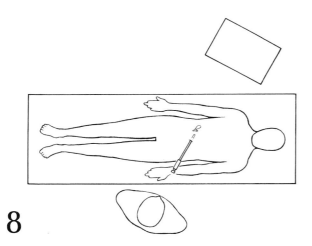

8

8 For the direction of instrument movement to correspond with what is seen on the television monitor, it is important for the surgeon to be positioned directly behind the laparoscope, with the instrument aimed directly toward the television monitor. This arrangement is important and is often not fully appreciated. When this position is not taken, the surgeon's movement to the right in the operating field will appear as a movement to the left on the monitor, making co-ordinated fine movements difficult.

This results in the placement of operative personnel differently from in open procedures. For example, in laparoscopic appendicectomies the surgeon should stand to the patient's left, with the laparoscope at the umbilicus pointing into the right lower quadrant with the monitor directly ahead of this to the right of the patient's feet. Given the length of the laparoscopic instruments, this also makes for a more comfortable working position for the surgeon.

Placement of additional ports

9a, b Once the viewing laparoscope is in place additional laparoscopic ports are almost always required. These are always placed under direct vision, viewing the peritoneal surface of the abdominal wall as the trocar is placed to avoid visceral injury. While viewing from the inside, the intended place of port placement is indented from the outside with the surgeon's finger. To plan more precisely for port placement, it is useful to use a 22-gauge needle with a local anaesthetic so that the intended path of port placement may be tested, especially when ports are placed near the epigastric vessels, the bladder or adhesions. Injection of local anaesthetic as the needle is slowly withdrawn also provides for excellent postoperative pain relief. An incision is then made in the skin in the direction of Langer's lines or in the direction of the surgical incision should conversion to an open procedure be required. As these ports are placed under direct vision, safety shields around the trocar point are not mandatory, but offer an added margin of safety. It should be emphasized that if difficulty is encountered in having an optimal angle of dissection or if more retraction is required, the surgeon should not hesitate to add additional ports as needed.

Retraction and exposure

Retraction and exposure are areas that pose some difficulty in laparoscopic surgery. The pneumoperitoneum tends to cause the colon and small bowel to fall more toward the side of the abdomen, helping particularly with exposure in the upper abdomen. The organ being removed may itself be grasped and used to help with the exposure. This is most commonly done in cholecystectomy where the fundus of the gallbladder is grasped and pushed as far as possible into the right upper abdomen, thereby rotating the liver cephalad and exposing the cystic and common duct. If atraumatic graspers are used, this technique of retracting the liver is particularly useful in upper abdominal surgery such as laparoscopic closure of a perforated duodenal ulcer or staging laparoscopy for patients with adenocarcinoma at the head of the pancreas. Particularly fragile organs, for example the inflamed appendix, may require more gentle means of retraction. It is useful to place a loop or snare of suture around the distal end of the appendix, tightening it to hold the tissue but not to cut into it. The free end of the suture may then be grasped and used to manipulate the appendix during the course of the dissection with minimal risk of perforation. Solid organs are often easily retracted with the use of specially designed fan retractors. These consist of a shaft that will fit through the laparoscopic trocar with broad deformable attachments that can be moved into position to retract the spleen or liver gently over a broad surface area.

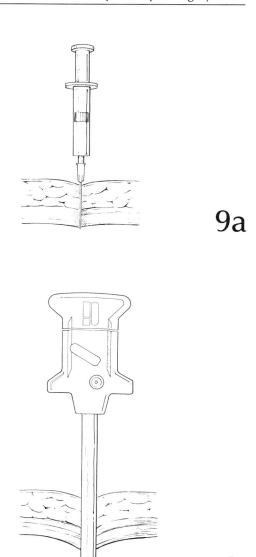

9a

9b

Positioning of the table is also important to allow gravity to assist as much as possible. This is employed to a much greater degree than is usually done in open surgery. The extreme angles used often require that the patient be especially well padded and secured to the operative table. The general principle is that the organ being dissected is elevated. For example, in laparoscopic cholecystectomy the patient is often put in the reverse Trendelenburg position with the right side up, causing the colon and small bowel to fall away from the area of dissection. In laparoscopic adrenalectomy where a medial visceral rotation may be used to gain access to the adrenal gland, the patient is often best positioned entirely on the side.

Principles of dissection

The principles of laparoscopic dissection do not differ fundamentally from methods used in open surgery. It is essential to maintain a dry field at all times, as the smallest oozing will obscure the field. Another important general principle is that dissection should be performed from inferior to superior to avoid blood running down and obscuring the field yet to be dissected. A variety of straight and curved dissectors is now available in configurations identical to those used in open surgery. Monopolar cautery is used quite extensively in an attempt to keep a dry field and a number of the dissecting instruments, including scissors and graspers, have attachments so that they may be used with the monopolar cautery.

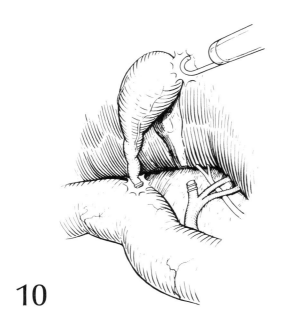

10

10 In addition, hooks with both L- and J-shaped tips are used to dissect gently small strands of tissue before they are cauterized.

Monopolar cautery represents a potential hazard because of the inadvertent conduction to adjacent viscera. This is more of a problem in laparoscopic than in open surgery as the entire length of the instrument may not be in the field of view and part of the instrument may inadvertently be in contact with an adjacent loop of bowel. In addition, the surgical field is generally kept quite dry, increasing the risk of conduction through the tissues themselves but decreasing conduction of current through surrounding fluid. For this reason, a number of bipolar instruments are being developed in which the current is conducted between the jaws of the instrument, minimizing the chance of such conduction injury. Use of laser energy for both cutting and cautery was popular earlier in the history of laparoscopic surgery and the term laser cholecystectomy was often used. Studies have shown that the laser is no more effective than electrocautery, and the cumbersome laser equipment and increased smoke generation within the abdomen make it less effective to use. Although there may be certain applications where laser energy is more effective, it has been abandoned by most general surgeons. Other technologies are being developed using ultrasound energy both to heat and mechanically disrupt tissue.

Suturing and stapling

Conventional suturing is less widely used in laparoscopic surgery as the refined movements to drive a needle through delicate tissue are more difficult to accomplish and continued improvements are being made in the needle holders themselves. For this reason surgeons turn to alternative means to achieve haemostasis or perform an anastomosis. Deformable metal clips, much like those used in open surgery, are widely used laparoscopically. These are available in self-reloading, multiple firing devices. Devices that fire a single staple to approximate two adjacent structures have been developed. These are similar in design to skin staplers and are used laparoscopically to, for example, attach a polypropylene mesh to the underlying fascia in a laparoscopic hernia repair.

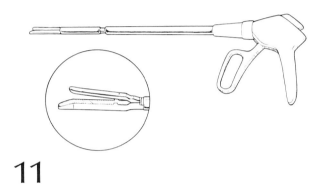

11

11 Stapling devices for performing gastrointestinal anastomoses have been miniaturized and adapted for laparoscopic use. This allows the division of bowel within the abdomen without the risk of stool leakage as well as the creation of anastomoses entirely within the abdominal cavity.

It should be noted that in most laparoscopic bowel resections much of the dissection is performed laparoscopically, then the ends of the bowel to be anastomosed are exteriorized through a small incision and the anastomosis itself performed extracorporeally using more conventional staplers or a suturing technique. Similar laparoscopic stapling devices have been developed that are in fact haemostatic and are extremely useful for dividing bowel mesentery and lung while providing haemostasis. Such stapling devices have even been successfully used to divide and control the splenic artery and vein.

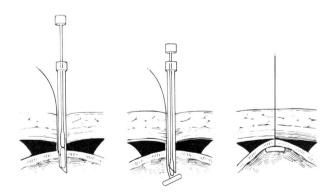

12

12 Other interesting means of suturing have been developed. One of the most novel is the T-fastener. This has been most widely used to secure the stomach or small bowel wall to the abdominal wall in the creation of a laparoscopic gastrostomy or jejunostomy. The device is analogous to that used to secure price tags to clothing: a needle containing a suture with a crossbar at the end is passed into the lumen of the viscus. The T-bar is then ejected within the lumen of the viscus and may be pulled up to secure the organ to the abdominal wall.

Retrieval of a specimen

Once the dissection of an organ has been completed in a laparoscopic procedure, the excised specimen must be removed from the abdomen. The specimen is often larger than the small incisions through the abdominal wall. The fascia around the umbilicus is easily stretched and may be incised with minimal additional discomfort to allow organ removal. In the case of the gallbladder, the neck is often exteriorized and the bile and stones removed to facilitate removal of the gallbladder wall through a 10-mm trocar site. Devices have also been developed to cut larger solid organs into smaller pieces, although in some cases this may interfere with adequate pathological staging of tumours. In laparoscopic hysterectomy the vagina is used to remove the specimen and in laparoscopic sigmoid colon resection the anus has been used for specimen removal, obviating the need for additional skin incisions.

Completion of procedure

At the completion of the procedure, it is important to inspect the operative field under reduced peritoneal pressure as the pneumoperitoneum may tamponade venous or portal bleeding. It is also important that the trocars are removed under direct vision with the laparoscope and the sites inspected to ensure that there is no bleeding. The camera is removed last. It is becoming increasingly recognized that it is important to close the fascia of trocar sites larger than 10 mm to avoid bowel herniation. In closing the fascia at the conclusion of an open surgical procedure, it would be unacceptable to leave a gap in the fascia that would admit a finger. The same principle applies to laparoscopic procedures. Hernation is probably less prevalent than it otherwise would be as many of the trocars are placed obliquely through the abdominal wall resulting in a flap valve effect once the trocars are removed. With the increasing use of ports up to 12–18 mm or even larger, the importance of fascial closure is becoming increasingly recognized. Long-acting local anaesthesia is injected at port site closures.

Postoperative care

If local anaesthesia has been used at the port sites, there is usually little discomfort after operation. Patients may exhibit referred shoulder pain, Kehr's sign, because of retained gas within the peritoneal cavity, although this rapidly resolves as the carbon dioxide is quickly resorbed. Postoperative pain may often be managed without the use of narcotics which may further minimize postoperative ileus. Laparoscopic procedures result in remarkably less ileus so that patients, even after colon resection, may be fed on the day of, or the day after, surgery. The reduced problem with ileus is thought to be due to less bowel manipulation, packing and tissue irritation. However, more recent studies have demonstrated that patients undergoing open procedures may be successfully fed much earlier than is the current practice. The decreased pain and diminished narcotic requirement after laparoscopic surgery makes the patient less anorexic immediately after surgery.

Although laparoscopic techniques are rapidly evolving with a plethora of new instrumentation and novel approaches to certain laparoscopic procedures, classic surgical techniques are valid. As opposed to operations being reinvented for laparoscopic techniques, the trend is toward laparoscopic technology evolving such that common surgical procedures, especially the more complex ones, may be performed using established techniques and principles.

Laparoscopic Nissen fundoplication

Glyn G. Jamieson FRACS, FACS
Dorothy Mortlock Professor of Surgery, University of Adelaide, Department of Surgery, Royal Adelaide Hospital, Adelaide, Australia

Robert Britten-Jones
Clinical Senior Lecturer and Senior Visiting Surgeon, Department of Surgery, Royal Adelaide Hospital, Adelaide, Australia

Operations which alter gastrointestinal function, but which do not require the removal of an organ or part of an organ, seem ideally suited to being undertaken laparoscopically. Fundoplication falls firmly into this category. The procedure was first reported in 1991 by Dallemagne who divided the short gastric vessels in performing the technique. The authors feel justified in calling their technique a Nissen fundoplication, as the anterior wall of the stomach is used without dividing the short gastric vessels as first described by Nissen.

Principles and justification

Indications

The indications for surgery and the objectives of the procedure are identical to the open technique. Whether the suturing which is achieved is as durable as the open technique is a question which will be answered only by long-term follow-up studies.

Contraindications

At present the relative contraindications to performing a fundoplication laparoscopically are a large fixed hiatus hernia and stricturing and shortened oesophagus. No doubt, with experience, these findings will be regarded as less of a problem.

Operation

A Veress needle is introduced immediately below the left costal margin in the mid-clavicular line and the abdomen is insufflated with CO_2 in the usual manner. The limit for intra-abdominal pressure is set at 10 mmHg as mediastinal emphysema can occur during this procedure. Although not usually a problem, patients can occasionally experience severe chest pain after surgery as a result of this complication.

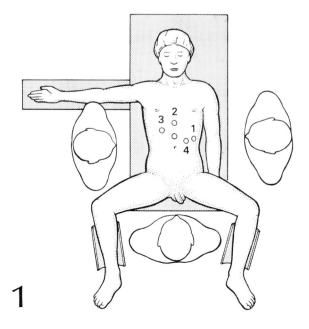

1 A 10-mm port is introduced just to the left of the midline (to avoid the falciform ligament) approximately two-thirds of the way from the xiphisternum to the umbilicus. The telescope ($0°$ or $30°$) with attached camera is introduced through this port. Additional ports are placed in (1) the left anterior axillary line below the costal margin (10-mm port), (2) just below and to the left of the xiphisternum (5-mm port), (3) below the right costal margin in the mid-clavicular line (10-mm port or 5-mm port), and (4) about 5 cm below the left costal margin in the mid-clavicular line (12-mm port). The surgeon sits between the patient's legs, which are supported in stirrups, and the table is tilted to a $30°$ head-up position.

2 A 5-mm probe or pair of grasping forceps is inserted through port (3) and the second assistant, standing on the patient's right, uses it under the left lobe of the liver to elevate it and retract it away from the oesophageal hiatus. A grasping forceps is then placed through port (2) for the surgeon's left hand, and a hook diathermy or pair of curved diathermy scissors is placed through port (4) for the surgeon's right hand. A further Babcock type grasping forceps is placed through port (1) and the first assistant, standing on the patient's left, uses this to grasp the stomach below the cardia and pull it downwards. A nasogastric tube is passed to ensure that the stomach is deflated.

The position of the hiatus is most easily found by opening the lesser omentum over the caudate lobe which takes the surgeon to the right side of the hiatus. The peritoneum and fascia in front of the hiatus is divided transversely with the diathermy hook or diathermy scissors, taking care to avoid the anterior vagus nerve(s), and then vertically downwards on either side over the pillars of the oesophageal hiatus. It is not as easy initially to find the oesophagus as might be expected. In fact, when carrying out the procedure for the first few times it may be helpful if an endoscope is passed, as the light clearly demonstrates the position of the oesophagus.

Attention is turned to cleaning the right pillar of the hiatus. Two manoeuvres may help in demonstrating the crus. The first is to place the grasping forceps through port (2) in the hiatus superiorly and to lift it craniad. The second is to have the assistant pull the stomach in the direction of the left iliac fossa. The region between the oesophagus to the left and the crus to the right is now dissected vertically for about 4–5 cm. The pair of grasping forceps through port (2) is used to displace the oesophagus to the left to aid in this dissection. The posterior vagus may be seen during this dissection but it is not as obvious as is sometimes stated, particularly if the dissection is kept close to the right wall of the oesophagus. Attention is now turned to the left pillar of the hiatus. Once again the two helpful manoeuvres are carried out with the assistant this time pulling the stomach towards the right iliac fossa. This time the grasping forceps is used to displace the oesophagus to the right while cleaning the tissue between the oesophagus and the left pillar of the hiatus.

In undertaking this dissection there is a tendency to pass through the hiatus into the thorax and care must be taken to avoid the pleura. The authors have found that they must continually try to keep the dissection as distal as possible (where it is more difficult) and not up in the

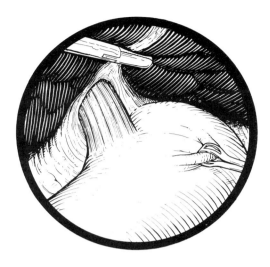

2

chest (where it is easier). This part of the dissection is not difficult, but making an opening behind the oesophagus does prove difficult on occasions. The problem is that the angle of entry of the various instruments means that when a pair of forceps is pushed behind the oesophagus, it tends to pass through the hiatus into the chest, or at least bury itself in the diaphragm.

Although port (1) is the most posteriorly placed port and in theory should be the best access for an instrument to pass behind the oesophagus, in practice the authors find that ports (2) or (3) are the best through which to carry out this manoeuvre. An instrument passed through the hiatus from port (1) will tend to be aimed at the heart, so it is also safer to proceed from right to left behind the oesophagus. Having an instrument with a curve or angle at the end facilitates this part of the procedure. When a passage has been created by an instrument behind the oesophagus, it is used to push the oesophagus anteriorly and the opening behind the oesophagus, the window, is gradually enlarged. Once again it must be emphasized that the dissection should be kept in the abdomen and not stray too much into the chest. It is important to dissect a moderately generous window behind the oesophagus of 4–5 cm in length, as this allows the stomach freer passage later in the operation. A nylon tape can be introduced percutaneously and slung around the oesophagus to emerge through the skin, or alongside one of the ports. Traction on this tape may help during passage of the stomach behind the oesophagus.

3 Attention is now turned to the stomach and a point is chosen on the anterior wall about 5 cm distal to the gastro-oesophageal junction and about halfway across towards the spleen. No dissection of the greater curvature or short gastric vessels is undertaken. The stomach is grasped with the forceps through port (1) and pushed upwards as high as possible to determine the mobility of the site chosen. If it appears tethered, then a trial and error process is used to find the most mobile part of the anterior wall of the stomach. This is then pushed to the left side of the oesophagus where grasping forceps with a ratchet are placed through port (3) and behind the oesophagus to pick up the anterior gastric wall.

As the stomach is drawn to the right, behind the oesophagus, the forceps through port (1) help to push the stomach from behind. It is this procedure which is made easier if a substantial window behind the oesophagus has been constructed.

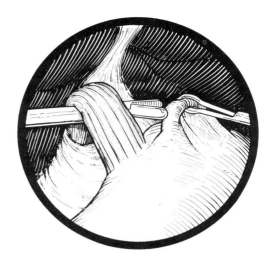

3

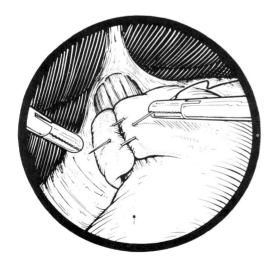

4

4 A pouch of anterior wall, approximately 3 cm in length, is brought behind the oesophagus and then the anterior wall to the left of the oesophagus is picked up and brought in apposition to the pouch. The nasogastric tube is removed and a 52-Fr bougie is passed down the oesophagus. Stitches can be inserted at this stage but early in their experience the authors found it helpful to insert staples to hold the two walls of the stomach together to facilitate subsequent insertion of sutures. A 12-mm port is introduced through port (2) and the stapler is introduced and two or three staples inserted. The stapler is removed and two needleholders are introduced. Three 3/0 polypropylene sutures are now inserted approximately 1 cm apart in order to create a wrap 2 cm in length. A mixture of intracorporeal and extracorporeal knot tying techniques are used. If staples have not been used to produce stomach wall apposition, it is easiest to insert the first suture and tie the knot extracorporeally. With the tissues held together, the remaining sutures can be placed and tied intracorporeally or extracorporeally.

The bougie is removed and replaced with a nasogastric tube. If there is any blood accumulation, the area is irrigated and the irrigating solution is sucked out. The ports are removed, the abdomen deflated and the skin incisions are closed.

5　The introduction of a traction tape around the oesophagus (see earlier) also facilitates the use of sutures to close the hiatus behind the oesophagus if this is thought necessary. Closure of the hiatus should be done before drawing the stomach around behind the oesophagus. Once again, one or two extracorporeal or intracorporeal sutures can be used.

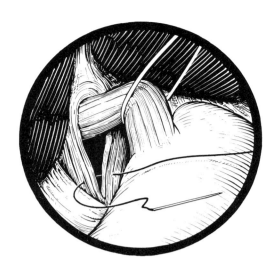

5

Postoperative care

Oral intake is commenced on the first postoperative day and patients are kept in hospital until the third or fourth postoperative day before discharge. It is likely that in future, with patients who can be instructed about the cautious introduction of a normal diet, discharge may occur earlier.

Outcome

The operation has been undertaken in 131 patients of ages ranging from 20 to 75 years, 74 of whom were men. The median operating time was 95 min (range 45–240 min). In 15 patients the procedure was converted to an open operation for technical reasons such as perioesophagitis and shortening, adiposity obscuring anatomy and large left lobe of the liver obscuring anatomy.

Follow-up in these patients is extremely short. Even

so, there have been several poor results which would have been unlikely to have occurred had the technique been performed as an open operation, e.g. acute incarceration of a paraoesophageal hernia (two patients), acute oesophageal obstruction (one patient). One patient died following a straightforward procedure because of acute thrombosis of her coeliac axis and superior mesenteric artery.

Conclusions

This is a documentation of the authors' initial experience with laparoscopic Nissen fundoplication and results will probably improve as experience grows and instrumentation is developed which is more specific for the technique. It is as yet too early to say that laparoscopic fundoplication will produce comparable results to open fundoplication, but the authors believe that eventually this is likely to be the case, particularly if the procedure is reserved for the uncomplicated and non-obese patient.

Illustrations by Marks Creative Consultants

Laparoscopic gastroenterostomy

L. K. Nathanson FRACS
Senior Lecturer, Department of Surgery, University of Queensland, Royal Brisbane Hospital, Queensland, Australia

History

The development of videolaparoscopy with small charge couple device cameras, high flow electronic CO_2 insufflators, the multipuncture approach and improved techniques of haemostasis have led to the practical application of therapeutic procedures within the abdomen. Laparoscopic suturing techniques were developed by Semm in gynaecology during the mid 1970s, but the limitation of straight needles and slow internal knotting coupled with the difficulty in acquisition of the right level of expertise with these techniques contributed to their limited appeal to many surgeons. With the development of simpler and more efficient techniques and improved needle holders, enteric anastomosis was evaluated initially with bilioenteric anastomosis, and later with gastrojejunostomy. The ongoing development of anastomotic stapling devices has ushered us rapidly into an era where laparoscopic enteric anastomosis can be readily achieved.

However, application of these techniques in the broader context of everyday intestinal surgery remains embryonic. Many of the cardinal principles of bowel surgery are skirted. Emphasis is made at this point that if these techniques are applied, for instance, to the opening of obstructed bowel for anastomotic bypass without proximal control of luminal contents, then extensive and dangerous peritoneal contamination will ensue. What may be accomplished using normal bowel does not translate automatically to what may be safely achieved in other pathological situations.

Instrumentation

Grasping forceps

Manipulation of bowel with instruments passing through cannulae fixed in positions by the abdominal wall requires patience and care. While the instrument jaws themselves may only apply a few grams of crushing force, as soon as the bowel is pulled or pushed the apex of contact between the forceps and the bowel very easily generates much larger forces, where perforation may result. Steps to minimize this hazard include the following. Before manipulation the bowel must be free of adhesions and mobile. Patient positioning and tilt of the operating table uses gravity to displace the bowel without the need for repeated manipulation. Both of the operator's hands should be used to improve tactile feedback, and with a third grasper in the hands of the assistant this allows a stepwise grasping and releasing of bowel to 'walk' efficiently along the bowel to the region of interest. (No hesitation should be felt about using a fifth access port if required.) The grasper must be kept in the field of view at all times while being moved to minimize the chance of bowel injury. On occasions the telescope may well be better inserted through one of the other ports as far away from the bowel as possible to facilitate an overall view of the proceedings. Very special care should be taken when handling obstructed dilated bowel, which is heavy as a result of its luminal fluid contents and has a thin friable wall as a result of dilatation.

The spring handled atraumatic grasping forceps, Babcock graspers and Dorsey bowel grasper are, at the present time, the best instruments for bowel manipulation. Frequently, the atraumatic grasping forceps slip when excessive traction is applied. Although at times this is irritating, it provides a safeguard against accidental bowel perforation. With due care dissecting forceps may be useful to retract bowel when applied to appendices epiploicae.

Needle holders and sutures

Basic techniques of endoscopic suturing are covered elsewhere in the text with mastery of internal knotting by square or reef knots being essential skills. The ability to grasp and manipulate standard curved needles is now possible with good quality laparoscopic needle holders incorporating tungsten carbide tip inlay in the jaws. Introduction of the curved needle requires the diameter of the larger 11-mm port. Suture and needle tangling in the port valve mechanism during insertion can be minimized by first backloading the suture and needle into a reducer tube. Once introduced, the orientation of the needle is best achieved by allowing it to drop onto a flat surface below the cannula site and then grasping it with the needle holder. Final orientation and obliquity of the needle shaft is adjusted by pressure applied via the grasping forceps in the surgeon's left hand. These grasping forceps ideally have a curved tip which allows tissue and needle grasping. The jaw hinge design may be single or twin action but must be engineered so that during internal knotting the loops of the suture wound around the shaft of the forceps during knot formation do not become jammed in the hinge mechanism as the loops of the knot slide down.

Suture grasping forceps used by the assistant should have a jaw finely engineered so that it grasps fine sutures without slipping but should also have rounded edges so that accidental cutting of the suture is avoided as traction is applied.

Bowel occlusion

Laparoscopic instrumentation for proximal and distal clamping of bowel is not yet available. One technique available at present is a sling of silicone or thick suture material which is introduced through the abdominal wall, passed around the bowel and back out through the abdominal wall to sling up and occlude the bowel lumen. This can be secured in place by an external clamp and has the added advantage of elevating the bowel and at the same time providing traction.

Principles and justification
Indications

Patients with gastric outlet obstruction as a result of chronic peptic ulceration are well suited to laparoscopic gastrojejunostomy. In a proportion of these patients the extent of fibrosis and distortion around the pylorus will be minimal allowing, if preferred, a pyloroplasty to be performed.

Another group is those patients having cholecystojejunostomy for malignant distal bile duct obstruction with incipient or established duodenal obstruction militating against simple endoscopic retrograde cholangiopancreatographic stenting. A proportion of patients initially stented will require bypass at a later stage due to recurrent stent obstruction or difficulties with stent replacement or the onset of duodenal obstruction later on in the course of their disease.

Some patients with pyloric gastric carcinoma and obstruction, where extensive metastatic spread or associated medical illness determine that resection is ill advised, are suitable for palliative bypass.

Care must be exercised in selection of patients with previous upper abdominal surgery. Distortion of anatomy and obliteration of tissue planes hamper laparoscopic dissection tremendously. Often, however, the extent and density of adhesions can only be assessed by a trial of laparoscopic dissection. Patients in this situation have to be aware of the possible need to complete the bypass as an open procedure.

Preoperative assessment and preparation

This is the same as for patients undergoing a similar procedure via a laparotomy incision with attention to nutrition, electrolytes and general assessment of medical fitness. An ultrasonographic scan of the upper abdomen is useful in patients who have had previous upper abdominal surgery to detect the extent of peritoneal adhesions and to find a point for initial laparoscopic access, away from any adhesions.

Operation

Patient positioning and port placement

1 Prophylactic intravenous antibiotics are administered after induction of anaesthesia. The patient is placed supine and nasogastric intubation is undertaken to decompress the stomach. Table tilt is not generally required. The surgeon stands on the patient's right side. The port in the mid zone to the right of the umbilicus should be so placed so that when occupied by a needle holder in the surgeon's right hand, the needle holder shaft lies parallel to the suture line on the stomach. This is an important point, as it allows simple insertion of the needle across the suture line, its subsequent grasping and re-introduction. The tissue grasping forceps in the surgeon's left hand inserted through the right upper quadrant port should arrive at the suture line at right angles to the needle holder. The placement of the third (assistant's) port should be out of the way of the other instruments and not block the laparoscopic view of the suture line. At least one of the accessory ports should be 11 mm in diameter to allow introduction of curved needles and large shaft instruments if required.

Initial inspection of the peritoneum is completed and, if gastric outlet obstruction is a result of chronic peptic ulceration, a truncal vagotomy is performed before commencing the gastroenterostomy.

The duodenojejunal flexure is then identified. This is achieved by carefully grasping the transverse colon and omentum with two atraumatic forceps and elevating it anterior and cephalad to the stomach. The assistant is then able to maintain this position with one atraumatic grasper, while the surgeon using two atraumatic graspers follows the small bowel up in a 'hand over hand' manner until the flexure is reached. The small bowel is then followed down and a suitable point chosen for the anastomosis. This should be checked by allowing the transverse colon to fall back to its normal position and the jejunum should easily pass around it up to the anterior wall of the stomach. This step is important as there is a tendency to underestimate the length of proximal small bowel required when viewing and handling it endoscopically.

Jamming loop knot

2a–c This knot is useful for constructing this anastomosis. It is fashioned outside the abdomen at the tail end of the suture using the steps illustrated. Care is taken not to over-tighten the knot at this stage as this impairs smooth tightening and locking of the loop inside the abdomen. The suture is introduced into the peritoneum by back-loading it into a reducer tube before insertion via the 11-mm port.

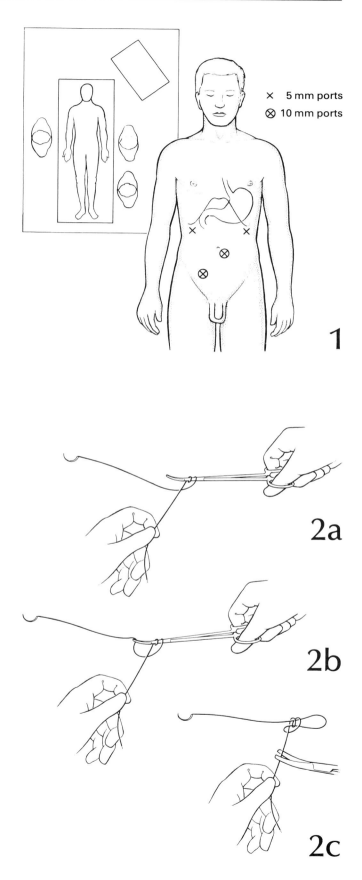

× 5 mm ports
⊗ 10 mm ports

1

2a

2b

2c

SUTURED ANASTOMOSIS

The assistant grasps the bowel and the serosa is scored on its antimesenteric aspect with high frequency electrocautery for 6 cm. A 6-cm line is marked on the antrum of the stomach in the position selected for the anastomosis. The marking of the length of the anastomosis in this manner must be judged with a calibrated instrument because experience has shown that this length of gastric suture line heals with a 2–3-cm diameter stoma. The diathermy marks also maintain the orientation of the jejunum and stomach during suturing.

The posterior layer is sutured first before opening the bowel. This is achieved with a single layer of continuous sutures, two each of about 15 cm in length. The author's preference is to use 3/0 polyglactin on a standard curved needle. The first suture is introduced into the peritoneum after tying its tail with the jamming loop knot.

Commencement of the posterior layer

3a, b Instillation of air into the stomach via the nasogastric tube occasionally improves exposure of the anterior wall of the stomach with displacement of the antrum from beneath the left lobe of the liver, facilitating suture placement in the stomach. The apex of the suture line is identified and the needle passed to incorporate the full thickness of bowel wall; the loop knot is then locked.

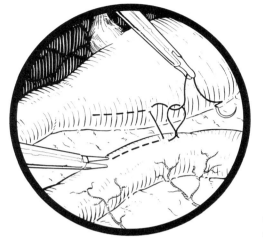

3a

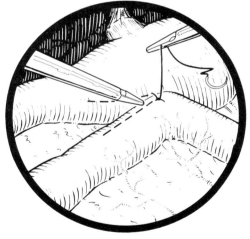

3b

Completion of posterior layer

4a–d With the assistant holding the suture and 'following' after each pass through tissue by the needle, the first suture completes the first half of the posterior layer and is then tied with either a reef or Aberdeen knot. The Aberdeen knot gives excellent security, providing three or more locking throws have been completed before the suture is pulled completely through the final loop and its tail trimmed. The second suture is then used to complete the posterior layer, tied and the tail cut long.

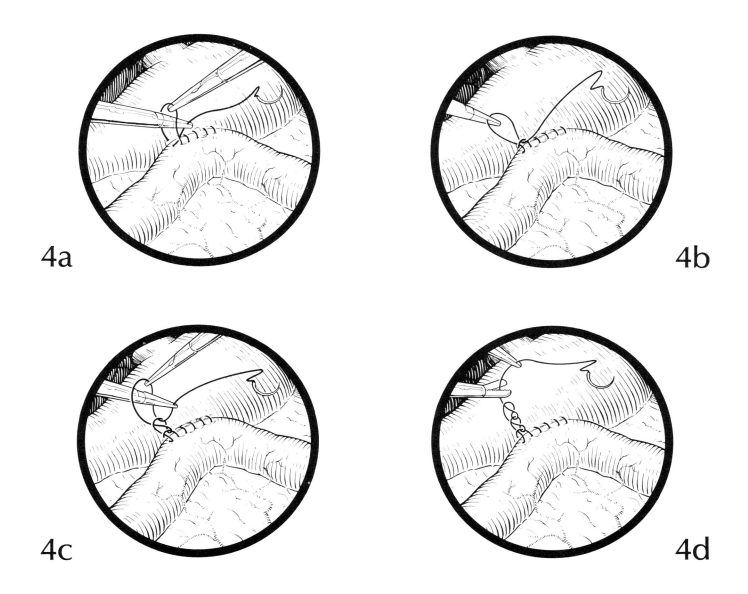

4a

4b

4c

4d

Opening the bowel

5   The jejunum is opened first, the muscle being divided by high frequency electrocautery. The mucosa is next divided using round nose scissors and any luminal contents are aspirated. Attention is then turned to the stomach which is first emptied of air and gastric juice by suction on the nasogastric tube. Monopolar high frequency electrocautery is used to open along the line of the serosa marked out initially. The control of bleeding from the rich blood supply of the stomach is most important to allow accurate suture placement and prevent postoperative suture line haemorrhage. Once the mucosa is reached this can be opened with dissecting scissors. Elevation of the anastomosis, by traction on the tail of the apical suture by the assistant, minimizes the spillage of gastric content by a combination of gravity and positive pressure of the insufflated CO_2 gas which often encourages the drainage of any gastric juice *up* the nasogastric tube rather than into the peritoneum. Care should be taken to ensure complete haemostasis at this time.

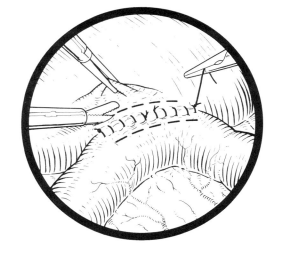

5

Anterior layer

6a, b   The anterior continuous layer is then commenced using the long tail of the posterior apical suture as a guide to the apex. Two sutures of 15 cm length are used, each initiated with the jamming loop knot and ended by using the Aberdeen knot or reef knot. Alternatively, after using the tail of the posterior suture as a guide to the placement of the final few sutures, the anterior suture can simply be tied to it using a reef knot.

The peritoneum is lavaged with warm Ringer lactate solution and aspirated dry. Peritoneal drainage is not routinely employed.

Comment

The entirely sutured anastomosis has some drawbacks in the context of gastroenterostomy. Because of the long suture line it takes time and patience to complete. Two sutures over this 6-cm anastomosis are also desirable to prevent the loosening of the tension on the tissue caused by alteration in bowel length with shortening of the suture line during peristaltic waves. Adequate haemostatic tension must be maintained after each pass of the needle by the assistant grasping the suture and elevating it upwards. Tissue approximation must be adequate to maintain haemostasis, especially with the renowned vascularity of the stomach.

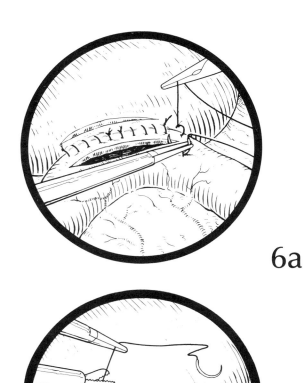

6a

6b

STAPLED AND SUTURED GASTROENTEROSTOMY

The combination of stapling combined with suture closure of the residual defect is attractive in the long 6-cm anastomosis. It allows rapid creation of the stoma and its only drawback lies with the expense of the disposable stapler and refill cartridge.

The ports are placed as for the sutured anastomosis except the 12-mm port for the stapler is used in the right upper quadrant.

External anchoring suture and enterotomy

7   An external anchoring suture placed through the stomach and jejunum at the efferent aspect of the anastomosis facilitates retraction and approximation of the jejunum and stomach. This is achieved with a 0 polypropylene suture on a straight needle inserted through the abdominal wall just above the right upper quadrant port. This is grasped using the needle holder, passed through the stomach and jejunum, and then passed back out through the abdominal wall to be anchored externally by an artery clip. The selected portion of jejunum is grasped by the assistant and an 8-mm enterotomy made using diathermy and scissors, followed by a similar enterotomy in the antrum of the stomach at the distal end of the proposed anastomosis.

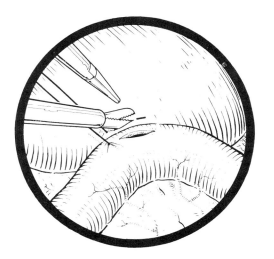

7

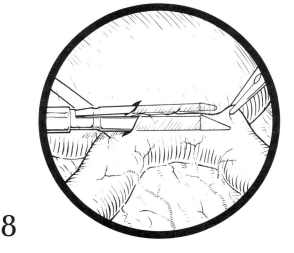

8

Application of stapler

8   The 60-mm Endo GIA stapler is introduced and inserted into the jejunum and then the stomach parallel to the greater curve, using the anchoring suture as countertraction, clamped, its position checked, and then fired. The suture line is inspected for haemostasis by inserting a sucker through the defect in the anastomosis, elevating it and then advancing the endoscope through to view the staple line from within. Possibly because of the three rows of staples used in the laparoscopic staplers, no bleeding from the staple line has been encountered.

If the 30-mm Endo GIA stapler is used two firings are required. The first is completed as described for the larger stapler. Once completed, the stapler is removed and a fresh bowel cartridge inserted. The reapplication of the stapler to extend the suture line takes care by the surgeon as the apex of the previous two rows of staples must be accurately found and the second firing must continue from this point if a devascularized segment of bowel is to be avoided.

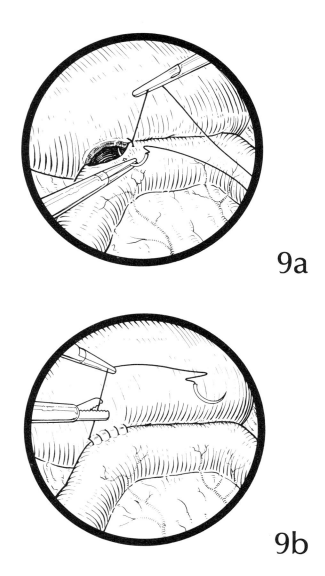

Suture of residual anastomotic defect

9a, b   Once the stapling has been completed the defect in the stomach and jejunum is closed with a continuous 3/0 polyglactin suture on a standard curved needle. A pretied jamming loop knot is used (see page 577) and, after passing through the apex of the suture line taking full-thickness stomach and jejunal wall, it is locked and then grasped and held in traction by the assistant. The sutures are placed 5 mm apart, incorporating full-thickness bites of stomach and jejunum. Completion of the suture line is with a reef or Aberdeen knot.

Comment

In practical terms the combination of suture closure of the residual defect after establishment of the bulk of the staple line using the stapler works well. Attempts at triangulation of the jejunal and stomach walls to staple closed the residual defect laparoscopically have been difficult. This is because, in attempting to ensure complete closure, a large portion of jejunal wall is included which results in jejunal luminal stenosis at the efferent end of the staple line. This process can likewise take a lot more time than initially estimated because of the difficulty experienced with holding up the edges of the open bowel during stapler application. In the author's hands planned suture closure is quicker and with present equipment more satisfactory.

Routine peritoneal drainage is not employed.

Postoperative care

Measures to minimize the risk of stomal ulceration are taken in all patients who have not undergone concomitant vagotomy. These usually entail the long-term use of alginates or H_2 receptor blockers.

Patients are encouraged to mobilize as soon as they have recovered from anaesthesia. With the exception of those with a long-standing preceding gastric outlet obstruction, the nasogastric tube is removed the next day and oral fluids commenced. Subsequent introduction of a solid diet is based on the wishes of the patient. Normal bowel function usually resumes by the third postoperative day and discharge from hospital is possible 4 days after surgery.

Outcome

The subjective assessment of benefits resulting from the laparoscopic approach suggests marked improvement in early postoperative recovery, with decreased need for analgesia, accelerated recovery of bowel function and decreased wound complications. The improvement, if any, in the rate of recovery of gastric emptying after prolonged obstruction remains to be proven.

Many aspects of sutured anastomosis require further instrumentation and refinement even to begin to approach the instrumentation available for open surgery. Simple atraumatic bowel clamps are needed. These should be able to be disconnected from their shaft once applied and so allow ports to be used for other instrumentation. Truly atraumatic bowel grasping forceps are required which function with little or no risk of perforating bowel (especially obstructed bowel). On the horizon are methods of suture fixation other than knots which can be rapidly applied and will greatly speed up this process.

The capacity to suture competently using the laparoscope is encouraged as it adds greatly to a surgeon's ability and confidence. Moreover, it increases the usefulness of the remarkable range of new stapling devices now becoming available.

Laparoscopic vagotomies

F. Dubois
Professor, CMC Pte de Choisy, Paris, France

History

Vagotomy is an old surgical procedure with Jaboulay possibly performing the first procedure in humans in Lyons in 1901[1]. Latarjet and Wertheimer[2], after experimental studies with regard to gastric innervation, reported their first 22 vagotomies in humans in 1922.

In 1943 Dragstedt and Owens[3] proposed that truncal vagotomy be used in the treatment of chronic duodenal ulcer. However, it became apparent that gastric denervation sometimes caused gastric stasis so that subsequently a gastric drainage procedure was added, initially a gastroenterostomy and later a pyloroplasty.

To avoid the side effects of total gastrointestinal denervation, and in particular diarrhoea, selective vagotomies were proposed by Jackson[4] in the USA and Franksson[5] in Sweden in 1948. In fact, the real promoters of these procedures in humans were Griffith and Harkins[6] in the USA, and Burge[7] in the UK.

Nevertheless, side effects still occurred, because of pyloric bypass, and to avoid them the concept of proximal gastric vagotomy or highly selective vagotomy arose, with conservation of the innervation of the pylorus and gastric antrum[8,9].

Over the past 20 years, highly selective vagotomy has become the standard surgical procedure in the treatment of chronic duodenal ulcer. Although the advent of H_2 blocking agents and omeprazole has left a very small place for surgical procedures, the rapid increase in popularity of laparoscopic surgery has made easier the acceptance of surgical procedures and all types of vagotomy can now be performed with this type of surgery.

Against this background, in 1989 we performed some laparoscopic highly selective vagotomies but changed to truncal vagotomies for the following reasons:

1. Highly selective vagotomy is difficult, takes a long time to perform and so is tiring for the surgeon when done laparoscopically.
2. The rate of recurrence of highly selective vagotomy is unacceptable (close to the natural rate of recurrence of the untreated ulcer).
3. The side effects of total vagotomy are much less than has often been stated.
4. Truncal vagotomy, particularly by the thoracoscopic approach, is a simple and safe procedure.

Anatomical background

1 A good knowledge of the anatomy of the vagus nerves is necessary for performing a vagotomy but gastric surgeons already have such knowledge. Originally, Delmas and Laux[10] described a perioesophageal plexus, which forms a large posterior trunk called the 'abdominal vagus trunk' with all its branches being collaterals.

However, as is well known to surgeons, in the region of the lower thoracic and abdominal oesophagus, where truncal vagotomy is performed, in most cases the vagus nerve exists as two trunks, a large posterior trunk and a smaller anterior trunk. Below the cardia, the anterior trunk produces a gastrohepatic branch and the anterior nerve of Latarjet which ends at the 'crow's foot' about 7 cm from the pylorus. The posterior trunk gives a large coeliac branch reaching the coeliac plexus and a smaller gastric branch: the posterior nerve of Latarjet.

Based on this anatomy, the following types of vagotomies have arisen:

1. Truncal vagotomy, dividing the trunks at the level of the oesophagus.
2. Selective vagotomy, dividing the anterior and posterior branches below the origin of the hepatic and coeliac branches.
3. Highly selective vagotomy, with division of the gastric branches proximal to the crow's foot, denervating the fundus and body of the stomach and preserving antral motility and pyloric function.

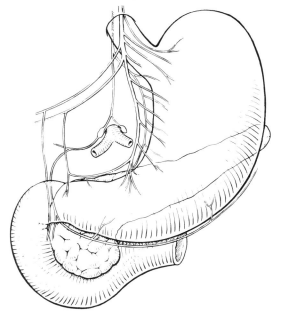

1

Preoperative

General anaesthesia is usual but high epidural anaesthesia is preferred by some. A nasogastric tube is placed.

A carbon dioxide pneumoperitoneum is electronically maintained at 12–14 mmHg.

The entire system, instruments, video and gas cylinder should be carefully checked before the procedure is started. Several video monitors are useful to aid the performance of the assistants.

The instruments used are those for standard laparoscopy.

Operation

The general conditions are the same as for other laparoscopic procedures.

The operation should take place in a fully equipped operating theatre and be carried out by a trained gastric surgeon because of the possible need to convert from a laparoscopy to an open procedure.

Position of the patient

The patient is placed in the lithotomy position with 30° reverse Trendelenburg. The surgeon is seated between the patient's legs and an assistant stands on each side of the patient.

2 The cannulae are inserted in the same way regardless of the type of vagotomy being performed.

In the normal subject, the optic system is introduced through a 10-mm trocar sheath above the umbilicus. The author uses a Z-shaped incision to avoid later dehiscence problems[11]. In obese patients the trocar should be inserted at a more craniad site.

The author usually works with a 0° laparoscope, but a 30° laparoscope can sometimes give a better view in the region of the cardia and it also seems to work better with obese patients. After a general inspection of the abdomen, and if the procedure seems feasible, further trocars are inserted.

1. A 5-mm trocar in a left sub-xiphisternal position for a retractor or for a suction–irrigation port: the exact location depends on the shape and volume of the falciform ligament and the size of the left hepatic lobe.
2. A 5-mm trocar in the right flank, for insertion of a pair of grasping forceps.
3. A 5-mm trocar below the left subcostal margin for insertion of another pair of grasping forceps.
4. A 10-mm trocar in the left flank for other instruments, e.g. dissector hook, scissors and clip appliers.

The position of the various cannulae is varied according to the practice of the operator, whether he is right or left handed, and the patient's configuration.

Two principles should constantly be borne in mind: first, to keep the cannulae as far as possible from each other to avoid the 'knitting needle' effect of the cannulae knocking into each other; second, to avoid approaching the organs from too oblique an angle. The next step depends on the type of vagotomy to be undertaken.

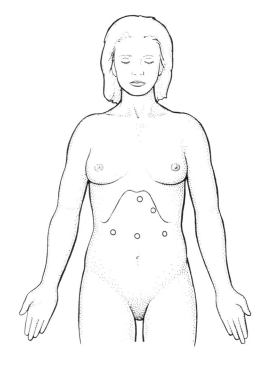

2

HIGHLY SELECTIVE VAGOTOMY (HSV)

The position of the stomach is made obvious by the insertion of a large endogastric tube (Faucher's tube). The stomach wall is grasped by a pair of forceps and pulled downward and to the left to expose the crow's foot. The left hepatic lobe is held craniad by a retractor. The procedure is then performed as follows.

Section of the neurovascular plane on the anterior aspect of the lesser curvature

3a, b The dissection, using scissors, hook or dissector, begins just above the crow's foot. The pedicles are severed after clipping or coagulating by bipolar cautery: this step should be performed carefully to avoid bleeding or damage to the nerve of Latarjet.

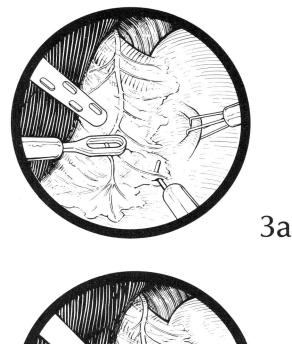

3a

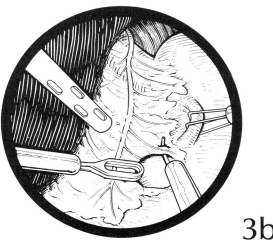

3b

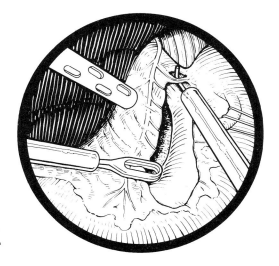

4

Section of the neurovascular pedicle

4 The neurovascular pedicle is dissected in front of the cardia and circular dissection of the lower oesophagus is performed for a distance of at least 2 cm.

Section of the neurovascular plane on the posterior aspect of the lesser curvature

5 For this step, the dissection can be carried out downwards from the cardia, upwards from the crow's foot, or a combination of both. It is helpful to enter the lesser sac first through the lesser omentum.

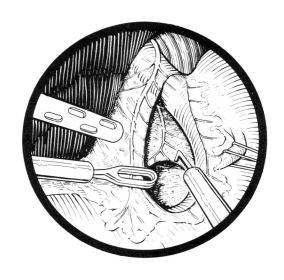

5

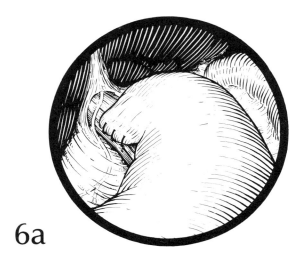

6a

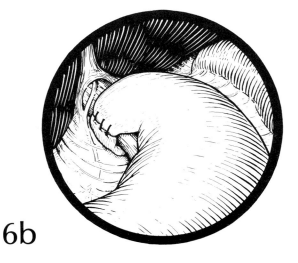

6b

6a, b The HSV is now completed and the lower oesophagus and the angle of His are freed. It is useful to perform an antireflux procedure, although most surgeons probably would not think this necessary.

The easiest antireflux mechanism to construct is an anterior flap of stomach which is sutured by three stitches or a running suture between the anterior wall of the fundus and the right side of the oesophagus and the right crus (Dor's procedure). If the oesophagus has been widely mobilized, it may be better to construct a posterior valve (Toupet's procedure) or a Nissen-Rossetti fundoplication.

OTHER SELECTIVE VAGOTOMIES

Since HSV takes a long time to perform well in both open and in laparoscopic surgery, two other types of vagotomies have been described which combine a posterior truncal vagotomy with an anterior selective denervation of the stomach.

The first is a procedure described in 1978 for open operation. It uses the anterior part of an HSV which is less difficult and time consuming than the posterior part.

A second procedure described in 1979 for open operation was an anterior seromyotomy of the lesser curvature of the stomach and posterior truncal vagotomy. The procedure was first performed laparoscopically in 1991 by Mouiel and Katkhouda[12].

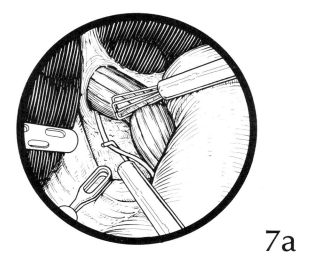

7a

7a, b The posterior truncal section is dealt with first. The anterior surface of the stomach is then stretched and the outline of the seromyotomy is marked with the hook coagulator, keeping the line 1.5 cm from the lesser curvature and extending from the level of the gastro-oesophageal junction to the level of the crow's foot. The hook is used to cut the serosa and the muscular layers, the two edges of the myotomy being held apart by forceps as the bluish mucosa appears. Usually four or five short vessels along the seromyotomy need to be clipped and transected to provide haemostasis.

After carefully verifying the integrity of the mucosa, if necessary by inflating the stomach, the seromyotomy is closed in an overlapping fashion by a continuous suture and reinforced by the application of a fibrin sealant.

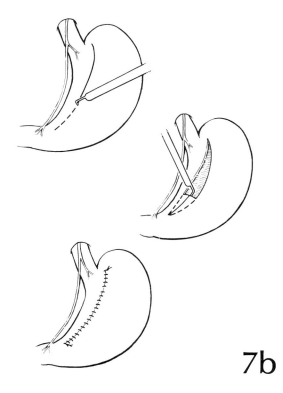

7b

LAPAROSCOPIC TRUNCAL VAGOTOMY

Initially this procedure commenced with the posterior vagotomy in the author's practice, but latterly the anterior vagotomy has been performed first.

8 The cardia is pulled downwards using a grasping forceps and the stretched peritoneum is opened in front of the oesophagus close to the hiatus.

The anterior and lateral aspects of the oesophagus are dissected free and one or several vagal trunks can be seen between the muscular fibres. They are freed by the hook and severed after haemostasis by electrocautery. The dissection has to be performed very carefully to avoid damaging the oesophageal wall.

When the oesophagus has been dissected in this way, it is usually easy to retract it to the left to find the posterior trunk with the hook.

For the posterior vagotomy, the white cord of the posterior vagus is easily recognized, freed with the hook, coagulated and cut. Some surgeons take a piece of the nerve for histological confirmation.

It is important to explore the back of the oesophagus and the right crus in case some smaller branches are found there.

In carrying out truncal vagotomies, the oesophagus is only partially mobilized and the angle of His is preserved. Therefore it is not necessary to add an antireflux procedure.

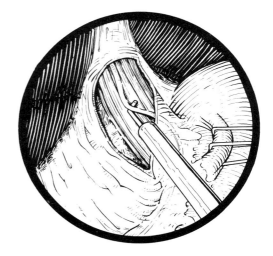

8

THORACOSCOPIC TRUNCAL VAGOTOMY

Description of this technique is appropriate as, although it is not a laparoscopic one, the equipment and methods are very similar.

For many years, Wittmoser (personal communication) has carried out thoracoscopic neurectomies and, in particular, vagotomies. He recommends two separate procedures at an interval of 3 weeks, combined with bilateral splanchnicectomy, in order to obviate spasm of the pylorus. We prefer a unilateral approach (usually left sided unless there are pleural adhesions) for bilateral truncal vagotomy.

Under general anaesthesia, a Carlens tube is passed so that the lung on the side to be explored can be collapsed. As for a posterolateral thoracotomy, the patient is placed on their right side with the surgeon standing behind and an assistant on the other side.

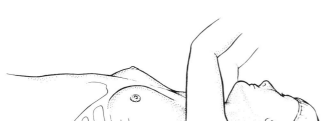
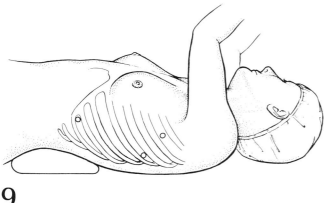

9 To induce a pneumothorax, a 1-cm incision is made through the eighth intercostal space in the posterior axillary line and a pair of blunt forceps is passed through the muscles so that the characteristic sound of air entering the chest indicates that the pleural space has been opened.

The forceps is replaced by a 10-mm trocar for the telescope and low pressure carbon dioxide insufflation is used to maintain the lung collapse and avoid the theoretical risk of air embolus.

The pleural cavity is explored and the two other 5-mm trocars are inserted under endoscopic view in the mid axillary line. A fourth 5-mm trocar is sometimes placed in the anterior axillary line as a retractor for the lung.

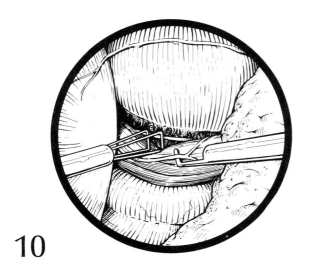

10 The operation begins by the division of adhesions, if any. The mediastinal pleura is opened with the coagulating hook or scissors, between the inferior pulmonary ligament and the aorta and the oesophagus can be seen immediately beneath this pleura. It is freed all round for about 5 cm and the vagus nerves are dissected with the hook, coagulated and divided.

At this level, the vagus is somewhat plexiform, made up of two big trunks and two or three smaller nerves.

If the opposite pleural cavity is opened, the pressure in the opposite lung tends to control gas leakage and the leak will be subsequently obstructed by the oesophagus.

There is seldom much bleeding as the perioesophageal space in this area is relatively avascular. As there is very little gaseous pressure, a certain degree of oozing from small veins is usual, though not troublesome.

No pleural drainage is required if there is no bleeding or leakage of air from the lung. In cases where bleeding or leakage of air occurs, a small drain is left and usually removed within 24–48 h.

Postoperative pain can be lessened by intercostal infiltration with local anaesthesia at the end of the procedure.

Postoperative care

A nasogastric tube is left in place for 24 h to avoid an acute gastric dilatation. It also allows measurement of the acidity of the aspirate to confirm the efficacy of the vagotomy.

Antibiotic prophylaxis is given with the premedication as well as thrombosis prophylaxis by heparin subcutaneously during the hospital stay.

Oral fluids are permitted as soon as the nasogastric tube is removed and alimentation is progressively introduced.

The postoperative course is usually uneventful.

Complications

A problem specific to truncal vagotomies is so called 'pylorospasm'. According to Dragstedt, it might be expected to occur in more than 40% of cases after total vagotomy, then necessitating some form of gastric drainage procedure.

Initially, a pyloric dilatation was thought to be necessary and was done routinely by an endoscopic balloon at the time of operation or immediately after. In fact it was noted that usually there was no pyloric spasm but a hypotonic antrum with a wide open pylorus. The routine use of dilatation has therefore been abandoned.

All patients are given cisapride postoperatively and after 21 days a barium meal is given. If there is gastric stasis, a balloon pyloric dilatation is then carried out, but this has been necessary in only two cases out of the last 20 thoracic vagotomies.

Outcome

It is too early to produce valid results for endoscopic vagotomies as all series are small and recent, and the treatment of duodenal ulcer needs to be evaluated after many years. However, a few observations can be made.

There is no reason why the route of access should influence the long-term results: it is mainly a problem of completeness of the vagotomy, and all types of vagotomies can be completed by laparoscopy or thoracoscopy.

HSV is a long and laborious procedure but posterior truncal vagotomy associated with an anterior selective gastric denervation is easier to perform. It is a worthwhile alternative for those surgeons who are reluctant to perform a total vagotomy. Bilateral truncal vagotomy is easy to perform by laparoscopy and even a little easier via thoracoscopy.

However, there is a risk of side effects, perhaps diarrhoea and, in particular, trouble with gastric emptying. The risk of persistent gastric atonia is 5–10%. Endoscopic pyloric selective dilatation can be reserved for this group of patients. The author considers that truncal vagotomies should be avoided in patients with chronic diarrhoea.

The postoperative course after laparoscopic vagotomy is usually uneventful. The author is of the opinion that this 'mini invasive' surgery should be considered as an attractive alternative to life-long medical therapy.

References

1. Hollender LF, Marrie A. *Highly Selective Vagotomy*. New York: Masson, 1979.

2. Latarjet MA, Wertheimer P. L'énervation gastrique. *J Med Lyon* 1921; 5 Nov: 1289.

3. Dragstedt LR, Owens FM. Sub-diaphragmatic section of the vagus nerves in the treatment of duodenal ulcer. *Proc Soc Exp Biol Med* 1943; 53: 152–4.

4. Jackson RG. Anatomic study of vagus nerves with a technique of transabdominal selective gastric vagus resection. *Arch Surg* 1948; 57: 333–52.

5. Franksson C. Selective abdominal vagotomy. *Acta Chir Scand* 1948; 96: 409–12.

6. Griffith CA, Harkins HN. Partial gastric vagotomy: an experimental study. *Gastroenterology* 1957; 32: 96–102.

7. Burge H. *Vagotomy*. London: Edward Arnold, 1964.

8. Johnston D, Wilkinson AR. Highly selective vagotomy without a drainage procedure in the treatment of duodenal ulcer. *Br J Surg* 1970; 57: 289–96.

9. Amdrup BM, Griffith CA. Selective vagotomy of the parietal cell mass. Part 1. *Ann Surg* 1969; 170: 207–14.

10. Delmas J, Laux G. *Système Nerveux Sympathique*. Paris: Masson, 1952; 337.

11. Semm K. *Atlas of Gynecologic Laparoscopy and Hysteroscopy*. Philadelphia: Saunders, 1977.

12. Mouiel J, Katkhouda N. Laparoscopic vagotomy in the treatment of chronic duodenal ulcer disease. *Probl Gen Surg* 1991; 8: 358–65.

Further reading

Benjamin SB, Glass RL, Cattau RL, Miller WB. Preliminary experience with balloon dilatation of the pylorus. *Gastrointest Endosc* 1984; 30: 93–5.

Cuschieri A. Laparoscopic vagotomy: gimmick or reality? *Surg Clin North Am* 1992; 72: 357–67.

Dubois F. Laparoscopic vagotomies. *Probl Gen Surg* 1991; 8: 348–57.

Steele RJC, Munro A. Successful treatment of gastric stasis following proximal gastric vagotomy using endoscopic balloon dilatation. *Endoscopy* 1989; 2: 120.

Taylor TV, Gunn AA, Macleod DAD, MacLennan I. Anterior lesser curve seromyotomy and posterior truncal vagotomy in the treatment of chronic duodenal ulcer. *Lancet* 1982; ii: 846–9.

Achalasia of the oesophagus: management by videoendoscopic surgery

Carlos A. Pellegrini MD, FACS

Professor and Chairman, Department of Surgery, University of Washington, Seattle, Washington, USA

Principles and justification

Achalasia of the oesophagus is a neuromuscular disorder which leads to oesophageal dilatation in the absence of a mechanical obstruction. Dilatation appears to be related to the inability of the oesophagus to generate adequate propulsive waves and sufficient relaxation in response to swallowing. The disease affects men more often than women, and its peak incidence is between 30 and 60 years. The cause is not known, but it is thought to be related to a degenerative or infectious process which causes the destruction of the ganglion cells of Auerbach's myenteric plexus and a hypertrophy of the circular muscle of the distal oesophagus. In areas where trypanosomiasis is endemic, such as Brazil, oesophageal dilatation similar to achalasia is seen in patients affected by Chagas' disease.

Exactly how the absence of Auerbach's plexus leads to the functional abnormality characteristic of achalasia is unclear. Physiological studies suggest that the cholinergic innervation of the sphincter is intact, but the non-cholinergic, non-adrenergic inhibitory innervation which mediates sphincter relaxation through nitric oxide, and perhaps vasoactive intestinal peptide and other peptides, has been lost. Patients with achalasia have a higher incidence of squamocellular carcinoma of the oesophagus, which has been thought to be secondary to stasis and prolonged contact of food with the mucosa.

Treatment for achalasia is aimed at decreasing resistance to flow through the lower oesophageal sphincter which improves oesophageal emptying. Calcium channel blockers are only partially effective. The best way to decrease resistance is by division or disruption of the circular muscle of the lower oesophagus. Extramucosal oesophagocardiomyotomy, described by Heller in 1913, effectively divides the circular muscle[1,2] but requires a thoracotomy or a laparotomy, which means that patients have to be hospitalized for 7–10 days and have residual discomfort for 6–8 weeks. Pressure-controlled balloon dilatation, which became available in the early 1970s, proved to be a relatively good method of disrupting the circular muscle layer. Although several series reported good results, this treatment is occasionally complicated by perforation[3] and it often leads to abnormal reflux or recurrent dysphagia. Since 1991 a thoracoscopic or laparoscopic approach has been used by the author to perform the Heller myotomy[4]. Using this approach, patients are hospitalized for 2–3 days, experience little discomfort, and are able to return to work within a week. It is a procedure that provides the benefit of myotomy with a level of discomfort similar to that of pneumatic dilatation.

Preoperative

Clinical

The earliest symptom is dysphagia, particularly for solids. Dysphagia progresses insidiously and it takes patients several months to notice that something is different. In fact, as the oesophagus gets larger it can accommodate more and more food, and the patients adapt to this new feeling. As the disease progresses, regurgitation becomes the most important feature. The presence of residual food in the oesophagus causes frequent episodes of aspiration and pneumonia. Because of the discomfort associated with eating, weight loss is common.

Radiology

Plain chest radiographs may show an air-fluid level in the oesophagus and a widening of the mediastinum in patients with advanced disease.

1 Upper gastrointestinal examination reveals a dilated oesophagus with a 'bird-beak' appearance at the gastro-oesophageal junction, quite different from the appearance of a benign or a malignant stricture.

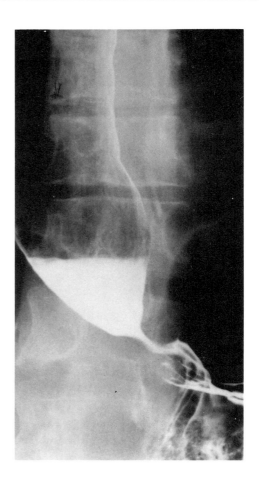

1

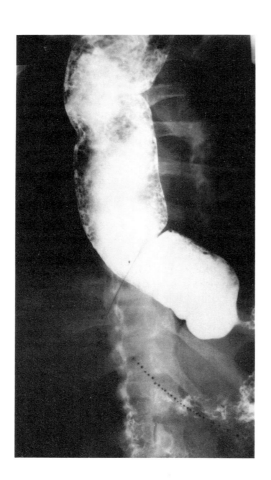

2

2 In later stages the oesophagus dilates and elongates, taking on the so-called 'sigmoid' appearance.

Endoscopy

Upper gastrointestinal endoscopy should always be performed to rule out a carcinoma. In patients with achalasia, this examination shows a dilated oesophagus often containing food particles from previous meals and oesophagitis, which is secondary to stasis. Any suspicious-looking mucosa should be biopsied.

Manometry

Achalasia is a functional disorder of the motor function of the oesophagus. Other disorders of oesophageal motility share some of its clinical features; thus, it is important to define the exact nature of the functional abnormality. This is best accomplished by manometry.

3 The most important finding is the inability to relax the lower oesophageal sphincter adequately in response to swallows. The second most common finding is the lack of peristaltic activity in the body of the oesophagus. Swallows elicit no response, or a low pressure, simultaneous, non-peristaltic contraction. Finally many, but not all, patients with achalasia have high pressure (i.e. over 30 mmHg) in the lower oesophageal sphincter.

Anaesthesia

Broad-spectrum antibiotics are given before surgery to decrease the risk of infection in case the mucosa is inadvertently entered during the operation. Patients should avoid solid food for the preceding 24 h to minimize the risk of aspiration. Nevertheless, because the large oesophagus can accumulate food and secretion, anaesthesia must be induced with care to prevent aspiration. If the operation is done via thoracoscopy, a double lumen endotracheal tube must be used to ventilate each lung independently.

Before starting the operation, a fibreoptic endoscope is introduced transorally into the oesophagus. This instrument plays an essential role in videoendoscopic surgery of the oesophagus. First, it helps to identify the oesophagus with minimal dissection of adjacent structures, and secondly, it provides a 'handle' with which to mobilize the oesophagus and bring the wall into the surgeon's field of view; thirdly, by tilting the tip of the instrument to one side or the other it assists the surgeon in separation of the edges of the myotomy, and it can estimate the percentage of the circumference that has been freed. Finally, and most importantly, it helps to determine the effectiveness of the operation by gauging the degree to which the obstruction at the cardio-oesophageal junction is relieved.

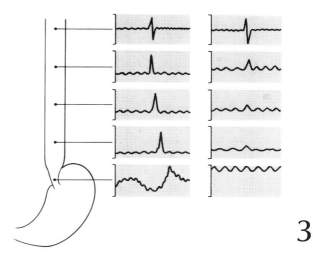

3

Operations

The availability of videoendoscopic techniques makes it possible today to perform a Heller myotomy, which relieves dysphagia better and more permanently than pneumatic dilatation without the need for a thoracotomy or a laparotomy. This operation can be accomplished by thoracoscopy[4] or laparoscopy[4,5]. The thoracoscopic approach is preferred as the entire oesophagus is easier to reach than through the abdominal approach. Moreover, when this operation is performed from the thoracic approach, the structures that support the antireflux mechanism are essentially left undisturbed, minimizing the need for an associated antireflux procedure. On the other hand, when a patient has had a previous thoracotomy, thoracoscopy is more complicated and the possibility of injury to the lung or other vital structures is increased. For these patients the laparoscopic approach is preferred. Both the thoracoscopic and laparoscopic approaches will be described.

THORACOSCOPIC HELLER MYOTOMY

4 The patient is placed on the right lateral decubitus over a bean bag. The left lung is allowed to collapse. The seventh intercostal space is marked in case an emergency thoracotomy has to be performed. Access to the chest is obtained using four (occasionally five) Thoracoports placed in a diamond-shaped pattern. The operation starts with a small incision in the third or fourth intercostal space slightly anterior to the posterior axillary line (A). A haemostat is carefully advanced into the chest, and a 5-mm port is inserted. Using a 5-mm telescope the thoracic cavity is examined to make sure the lung is adequately collapsed, and to determine the best site for the remaining ports. A 10-mm port is placed through the fifth or sixth intercostal space, approximately 5 cm behind the posterior axillary line, near the tip of the scapula, under direct vision (B). A 10-mm telescope is now placed through this port, which will be the 'telescope port' for most of the operation. A lung retractor is then introduced through the first port (which may now be converted to 10 mm if needed). The lung is pulled upward and a second 10-mm port is then positioned through the seventh intercostal space in the midaxillary line (operating port) (C). A 5-mm port is inserted through the sixth intercostal space in the anterior axillary line (retraction-separation port) (E). A fifth trocar is occasionally required for an instrument to depress the diaphragm or for instruments used in the surgeon's left hand (D). After the lung is fully collapsed by the anaesthetist it is further retracted upwards using the Endo-Retract, or a three-pronged (Storz) retractor.

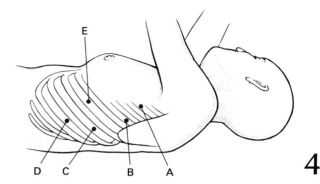

4

5 With traction on the inferior lobe, the inferior pulmonary ligament is divided. This exposes the pleura overlying the groove between the pericardium and the aorta, and this is then divided using electrocautery. The oesophagus lies deep in the groove, partially obscured by the descending aorta.

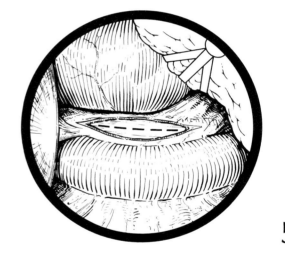

5

6 The tip of the oesophagoscope is advanced to an area near the gastro-oesophageal junction. Tilting the tip of the oesophagoscope, the oesophagus is lifted upwards from its mediastinal bed and placed directly within view of the surgeon. After dissecting fat and connective tissue from the surface of the oesophagus, the oesophageal myotomy is begun using the hook electrocautery at a point midway between the inferior pulmonary vein and diaphragmatic hiatus.

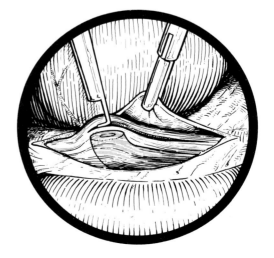

6

7 The myotomy is carried down through the circular layer using a 90° angled hook until the submucosal plane is reached. At this point, the myotomy is lengthened in both directions using the bipolar Shaw scissors or hook cautery, taking care not to penetrate the mucosa. The bipolar scissors are useful for this step since they remain effortlessly in the appropriate plane and coagulate the vessels while cutting the muscle.

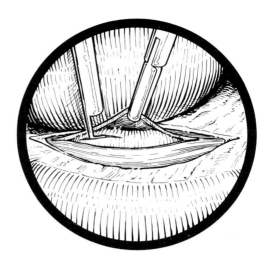

7

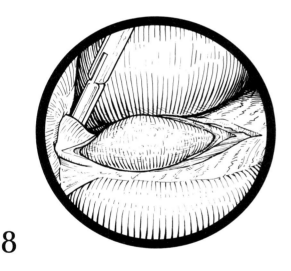

8

8 When performing the lowest (most caudad) extent of the myotomy, the diaphragm should be pushed downwards and the oesophagus pulled up with graspers. Meanwhile, the endoscopist reports how much farther the dissection must go in order to divide the sphincter completely.

It is often necessary to suction gas from the stomach via the endoscope because gastric distension pushes the left hemidiaphragm upwards, obscuring the view of the hiatus. As the stomach is reached the orientation of the muscle fibres changes, the vascular supply to the muscle becomes more abundant, and the mucosa becomes thinner, so extra care must be taken at this point to avoid bleeding and mucosal injury. The myotomy is carried approximately 0.5 cm onto the stomach or as far as is needed to relieve the obstruction. The completion of the myotomy is evident to the endoscopist as the lumen at the gastro-oesophageal junction suddenly becomes widely patent.

After the myotomy is complete, blunt dissection with graspers is usually necessary to separate the edges of the muscle and allow the mucosa to pouch through. Approximately 30–40% of the circumference of the oesophageal mucosa should be visible at the end of the dissection to prevent healing of the myotomy. Finally, a 28-Fr angled chest tube is placed through the lowest trocar site (usually a 10-mm port site) and is left to underwater drainage.

LAPAROSCOPIC HELLER MYOTOMY

9 Pneumoperitoneum is first established by inserting a needle in the right upper quadrant and access to the abdomen is obtained by four or occasionally five trocars. First, a 5-mm trocar is placed in the right upper quadrant (A). This allows examination of the abdomen and placement of additional trocars under direct view. Next, a 10-mm trocar is placed in the midline, 3–4 cm above the umbilicus (B) (camera port), and another in the left upper quadrant at the anterior axillary line (C) (operating port). Additional trocars are placed in the right upper quadrant (retracting ports) as needed (D and E).

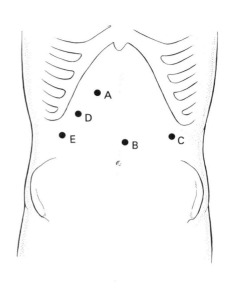

9

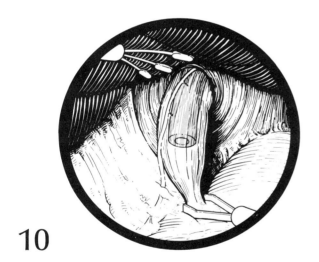

10

10 The left lobe of the liver is retracted upwards using the Endo-Retract retractor. Occasionally, the triangular ligament and part of the coronary ligament of the liver are in the way and must be divided. Most often, however, lifting the left lobe of the liver provides adequate exposure of the diaphragmatic hiatus. At this point in the operation a 30° telescope is required because the operator must have a more perpendicular view of the anterior wall of the oesophagus. The oesophagus is dissected away from the hiatus by dividing the overlying peritoneum and the phreno-oesophageal membrane. Both vagi are easily seen and should be preserved. This, and subsequent manoeuvres, require downward traction on the stomach, which can be achieved using an Endo-Babcock clamp.

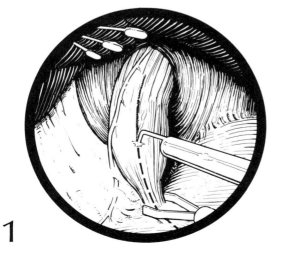

11

11 A point on the anterior surface of the oesophagus several centimetres above the gastro-oesophageal junction is selected for the myotomy and, using cautery, a line is marked on the surface of the oesophagus parallel to the anterior vagus nerve.

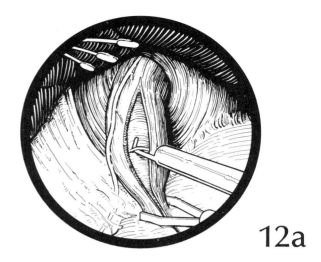

12a

12a, b The myotomy is begun at a convenient point using the hook cautery and is carried down to the submucosal space as described in the preceding section (*see* page 597). The endoscope is essential to lift the anterior aspect of the oesophagus and to determine the length of the myotomy.

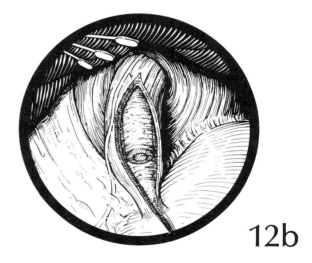

12b

Postoperative care

After surgery the patients are left fasting for the first 24 h. Antibiotics are discontinued at this time. If there is no evidence of air leak and the chest radiograph shows good expansion of the lung, the chest tube is removed. If the patient has no nausea, and the abdomen is not tender, the nasogastric tube is also removed at this time. Once the chest tube is removed, analgesics are rarely required.

Food is given as soon as the nasogastric tube is removed and patients are kept on a mechanically soft diet for the first few days. In most instances they are ready to leave the hospital on the second postoperative day. If the mucosa was entered during the operation, the patient should be left fasting for 6–7 days and the area checked for leaks with an oesophagogram before the patient is fed.

Long-term follow-up involves re-evaluation by manometry within 2–3 months of the operation to determine the effectiveness of the procedure in terms of changes of the lower oesophageal sphincter pressure. In addition, 24-h pH monitoring should be performed to determine the amount of reflux that is occurring[6]. Because the pressure of the lower oesophageal sphincter has been substantially decreased, some of these patients may have abnormal gastro-oesophageal reflux on pH testing despite the fact that they are asymptomatic. Patients found to have abnormal reflux are placed on H_2 blockers and are re-evaluated 1 year later with endoscopy and 24-h pH monitoring.

Complications

Bleeding

Bleeding can occur at the site of entry of the trocars, particularly in the chest. Laceration of one of the intercostal vessels usually requires ligature of the vessel under direct or video-assisted vision. Bleeding can also occur while dissecting the perioesophageal tissue, or performing the myotomy. Even small amounts of bleeding have substantial detrimental effects in videoendoscopic surgery. This is because blood obscures the area of operation, absorbs light and decreases visibility. Furthermore, bleeding from near the telescope trocar site causes blood to drip along the telescope, and when it reaches the lens it obscures the view, requiring removal of the telescope and cleaning. Thus, any bleeding has to be controlled immediately.

Mucosal injury

A small laceration of the oesophageal mucosa may occasionally occur. This is more likely to happen near the gastro-oesophageal junction where the plane that separates the muscular coat of the oesophagus from the mucosa becomes less apparent. The mucosal defect can easily be closed with a stitch of 4/0 polyglyconate or other slowly reabsorbable material. Because of the proximity to the stomach, it may be possible to buttress this closure with the gastric fundus which is attached with a stitch to the oesophageal muscle at each side of the edges of the myotomy. If the surgeon has experience with videoendoscopic suturing, the repair can be done without opening the chest or abdomen. On the other hand, if this is not possible, a small thoracotomy or laparotomy should be performed. The oesophagus and the tear are easily visible as they have been previously exposed and dissected, and the closure can be accomplished expeditiously in most cases.

An area of the mucosa may slough after the operation. This may occur because of thermal injury to the mucosa during the course of the dissection, which may necrose and slough a few days later. This complication has not been observed in any of the author's patients, but it has been reported elsewhere. This must be treated like a delayed oesophageal perforation (see chapter on pp. 244–255).

Residual or recurrent dysphagia

Residual dysphagia occurs most commonly when the myotomy is not carried far enough into the stomach. This problem was initially encountered in patients approached thoracoscopically. Since the progress of the myotomy is monitored by endoscopy and the endoscopic view determines when the last bundle of muscle is divided, the author has not had this problem. Recurrent dysphagia may be seen in patients in whom the myotomy heals (that is why the edges must be separated to free at least 40% of the circumference of the oesophagus), or if a stricture develops in the area. Strictures may be secondary to abnormal gastro-oesophageal reflux.

Abnormal gastro-oesophageal reflux

Since the operation divides the lower oesophageal sphincter, there is always a chance for gastro-oesophageal reflux to occur. When the operation is done thoracoscopically the structures that support the cardia are disturbed less than when the operation is done transabdominally, and several series have shown that an associated antireflux procedure is not needed[2,7]. The author advocates testing of patients with 24-h pH monitoring and treatment of those found to have abnormal reflux even if they are asymptomatic.

References

1. Skinner DB. Myotomy and achalasia. *Ann Thorac Surg* 1984; 37: 183–4.

2. Ellis FH Jr, Crozier RE, Watkins E Jr. Operation for esophageal achalasia: results of esophagomyotomy without an antireflux operation. *J Thorac Cardiovasc Surg* 1984; 88: 344–51.

3. Sauer L, Pellegrini CA, Way LW. The treatment of achalasia. A current perspective. *Arch Surg* 1989; 124: 929–32.

4. Pellegrini CA, Wetter LA, Patti M *et al*. Thoracoscopic esophagomyotomy: initial experience with a new approach for the treatment of achalasia. *Ann Surg* 1992; 216: 291–9.

5. Shimi S, Nathanson LK, Cuschieri A. Laparoscopic cardiomyotomy for achalasia. *J R Coll Surg Edinb* 1991; 36: 152–4.

6. DeMeester TR, Wang CI, Wernly JA *et al*. Technique, indications and clinical use of 24-hour esophageal pH monitoring. *J Thorac Cardiovasc Surg* 1980; 79: 656–70.

7. Shoenut JP, Wieler JA, Micflikier AB, Teskey JM. Esophageal reflux before and after isolated myotomy for achalasia. *Surgery* 1990; 108: 876–9.

Endoscopic oesophagectomy

Gerhard F. Buess MD, FRCS(Ed)
Professor of Surgery, Eberhard-Karls University, Schnarrenberg Clinic, Tübingen, Germany

Guy J. Maddern PhD, MS, FRACS
Jepson Professor of Surgery, University of Adelaide, The Queen Elizabeth Hospital, Australia

History

Because of the perceived invasiveness of a combined abdominal and thoracic approach for resection of oesophageal cancer, the use of transhiatal oesophagectomy has gained in popularity. This has occurred despite any evidence of a reduction in pulmonary complications with the use of a transhiatal approach. The transhiatal approach, while avoiding a thoracotomy, is not without complications, which may include significant intraoperative blood loss, a high rate of pleural openings and trauma to the recurrent laryngeal nerve. In an attempt to minimize such operative trauma the technique of endoscopic oesophagectomy without thoracotomy has been devised using endoscopic dissection of the oesophagus. The technique had its first application in humans in 1989 after extensive animal studies[1-3].

At present only anecdotal reports of thoracoscopic dissection of the oesophagus exist. It has, however, been well established in animal models and may be used in the future to allow safe mobilization of large oesophageal carcinomas or perhaps to construct primary intrathoracic anastomoses.

Preoperative

Assessment

Endoscopic dissection of the oesophagus can be performed to treat both benign and malignant oesophageal disease. Preoperative assessment, investigation and management is the same as employed for the more conventional surgical techniques. Endoscopic findings are vitally important to the intraoperative approach to the tumour. While computed tomography is often of little help in assessing oesophageal wall penetration and infiltration of surrounding structures, the authors have found endoscopic transluminal ultrasonography to be the most precise diagnostic method for accurately assessing the T stage of oesophageal cancer and for guiding operative planning for this procedure.

Operation

The operation is performed simultaneously by two teams of surgeons, one team performing the abdominal phase and the other the cervical incision and endoscopic dissection.

1 The patient is placed in the supine position with the thorax elevated on the right with a 5-cm thick support which permits skin preparation in the posterior axillary line in case rapid conversion to an anterolateral thoracotomy is required. The patient's head is rotated to the right, and the patient is draped so that the mediastinal operating team is isolated from the anaesthetic area, using a frame covered with sterile drapes.

In cervical oesophageal cancer, resectability should be verified before the abdominal phase of the operation is started. In patients with a distal tumour, resectability is determined by a laparotomy before commencement of the cervical operative phase.

The abdominal phase of the operation has been described in the chapter on pp. 178–188 and follows

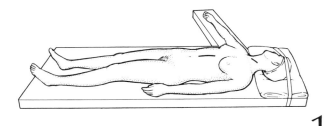

1

conventional surgical techniques. The left cervical incision runs from the level of the thyroid cartilage down to the cervical notch. The cervical oesophagus is mobilized in the usual fashion, as described on pp. 45–51, and encircled with a silicone tube without traumatizing the left recurrent laryngeal nerve.

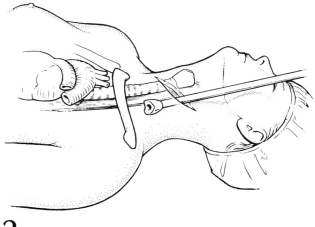

2

2 The space for the endoscopic operation is created by mechanical separation of tissue planes. Initially space must be prepared by open dissection; once sufficient access has been created the tip of the mediastinoscope is introduced.

3 The mediastinoscope has been specifically developed for this procedure by Wolfe AG, Germany. It incorporates a modified bell-shaped dilating cone that permits easy passage along the oesophagus while maintaining the central position of the oesophagus. An 8 × 12-mm working channel and an eyepiece with an oblique offset allows the surgeon to work both sitting and standing, and an integrated lens irrigation system permits frequent cleaning while maintaining vision and not requiring instrument removal.

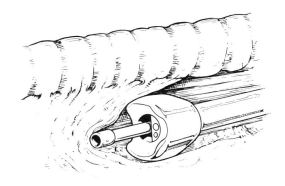

3

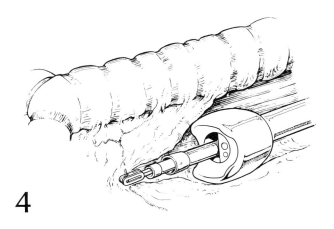

4

4 In addition, new endoscopic instruments have been developed for achieving haemostasis. In the near future an endoscopic clipping instrument will allow the simultaneous application of two resorbable polydioxanone clips and the division of the clipped structure with an integrated cutting device. A prototype of a bipolar water-rinsed endoscopic coagulation forceps with integrated scissors is now used for the dissection and coagulation of exposed blood vessels without a change of instruments.

5 The central instrument channel can also be used to introduce a combined sucker/diathermy instrument. The non-insulated tip of the sucker is fashioned in such a way that vascular pedicles are centralized during dissection and coagulation. Through the central canal of the combined sucker, instruments such as hooks, scissors, or forceps can be introduced.

By pulling these instruments back 5 cm, suction can be activated. The instrument channel of the endoscope also serves as access for more conventional endoscopic instruments, such as a single clip applicator.

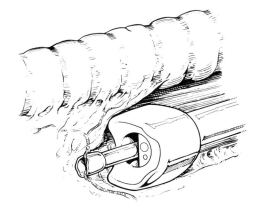

5

6 An assistant provides traction on the oesophageal sling and activates the diathermy and lens irrigation, and a scrub nurse stands behind the surgeon to pass the instruments.

After inserting the mediastinoscope via the cervical incision into the retropharyngeal space, the oesophageal dissection continues just outside the plane of the longitudinal oesophageal muscle. Using blunt dissection the loose areolar tissue surrounding the oesophagus is separated, revealing vascular structures which are grasped by insulated forceps and coagulated by monopolar diathermy.

The instrument is initially guided by a finger and may be helped by using a small right-angled retractor. In the first instance the instrument is passed along the posterior oesophagus, and by a combination of suction and blunt dissection the loose areolar plane between the oesophagus and surrounding structures is separated while staying close to the longitudinal oesophageal muscle. Mechanical dilatation with the 'olive' on the tip of the mediastinoscope provides space for the operation to proceed. Fibrous bridges of connective tissue attached to the oesophagus, even if avascular, should be cut with scissors, otherwise muscle fibres are avulsed from the oesophagus. When vessels are seen they should be controlled by coagulation using the blunt tip of the suction diathermy before division; when greater than

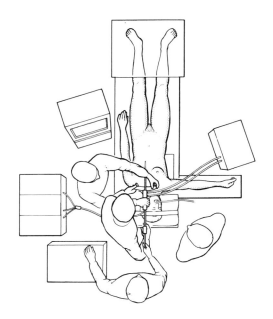

6

1 mm in diameter they must first be compressed by the monopolar or bipolar diathermy forceps and coagulated or ligated between clips. A similar procedure follows for the left side of the oesophagus, with visualization of the left aortic arch and descending aorta.

The anterior dissection positions the mediastinoscope between the trachea and the oesophagus, with the posterior wall of the trachea and the ridges of the cartilaginous tracheal ring seen anteriorly. On the right side the laterally situated azygos vein is normally not exposed. Drainage is not required if the pleura is breached, providing there is adequate haemostasis.

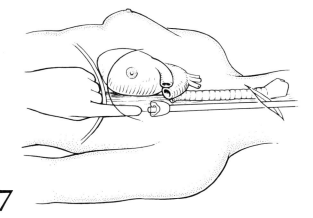

7

Tumour dissection

7 Fibrous tissue encountered around the tumour is often more dense. This necessitates a wider excision away from the oesophageal muscle fibres. With tumours of the distal one-third of the oesophagus, tumour dissection is alternately performed by the mediastinal and abdominal surgeons. With large tumours the additional information provided by the abdominal surgeon's digital assessment improves the safety of the mediastinal surgeon's dissection.

8 Once initial preparation is complete, the abdominal surgeon places a plastic tube within view of the mediastinoscope. This is grasped by the jaws of the grasping forceps and the mediastinoscope is withdrawn to the neck. With the mediastinal oesophagus now firmly sutured to the plastic tube, the nasogastric tube is withdrawn and the oesophagus transected with a GIA stapler 3 cm distal to the inferior thyroid artery.

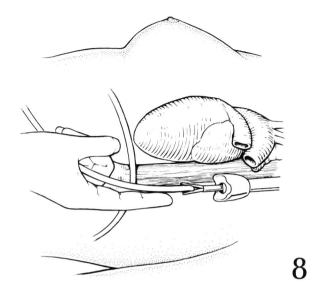

8

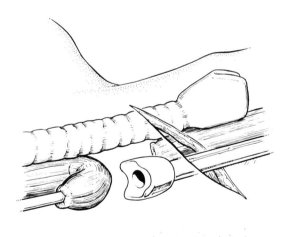

9 With gentle tension on the plastic tube the oesophagus folds on itself. The mediastinoscope is inserted to follow this process visually. Any remaining oesophageal attachments can be readily identified, exposed and divided. The oesophagus is delivered into the abdomen.

10 The posterior mediastinum is then displayed by the abdominal surgeon inserting a swab mounted on a grasping forceps up to the tracheal bifurcation. By following the swab with the mediastino-scope as it is slowly withdrawn, an optimal view of the oesophageal bed is obtained with the aim of complete haemostasis.

The abdominal surgeon then resects the oesophagus and fashions a gastric tube, as described in the chapter on pp. 142–153. With a plastic tube securely sutured to the stomach, the mediastinoscope is used to pull the plastic tube up to the neck, avoiding twisting of the stomach.

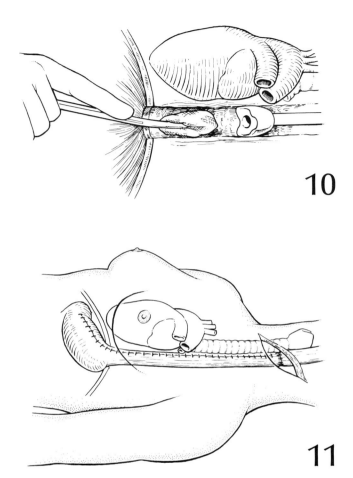

11 With the upper part of the stomach positioned at the suprasternal notch, a tension-free anastomosis to the cervical oesophagus is fashioned using an end-to-end technique. On completion drains are inserted in the region of the cervical anastomosis and subphrenic region.

Postoperative care

In the immediate postoperative period intensive monitoring is performed in the intensive care unit with vigorous treatment of cardiopulmonary dysfunction. Routine perioperative antibiotics, careful ventilation and fluid replacement, regular abdominal and thoracic ultrasonography and thoracic radiography are required for postoperative management. Shortly after extubation on the first or second day the patient can be transferred to the ward under close surveillance. Between the seventh and tenth day after operation the anastomosis is checked by a Gastrografin swallow, followed by gradual oral intake.

References

1. Buess GF, Becker HD, Naruhn MB, Mentges BR. Endoscopic esophagectomy without thoracotomy. *Probl Gen Surg* 1991; 8: 478–86.

2. Kipfmuller K, Naruhn M, Melzer A, Kessler S, Buess G. Endoscopic microsurgical dissection of the esophagus: results in an animal model. *Surg Endosc* 1989; 3: 63–9.

3. Buess G, Becker HD, Lenz G. Perivisceral endoscopic oesophagectomy. In: Cuschieri A, Buess G, Perissat J, eds. *Operative Manual of Endoscopic Surgery*. Part 2. Heidelberg: Springer, 1992; 149–65.

List of products

Allis' clamps, Codman, Massachusetts, USA

Babcock's forceps, Codman, Massachusetts, USA

Dacron, Du Pont, Wilmington, USA
Dexon, Davis & Geck, Gosport, UK/Davis & Geck International, c/o Cyanamid International, Wayne, New Jersey, USA

EEA stapler, Auto Suture Co. UK, Ascot, UK/US Surgical Corporation, Connecticut, USA
Endo-Babcock, Auto Suture Co. UK, Ascot, UK/US Surgical Corporation, Connecticut, USA
Endo-Retract, Auto Suture Co. UK, Ascot, UK/US Surgical Corporation, Connecticut, USA
Ethibond, Ethicon, Edinburgh, UK/Ethicon Inc, Somerville, New Jersey, USA

Gastrografin, Schering Health Care, UK
GIA stapler, Auto Suture Co. UK, Ascot, UK/US Surgical Corporation, Connecticut, USA

ILS stapler, Ethicon Endosurgery, Edinburgh, UK/Ethicon Endosurgery, Cincinatti, Ohio, USA

Ligaclip, Ethicon Endosurgery, Edinburgh, UK/Ethicon Endosurgery, Cincinatti, Ohio, USA

Marlex, C P Bard, Massachusetts, USA
Maxon, Davis & Geck, Gosport, UK/Davis & Geck International, c/o Cyanamid International, Wayne, New Jersey, USA
Mousseau-Barbin tube, Porges Catheter Corporation, New York, USA

Prolene, Ethicon, Edinburgh, UK/Ethicon Inc, Somerville, New Jersey, USA

Rigiflex dilator, Rigiflex Inc, Belmont, Massachusetts, USA

Satinsky clamp, Codman, Massachusetts, USA
SGIA 50 stapler, Auto Suture Co. UK, Ascot, UK/US Surgical Corporation, Connecticut, USA
Shaw scissors, Hemostatic Surgery Corporation, San Francisco, USA

TA 55 stapler, Auto Suture Co. UK, Ascot, UK/US Surgical Corporation, Connecticut, USA
TA 90 stapler, Auto Suture Co. UK, Ascot, UK/US Surgical Corporation, Connecticut, USA
Thoracoports, Auto Suture Co. UK, Ascot, UK/US Surgical Corporation, Connecticut, USA

Vicryl, Ethicon, Edinburgh, UK/Ethicon Inc, Somerville, New Jersey, USA

Index